Age-Adjusted Psychiatric Treatment for the Older Patient

Howard H. Fenn
James A. Bourgeois
Catharine Birtley Fenn
Editors

Age-Adjusted Psychiatric Treatment for the Older Patient

Springer

Editors
Howard H. Fenn
VA Health Care System
Palo Alto, CA, USA

Department of Psychiatry
and Behavioral Sciences
Stanford University
Stanford, CA, USA

Catharine Birtley Fenn
Menlo Park, CA, USA

James A. Bourgeois
Psychiatry and Behavioral Sciences
University of California, Davis
Sacramento, CA, USA

ISBN 978-3-031-53975-6 ISBN 978-3-031-53976-3 (eBook)
https://doi.org/10.1007/978-3-031-53976-3

This Springer imprint is published by the registered company Springer Nature Switzerland AG
The registered company address is: Gewerbestrasse 11, 6330 Cham, Switzerland

Paper in this product is recyclable.

Dedicated to
W. Thomas Birtley
Arthur Cary Fenn, MD

Preface

> Willy Loman never made a lot of money. His name was never in the paper. He's not the finest character that ever lived. But he's a human being, and a terrible thing is happening to him. So attention must be paid. He's not to be allowed to fall into his grave like an old dog. Attention, attention must be finally paid to such a person. You called him crazy—
> [From Act 1, *Death of A Salesman*, a play in two acts by Arthur Miller, (Miller A. Death of a Salesman, Viking Penguin, Inc. 1949)]

In this classic American tragedy, Linda, the wife of Willy Loman, is talking to her two self-involved sons about the decline of her husband of over 40 years. Willy is in his mid-60s and has spent over 30 years as an on-the-road salesman. He is struggling now with diminished career options, displacement by younger salesmen, financial stressors, and failing health. He is pained by unfulfilled expectations for his two irresponsible, grown sons. He has managed stressors primarily by distorting or ignoring reality with unrealistic fantasies of success. Linda reveals that she found a hose with which Willie has been planning suicide with gas, but she has kept this secret so as not to humiliate him.

Near the end of the play, Willy's fantasies begin to morph into delusions. He hallucinates a figure from his past who reminds him of missed opportunities.

In the last scene, Willy dies off-stage in a burst of self-destructive behavior, planting a garden in the middle of the night. His cause of death is never revealed, but an acute myocardial infarction or stroke are most likely.

With an *age-adjusted* approach to his psychiatric condition, perhaps Willy might have responded to gentle questions and concern from his primary care clinician, who might have identified suicidal impulses, and would have encouraged more adaptive coping, or referred him to a pastor or a psychotherapist. If Willy were living in the current age of pharmacotherapy, his mood and outlook could have improved with 100 mg daily of sertraline. A small dose of 1 mg risperidone daily might have ameliorated the severity of delusions. A thorough medical work-up could have diagnosed coronary artery disease, hypertension, and hyperlipidemia, prompting preventive interventions such as healthier diet, lipid-lowering atorvastatin, lisinopril, and possibly an anticoagulant.

Willy might have stabilized psychiatrically and medically. He could have retired and lived into his 80s. Even if he eventually developed a vascular major neurocognitive disorder (MNCD) with neuropsychiatric symptoms

(NPS), he could have been treated with interventions to minimize any adverse effects.

These are the goals, using *age-adjusted* psychiatric treatment, to which the chapters in this book aspire. But that is not the tragedy that Arthur Miller wrote.

Anyway, who would be interested in a play entitled *Life of a Salesman*?

Palo Alto, CA, USA — Howard H. Fenn
Sacramento, CA, USA — James A. Bourgeois
Menlo Park, CA, USA — Catharine Birtley Fenn

Caveat: Medication Use

Many medications discussed in this book are recommended for psychiatric symptoms beyond any initial US FDA-approved indications. This *off-label* use, based upon clinical experience and randomized clinical trials, is inherent in geriatric psychiatry practice. In part, this is because the necessary medication trials have often not included geriatric subjects. For example, many medications used to treat behavioral and psychiatric symptoms of dementia (BPSD) have US-FDA indications only for bipolar disorder, psychosis, and/or depressive disorders. Whether with FDA indication or not, the *age-adjusted* ethic encourages *carefully dosed and closely monitored* treatment for a wide range of psychiatric illnesses.

Psychiatric diagnoses are consistent with the Diagnostic and Statistical Manual of Mental Disorders: DSM-5-TR, American Psychiatric Publishing; 2022.

Acknowledgments

Our Appreciation to

Herbert Ochitill, MD, enduring colleague and friend, for consultation and support throughout this process.

Contents

Contributors

Ana Jessica Alfaro VA Palo Alto Health Care System, Geriatric Research, Education and Clinical Center (GRECC), Palo Alto, CA, USA

Department of Psychiatry and Behavioral Services, Stanford University School of Medicine, Palo Alto, CA, USA

Zainab Bhojani Ontario Shores Centre for Mental Health Sciences, Whitby, ON, Canada

Schulich School of Medicine and Dentistry, London, ON, Canada

Geriatric Psychiatry, London Health Sciences Centre, London, Ontario, Canada

Mervin Blair Ontario Shores Centre for Mental Health Sciences, Whitby, ON, Canada

Lawson Health Research Institute/Parkwood Institute, London, ON, Canada

Ian O. Bledsoe UCSF Weill Institute for Neurosciences, San Francisco, CA, USA

Department of Neurology, University of California, San Francisco, San Francisco, CA, USA

Dawn Bruijnzeel University of Florida College of Medicine, Gainesville, FL, USA

North Florida South Georgia VA Medical Center, Gainesville, FL, USA

Elizabeth B. Bruns Department of Psychiatry and Behavioral Sciences, University of California, San Francisco, San Francisco, CA, USA

UCSF Weill Institute for Neurosciences, San Francisco, CA, USA

Amer M. Burhan Ontario Shores Centre for Mental Health Sciences, Whitby, ON, Canada

Department of Psychiatry, Temerty School of Medicine, University of Toronto, Whitby, ON, Canada

Erin Cassidy-Eagle Department of Psychiatry and Behavioral Services, Stanford University School of Medicine, Palo Alto, CA, USA

Christa DeFries Talkiatry, New York City, NY, USA

Maria Farooqi Veterans Affairs Palo Alto Health Care System, Palo Alto, CA, USA

Howard H. Fenn Department of Psychiatry and Behavioral Sciences, Stanford University, Stanford, CA, USA

VA Health Care System, Palo Alto, CA, USA

Sheena Ghodasara Division of Geriatric Psychiatry, Department of Psychiatry, Western University and London Health Sciences Centre, London, ON, Canada

Western University, London, ON, Canada

Division of Geriatric Psychiatry, Department of Psychiatry, London Health Sciences Centre, London, ON, Canada

Geriatric Psychiatry, Halton Health, Halton, Ontario, Canada

Christine E. Gould VA Palo Alto Health Care System, Geriatric Research, Education and Clinical Center (GRECC), Palo Alto, CA, USA

Department of Psychiatry and Behavioral Services, Stanford University School of Medicine, Palo Alto, CA, USA

Psychology Service, VA Palo Alto Health Care System, Palo Alto, CA, USA

Daphne Goveas Lawson Health Research Institute/Parkwood Institute, London, ON, Canada

Rita Hitching University of Newcastle, Newcastle, NSW, Australia

School of Medicine and Public Health, University of Newcastle, Newcastle, NSW, Australia

Poh Choo How Department of Psychiatry and Behavioral Sciences, University of California, Davis, Sacramento, CA, USA

Mike Kelly Coalinga State Hospital, Coalinga, CA, USA

Leah McGowan McGowan Family Law, P.C., Woodside, CA, USA

Amanda Mihalik-Wenger University of Washington, Department of Psychiatry, Seattle, WA, USA

University of Florida, College of Medicine, Gainesville, FL, USA

Meena Nuthi NFSG VAMC, Gainesville, FL, USA

University of Florida, College of Medicine, Gainesville, FL, USA

Malcom Randall VA Medical Center, Gainesville, FL, USA

Chinyere I. Ogbonna Addiction Medicine and Recovery Services, Kaiser Permanente San Jose, San Jose, CA, USA

Boski Patel Department of Psychiatry, The Permanente Medical Group, Kaiser Permanente, Northern California, Santa Clara, CA, USA

James Patience Parkwood Institute, London, ON, Canada

Talia Puzantian Keck Graduate Institute School of Pharmacy and Health Sciences, Claremont, CA, USA

Caroline A. Racine UCSF Weill Institute for Neurosciences, San Francisco, CA, USA

Department of Neurological Surgery, University of California, San Francisco, San Francisco, CA, USA

Kate Marie Richards Department of Psychiatry and Behavioral Sciences/ Department of Family and Community Medicine, UC Davis Health, Sacramento, CA, USA

Elyse Ross Division of Geriatric Psychiatry, Department of Psychiatry, Western University and London Health Sciences Centre, London, ON, Canada

Division of Geriatric Psychiatry, Department of Psychiatry, Dalhousie University, Halifax, Nova Scotia, Canada

Andreea L. Seritan Department of Psychiatry and Behavioral Sciences, University of California, San Francisco, San Francisco, CA, USA

UCSF Weill Institute for Neurosciences, San Francisco, CA, USA

Yelizaveta Sher Division of Medical Psychiatry, Psychiatric and Psychological Services, Adult Cystic Fibrosis Program, Stanford University and Medical Center, Stanford, CA, USA

William B. Smith Department of Psychiatry and Behavioral Sciences, University of California, San Francisco, San Francisco, CA, USA

UCSF Weill Institute for Neurosciences, San Francisco, CA, USA

Barbara R. Sommer Department of Psychiatry and Behavioral Sciences, Stanford University, Palo Alto, CA, USA

Shannon Suo Call Psych, Sacramento, CA, USA

Uma Suryadevara College of Medicine, University of Florida, Gainesville, FL, USA

North Florida South Georgia VA Medical Center, Gainesville, FL, USA

Malcom Randall VA Medical Center, Gainesville, FL, USA

Vittavat Termglinchan Department of Medicine, Clinical Excellence Research Center, Stanford School of Medicine, Stanford, CA, USA

Sama Thiab Lawson Health Research Institute/Parkwood Institute, London, ON, Canada

Peter J. Ureste Department of Psychiatry and Behavioral Sciences, University of California, San Francisco, San Francisco, CA, USA

UCSF Weill Institute for Neurosciences, San Francisco, CA, USA

Thelepa Vaithianathan Ontario Shores Centre for Mental Health Sciences, Whitby, ON, Canada

Justin Wenger Seattle VA Medical center, Seattle, WA, USA

University of Florida, College of Medicine, Gainesville, FL, USA

Glen Xiong Department of Psychiatry and Behavioral Sciences, University of California, Davis, Sacramento, CA, USA

Ira Yenko VA Palo Alto Health Care System, Geriatric Research, Education and Clinical Center (GRECC), Palo Alto, CA, USA

1 Introduction

Howard H. Fenn, Catharine Birtley Fenn, and James A. Bourgeois

Abstract

The principles of age-adjusted clinical practice and the goals of this book are discussed. The need for a review from this perspective is supported by evidence from clinical experience and scientific literature of excessive polypharmacy, deprescribing initiatives, and non-pharmacological interventions. It is emphasized that the theme of the book is to better accommodate medication use with the physiological changes of aging as well as to include non-pharmacological interventions in geriatric treatment planning.

The principles of *age-adjusted* treatment are not new. The advice for prescribing to the aging patient has always been to "start low, go slow." This book fleshes out that dictum, based upon research evidence, clinical experience, and trends we have noticed in the literature. Over the years, however, we have observed and participated in practices which, though common, can be counter-productive to the geriatric patient. Examples are as follows:

- Focusing on psychiatric symptoms without attention to contributing factors
- Minimizing the impact of chronic pain, sleep deprivation, sensory limitations, personal loss, physical limitations, infection, dehydration, and drug–drug interactions
- Starting medications before trying non-pharmacological interventions
- Overlooking prior treatments, their efficacy, adverse effects, or outcomes
- Re-prescribing psychotropic medications without reviewing indications or effectiveness
- Employing doses and formulations without adjustments for aging pharmacokinetics and pharmacodynamics
- Carrying forward psychiatric diagnoses without re-evaluating their validity

H. H. Fenn (✉)
VA Health Care System, Palo Alto, CA, USA

Department of Psychiatry and Behavioral Sciences, Stanford University, Stanford, CA, USA
e-mail: hhfenn@aol.com, howard.fenn@va.gov

C. B. Fenn
Menlo Park, CA, USA

J. A. Bourgeois
Department of Psychiatry and Behavioral Sciences, University of California, Davis, Sacramento, CA, USA
e-mail: jbourgeois@ucdavis.edu

H. H. Fenn et al. (eds.), *Age-Adjusted Psychiatric Treatment for the Older Patient*,
https://doi.org/10.1007/978-3-031-53976-3_1

An *age-adjusted* approach seeks to:

- First rule out or treat any systemic medical conditions associated with the psychiatric symptoms
- Search history for prior psychiatric symptoms, treatments, responses, and outcomes
- Consider delirium as a possible contributor before focusing on other psychiatric syndromes, especially in frail patients with preexisting neurocognitive disorders
- Use lower-than-usual medication doses for geriatric patients who may have a therapeutic response at lower doses
- Avoid delirium-promoting CNS active agents (e.g., benzodiazepines, Z-drugs, anticholinergics, antihistamines) when treating *other* psychiatric illnesses
- Include *non*-pharmacological modalities as first-line options
- Change medications or doses one at a time
- Avoid unnecessary polypharmacy

This approach is not characterized as *holistic, integrative, alternative, or non-traditional.* Rather, it endorses medication interventions when needed as part of a comprehensive treatment plan. A combination of psychotherapeutic interventions, non-pharmacological modalities, *and* judiciously managed medications can improve quality of life and avoid the adverse effects of aging on medication use.

Each chapter begins with a complex case example, based upon clinical experience, which illustrates the topic. It then reviews current evidence-based evaluation and treatments. *Age-Adjusted Recommendations,* distilled from the literature, are offered at the end of each chapter. The intent is to provide actionable advice to *supplement*, but not *supplant,* good clinical judgment which can improve quality of life by managing psychiatric symptomatology and minimizing adverse results.

A growing body of evidence in medical literature supports this theme. Greater than 50% of patients aged 57–85 years use five or more medications according to the National Institute on Drug Abuse (NIDA) (Charlesworth et al. 2015). Many risks of inappropriate polypharmacy have been articulated (Rothchild 2021). Excessive use of psychotropic medications for residents of nursing homes and other geriatric treatment settings is well known (Cool et al. 2014). As a result, *deprescribing* protocols, applicable to the aged patient, have been developed (Martinez et al. 2017). Benefits of cognitive-behavioral therapies (CBT) and other supportive therapy models (STM) have been validated by RCT evidence as safe and effective interventions for many psychiatric illnesses (Ruesch et al. 2017). Finally, telemedicine, technology-assisted monitoring, and digital technologies are facilitating early detection of behavioral symptoms, cognitive deficits, and other markers of decline (Gould et al. 2020).

This topic is timely. In societies across the globe, the proportion of aging adults is growing faster than any other age group, due to declining fertility rates combined with longer life expectancy (World Health Organization 2012). Regrettably, the number of health care practitioners per capita with specialized geriatric training has not kept up with this increasing need (Grady and Singleton 2011).

Experienced clinicians as well as trainees from various disciplines, generalists, and geriatric specialists, will all inevitably treat greater numbers of aged patients who have psychiatric symptoms. This enlarging group of health care practitioners is the audience to whom this book is directed.

References

Charlesworth CJ, Smit E, Lee DS, et al. Polypharmacy among adults aged 65 years and older in the United States: 1988–2010. J Gerontol A Biol Sci Med Sci. 2015;70(8):989–95.

Cool C, Cestac P, Labrode C, et al. Potentially inappropriate drug prescribing and associated factors in nursing homes. J Am Med Dir Assoc. 2014;15(11):850.e1.

Gould CE, Loup J, Kuhn E, et al. Technology use and preferences for mental health self-management interventions among older veterans. Int J Geriatr Psychiatry. 2020;35(3):321–30.

Grady B, Singleton M. Telepsychiatry "coverage" to a rural inpatient psychiatric unit. Telemedicine e-Health. 2011;17(8):603–8. https://doi.org/10.1089/tmj.2011.0031.

Martinez YV, Renom-Guiteras A, Reeves D, et al. A set of systematic reviews to help reduce inappropriate prescribing to older people: study protocol. BMC Geriatr. 2017;17(Suppl 1):231.

Rothchild AJ. The pitfalls of psychotropic polypharmacy. J Clin Psychopharmacol. 2021;41(3):227–32.

Ruesch M, Helmes A, Bengel J. Cognitive-behavioral group therapy for patients with physical diseases and comorbid depressive or adjustment disorders on a waiting list for individual therapy: results from a randomized controlled trial. BMC Psychiatry. 2017;17(1):1–3.

World Health Organization. Health topics: ageing. 2012. www.who.int/topics/ageing/en. Accessed 28 Mar 2018.

Part I

Foundations of Evaluation and Treatment

2 Geriatric Pharmacology Overview

Poh Choo How, Barbara R. Sommer, and Glen Xiong

Abstract

This age of pharmacology and geriatric psychiatry requires an appreciation for the pharmacology of aging. Suboptimal prescribing, which affects 25% of those aged 65–69 years and 45% of those aged 70–79 (Charlesworth et al., J Gerontol A Biol Sci Med Sci 70:989–995, 2015), can result in increased risk of adverse effects.

This chapter reviews common medication adverse effects and risks as well as approaches which can minimize their frequency and severity. The *effectiveness* of pharmacological treatments for specific conditions is covered in the other chapters. We review factors such as inappropriate polypharmacy, as well as unnecessary, ineffective, or harmful medications and their potential for harm. Risks are significant especially for geriatric patients, for whom the physiological changes of aging, in combination with the high prevalence of chronic medical conditions, alter (1) the ways that medications are processed *by the body* (pharmacokinetics) and (2) the effects of medications *on the body* (pharmacodynamics).

P. C. How (✉) · G. Xiong
Department of Psychiatry and Behavioral Sciences, University of California, Davis, Sacramento, CA, USA
e-mail: phow@ucdavis.edu; gxiong@ucdavis.edu

B. R. Sommer
Department of Psychiatry and Behavioral Sciences, Stanford University, Palo Alto, CA, USA
e-mail: brsommer@stanford.edu

Case Example: Drug–Drug Interactions and Adverse Effects

A 65-year-old computer scientist complained of forgetfulness, distractibility, slight gait instability, intermittent paresthesias of one lower extremity, and "mental fogginess." He sought neurological consultation to rule out Alzheimer's disease. The symptoms began within the previous 5 years but worsened over the past year. His mood was demoralized and apprehensive, as these symptoms impacted his work performance.

He had been treated for bipolar II disorder for 15 years, ever since an episode of dysphoria and apparent "hyperactivity," which in hindsight was because he increased his time at work, in the context of a prolonged, contentious divorce. Details of the original mood episode had not been re-examined, and the patient had not experienced any subsequent mood symptoms. His prescriber continued the original medication regimen for prevention of relapse: carbamazepine (CBZ) 400 mg twice daily and lamotrigine 400 mg daily. Fluoxetine 20 mg daily was added to his regimen 1 year earlier to treat the presumed relapse of bipolar II disorder, major depressive episode, and the fluoxetine was increased to 40 mg daily when dysphoria did not resolve.

H. H. Fenn et al. (eds.), *Age-Adjusted Psychiatric Treatment for the Older Patient*,
https://doi.org/10.1007/978-3-031-53976-3_2

At consultation, the CBZ level was found to be 16 mcg/mL (therapeutic range 4–12). The lamotrigine level was thought to be subtherapeutic because its hepatic metabolism had been induced by carbamazepine. A neurological examination found no evidence of stroke, focal findings, nor of a neurodegenerative disorder. A Montreal Cognitive Assessment (MoCA) was scored at 29/30. It was hypothesized that subjective cognitive symptoms, intermittent incoordination, and paresthesias were related to CBZ toxicity.

Carbamazepine was tapered and discontinued over the course of 2 months. No mood symptoms re-emerged; he became less depressed and apprehensive as his "mental fogginess" and functioning improved. Paresthesias were resolved. Fluoxetine was tapered to 10 mg daily, and lamotrigine was discontinued.

Discussion

CBZ is an autoinducer of CYT P450 3A4, which can increase drug metabolism and reduce the serum level of lamotrigine (Table 2.1). In this case, the addition fluoxetine (an CYP 450 3A4 inhibitor) *inhibited* CBZ metabolism, raising its concentration and related adverse effects of sedation and ataxia. The prior diagnosis of bipolar II disorder was re-examined, and no history of hypomania or mania could be confirmed. A new diagnosis of *adjustment disorder with mixed anxiety and depressed mood* was offered. Discontinuation of CBZ did not result in a relapse of depressive symptoms, hypomania, or other evidence of bipolar II disorder. This permitted tapering and discontinuation of fluoxetine and lamotrigine. The patient began engaging in Cognitive Behavioral Therapy (CBT) which helped him manage stressors at work.

Table 2.1 Drug–drug interactions and adverse effects of polypharmacy in older adults

General adverse effects of polypharmacy

- Reduced adherence to treatment regimen
- Drug–drug interactions (see specifics below)
- Diminished ability for daily functioning
- Cognitive impairment
- Falls
- Malnutrition
- Urinary symptoms

Medications/ drug–drug interactions	Effects
Proton-pump inhibitors	Decreased absorption of other medications (can administer at different times to avoid interaction)
NSAIDs, diuretics, ACE inhibitors, and lithium	Decreased renal clearance of lithium and increased risk of lithium toxicity
SSRIs and opioids	Increased risk of serotonin syndrome
SSRIs and NSAIDs/ anticoagulants	Increased risk of GI and CNS bleeds
SSRIs and antipsychotics	Decreased metabolism of antipsychotics due to CYT P450 inhibition, increased half-lives of antipsychotics
Opioids and antipsychotics	Increased risk of CNS and respiratory depression
Carbamazepine	Increased and decreased levels of other medications
Valproic acid and lamotrigine	Decreased metabolism and increased half-life of lamotrigine, increased risk of Stevens-Johnson syndrome
Benzodiazepines	Increased risk of falls, fractures, cognitive impairment
Benzodiazepines and opioids	Increased risk of respiratory depression
Tricyclic antidepressants	Increased risk of delirium due to anticholinergic effects
Beta-blockers	Increased risk of bradycardia, orthostatic hypotension, loss of consciousness
Steroids	Increased risk of depressive disorder and other mood changes

Sources: Charlesworth et al. (2015), Lea et al. (2013) and Obreli-Neto et al. (2012)

Pharmacokinetics in Aging

The processes by which the body manages a drug constitute *pharmacokinetics*. Age-related changes impact metabolism, distribution, and elimination, and to a much lesser extent absorption. (Summarized in Table 2.2).

Absorption

Differences in drug solubility and changes in gastrointestinal (GI) function in aging individually affect the absorption of orally administered medications. Most medications are poorly soluble, and absorption is decreased in the aged by a combination of lower saliva production and decreased gastric acid secretion, leading to increased gastric pH (Carlo and Alpert 2015). The anticholinergic burden of medications can contribute to dry mouth, which affects sublingual and oral-dissolving tablet formulations. Co-administration of proton-pump inhibitors, antacids, and antihistamines can also diminish absorption.

Some medications need to be administered with food to stimulate gastric secretions and

Table 2.2 Pharmacokinetic changes with aging

Pharmacokinetic process	Drug–drug interactions	Implications	Clinical applications
Absorption ↓ Gastric emptying time ↓ Intestinal motility ↓ Gastric acid secretion ↑ Gastric pH	Antacids, proton-pump inhibitors, and H2 blockers increase gastric pH Anticholinergic burden (AB) of contributing to dry mouth, low saliva production	Reduced medication absorption, longer time to steady state or effective serum drug levels	Longer interval before titration and dose changes Use different medication formulations to promote absorption Changing medication administration time so as not to overlap with proton-pump inhibitors or antacids
Distribution ↓ *Vd* of hydrophilic drugs ↑ *Vd* of hydrophobic drugs Hypoalbuminemia decreases *Vd* of protein-bound medications leading to increased levels of free medications	Diuretics further decrease VOD of hydrophilic medications	Increase/decrease *Vd*	Dosage adjustment required with increase in age Close monitoring of free medication levels, especially medications with narrow therapeutic indices (e.g., lithium) Monitor for changes in *Vd* with dehydration, diuresis, third-spacing (e.g., ascites, pleural effusion), vomiting, and diarrhea
Metabolism ↓ Hepatic mass and microsomal metabolic capacity	Many medications are inhibitors and inducers of CYT P450 activity Some drugs bypass the phase I process and go directly to phase II (e.g., lorazepam, oxazepam, temazepam, and lamotrigine) Some drugs bypass liver enzymes altogether and are excreted directly through the kidney (e.g., lithium)	Increased/decreased drug metabolism Increased/decreased medication concentration and half-life	Close monitoring of drug levels Decrease polypharmacy and check for drug–drug interactions Dosage reduction of hepatically metabolized medications Administer active metabolite when appropriate/available Consider consultation with a pharmacist
Elimination ↓ GFR with age	Use of NSAIDs and antihypertensive drugs further affect renal function	Decreased elimination of medications, leading to longer half-lives	Dose reduction in patients with renal failure

enhance absorption (e.g., ziprasidone, lurasidone). Gastric emptying time and intestinal motility also decrease in the aged individual and can be further reduced by anticholinergic and opioid medications or pro-kinetic agents (Carlo and Alpert 2015). Poor nutritional status can impede the absorption of medications especially in frail elderly and nutritionally compromised patients who have a lower expression of epithelial transporters. Medical co-morbidities which interfere with absorption include poorly controlled heart failure (due to decreased GI blood flow, hepatic congestion, and GI edema), diabetic gastroparesis, and Parkinson's disease.

Aging thereby delays absorption and attainment of steady-state levels although eventually serum levels may be comparable to those in younger individuals. Medications may need to be titrated more slowly to avoid large increases in serum levels. Long-acting injectable (LAI) APs are beneficial because absorption of oral medications is potentially decreased, along with poor medication adherence. LAIs were found to be superior to oral antipsychotics to prevent re-hospitalization in geriatric patients with schizophrenia (Lin et al. 2020).

Distribution

Volume of distribution (*Vd*) comprises the specific body compartments to which a medication is distributed. During aging, there is an increase in the percentage of body fat (on average 30% more than in young adults) and thus an increase in the *Vd* for *hydrophobic* medications (Carlo and Alpert 2015). As a result, hydrophobic medications (e.g., long-acting injectable antipsychotics) take a longer time to reach steady-state levels and are eliminated at a slower rate. In contrast, a decrease in the percentage of body water in geriatric individuals results in a decrease in the *Vd* for *hydrophilic* medications (e.g., lithium carbonate). Thus, lower doses, and dose reductions, of *hydrophilic* medications may be required to achieve therapeutic levels in older adults. Close monitoring of changes in *Vd* is warranted because older adults are more susceptible to medication toxicity from sudden changes in fluid dynamics (Table 2.2).

Many medications are highly protein bound by albumin and alpha-1-glycoprotein. Changes in protein binding can lead to increase in free (active) medication fractions which result in clinical effects. For example, valproic acid (VPA) is highly bound to albumin. Routine laboratory studies of VPA calculate levels of this protein-bound medication which is not significantly different from free medication levels when albumin levels are normal. In cases of protein malnutrition with hypoalbuminemia, VPA levels may *appear* abnormally low or subtherapeutic, even though *free* medication levels may be disproportionately elevated (Dore et al. 2017). This may lead clinicians to raise the VPA dose, which ultimately increases the free fraction concentration and the risk of VPA toxicity. In the setting of hypoalbuminemia, *free* VPA levels are more clinically useful because they reflect a more accurate picture of VPA activity.

Metabolism

Most medications are metabolized by the liver through *phase I oxidation* via cytochrome P450 enzymes, followed by *phase II glucuronidation* which further increases their solubility in order to be excreted by the kidney. Phase II metabolism is not generally affected by *normal* aging but is significantly reduced in *frail* geriatric individuals (Khan and Roberts 2018).

Hepatic mass decreases by up to 20% in the aged, and cellular metabolic activity in liver microsomes diminishes (Stader et al. 2019); both changes compromise medication metabolism. Hepatic insufficiency further lowers the rate of medication metabolism and increases the risk of accumulation of unmetabolized medications (increased half-life) and adverse reactions. In such cases, medication metabolites with bioactive properties (e.g., paliperidone, desvenlafaxine), may offer advantages over their respective parent medications.

Antiepileptics, among other medications, can induce and/or inhibit cytochrome P450 enzymes. If two or more medications are present, medication levels and half-lives can be difficult to assess; pharmacist consultation and drug–drug interaction (DDI) applications provide guidance to minimize risk of adverse DDIs.

Elimination

Renal mass decreases by 20–30% by the seventh decade of life, and glomerular filtration rate (GFR) decreases by 35% (Stader et al. 2019). This increases half-lives of medications and metabolites eliminated through the kidney, and requires dose adjustment, especially in those with renal pathology. Extra caution is warranted for nephrotoxic medications that can decrease GFR (e.g., nonsteroidal anti-inflammatory drugs, angiotensin-converting enzyme inhibitors) or contribute to dehydration (e.g., diuretics).

Pharmacodynamics in Aging

The effects that medications exert on the body constitute *pharmacodynamics*. Age-related changes modify pharmacodynamics in ways that either enhance or decrease the impact of the medication. This is mediated by medication binding to targeted receptors, enzymes, or other proteins with biological functions and second messenger systems. Differences due to age can be attributed to changes in the affinity of the receptor to the medication and the number and rate of turnover of receptors available for medication binding.

Although there is a great variation among individuals, receptor density in general *declines* with normal aging (Knudsen 2003). For pharmacodynamic reasons, lower initial starting doses and lower target doses in older patients can often achieve the same therapeutic effects as higher doses in younger patients. For example, half the target dose of benzodiazepines may achieve sedation in individuals ≥65 years of age compared to younger patients (American Geriatrics Society Beers Criteria Update Expert Panel 2019).

Lower receptor density in the aged individual can increase susceptibility to adverse medication effects. Reduction in cholinergic receptors in the central nervous system, for example, can make geriatric patients more likely to experience central adverse reactions to anticholinergic drugs (e.g., cognitive impairment, delirium). In the case of antipsychotics (APs), lower target doses are also recommended due to increased risk of extrapyramidal symptoms and associated falls. Reducing AP doses by up to 40% has been shown to increase D2 receptor availability and overall cognitive abilities in geriatric patients with schizophrenia while maintaining adequate symptom management (Rajji et al. 2017). For antidepressants also, lower target doses decrease the risk of cognitive impairment, falls, bleeding, syndrome of inappropriate antidiuretic hormone (SIADH), and cardiovascular events (Darowski et al. 2009).

Blood–Brain Barrier (BBB)

Tightly apposed endothelial cells, specialized to impede constituents in the peripheral circulation from entering the cerebrospinal fluid (CSF), constitute the BBB. This structure serves not only as a wall separating the brain from substances in the periphery but is an important contributor to normal neuronal function (Marques et al. 2013). When intact, around 98% of small molecules cannot get into the brain, excluding many that could otherwise treat central nervous system (CNS) diseases, though psychotropic medications, which often consist of small, lipid-soluble molecules, usually cross through the BBB easily (Pardridge 2007; Zlokovic 2008).

Aging is the most common risk factor for disruptions of the BBB, which may occur even in the absence of co-morbidities such as hypertension (Montagne et al. 2015). Some studies of aging wild-type mice show an influx of pro-inflammatory substances such as *tumor necrosis factor alpha* (TNF-α), and it has been hypothesized that in humans, a permeable BBB may ultimately lead to neurogenerative disorders such as Alzheimer's disease (AD) and vascular dementia (Elahy et al. 2015; Zlokovic 2008). A study of aged adults found that BBB leakage begins specifically in the hippocampal region and is more marked in those with mild cognitive impairment than in subjects with normal cognition (Montagne et al. 2015). Neurodegenerative disorders may in turn increase BBB permeability further, thus creating a feedback loop (Elahy et al. 2015). Continued disruptions to the BBB may increase the risk of peripherally acting medications to freely enter the cerebrospinal fluid (CSF). Theoretically, peripherally acting anticholinergic medications, such as glycopyrrolate, could give rise to similar CNS effects as atropine (Zlokovic 2008).

Psychotropic Medications in Geriatrics: Adverse Events and Safety

Drug–drug interactions and inappropriate polypharmacy can increase the risk of adverse effects in the geriatric patient due to declining hepatic metabolism, diminished renal function, and/or changes in pharmacodynamics due to decreased brain volume. Polypharmacy has been associated with a decline in cognitive, physical, and emotional capabilities (Khezrian et al. 2019). The Beers Criteria offer guidelines of Potentially Inappropriate Medication (PIM) use in older adults. Table 2.3 summarizes common adverse events associated with psychotropic medications in older adults, for example, difficulty of swallowing in the oldest-old and frail patient but can have serious consequences in terms of choking and proper delivery of medications. Some formulations, such as wafers for mirtazapine, liquid/citrate solutions for lithium, for example, or tinier doses should be considered.

Antidepressants (ADs)

Prescriptions for antidepressants among individuals aged 65 and older have increased significantly since 2001, raising concerns about inappropriate use (Maust et al. 2017). A cohort study of >60,000 individuals ≥65 years of age reported that use of *any* AD was associated with higher all-cause mortality, attempted suicide/self-harm, stroke/transient-ischemic attacks, fracture, and epilepsy/seizures compared to when ADs *were not used* (Coupland et al. 2011).

Improvement in symptoms of depression or anxiety, as seen as adjustment disorders, can often be accomplished with non-pharmacological approaches (see Chaps. 14 and 15). In addition, aging adults and the oldest-old are vulnerable to medications which may have a direct effect on mood and behavior, such as corticosteroids (mood effects), beta-adrenergic blockers (reduced energy), or benzodiazepines and opioids (sedation, delirium) (Nørgaard et al. 2020).

Various ADs have been associated with specific adverse events (Table 2.3). Monoamine oxidase inhibitors (MAOIs) should be avoided in aging adults due to the risk of hypertensive crises, especially in combination with tyramine-rich foods. Similar caution accrues to tricyclic antidepressants (TCAs) due to strong anticholinergic properties, sedation, and orthostatic hypotension (risk of falls), although doxepin at a dose of ≤6 mg/day is considered safe (American Geriatrics Society Beers Criteria Update Expert Panel 2019). The selective serotonin reuptake inhibitor (SSRI) paroxetine has relatively high anticholinergic properties among SSRIs. Some SSRIs, such as fluoxetine, paroxetine, and fluvoxamine, are strong inhibitors of cytochrome P450 enzymes, and can prolong the half-life of their substrates. Sertraline, citalopram, and escitalopram are weaker inhibitors of cytochrome P450 enzymes and have lower risk of causing drug–drug interactions compared to other SSRIs.

Vortioxetine has an efficacy and side effect profile similar to other SSRIs. This medication may decrease the rate of age-related cognitive impairment and enhance the treatment of depressive disorders in patients with Alzheimer's disease (Cumbo et al. 2019; Deardorff and Grossberg 2014; Lenze et al. 2020). A trial of vortioxetine vs. sertraline in elderly patients with MDD found no differences in efficacy or safety (Borhannejad et al. 2020). Vilazodone and levomilnacipran have comparable safety and tolerability profiles compared to SSRIs and SNRIs, respectively. Significant safety concerns in the aging patient have *not* been reported for esketamine nasal spray although the study was funded by the manufacturer (Ochs-Ross et al. 2019).

Table 2.3 Cautions and common adverse events of psychotropic medications

Category of medication	Adverse effects/increased risk of
Antidepressants	Serotonin syndrome SIADH/hyponatremia (SIADH can also be due to polydipsia) Falls Cardiac complications Serotonin syndrome Sexual side effects Gastrointestinal bleeding Discontinuation syndrome
MAOIs	Hypertensive crisis when combined with tyramine-rich foods
TCAs	Anticholinergic adverse effects, delirium risk, sedation, and orthostatic hypotension
SSRIs	GI bleeds, falls, and hip fractures Many are inhibitors of CYT P450, increases half-life of other drugs (drug–drug interactions) Avoid paroxetine due to anticholinergic properties and increased risk of antidepressant discontinuation syndrome due to short half-life (REF)
SNRIs	GI bleeds, falls, and hip fractures (use duloxetine with caution in those with renal failure; avoid in hepatic disease) Antidepressant discontinuation syndrome
Bupropion	Dose adjustments needed in renal and hepatic failure
Mirtazapine	Dose adjustments needed in renal and hepatic failure
Antipsychotics	Stroke and mortality in those with a neurocognitive disorder Sedation Cognitive impairment Falls Neutropenia Orthostatic hypotension Cardiac complications Metabolic syndrome
First generation (FGA)	EPS, NMS, TD, dystonia, QTc prolongation with haloperidol
Second generation (SGA)	Metabolic syndrome Quetiapine has serotonin partial agonist activity and can increase the risk of serotonin syndrome when combined with serotonergic antidepressants QTc prolongation with risperidone, ziprasidone, quetiapine, clozapine
Mood stabilizers	Sedation Cognitive impairment
Lithium	Decreased *Vd* with age, monitor levels and renal function closely, delirium risk, hypo/hyperthyroidism, hyperparathyroidism
Antiepileptic agents	Hyperammonemic encephalopathy (valproic acid/VPA) Hyponatremia/SIADH (carbamazepine, oxcarbazepine, VPA) Increased blood levels of other medications
Benzodiazepines and Z-drugs	Cognitive impairment, falls, fractures, delirium, and motor vehicle accidents
Opioids	Sedation, respiratory depression
Stimulants	Cardiac complications and mortality
Cognitive enhancers/ cholinesterase inhibitors	Mortality (especially rivastigmine). May precipitate mania/psychosis
Anticholinergics	Delirium, cognitive impairment, urinary retention, constipation, dry mouth, blurred vision

Sources: Coupland et al. (2011), Gorgas et al. (2019) and American Geriatrics Society Beers Criteria Update Expert Panel (2019)

Adverse Effects in Antidepressants

Serotonin syndrome (SS) or serotonin toxicity. The pathophysiology of aging suggests increased vulnerability to SS due to an increased polymorphism and declines in expression and inducibility of CYT P450 enzymes. Impaired renal function and a reduction of renal clearance can result in hyper-serotonergic states with the use of serotonergic agents.

Medications which directly or indirectly increase central serotonin neurotransmission at postsynaptic receptors, 5-hydroxytryptamine 1A (5-HT1A) and 5-hydroxytryptamine 2A (5-HT2A) can produce SS. Psychotropic and non-psychotropic medications (such as tramadol) impact serotonin receptors, resulting in excessive levels of serotonin (Hede and Devillé 2019). SS can be precipitated when multiple serotonergic agents are combined or with high doses of a single serotonergic agent. Timing of dosage, frequency of administration, drug–drug interactions, and drug overdose, as well as inadequate washout periods between serotonin-enhancing medications, can contribute to excess serotonin levels (Wang et al. 2016).

Because it is a direct response to increased levels of serotonergic activity, SS can be identified with a thorough review of medications. SS often presents on a continuum with nonspecific clinical stages, but if not noticed and managed early, its progression can lead to organ failure and death (Boyer and Shannon 2005).

The *Hunter Toxicity Criteria* specify symptoms which identify SS (Dunkley et al. 2003), and Table 2.4 summarizes the stages of SS from mild, moderate, to severe. While SS remains a clinical diagnosis (Francescangeli et al. 2019), rigid adherence to the diagnositc criteria may leave SS undetected in old age where it may manifest as nonspecific and common symptoms such as confusion, anxiety, or restlessness.

The differential diagnosis of SS is extensive (Table 2.4), and initial treatment is focused on supportive measures in a medical emergency/inpatient hospital setting. Serotonergic medication(s) should be discontinued, and rarely, serotonin antagonists, such as cyproheptadine, may be needed.

Table 2.4 Symptoms and stages of serotonin syndrome

Symptoms of serotonin syndrome		
Delirium	Autonomic instability	Neuromuscular hyperactivity
Agitation Pressured speech Confusion	Tachycardia Shivering Mydriasis Diaphoresis	Hyperreflexia Clonus Tremor Mydriasis
Risk factors History of exposure to a serotonergic medication Presence of one or more of the following: 1. Spontaneous clonus 2. Inducible clonus with agitation and diaphoresis 3. Ocular clonus with agitation and diaphoresis 4. Tremor and hyperreflexia 5. Hyperthermia with temperature over 38 °C/100.4 °F		
Differential diagnosis • Neuroleptic malignant syndrome • Malignant hyperthermia • Toxic levels of sympathomimetics, anticholinergics, lithium, and other substances • Alcohol/other sedative-hypnotic withdrawal • Meningitis		
Stages of serotonin syndrome		
Mild	Mild symptoms of neuromuscular excitation and autonomic dysfunction that do not necessarily lead to delirium. Symptoms of toxicity can begin within 1 h of a precipitating event, such as an overdose, in approximately 30% of patients, and within 6 h in 60% (Boyer and Shannon (2005)	
Moderate	Worsening neuromuscular symptoms such as opsoclonus (uncontrolled eye movements—rapid, involuntary, unpredictable, conjugate, and fast), agitation, hypertension, hyperthermia (>40 °C/104 °F), delirium, hyperactive bowel sounds and diarrhea, nausea, and vomiting	
Severe	Severe neuromuscular excitation: Rigidity, respiratory failure, tonic-clonic seizures, altered cognition and arousal (manifested as coma or delirium), autonomic dysfunction with severe hyperthermia (>40 °C, >104 °F), and blood pressure fluctuation. Without treatment of the rigidity, hyperthermia can lead to rhabdomyolysis (manifest by high CPK), cell damage, myoglobinuria, renal failure, metabolic acidosis, acute respiratory distress syndrome, disseminated intravascular coagulation, and death. In SS, spontaneous/induced clonus and hyperreflexia are both more pronounced in the lower extremities	

Sources: Boyer and Shannon (2005), Dunkley et al. (2003) and Fink and Taylor (2001)

Syndrome of Inappropriate Antidiuretic Hormone (SIADH) and hyponatremia. SSRIs, SNRIs, TCAs, and mirtazapine are associated with hyponatremia and SIADH in the geriatric patient. Antidepressant-associated hyponatremia is more likely present when ADs are combined with an antihypertensive agent or more than one hypoglycemic agent (Grover et al. 2018). The prevalence of SIADH among those taking an antidepressant ranges as high as 15–20% depending on the agent and parameters used to define hyponatremia (Greenblatt and Greenblatt 2016). Medication-induced hyponatremia is usually caused by SIADH, confirmed by low serum osmolality and high urine osmolality. Other causes such as psychogenic polydipsia, heart failure, nephrotic syndrome, and acute kidney injury should also be considered.

SSRIs, several other antidepressant categories, and non-antidepressant serotonergic agents may also increase the risk of hyponatremia in geriatric patients. Risk factors for SIADH in response to AD treatment include older age (>85 years), female sex, and low body mass index (Greenblatt and Greenblatt 2016; Leth-Møller et al. 2016). Concomitant diuretic use, baseline low-normal plasma sodium levels, and lung and CNS cancers are also risk factors for SIADH. The geriatric patient has an increased risk of falls, seizures, cognitive deficits, all of which can also be associated with hyponatremia (≤125 mEq/L) (Mendez and Cummings 2003). Antidepressant-induced hyponatremia/SIADH can present with delirium.

The mean time to onset of hyponatremia from SSRIs is 2–4 weeks following initiation (Leth-Møller et al. 2016). Mild cases of hyponatremia can usually be managed with fluid restriction and discontinuation of the provocative medication. Most cases resolve within 2 weeks of stopping the offending medication (Kirby and Ames 2001).

Cardiac complications. Citalopram, and to a lesser degree its enantiomer escitalopram, among all SSRIs, pose a risk of QTc prolongation, in a dose-dependent manner (over 30 mg/day of citalopram or 15 mg/day of escitalopram), which can increase the risk of fatal arrhythmias such as *Torsades de Pointes* (TdP) (Beach et al. 2018). The US FDA issued a black box warning for citalopram and lowered the recommended maximum dose to 20 mg/day for individuals older than 60 years (US Food and Drug Administration 2017). Hepatic impairment, poor CYP2C19 metabolism, or the presence of CYP2C19 inhibitor medications raises the risk. Although 10–20 mg/day of citalopram can induce QTc prolongation, the actual risk of *Torsades de Pointes* (TdP) may not be clinically significant (Beach et al. 2018). Some studies report that citalopram doses >40 mg daily did not demonstrate a greater risk of arrhythmia or mortality compared to doses <20 mg daily (Zivin et al. 2013). Nonetheless, it is still recommended to discontinue citalopram in individuals with EKG evidence of severely long QTc or other evidence of cardiac conduction system disease. The geriatric patient with persistent QTc intervals greater than 500 ms and other relative contraindications (e.g., hypomagnesemia, hypokalemia, recent myocardial infarction, decompensated heart failure) should not receive citalopram. Except for citalopram and escitalopram, patients taking SSRIs had lower rates of cardiac events and dysrhythmias compared to those taking MAOIs, TCAs, and SNRIs (Beach et al. 2018). Trazodone can have adverse cardiovascular effects, including orthostasis, and rarely, extrapyramidal symptoms and syncope at high doses (Mayor et al. 2015).

Falls. Among aging adults, falls constitute the fifth leading cause of death, due to fractures, head trauma, and institutionalization (Van Swearingen and Studenski 2014). Ten to fifteen percent of falls cause major injuries in this population (Lord et al. 2017), especially during an inpatient stay. SSRIs may increase fall risk in the aged with odds ratios of 1.6–1.9 (Lenze et al. 2017), but some authors suggest that an association of increased fall risk with SSRIs does not constitute a cause and effect (Gebara and Lenze 2015). Orthostasis, sedation, or decreased postural control (Kvelde et al. 2015) may contribute to falls, gait instability, agitated confusion, urinary incontinence, and urinary frequency (Murray et al. 2007).

Serotonin/norepinephrine reuptake inhibitors (SNRIs) are included in updated Beers Criteria, with the recommendation to avoid them in patients with a history of falls or fractures (American Geriatrics Society Beers Criteria Update Expert Panel 2019).

Discontinuation syndrome. Insomnia, nausea, imbalance, sensory disturbances, and hyperarousal can emerge following discontinuation of SSRIs (Harvey and Slabbert 2014). These subtle changes in mood, sleep, and appetite may be mistaken for signs of a depressive disorder relapse and/or an anxiety disorder. Delirium and psychosis associated with discontinuation of antidepressants have been reported. Discontinuation symptoms typically last about a week are often mild and self-limited. This time course can facilitate their differentiation from a recurrence of the original target symptoms of depression or anxiety. Risk factors include use of SNRIs (due to sudden withdrawal of added noradrenergic stimulation) and anti-depressants with shorter half-lives (e.g., fluvoxamine, paroxetine), although there are also case reports of discontinuation syndrome after stopping SSRIs with longer half-lives (Harvey and Slabbert 2014).

Gastrointestinal (GI) bleeding and hemorrhagic stroke (HS). SSRIs are associated with an increased risk of bleeding, especially gastrointestinal bleeding [OR 1.55 (95% CI 1.32–1.81)] (Laporte et al. 2017). This risk increases with the use of nonsteroidal anti-inflammatory drugs and low dose aspirin (Yuan et al. 2006). Furthermore, the use of SSRIs in conjunction with oral anticoagulants (OACs) in older adults can be lethal. Warfarin, the most prescribed OAC globally, shows significant risk of drug–drug interactions with fluoxetine and fluvoxamine (Spina et al. 2020).

Medications which inhibit serotonin and/or noradrenaline reuptake have been shown to increase the risk of HS in patients aged 65 years and older (Shafer et al. 2019). One case-control study of 4059 cases and 40,590 controls found an increased risk of HS in SSRIs (OR 1.39, 95% CI 1.22–1.58), selective serotonin/norepinephrine reuptake inhibitors (SNRIs) (1.69, 1.35–2.11), norepinephrine and specific serotonergic ADs (1.44, 1.22–1.69), and norepinephrine reuptake inhibitors (3.81, 1.54–9.43), compared with tri- and tetracyclic antidepressants. Patients with a high baseline risk of bleeding and depression had the greatest risk.

Sexual side effects. Adverse effects such as decreased libido, anorgasmia, erectile dysfunction, and delayed ejaculation are common reactions to SSRIs and SNRIs with rates ranging from 20 to 70%, though these adverse effects may be under-reported (Serretti and Chiesa 2009). *Chronic* use of serotonergic antidepressants increases the risk of sexual dysfunction. Non-serotonergic and newer antidepressants are less likely to produce these adverse effects. For example, rates of sexual dysfunction reported with bupropion, a noradrenergic and dopaminergic reuptake inhibitor, are comparable to placebo (~15%) and the rates of mirtazapine, an alpha-2-antagonist, are slightly above placebo (~20%). Evidence shows that switching from an SSRI to vortioxetine can lead to improvement in sexual dysfunction although these studies were done by the manufacturer (Jacobsen et al. 2019).

Other adverse effects associated with antidepressants. Duloxetine requires dose adjustments for patients with mild renal failure and is to be avoided in patients with a Glomerular Filtration Rate (GFR) of <30 mL/min and those with hepatic insufficiency. Mirtazapine and bupropion require dose adjustments in patients with renal and hepatic impairment. Bupropion is associated with an increased risk for seizures, although not specific to the aged. It also has a risk of inducing or worsening psychotic symptoms due to its dopaminergic and noradrenergic properties.

Antipsychotics (APs)

Geriatric patients have decreased D2-receptor density and increased risk of adverse effects from dopamine antagonism, necessitating close symptom monitoring and lower AP doses (Tsuboi et al. 2011). APs in aging adults have been associated with worsening cognitive impairment and sedation due to longer treatment durations, baseline cognitive impairment, metabolic adverse effects, and anticholinergic properties of APs

(MacKenzie et al. 2018; Tsuboi et al. 2011; Wolf et al. 2016). Antipsychotics are considered Potentially Inappropriate Medications (PIMs) in major neurocognitive disorders (MNCD) and carry an FDA black box warning due to an increased risk for stroke, cognitive impairment, and mortality in this population (American Geriatrics Society Beers Criteria Update Expert Panel 2019). *Brexpiprazole* has been approved by the US FDA for agitation associated with dementia due to Alzheimer's disease. For further discussion, see Chap. 9 *Psychotic Symptoms and Syndromes*.

Categories of Adverse Effects in APs

Neuroleptic Malignant Syndrome (NMS). This life-threatening, rare syndrome can occur within 72 h after starting a dopamine antagonist, especially a first-generation antipsychotic (FGA) with geriatric patients on high dosages at particular risk. Mood stabilizers (e.g., lithium, carbamazepine), antidepressants (e.g., paroxetine, sertraline, amitriptyline), and antiemetic agents (e.g., metoclopramide) (Tse et al. 2015) have also been implicated.

Symptoms include hyperthermia of >100.4 °F on at least two measurements, along with profuse diaphoresis, tremor, sialorrhea, akinesia, generalized rigidity, dystonia, trismus, myoclonus, dysarthria, dysphagia, hemodynamic instability, and delirium. Laboratory studies include elevated creatine kinase (CK) and potassium from the leakage of these intracellular substances into the bloodstream because of rhabdomyolysis and decreased serum iron. Interventions should include abrupt discontinuation of antipsychotics, emergency stabilization, supportive treatment in a hospital with intravenous fluids to facilitate elimination of CK and protect against kidney injury, and cooling blankets to normalize decrease hyperthermia. Rarely, the use of dopamine agonists such as dantrolene and bromocriptine may be required.

Extrapyramidal Symptoms (EPS). Extrapyramidal symptoms can be divided into early (acute dystonia, akathisia, Parkinsonism) and later-onset (tardive dyskinesia [TD]), and often prompt medication discontinuation (Divac et al. 2014). Dystonic reactions due to APs are characterized by rigidity in a specific muscle group, which can be life threatening when respiratory muscles are involved. Intramuscular diphenhydramine or benztropine for immediate muscle relaxation can ameliorate the rigidity, although anticholinergics raise the risk of delirium in geriatric patients. Akathisia, characterized by motor restlessness, responds to AP dose reduction, treatment with beta-adrenergic blockers, and/or benzodiazepines.

Parkinsonism can emerge a few days to several months after AP initiation. The increased risk of parkinsonian symptoms is due in part to loss of dopamine production with increasing age, which underscores the need for an age-adjusted approach to FGA and second-generation APs (SGAs) for the oldest-old and frail. Switching to SGAs is often recommended because SGAs have a lower risk of EPS compared to FGAs, although the risks are not negligible (Gurevich et al. 2012). The rates of AP-induced parkinsonism are 55% with haloperidol (FGA) and 26% with olanzapine (SGA) (Divac et al. 2014).

TD appears after months or years of AP treatment and is difficult to resolve; anticholinergic drugs are not recommended. There is limited evidence for the efficacy of vitamin supplementation (Soares-Weiser et al. 2018). Switching to an SGA, dose reduction or gradual discontinuation are options. Parsimonious use of APs combined with social interaction can help reduce risk of TD, EPS, and mortality (Ballard et al. 2016).

If EPS emerges, lowering AP doses, switching to an SGA, or a lower potency FGA are recommended over the use of anticholinergic medications such as diphenhydramine and benztropine. Highly anticholinergic APs such as chlorpromazine are not recommended. Clozapine, which is highly anticholinergic, is not commonly used in geriatric patients, but can be of benefit for psychosis in Parkinson's disease or major neurocognitive disorder with Lewy bodies, due to its relatively mild EPS profile (Weintraub and Hurtig 2007). Lower clozapine doses minimize the risk of neutropenia, constipation, and lowering the seizure threshold.

Cardiac Complications. Antipsychotics are associated with cardiotoxic effects including myocarditis, cardiomyopathy, tachycardia (related to anticholinergic properties of APs), and QTc prolongation leading to an overall increased risk of sudden cardiac deaths (Sweeney et al. 2020). Ziprasidone and intravascular haloperidol carry higher risks of QTc prolongation compared to other APs. Most APs have the potential to cause myocarditis; clozapine carries the highest risk.

Falls. APs are associated with an increased risk of falls due in part to sedation, postural instability, shuffling gait, parkinsonism, EPS, and orthostatic hypotension (Fraser et al. 2015; Mehta et al. 2010). No significant differences in fall risk have been confirmed between FGAs and SGAs. Slow titration when increasing doses, smaller dose increases, monitoring with the Abnormal Involuntary Movement Scale (AIMS), and orthostatic vital signs are recommended.

Other adverse events associated with antipsychotics. AP use is associated with lowered seizure threshold (especially with low potency APs; e.g., clozapine, chlorpromazine) (Lertxundi et al. 2013). Clozapine serum levels should be monitored regularly to ensure a range of 350–900 mcg/L (or norclozapine levels of 25–400 mcg/L). While clozapine-induced neutropenia has been well-studied, other APs can also reduce neutrophil counts (Ingimarsson et al. 2016). SGAs may also exacerbate or cause SIADH in the aged, and close monitoring of sodium levels is recommended when starting or increasing doses (Lam 2009). Lower potency APs are associated with the development of metabolic syndrome which contributes to cardiac risks and mortality through weight gain, diabetes mellitus, and hyperlipidemia (MacKenzie et al. 2018).

Mood Stabilizers

Antiepileptic drugs (AEDs) contribute to a risk of sedation and falls and are recommended primarily for seizures, bipolar disorder, and depressive disorders (American Geriatrics Society Beers Criteria Update Expert Panel 2019). Carbamazepine (CBZ) is an autoinducer of CYP3A4 and can decrease the half-lives of drugs metabolized by CYT P450 3A4. Carbamazepine (CBZ), oxcarbazepine, and VPA may exacerbate or cause hyponatremia/SIADH. CBZ also carries a risk of hepatotoxicity and blood dyscrasias.

Valproic acid (VPA) is an inhibitor of the phase II enzyme that metabolizes lamotrigine (LTG) and can result in elevated serum level of LTG; the dose of LTG must be adjusted accordingly (often lower) when prescribed with VPA. Aged patients are susceptible to hepatotoxicity, hyperammonemia encephalopathy, bleeding, and pancreatitis related to VPA; frequent laboratory monitoring of medication levels, ammonia levels, and liver-associated enzymes is warranted (Mittal et al. 2009). *Free VPA* levels provide an accurate picture of the levels of active medication and can help guide dosing and avoid toxicity when there is hypoalbuminemia. Long-term use of VPA is associated with accelerated brain volume loss and possibly worsening cognitive impairment in Alzheimer's disease (Fleisher et al. 2011).

Lamotrigine (LTG) has antiepileptic, mood stabilizing, and anti-depressive effects and is indicated for the treatment of seizure disorder and bipolar II disorder. LTG in aging adults is also associated with an increased risk of falls and other nonspecific side effects (e.g., sleep disturbance, weight loss, and rash). When rashes emerge, LTG is routinely discontinued, and as a result there is sparse information about the incidence of Stevens-Johnson syndrome (Sajatovic et al. 2011).

Lithium, a mood stabilizer with first-order kinetics, is eliminated solely through the kidneys and should not be prescribed with medications that affect renal clearance, such as ACE inhibitors, loop diuretics, or NSAIDs. Lithium can cause nonspecific T-wave changes on electrocardiogram, and a baseline EKG should be obtained prior to initiation of therapy in older adults. It has been associated with hypercalcemia, nephrogenic diabetes insipidus, hyperparathyroidism, and hypothyroidism and should be monitored closely for electrolyte abnormalities, renal and thyroid/parathyroid function, and lithium levels.

Signs and symptoms of lithium toxicity may not appear until 1–2 days after toxic levels are reached; thus, early dosing and monitoring of levels are needed prior to dosage adjustment. Lower starting and target doses (Shulman et al. 2018) with lower lithium concentrations may be better tolerated and may maintain mood stability in the aged (Tondo et al. 2019).

Benzodiazepines and Z-Drugs

In September 2020, the US FDA updated a boxed warning for the use of benzodiazepines to "… address the serious risks of abuse, addiction, physical dependence, and withdrawal reactions" in this class of medications (US Food and Drug Administration 2020). Benzodiazepines and non-benzodiazepine and benzodiazepine-receptor agonist hypnotics (or Z-drugs) are considered PIMs (see Table 2.2). Benzodiazepines for aging adults increase the risks of cognitive impairment, including major neurocognitive disorder, falls, and mortality. Minimal doses of benzodiazepines may be considered in cases of seizure disorder, catatonia, alcohol or benzodiazepine withdrawal, or for initiation of anesthesia for procedures. See Chap. 7 *Substance Use Disorders*. Alternatives to benzodiazepines and Z-drugs for insomnia include non-pharmacological and pharmacological treatments. For further discussion, see Chap. 8 *Sleep*.

Opioids

The Beers Criteria recommend avoiding opioids in patients with a history of falls or fractures, except in the context of severe acute pain, with a duration not exceeding 2 weeks. Opioids have been associated with an increased risk of fractures in the aged patient (Hunnicutt et al. 2018). Combining antidepressants (ADs) with opioids increases the risk of serotonin syndrome, as many opioids have serotonin agonistic properties by increasing serotonin release and decreasing serotonin reuptake and and serotonin receptor activation (Francescangeli et al. 2019). Opioids combined with APs increase the risk of CNS depression.

Stimulants

These medications are used as adjunctive treatment for treatment-resistant depression (TRD) in aging adults. Methylphenidate has been effective for TRD when combined with citalopram short term (Smith et al. 2021). Common adverse effects include insomnia, irritability, headache, weight loss, and decreased appetite. Among aged adults, stimulants are associated with increased incidence of cardiovascular events (e.g., myocardial infarction, stroke, or transient-ischemic attacks, arrhythmias) especially within 30 days of initiation (Tadrous et al. 2021), calling for close monitoring.

Cognitive Enhancers

Cholinesterase inhibitors (e.g., rivastigmine, donepezil, and galantamine) and memantine have been FDA-approved for the treatment of cognitive impairment in Alzheimer's disease and other related neurocognitive disorders. Analysis of adverse effects of cholinesterase inhibitors in the United States and Canada indicates a higher risk of death with rivastigmine [ROR 3.42 95% CI (2.94–3.98)] compared to donepezil and galantamine, along with increased risk of falls (rivastigmine), syncope (donepezil), seizures (donepezil), and loss of consciousness (galantamine) (Ali et al. 2015). A meta-analysis of RCTs of memantine treatment for Alzheimer's disease demonstrated an increased risk for somnolence without an increase in serious adverse events and death (Jiang and Jiang 2015).

Cholinesterase inhibitors may increase the risk of precipitating mania and/or psychosis. One case report noted mania with psychotic features after the use of donepezil in a patient with Alzheimer's disease and in the absence of preexisting bipolar disorder (Hategan and Bourgeois 2016). *Aducanumab*, a monoclonal antibody which targets tau, approved by the US FDA in 2022, is discussed in Chap. 5 *NPS and Neurocognitive Disorders*.

Anticholinergics

Aging adults are prescribed a wide range of medications with anticholinergic properties. These include antidepressants, antipsychotics, antihistamines, muscle relaxants (e.g., cyclobenzaprine), and medications to address urinary incontinence (e.g., oxybutynin, tolterodine, and trospium). All add to the anticholinergic and cognitive burden (Salahudeen et al. 2015). Diphenhydramine, benztropine, and trihexyphenidyl are often used to prevent or reduce extrapyramidal symptoms of APs, although medications with strong anticholinergic properties are considered PIMs due to their increased risk of subsequent neurocognitive disorder (Heser et al. 2018). A study of over 700,000 geriatric patients found that anticholinergic drug use was more common among *cholinesterase inhibitor* users compared to non-users, especially among males, resulting in antagonistic pharmacodynamic effects and limitations of medication efficacy (Johnell and Fastbom 2008).

Medical Evaluation and Laboratory Monitoring

Comprehensive medical, psychiatric, and neurocognitive examination, determination of prior falls, and baseline laboratory testing should precede initiation of a new psychotropic medication (Table 2.5). Liver and renal function should be checked every 12 months for patients taking anti-

Table 2.5 Laboratory testing and monitoring for antipsychotics and mood stabilizers

	At baseline, prior to initiation of medication	Every 3–6 months	Every 6–12 months	Additional considerations
Medication reconciliation		✓	✓	At every visit
Vital signs	✓	✓	✓	At every visit
Comprehensive metabolic panel	✓		✓	Every 3 months if taking ≥3 medications or medications with known hepatotoxic or renotoxic side effects Consider more frequent evaluation of sodium levels in older adults on SSRIs
Complete blood count	✓		✓	More frequently if taking medications known to cause blood dyscrasias (e.g., mood stabilizers, antipsychotics)
Thyroid stimulating hormone and free T4	✓		✓	Increase frequency if on lithium
Lipid panel	✓		✓	Every 3–6 months if on antipsychotics
Hemoglobin A1C	✓		✓	Every 3–6 months if on antipsychotics
Urinalysis	✓			As needed for new onset delirium, irritability, changes to baseline mental status
Urinary toxicology	✓			As needed for new onset delirium, irritability, changes to baseline mental status
Electrocardiogram	✓		✓	As needed with new cardiovascular symptoms
Steady-state medication levels	✓ (If already on medication)	✓		With every dosage, addition, or removal of other medications (due to risk of drug–drug interaction)

Sources: Zeier et al. (2013) and Cullison et al. (2014)

psychotics and mood stabilizers (Cullison et al. 2014; Zeier et al. 2013) and more frequently if the patient is taking ≥3 medications or taking a medication with known hepatotoxic or renotoxic effects. Steady-state levels of medications requiring close monitoring (e.g., lithium, valproic acid), should be at initiation, dose changes, and addition or removal of other medications. For further discussion, see Chap. 4: *Laboratory Studies, Neuroimaging, and Neuropsychological Testing.*

The number of prescribers and prescriptions increases with age (Charlesworth et al. 2015), and geriatric patients may be unable to report or confirm the resulting adverse effects. Family members, credible observers, and caregivers, along with medication reconciliation and coordination of care can fill the information gap. Follow-up should include scrutiny for confusion, irritability, changes in appetite, routines, activities, or vague changes (e.g., patients "not being themselves"). Risks and benefits of ongoing or new treatments, dose adjustments, and drug–drug interactions should be reviewed. An integrated care approach can significantly decrease inappropriate polypharmacy and adverse effects of AP treatment in older adults with schizophrenia, in part due to more frequent assessments of EPS, metabolic disturbances, fall risk, and cognitive impairment (Abdool et al. 2019).

Age-Adjusted Prescribing Strategies

Signs of Polypharmacy

Several factors contribute to over-prescription of medications (Table 2.6). The ARMOR protocol facilitates evaluation of polypharmacy in elderly patients; the POM method helps assess patient function and overall clinical status. Other strategies are reviewed below.

Table 2.6 Over-prescription, consequences, and recommendations

Risk factors for over-prescription
• Old-old age (≥80 years)
• Polypharmacy (≥5 medications)
• Higher number of co-morbid medical conditions
• Higher number of outpatient prescribers
• Higher number of urgent care and emergency department visits
• Prescriptions for an antidepressant without face-to-face or telemedicine contact (e.g., electronically through EMR or via telephone)
Consequences of over-prescription
• Increased risk of adverse drug reactions
• Reduced medication adherence
• Increased risk of serious drug–drug interactions
• Increased health care cost
• Reduced functional ability and ability to perform independent activities of daily living, increased risk of living in a nursing home
• Increased risk of geriatric syndromes (e.g., cognitive impairment, falls, malnutrition, urinary incontinence)
Recommendations for reducing polypharmacy
• Evaluate polypharmacy in aging persons using the **ARMOR** protocol
• **A**ssess all medications, especially those on the beers criteria
• **R**eview medication regimen for adverse effects and drug–drug and drug–disease interactions
• **M**inimize number of non-essential medications
• **O**ptimize medications for renal and hepatic clearance using physiological data such as heart rate and serum drug levels. Consider tapering antidepressants and avoid duplication of medication properties
• **R**eassess patient for function, cognition, compliance, and overall clinical status. Consider the prescribing optimization method (POM) comprising 6 questions:
Is undertreatment present and addition of medication indicated?
• Does the patient adhere to their medication schedule?
• Which medications can be withdrawn or are inappropriate?
• Which adverse effects are present?
• Which clinically relevant interactions are to be expected?
• Should the dose, frequency, and/or form of the medication be adjusted?

Sources: Bobo et al. (2019), Drenth-van Maanen et al. (2009), Haque (2009)) and Levy (2017)

Deprescribing

Lack of coordination among clinicians, multiple prescribers, and incomplete scrutiny of medication regimens can contribute to excessive or duplicated pharmacologic properties, contributing to falls, all-cause mortality, and hospitalization (Kua et al. 2019). But *deprescribing* has its own risks: drug discontinuation syndromes, relapse of the original symptoms, and return or worsening of the medical condition(s) (Reeve et al. 2018). Successful deprescribing strategies include close monitoring during and after medication withdrawal to minimize the risk of withdrawal syndromes, particularly with a medication taken for an extended period and/or in high doses (see Table 2.6). Inpatient hospitalization should be considered when rapid tapering is required due to severe adverse effects. Gradual deprescribing is preferred, with close monitoring at each decrement of dosing. Collaboration with other health care professionals, including pharmacists and nurses, within a collaborative care model is recommended (Abdool et al. 2019).

Switching Medications

Lack of an adequate response to a medication or intolerability due to adverse effects may require a change. For serious adverse reactions (e.g., serotonin syndrome, neuroleptic malignant syndrome, catatonia, and toxicity), the medication should be discontinued immediately. Hospitalization should be considered when there is a need to switch medications, especially in the presence of complicated regimens, life-threatening conditions, multiple medical co-morbidities, severe symptoms, frailty, and questionable medication adherence.

Medication Reconciliation

At various "junctions" in health care (e.g., hospitalization, switch in prescribers, change in living situations, surgical procedure, and specialty consultation), a clinician may prescribe new medications, change dosages, and alter regimens. Often this may be done in the absence of communication with the other prescribers. These changes should be in the context of the whole regimen, and appropriate indications, duplication of therapies, incompatibilities, adverse interactions, and contraindications are reviewed. Collaboration with clinical pharmacists can also identify those medications without appropriate indications (Dolder et al. 2008; Wolf et al. 2015).

Specific Medication Strategies

Antipsychotic discontinuation and assessment. APA practice guidelines (Reus et al. 2016; American Psychiatric Association 2016) suggest tapering APs within 4 months of initiating treatment if there is no response to an adequate dose, unless there is a history of symptom recurrence during previous tapering trials. Monthly assessment for withdrawal dyskinesias, recurrence of EPS, and drug-induced parkinsonian symptoms are recommended during tapering and for 4 months following AP discontinuation (Reus et al. 2016). The Antipsychotic Discontinuation in Alzheimer's Disease (ADAD) trial reported that patients who initially responded to risperidone over 16 weeks of open label treatment had a two-to-four times greater risk of reemergence of symptoms at 16–32 weeks after risperidone discontinuation vs. risperidone continuation (Devanand et al. 2012).

Antidepressant (AD) switching. It is appropriate to substitute one AD for another from *the same* medications class when

- A patient with mild or moderate depressive disorder does not respond to an AD.
- The medication has been taken for a prolonged period (months or years) and/or at a high dose without apparent benefit.
- There is an increased risk of symptom relapse, drug–drug interactions, or the patient has multiple co-morbidities.
- The patient is among the oldest-old or frail.

A medication from another class of antidepressants should be tried for major depressive episodes (Boyce et al. 2020) which have not responded to the first medication. SSRIs/SNRIs with shorter half-lives (e.g., paroxetine and fluvoxamine) require a slow taper to avoid the risk of discontinuation syndrome. SSRIs with long half-lives such as fluoxetine may not require a taper. However, *adding* a second antidepressant or other serotonergic agent to another serotonergic agent can increase the risk of serotonin syndrome. In a cohort study which studied antidepressant prescribing in older individuals, 11% of subjects were switched to a different antidepressant within 12 months of treatment (Gadzhanova et al. 2018). For further discussion, see Chap. 11 *Depressive Disorders.*

Delirium and psychotropic medications. Geriatric patients are vulnerable to delirium, especially within intensive care units (ICU). A review of 10 systematic reviews reported that quetiapine and dexmedetomidine performed significantly better than placebo in the treatment of *hyperactive* delirium in people with COVID-19 infections in ICU settings (Ostuzzi et al. 2020a). For further discussion, see Chap. 6 *Delirium.*

Conclusions

Geriatric patients are at risk for inappropriate polypharmacy, drug–drug interactions, overmedication, and untherapeutic or excessive serum drug levels. Complex medication regimens, with different prescribers treating various medical comorbidities and symptoms, can lead to unrecognized adverse effects, poor adherence, and ineffectiveness. Good prescribing principles encourage the routine scrutiny of medication regimens to avoid duplicating medication properties and unnecessary complexity. An *age-adjusted* approach includes the initiation of the lowest effective medication doses, slow titration/tapering, and changing one dose or medication at a time. This practice facilitates the identification of untoward effects and assessment of effectiveness by minimizing confounding variables.

Age-Adjusted Recommendations

- Observe for adverse drug reactions in geriatric patients due to declining renal and hepatic functions, changes in the blood–brain barrier, or reduced receptor function.
- Scrutinize aging adults for *atypical* symptoms of adverse drug reactions due to overmedication, polypharmacy, and drug–drug interactions.
- Adhere to principles of *age-adjusted* prescribing:
  - Start at a low dose and maintain the lowest *effective* dose.
  - Change one drug or dosage at a time.
  - Titrate up or taper down gradually.
  - Monitor drug levels, renal and liver functions, and adverse effects routinely.
  - Evaluate for potential drug–drug interactions.
  - Avoid deliriogenic medications.
  - Re-assess the total medication regimen regularly, especially with multiple prescribers.

Minimize inappropriate polypharmacy and unnecessary prescribing:

- Begin with non-pharmacological interventions.
- Switch medications that have limited effectiveness or are poorly tolerated.
- *De-prescribe* medications which add unnecessary or overlapping pharmacological properties and which contribute to adverse drug–drug interactions.
- Re-evaluate medications which have been inherited from other prescribers; assess for uncertain or unnecessary indications.
- Observe for medication withdrawal/discontinuation phenomena.

References

Abdool PS, Supasitthumrong T, Patel K, et al. Using an integrated care pathway for late-life schizophrenia improves monitoring of adverse effects of antipsychotics and reduces antipsychotic polypharmacy. Am J Geriatr Psychiatry. 2019;27(1):84–90.

Ali TB, Schleret TR, Reilly BM, et al. Adverse effects of cholinesterase inhibitors in dementia, according to the pharmacovigilance databases of the United States and Canada. PLoS One. 2015;10(12):e0144337.

American Geriatrics Society Beers Criteria Update Expert Panel. American Geriatrics Society 2019 updated AGS beers criteria for potentially inappropriate medication use in older adults. J Am Geriatr Soc. 2019;67(4):674–94.

American Psychiatric Association. The American Psychiatric Association practice guideline on the use of antipsychotics to treat agitation or psychosis in patients with dementia. Washington, DC: American Psychiatric Publishing Inc.; 2016.
Ballard C, Orrell M, Yong Zong S, et al. Impact of antipsychotic review and nonpharmacological intervention on antipsychotic use, neuropsychiatric symptoms, and mortality in people with dementia living in nursing homes: a factorial cluster-randomized controlled trial by the Well-being and health for people with dementia (WHELD) program. Am J Psychiatry. 2016;173(3):252–62.
Beach SR, Celano CM, Sugrue AM, et al. QT prolongation, Torsades de pointes, and psychotropic medications: a 5-year update. Psychosomatics. 2018;59(2):105–22.
Bobo WV, Grossardt BR, Lapid MI, et al. Frequency and predictors of the potential overprescribing of antidepressants in elderly residents of a geographically defined U.S. population. Pharmacol Res Perspect. 2019;7(1):e00461.
Borhannejad F, Behnam Shariati B, Sina Naderi S, et al. Comparison of vortioxetine and sertraline for treatment of major depressive disorder in elderly patients: a double-blind randomized trial. J Clin Pharm Ther. 2020;45(4):804–11.
Boyce P, Hopwood M, Morris G, et al. Switching antidepressants in the treatment of major depressive disorder: when, how, and what to switch to? J Affect Disord. 2020;261:160–3.
Boyer EW, Shannon M. The serotonin syndrome. N Engl J Med. 2005;352:1112–20.
Carlo AD, Alpert JE. Geriatric psychopharmacology: pharmacokinetic and pharmacodynamic considerations. Psychiatr Ann. 2015;45(7):336–41.
Charlesworth CJ, Smit E, Lee DS, et al. Polypharmacy among adults aged 65 years and older in the United States: 1988–2010. J Gerontol A Biol Sci Med Sci. 2015;70(8):989–95.
Coupland CA, Dhiman P, Barton G, et al. A study of the safety and harms of antidepressant drugs for older people: a cohort study using a large primary care database. Health Technol Assess. 2011;15(28):1–202.
Cullison SK, Resch WJ, Thomas CJ. How should you use the lab to monitor patients taking a mood stabilizer? Curr Psychiatr Ther. 2014;13(7):51–5.
Cumbo E, Cumbo S, Torregrossa S, Migliore D. Treatment effects of vortioxetine on cognitive functions in mild Alzheimer's disease patients with depressive symptoms: a 12 months, open-label, observational study. J Prev Alzheimers Dis. 2019;6(3):192–7.
Darowski A, Chambers SC, Chambers DJ. Antidepressants and falls in the elderly. Drugs Aging. 2009;26(5):381–94.
Deardorff JD, Grossberg GT. A review of the clinical efficacy, safety and tolerability of the antidepressants vilazodone, levomilnacipran and vortioxetine. Expert Opin Pharmacother. 2014;15(17):2525–42.
Devanand DP, Mintzer J, Schultz S, et al. The antipsychotic discontinuation in Alzheimer disease trial: clinical rationale and study design. Am J Geriatr Psychiatry. 2012;20(4):362–73.
Divac N, Prostran M, Jakovcevski I, Cerovac N. Second-generation antipsychotics and extrapyramidal adverse effects. Biomed Res Int. 2014;2014:6563870.
Dolder C, Szymanski B, Wooton T, McKinsey J. Pharmacist interventions in an inpatient geriatric psychiatry unit. Am J Health Syst Pharm. 2008;65(19):1795–6.
Dore M, San Juan AE, Frenette AJ, et al. Clinical importance of monitoring unbound valproic acid concentration in patients with hypoalbuminemia. Pharmacotherapy. 2017;37(8):900–7.
Drenth-van Maanen AC, van Marum RJ, Knol W, et al. Prescribing optimization method for improving prescribing in elderly patients receiving polypharmacy. Drugs Aging. 2009;26(8):687–701.
Dunkley EJC, Isbister GK, Sibbritt D, et al. The hunter serotonin toxicity criteria: simple and accurate diagnostic decision rules for serotonin toxicity. QJM. 2003;96(9):635–42.
Elahy M, Jackaman C, Mamo JC, et al. Blood–brain barrier dysfunction developed during normal aging is associated with inflammation and loss of tight junctions but not with leukocyte recruitment. Immun Ageing. 2015;12:2.
Fink M, Taylor MA. The many varieties of catatonia. Eur Arch Psychiatry Clin Neurosci. 2001;251(S1):I8–13.
Fleisher AS, Truran D, Mai JT, et al. Chronic divalproex sodium use and brain atrophy in Alzheimer disease. Neurology. 2011;77(13):1263–71.
Francescangeli J, Karamchandani K, Powell M, Bonavia A. The serotonin syndrome: from molecular mechanisms to clinical practice. Int J Mol Sci. 2019;20(9):2288.
Fraser LA, Liu K, Naylor KL. Falls and fractures with atypical antipsychotic medication use: a population-based cohort study. JAMA Intern Med. 2015;175:450–2.
Gadzhanova S, Roughead EE, Pont LG. Antidepressant switching patterns in the elderly. Int Psychogeriatr. 2018;30(9):1365–74.
Gebara MA, Lenze EJ. A meta-analysis investigating falls in older adults taking selective serotonin reuptake inhibitors confirms an association but by no means implies causation response. Am J Geriatr Psychiatry. 2015;23(10):1098–9.
Gorgas MQ, Torres F, Vives R, et al. Effects of selective serotonin reuptake inhibitors and other antidepressant drugs on the risk of hip fracture: a case–control study in an elderly Mediterranean population. Eur J Hosp Pharm. 2019;28(1):28–32.
Greenblatt HK, Greenblatt DJ. Antidepressant-associated hyponatremia in the elderly. J Clin Psychopharmacol. 2016;36(6):545–9.
Grover S, Shouan A, Mehra A, et al. Antidepressant-associated hyponatremia among the elderly: a retrospective study. J Geriatr Ment Health. 2018;5(2):115.
Gurevich A, Guller V, Berner YN, Tal S. Are atypical antipsychotics safer than typical antipsychotics for treating behavioral and psychological symptoms of dementia? J Nutr Health Aging. 2012;16(6):557–61.

Haque H. ARMOR: a tool to evaluate polypharmacy in elderly persons. Ann Longterm Care. 2009;17(6):26–30.
Harvey BH, Slabbert FN. New insights on the antidepressant discontinuation syndrome. Hum Psychopharmacol. 2014;29(6):503–16.
Hategan A, Bourgeois JA. Donepezil-associated manic episode with psychotic features: a case report and review of the literature. Gen Hosp Psychiatry. 2016;38(115):e1–115.e4.
Hede V, Devillé C. Treating psychiatric symptoms and disorders with non-psychotropic medications. Dialogues Clin Neurosci. 2019;21(2):193–201.
Heser K, Luck T, Röhr S, et al. Potentially inappropriate medication: association between the use of antidepressant drugs and the subsequent risk for dementia. J Affect Disord. 2018;226:28–35.
Hunnicutt JN, Hume AL, Liu SH, et al. Commonly initiated opioids and risk of fracture hospitalizations in United States nursing homes. Drugs Aging. 2018;35:925–36.
Ingimarsson O, Haraldsson M, Jonsdottir H, Maccabe JH. Neutropenia and agranulocytosis during treatment of schizophrenia with clozapine versus other antipsychotics: an observational study in Iceland. BMC Psychiatry. 2016;16(1):1–8.
Jacobsen P, Zhong W, Nomikos G, Clayton A. Paroxetine, but not vortioxetine, impairs sexual functioning compared with placebo in health adults: a randomized, controlled trial. J Sex Med. 2019;16(10):1638–49.
Jiang J, Jiang H. Efficacy and adverse effects of memantine treatment for Alzheimer's disease from randomized controlled trials. Neurol Sci. 2015;36:1633–41.
Johnell K, Fastbom J. Concurrent use of anticholinergic drugs and cholinesterase inhibitors. Drugs Aging. 2008;25(10):871–7.
Khan MS, Roberts MS. Challenges and innovations of drug delivery in older age. Adv Drug Deliv Rev. 2018;135:3–38.
Khezrian M, McNell CJ, Myt PK, Murray AD. The association between polypharmacy and late life deficits in cognitive, physical and emotional capability: a cohort study. Int J Clin Pharm. 2019;41:251–7.
Kirby D, Ames D. Hyponatremia and selective serotonin re-uptake inhibitors in elderly patients. J Geriatr Psychiatry. 2001;16:494–3.
Knudsen GM. Assessment of neuroreceptor changes in healthy aging and in Alzheimer's disease with emission tomography. Int Congr Ser. 2003;1252:299–308.
Kua CH, Mak VS, Huey Lee SW. Health outcomes of deprescribing interventions among older residents in nursing homes: a systematic review and meta-analysis. J Am Med Dir Assoc. 2019;20(3):362–73.
Kvelde T, Lord S, Close JCT, et al. Depressive symptoms increase fall risk in older people, independent of antidepressant use, and reduced executive and physical functioning. Arch Gerontol Geriatr. 2015;60(1):190–5.
Lam YWF. SIADH caused by multiple atypical antipsychotics. Psychopharmacology. 2009;20(7):2.
Laporte S, Chapelle C, Caillet P, et al. Bleeding risk under selective serotonin reuptake inhibitor (SSRI) antidepressants: a meta-analysis of observational studies. Pharmacol Res. 2017;04(119):19–32.
Lea M, Rognan SE, Koristovic R, Wyller TB, & Molden E. Severity and Management of Drug–Drug Interactions in Acute Geriatric Patients. Drugs & Aging, 2013;30(9):721–27. https://doi.org/10.1007/s40266-013-0091-y.
Lenze EJ, Stark S, Avidan MS. Alternative facts? Antidepressants and falls in older adults. Am J Geriatr Psychiatry. 2017;25(12):1337–8.
Lenze EJ, Stevens A, Waring JD, et al. Augmenting computerized cognitive training with vortioxetine for age-related cognitive decline: a randomized controlled trial. Am J Psychiatry. 2020;177(6):548–55.
Lertxundi U, Hernandez R, Medrano J, et al. Antipsychotics and seizures: higher risk with atypicals? Seizure. 2013;22(2):141–3.
Leth-Møller KJ, Hansen AH, Torstensson M, et al. Antidepressants and the risk of hyponatremia: a Danish register-based population study. BMJ Open. 2016;6(5):e0112200.
Levy HB. Polypharmacy reduction strategies. Clin Geriatr Med. 2017;33:177–87.
Lin CH, Chen FC, Chan HY, Hsu CC. A comparison of long-acting injectable antipsychotics with oral antipsychotics on time to rehospitalization within 1 year of discharge in elderly patients with schizophrenia. Am J Geriatr Psychiatry. 2020;28(1):23–30.
Lord S, Galna B, Yarnall AJ, et al. Natural history of falls in an incident cohort of Parkinson's disease: early evolution, risk and protective features. J Neurol. 2017;264(11):2268–76.
MacKenzie NE, Kowalchuk C, Agarwal SM, et al. Antipsychotics, metabolic adverse effects and cognitive function in schizophrenia. Front Psychiatry. 2018;9:622.
Marques F, Sousa JC, Sousa N, Palha JA. Blood–brain-barriers in aging and in Alzheimer's disease. Mol Neurodegener. 2013;8(1):1–9.
Maust DT, Blow FC, Wiechers IR, et al. National trends in antidepressant, benzodiazepine, and other sedative-hypnotic treatment of older adults in psychiatric and primary care. J Clin Psychiatry. 2017;78(4):363–71.
Mayor JS, Pacheco A, Esperança S, Silva AO. Trazodone in the elderly: risk of extrapyramidal acute events. Case Rep. 2015;2015:bcr2015210726.
Mehta S, Chen H, Johnson ML, Aparasu RR. Risk of falls and fractures in older adults using antipsychotic agents: a propensity-matched retrospective cohort study. Drugs Aging. 2010;27(10):815–29.
Mendez MF, Cummings JL. Dementia: a clinical approach. Philadelphia: Elsevier Science Publishing Company; 2003. p. 48–438.
Mittal V, Muralee S, Tampi RR. Valproic acid-induced hyperammonemia in the elderly: a review of the literature. Case Rep Med. 2009;2009:802121.
Montagne A, Barnes SR, Sweeney MD, et al. Blood–brain barrier breakdown in the aging human hippocampus. Neuron. 2015;85(2):296–302.

Murray GR, Cameron ID, Cumming RG. The consequences of falls in acute and subacute hospitals in Australia that cause proximal femoral fractures. J Am Geriatr Soc. 2007;55:577–82.
Nørgaard A, Jensen-Dahm C, Gasse C, et al. Association of benzodiazepines and antidepressants with 180-day mortality among patients with dementia receiving antipsychotic pharmacotherapy: a nationwide registry-based study. J Clin Psychiatry. 2020;81(4):19m12828.
Obreli-Neto PR, Nobili A, Júnior DP, et al. Incidence and predictors of adverse drug reactions caused by drug–drug interactions in elderly outpatients: a prospective cohort study. J Pharm Sci. 2012;15(2):332–43.
Ochs-Ross R, Daly EJ, Zhang Y, et al. Efficacy and safety of esketamine nasal spray plus an oral antidepressant in elderly patients with treatment-resistant depression. Am J Geriatr Psychiatry. 2019;28(2):121–41.
Ostuzzi G, Gastaldon C, Papola D, et al. Pharmacological treatment of hyperactive delirium in people with COVID-19: rethinking conventional approaches. Ther Adv Psychopharmacol. 2020a;10:2045125320942703.
Pardridge WM. Blood–brain barrier delivery. Drug Discov. 2007;12(1–2):54–61.
Rajji TK, Benoit HM, Nakajima S, et al. Cognition and dopamine D-2 receptor availability in the striatum in older patients with schizophrenia. Am J Geriatr Psychiatry. 2017;25(1):1–10.
Reeve E, Moriarty F, Nahas R, et al. A narrative review of the safety concerns of deprescribing in older adults and strategies to mitigate potential harms. Expert Opin Drug Saf. 2018;17(1):39–49.
Reus VO, Focthmann LJ, Eyler AE, et al. The American Psychiatric Association practice guideline on the use of antipsychotics to treat agitation or psychosis in patients with dementia. Am J Psychiatry. 2016;173(5):543–6.
Sajatovic M, Gildengers A, Al Jurdi RK, et al. Multisite, open-label, prospective trial of lamotrigine for geriatric bipolar depression: a preliminary report. Bipolar Disord. 2011;13(3):294–302.
Salahudeen MS, Duffull SB, Nishtala PS. Anticholinergic burden quantified by anticholinergic risk scales and adverse outcomes in older people: a systematic review. BMC Geriatr. 2015;15(1):1–14.
Serretti A, Chiesa A. Treatment-emergent sexual dysfunction related to antidepressants: a meta-analysis. J Clin Psychopharmacol. 2009;29(3):259–66.
Shafer W, Princk C, Kollhorst B, Schink T. Antidepressants and the risk of hemorrhagic stroke in the elderly: a nested case-control study. Drug Saf. 2019;42(9):1081–9.
Shulman KI, Almeida OP, Herrmann N, et al. Delphi survey of maintenance lithium treatment in older adults with bipolar disorder: an ISBD task for report. Bipolar Disord. 2018;21:117–23.
Smith KR, Kahlon CH, Brown JN, Britt RB. Methylphenidate use in geriatric depression: a systematic review. Int J Geriatr Psychiatry. 2021;36(9):1304–12.
Soares-Weiser K, Maayan N, Bergman H. Vitamin E for antipsychotic-induced tardive dyskinesia. Cochrane Database Syst Rev. 2018;1:CD000209.
Spina E, Barbieri MA, Cicala G, et al. Clinically relevant drug interactions between newer antidepressants and oral anticoagulants. Expert Opin Drug Metab Toxicol. 2020;16(1):31–44.
Stader F, Siccardi M, Battegay M, et al. Repository describing an aging population to inform physiologically based pharmacokinetic. Clin Pharmacokinet. 2019;58(4):483–501.
Sweeney M, Whiskey E, Patel RK, et al. Understanding and managing cardiac side-effects of second-generation antipsychotics in the treatment of schizophrenia. BJPsych Adv. 2020;26(1):26–40.
Tadrous M, Shakeri A, Chu C, et al. Assessment of stimulant use and cardiovascular event risks among older adults. JAMA Netw Open. 2021;4(10):e2130795.
Tondo L, Tondo L, Alda M, et al. Clinical use of lithium salts: guide for users and prescribers. Int J Bipolar Disord. 2019;7(1):1–10.
Tse L, Barr AM, Scarapicchia V, Vila-Rodriguez F. Neuroleptic malignant syndrome: a review from a clinically oriented perspective. Curr Neuropharmacol. 2015;13(3):395–406.
Tsuboi T, Suzuki T, Uchida H. A tipping point in drug dosing in late-life schizophrenia. Curr Psychiatry Rep. 2011;2011(13):225–33.
US Food and Drug Administration. FDA drug safety communication: revised recommendations for Celexa (citalopram hydrobromide) related to a potential risk of abnormal heart rhythms with high doses. 2017. https://www.fda.gov/drugs/drug-safety-and-availability/fda-drug-safety-communication-revised-recommendations-celexa-citalopram-hydrobromide-related. Accessed 11 Oct 2020.
US Food and Drug Administration. FDA requiring boxed warning updated to improve safe use of benzodiazepine drug class. 2020. https://www.fda.gov/drugs/drug-safety-and-availability/fda-requriting-boxed-warning-updated-improve-safe-use-benzodiazepine-drug-class. Accessed 11 Oct 2020.
Van Swearingen JM, Studenski SA. Aging, motor skill, and the energy cost of walking: implications for the prevention and treatment of mobility decline in older persons. J Gerontol A Biol Sci Med Sci. 2014;69(11):1429–36.
Wang RZ, Vashistha V, Kaur S, Houchens NW. Serotonin syndrome: preventing, recognizing and treating it. Cleve Clin J Med. 2016;83(11):810–7.
Weintraub D, Hurtig HI. Presentation and management of psychosis in Parkinson's disease and dementia with Lewy bodies. Am J Psychiatry. 2007;164(10):1491–8.
Wolf C, Pauly A, Mayr A, et al. Pharmacist-led medication reviews to identify and collaboratively resolve drug-related problems in psychiatry—a controlled, clinical trial. PLoS One. 2015;10(11):e0142011.
Wolf A, Leucht S, Pajonk FG. Do antipsychotics lead to cognitive impairment in dementia? A meta-analysis

of randomized placebo-controlled trials. Eur Arch Psychiatry Clin Neurosci. 2016;267(3):187–98.

Yuan Y, Tsoi K, Hunt RH. Selective serotonin reuptake inhibitors and risk of upper GI bleeding: confusion or confounding? Am J Med. 2006;119(9):719–27.

Zeier K, Connell R, Resch W, Thomas CJ. Recommendations for lab monitoring of atypical antipsychotics. Curr Psychiatr Ther. 2013;12(9):51–4.

Zivin K, Pfeiffer PN, Bohnert ASB, et al. Evaluation of the FDA warning against prescribing citalopram at doses exceeding 40 mg. Am J Psychiatry. 2013;170(6):642–50.

Zlokovic BC. The blood–brain barrier in health and chronic neurodegenerative disorders. Neuron. 2008;57(2):178–201.

3 Essential Medical Evaluation

Vittavat Termglinchan, Maria Farooqi, Howard H. Fenn, Thelepa Vaithianathan, Sheena Ghodasara, Elyse Ross, and Amer M. Burhan

Abstract

Geriatric has been defined as 65 years or older since 1935 when life expectancy in the United States was 58 years (Social Security Administration, Life expectancy for social security. Social Security History, 2023). Mean life expectancy in the United States has since increased, by some measures to 79 years. As a result, a larger proportion of the population now can be considered *geriatric*.

Eighty six percent of individuals over 65 years have at least one chronic systemic medical illness, and more than 50% have at least two chronic conditions (National Center for Health Statistics, Percent of U.S. adults 55 and over with chronic conditions, 2015). Systemic medical illnesses in this age-group often include psychiatric symptomatology, such as depressive symptoms in cardiac disease, or psychotic symptoms in major neurocognitive disorder (MNCD). A thorough medical evaluation, therefore, is indicated for geriatric patients admitted to a long-term care (LTC), skilled nursing facility (SNF), or psychiatric unit, as well as for those presenting for outpatient psychiatric care.

The reader is referred to many excellent textbooks of geriatric medicine and to online resources for up-to-date guidance in medical diagnosis and treatment.

This chapter provides a brief overview of systemic medical conditions and medical

V. Termglinchan
Department of Medicine, Clinical Excellence Research Center, Stanford School of Medicine, Stanford, CA, USA
e-mail: vittavat@stanford.edu

M. Farooqi
Veterans Affairs Palo Alto Health Care System, Palo Alto, CA, USA
e-mail: Maria.Farooqi@va.gov

H. H. Fenn
VA Health Care System, Palo Alto, CA, USA

Department of Psychiatry and Behavioral Sciences, Stanford University, Stanford, CA, USA
e-mail: hhfenn@aol.com, howard.fenn@va.gov

T. Vaithianathan
Ontario Shores Centre for Mental Health Sciences, Whitby, ON, Canada
e-mail: vaithianathant@ontarioshores.ca

S. Ghodasara
Geriatric Psychiatry, Halton Health, Milton, ON, Canada
e-mail: sghodasara@haltonhealthcare.com

E. Ross
Division of Geriatric Psychiatry, Department of Psychiatry, Dalhousie University, Halifax, Nova Scotia, Canada
e-mail: elysec.ross@nshealth.ca

A. M. Burhan (✉)
Ontario Shores Centre for Mental Health Sciences, Whitby, ON, Canada

Psychiatry at Temerty School of Medicine, University of Toronto, Whitby, ON, Canada
e-mail: burhana@aontarioshores.ca

H. H. Fenn et al. (eds.), *Age-Adjusted Psychiatric Treatment for the Older Patient*,
https://doi.org/10.1007/978-3-031-53976-3_3

events common to geriatric patients who are in a long-term care facility (LCF), Skilled Nursing Facility (SNF), psychiatric unit, or similar unit, as well as those seen in outpatient settings. It offers recommendations for prompt recognition and referral to specialty care or urgent medical care. The goal is to reduce systemic medical complications, avert prolonged stays, and minimize the severity and duration of the conditions and associated psychiatric/behavioral symptoms.

Case Example: Agitation Due to Urinary Retention Attributed to an Exacerbation of Schizophrenia

A 68-year-old destitute man with a 45-year history of schizophrenia and acute psychotic exacerbation was treated in an acute psychiatric unit where he stabilized after with 5 mg olanzapine at bedtime. After 5 days, he was transferred to a long-term care unit (LTC). At the time of transfer, he was calm, compliant, but his thought processes were disorganized, and he was isolative.

Three days after admission to LTC, the patient became agitated and irritable. He rocked in bed and paced his room. He stopped eating and drank very little. The on-call physician, assuming the agitation was a symptom of psychotic exacerbation, increased the dose of olanzapine to 10 mg at bedtime. The next day the patient began screaming obscenities and was threatening to the staff. Haloperidol 2 mg every 2 h for agitation was ordered, and the patient received a total of 8 mg over 12 h. By the end of the day, he was yelling, swinging his arms, and walking constantly. He was started on a dose of 1 mg benztropine twice daily, on the assumption he was experiencing akathisia. He was not cooperative with a MoCA.

That night he developed visual hallucinations of people and animals in his room, which he had never had before. He could not sleep. He pointed to his lower abdomen, complaining of "pain down there." The on-call physician examined him, found no abdominal rigidity or tenderness, and ordered 12.5 mg of diphenhydramine for sleep. The patient screamed through the night and had other vague somatic complaints. Another physical examination now revealed dry hot skin and dry mucous membranes. A bladder scan showed urinary retention, and urinary catheterization produced a post-void residual (PVR) of approximately 800 cc. Auscultation of the abdomen showed no bowel sounds, and palpation of the abdomen as well as digital rectal exam revealed a large amount of feces, which was confirmed by X-ray. He had not had a bowel movement for 3 days.

Relevant Laboratory Results:

Sodium: 146 mEq/L (normal range 136–145 mEq/L)

Potassium: 3.5 mEq/L (normal range 3.5–5.0 mEq/L)

Blood urea nitrogen BUN: 20 mg/dL (normal range 8–20 mg/dL)

Serum creatinine: 1.40 mg/dL (normal range for men 0.70–1.30 mg/dL)
GFR: 55 mL/min/1.73 m^2 (normal range >60 mL/min/1.73 m^2)

Ammonia: 60 μg/dL (normal range 40–70 μg/dL)

TSH: 0.6 mU/L (normal range 0.4–5.3 mU/L)

Vitamin B12: 350 pg/mL (normal range 200–800 pg/mL)
Folate: 1.7 mg/mL (normal range: 1.8–9.0 ng/mL)
Hemoglobin: 14.0 g/dL (normal range for men over 60 13.2–17.5 g/dL)
Fasting glucose: 75 mg/dL (normal range 70–110 mg/dL)
Creatine kinase: 210 IU/L (normal range <190 IU/L)

Urinalysis: no bacteria or WBCs, trace protein

The working diagnosis was changed to *delirium* secondary to anticholinergic toxicity, with acute urinary retention, in a setting of benign prostatic hypertrophy (BPH). All medications with anticholinergic properties were discontinued. Over the next 2 days, enemas evacuated his bowels, and bowel movements became more regular. Voiding was encouraged prior to bedtime, and a sitter assigned at night. A dose of aripiprazole 2 mg at bedtime and a laxative were started.

He became calmer, less irritable, and more cooperative. He continued to display rambling speech and a thought disorder. His MoCA scored 25/30. He urinated frequently, ate meals with others, and had small hard bowel movements.

Discussion

Agitation and distress in an aging patient with schizophrenia were mis-identified as a symptom of his psychotic episode. An increased dose of olanzapine, with its anticholinergic properties, combined with benztropine and diphenhydramine to produce a significant anticholinergic burden (AB). These interventions precipitated delirium, urinary retention, and constipation. The patient had not been carefully assessed for BPH, night-time awakenings, bowel habits, or prior episodes of urinary retention. When he developed physiological symptoms of anticholinergic overload, he had difficulty expressing his complaints.

A Comprehensive Geriatric Assessment (CGA)

This interdisciplinary diagnostic process includes laboratory, other investigations, thorough history, and physical examination (see Table 3.1). A meta-analysis of 22 RCTs (representing more than 10,000 geriatric patients) reported that patients who underwent CGA, at a median follow-up of 1-year, were more likely to be alive and living independently in their own homes (odds ratio 1.16; 95% CI 1.05–1.28; $p = 0.003$) than those who had not. The mortality rate of patients who received CGA was also less (odds ratio 0.76; CI 0.64–0.90; $p = 0.001$) (Ellis et al. 2011). Another study of patients over 65 years old with neurocognitive disorders, low socioeconomic status, and a history of poor outpatient follow-up reported that frequent laboratory abnormalities were discovered upon admission (Elsawy and Higgins 2011).

Minimum screening investigations recommended for asymptomatic geriatric patients who are admitted to psychiatric units include (1) serum glucose, (2) electrolytes, (3) blood urea nitrogen (BUN), (4) creatinine, and (5) urinalysis (Ellis et al. 2011; Elsawy and Higgins 2011). The American Association of Emergency Physicians (AAEP) guidelines recommend further systemic medical work-up for new psychiatric symptoms with onset after age 45 (Wilson et al., 2017). For further discussion, see Chap. 4 *Laboratory Studies, Neuroimaging, and Neuropsychological Testing* (Table 3.1).

Secondary Prevention

Heightened vigilance and assessments for systemic medical conditions and adverse events can help prevent complications and avoid misdiagnosis and delayed treatment (Table 3.2).

Common Medical Conditions in Long-Term Care or Similar Facilities

Chronic Pain

Chronic pain can contribute to neuropsychiatric (NPS) symptoms, impaired physical function, immobility, falls, agitation, diminished appetite, sleep disruption, depressed mood, anxiety, distractibility, and delirium. The range of beneficial non-pharmacological treatments for chronic pain includes physical therapy, acupuncture, chiropractic manipulation, and massage. Psychoeducational interventions include cognitive-behavioral therapy (CBT) and meditation, which have minimal side effects and can facilitate reduction in medication doses.

Low Back Pain

Nonpharmacologic treatments include superficial heat, deep heat, superficial cooling, biofeedback, and transcutaneous electrical nerve stimulation, along with exercises, physical therapy, postural/exercise/mindfulness protocols, acupuncture, and chiropractic care. Pharmacologic treatment includes topical analgesics (e.g., topical methyl salicylates, capsaicin cream, diclofenac gel, lidocaine cream, lidocaine patch), intra-articular injections, and scheduled acetaminophen.

Table 3.1 Common laboratory investigations in geriatric inpatients

Clinical presentation	Condition to work-up	Investigation
Depressive disorder, fatigue	Anemia, hypothyroidism	CBC, TSH
Depressive disorder while on lithium	Hypothyroidism	TSH
Cognitive impairment	Hypothyroidism, vitamin deficiencies, neurosyphilis	TSH, B12 level, folate level, vitamin D level, syphilis screen, neuroimaging LP for CSF biomarkers (amyloid-beta and tau) if suspected Alzheimer's disease
New onset psychotic disorder	Hypo or hyperthyroidism, neurocognitive disorder, delirium, B12 deficiency	CBC, metabolic panel, liver-associated enzymes, TSH, vitamin D, vitamin B12, folate, neuroimaging, urine drug screen, urinalysis, HIV, other infectious causes
Sleep disturbance, daytime sleepiness	Sleep apnea	Polysomnography
Manic/hypomanic episode	Hyperthyroidism, neurocognitive disorder, B12 deficiency, corticosteroid exposure	TSH, neuroimaging, B12 level
Alcohol intoxication/ withdrawal	History of alcohol abuse	LAE

Table 3.2 USPSTF (US Preventive Services Task Force) Recommendations for secondary prevention

Investigation	Recommendation
AAA ultrasonography	Once between age 65 and 75 in men who have never smoked
Depression screening	Yearly
Fecal occult blood test (), fecal immunochemical test (FTT), sigmoidoscopy, or colonoscopy for colon cancer screening	Age 50 to age 75 Yearly for FOBT and FIT Every 5 years for sigmoidoscopy Every 10 years for colonoscopy
HIV screening	At least once in person aged more than 65 years old with risk factors for HIV
	Yearly in persons aged 55–80 with more than or equal to 30 pack years of smoking and currently smoke or have quit in the past 15 years
Mammography	Every 2 years in women aged 50–74
Osteoporosis screening	In women aged 65 years and older

Adapted from USPSTF recommendations for secondary prevention (US Preventive Services Task Force 2023)
FOBT fecal occult blood test, *FIT* fecal immunochemical test

Opioids and NSAIDs are not medications of choice in frail older adults.

Osteoarthritis

Osteoarthritis is the second most common chronic systemic medical condition among aging adults in the US and a frequent cause of chronic pain and disability (Federal Interagency Forum on Aging-Related Statistics 2016). Approximately 50% of oldest-old adults (85 years and above) had a diagnosis of osteoarthritis in one study (Collerton et al. 2009). The prevalence of osteoarthritis may be higher in females than males.

As the population ages, the rate of severe hip and knee osteoarthritis will likely increase (Anderson and Loeser 2010). Joint replacement surgery may be the best option for healthy aging adults when its benefits outweigh the risks. In general, when patients with chronic intractable pain fail conservative treatments, referral to a pain management specialist or to a surgical specialist is appropriate. For further discussion, see Chap. 5 *NPS and Neurocognitive Disorders* and Chap. 15 *Psychotherapeutic Interventions* (Table 3.3).

Falls

In 2015, more than one in four older adults in the US reported falling, and more than 28,000 older adults died as a result of falls (Centers for Disease Control and Prevention 2020b). Injuries after falls in the elderly are more common due to the higher prevalence of chronic systemic medical conditions such as osteoporosis (Morley et al. 2013). Fall risk is estimated to be especially high within inpatient geriatric psychiatry units (Blair and Gruman 2005). In one study, 84 out of 144 psychiatric inpatients experienced falls, often in the evening, with locations in the bedroom, bathroom, and hallway, where many (about 58%) were unwitnessed (Edelstein and Brown 2000). The following three questions, help screen for future risk (Ganz and Latham 2020):

- Do you feel unsteady standing or walking?
- Do you worry about falling?

Have you fallen in the past year; if yes, how many times, and were you injured?

Instruments to screen for fall risk include:

The STEADI (Stopping Elderly Accidents, Deaths and Injuries) initiative includes educational materials and tools to improve fall prevention (Centers for Disease Control and Prevention 2020b). Its three core elements comprise *Screen, Assess, and Intervene* to reduce fall risk by giving older adults tailored interventions. When patient screens *not at risk*, STEADI initiative recommends education on fall prevention, referral to physical therapy, evidence-based physical exercise, or fall prevention program; e.g., Tai Chi (Hu et al. 2016).

- *Timed Up and Go (TUG)* is a brief questionnaire that can be completed by older adult in ≥12 s (Centers for Disease Control and Prevention 2017).

Interventions for moderate fall risk include:

- *Prevention of orthostatic hypotension.* Regular blood pressure assessment is the most cost-effective test in the investigation of falls (Gangavati et al. 2011). A sustained reduction of BP (at least 20 mmHg) in systolic blood pressure within 3 min of positional change (i.e., reclining to sitting or sitting to standing), common in older adults, is often precipitated by dehydration, certain medications, and prolonged bed rest. Adjusting doses of medications that can cause orthostatic hypotension (e.g., diuretics, beta-blockers, alpha-blockers, quetiapine, and trazodone), adequate hydration, compression stockings, and changing positions slowly can all benefit.
- *Exercise:* A meta-analysis of 59 randomized trials, which included both healthy patients and those with chronic systemic medical conditions, supported the benefits of exercise to prevent falls in patients with elevated risk of falls. Balance training, for example, was achieved by progressively reducing the base of support, removing upper limb support, and moving the center of gravity to challenge balance (Sherrington et al. 2019). The rate of falls was 23% (CI 17–29) lower among the participants in the exercise groups than the control groups; the participants in the exercise groups had 0.20 fewer falls per person per year.
- *Assessment for medical and environmental contributors:* If the patient screens *at risk* for falls, CDC recommends assessment of lower extremities for neuropathy, evaluation of footwear, and assessment for comorbidities such as depressive disorders, osteoporosis, and/or visual impairment. In addition, modifications

Table 3.3 Chronic pain: non-pharmacological and pharmacological approaches

Non-pharmacological treatments	Pharmacological treatments
• Superficial heat, deep heat, superficial coding • Biofeedback and transcutaneous electric nerve stimulation • Physical therapy • Acupuncture • Chiropractic care	• Topical analgesics (e.g., topical methyl salicylates, capsaicin cream, diclofenac gel, lidocaine cream, and lidocaine patch) • Scheduled acetaminophen • Intra-articular injections

of the environment along with training in the use of technical and mobility aids can help. One study found that reduction of environmental risks significantly reduced the rate of falls in a randomized group of aged adults versus a control group [incidence rate ratio (IRR) = 0.63, CI = 0.43–0.94, p = 0.009] (Nikolaus and Bach 2003).

Modifiable fall risks include:

1. Home hazards such as throw rugs, poor lighting, slippery tub floor.
2. Medication regimens increase fall risk. Drugs and their combinations associated with increased falls risk should be reviewed, such as benzodiazepines, antihypertensives, opioids, some antidepressants, anticholinergics, and diuretics.

Osteoporosis and Osteopenia

Osteopenia is normal loss of bone density with aging, but many old-oldest adults have *osteoporosis*, a more severe weakening of the bone. *Osteoporosis* is associated with an increased rate of bone fractures, while *osteopenia* is not. According to the National Osteoporosis Foundation, as many as half of all women over the age of 50 will break a bone because of osteoporosis (National Osteoporosis Foundation 2020), as will 27% of men over 50 (National Osteoporosis Foundation 2015). The USPSTF recommends bone density screening for women over age 65 (US Preventive Services Task Force 2023; US Preventive Services Task Force et al. 2018). The recommendation for osteoporosis screening in men has not been clearly delineated (US Preventive Services Task Force et al. 2018). Elemental calcium 1200 mg/day (diet plus supplement) for women age ≥50 and men age ≥70 or 1000 mg/day for men age <70 is recommended. Vitamin D 800–1000 IU/day is also recommended if a deficiency of vitamin D has been identified (Guirguis-Blake et al. 2018); vitamin D3 (cholecalciferol) is the preferred form of supplementation (Ross et al. 2011).

Bisphosphonates are used successfully for osteoporosis, the major underlying cause of fractures, especially in postmenopausal women and older adults. These medications carry a rare risk of osteonecrosis of the jaw (ONJ). Alendronate is the most prescribed; other oral bisphosphonates, such as risedronate and ibandronate, and zoledronic acid in IV formulation pose a much higher risk of this condition than oral formulations of bisphosphonates. Clinical vigilance, good oral hygiene, and assessments every 3 months with panoramic jaw radiography can detect signs of ONJ early (Shannon et al. 2011).

Urological Symptoms

Involuntary leakage of urine may be considered *urinary incontinence* if a urinary tract infection (UTI) can be ruled out. Further steps include a review of the patient's medication regimen to identify categories of medications which impact urinary function, such as anticholinergics and diuretics. If urinary incontinence has worsened with initiation or up-titration of these medications, tapering dosages or deprescribing can improve urinary function.

If *nocturia* is present, lifestyle changes such as limiting caffeine, alcohol, and fluid intake in the evening are the first step. Pelvic floor muscle exercises, biofeedback to supplement pelvic muscle exercises, bladder training, and weight loss can benefit. The abrupt onset of urinary incontinence, constant pelvic pain, or hematuria suggest referral to a urologist to consider neoplastic or neurologic disease if a urinary tract infection can be ruled out (Reuben et al. 2019) (Table 3.4).

Urinary retention is estimated to occur in one out of three men over the age of 80 (Emberton and Anson 1999). The inability to empty the bladder leads to a spectrum of symptoms from urinary urgency and incontinence and has been associated with poorer outcomes, including urinary tract infection, suprapubic discomfort, with higher mortality rates (Smith and Albazzaz 1996). Renal failure can result from obstructive uropathy and can lead to delirium. *Urinary*

Table 3.4 Management of urinary incontinence

Steps	Recommendation
Step 1	Medication should be reconciled, de-prescribed, or dose adjusted. Such as medications including anticholinergics, diuretics, and cholinesterase inhibitors, especially if urinary incontinence is worsened with recent initiation or up-titration of these medications
Step 2	Non-pharmacological approaches to limit caffeine and alcohol intake, and fluid intake after dinner to minimize nocturia
Step 3	Pharmacotherapy by primary care physician or consultation with urologist. This comes with side effects, so should be managed along with medical and/or urology teams

Adapted from Samuelsson et al. (2015)

urgency, often associated with urinary retention, is an independent risk factor for falls (Boele van Hensbroek et al. 2009), because aging adults with unstable gait may rush to the bathroom.

Hypertension (HTN)

Hypertension is the most common chronic disease of older adults (Federal Interagency Forum on Aging-Related Statistics 2016). *Isolated systolic* hypertension is the most prevalent form of hypertension, present in approximately two-thirds of hypertensive individuals above 60 years of age (Izzo et al. 2000). Studies have demonstrated clinical benefits in treating isolated systolic hypertension, with reductions in overall cardiovascular disease morbidity and mortality.

Evidence supports tighter blood pressure (BP) control in ambulatory community-dwelling patients if it is well-tolerated. In 2014, the Eighth Joint National Committee (JNC 8) recommends BP goal of less than 150/90 mmHg for adults over 60 years (Armstrong and Joint National Committee 2014). Other randomized controlled trials (RCTs) have demonstrated the benefit of stricter BP control; American Heart Association (AHA) and American College of Cardiology (ACC) along with American Geriatric Society and other professional societies offered in 2017 a guideline to target optimum systolic BP at less than 130 mmHg for older adults age more than 65 years living in a noninstitutionalized ambulatory community-dwelling setting (Table 3.5) (Whelton et al. 2018).

Table 3.5 AGS and ADA recommendations for glycemic treatment

Patient health	HBA1C goal
Functional, cognitively intact, and have significant life expectancy (healthy)	<7.5% (7.0–7.5%)
Complex/intermediate[a]	7.5–8.0%
Very complex/poor health[b]	8.5–9.0%

[a]Multiple (3 or more) coexisting chronic illness, or 2 or more instrumental activities of daily living impairment, or mild to moderate cognitive impairment

[b]Long-term care, or end-stage chronic illnesses, or moderate to severe cognitive impairment, or 2 or more activities of daily living dependencies (American Diabetes Association 2020; Reuben et al. 2019)

The Hypertension in the Very Elderly Trial (HYVET) and Systolic Blood Pressure Intervention Trial (SPRINT) included frail older adults living independently. Both trials were stopped early because benefits were observed (HYVET discontinued after 1.8 years and SPRINT after 3.26 years) (Beckett et al. 2018; SPRINT Research Group et al. 2015).

BP-lowering therapy is one of the few interventions shown to reduce mortality risk in frail older individuals. RCTs in noninstitutionalized community-dwelling older persons have also demonstrated that improved BP control *does not* exacerbate orthostatic hypotension and has no adverse impact on risk of injurious falls. However, SPRINT excluded those with low (<110 mmHg) standing systolic BP on study entry. Older persons need to be monitored for orthostatic hypotension during treatment (Whelton et al. 2018).

In summary, RCTs have demonstrated that in community-dwelling older adults, even adults >80 years, goals during antihypertensive treatment are not different from those for persons <65 years, but with a high comorbidity burden, careful titration of anti-hypertensives is needed. Unfortunately, large RCTs have often not included older persons who live in nursing homes, or those with dementia.

Guidelines for hypertension control include:

- <130 mmHg systolic for older adults age >65 years in a noninstitutionalized ambulatory community-dwelling setting (Whelton et al. 2018)
- <150/90 mmHg for older adults >60 years (Armstrong and Joint National Committee 2014)
- <140/90 mmHg for older adults >60 years old with diabetes mellitus and/or CKD (Armstrong and Joint National Committee 2014).

Diabetes Mellitus (DM)

The psychosocial stressors of unmanaged DM include chronic neuropathic pain, loss of ambulation, and dependence on others. Regular foot examinations minimize the risk of amputations, especially in older adults with visual impairment.

According to American Geriatric Society (AGS) and American Diabetes Association (ADA), goals of glycemic treatment in older adults must be individualized (American Diabetes Association 2020). Diabetic medications such as sulfonylureas and insulin carry a substantial risk of hypoglycemia and should be weighed carefully in vulnerable older adults. Aging adults who are functional, cognitively intact, and have significant life expectancy should receive diabetic care with similar goals to those for younger adults [e.g., hemoglobin A1C (HgBA1C) goal <7.5%]. If there are multiple coexisting chronic illnesses, HgBA1C goal should be liberalized (see Table 3.5).

Stroke and Neuropsychiatric Symptoms

Every year, more than 795,000 people in the United States suffer stroke, and about 610,000 of these are first strokes (Centers for Disease Control and Prevention 2020c). Nearly two-thirds of patients with strokes were over the age of 65. Neuropsychiatric symptoms (NPS) occur in about 30% of patients who experience stroke (Ferro et al. 2016). Approximately 87% of strokes are *ischemic* in etiology, with the rest primarily *hemorrhagic* (Benjamin et al. 2019).

Time of onset of symptoms, when the patient was last seen "normal" or at her/his baseline, is crucial, as there is limited time available for effective interventions (e.g., anti-platelets, anti-coagulants, thrombolysis, and thrombectomy). Thrombolytics are effective only if the stroke is recognized and diagnosed within 3 h (or 4.5 h in specific cases) of the first symptoms. The ***FAST*** (Face Arm Speech Test) (Centers for Disease Control and Prevention 2020d) (see Table 3.6) can prompt urgent transfer for stroke management to the closest ED; no work-up need delay this because ***FAST*** can take 30 s or less.

Stroke reduces mobility in more than half of stroke survivors age ≥65 leading to significant psychiatric sequelae. The onset of right-sided weakness with aphasia is also common, suggesting an acute neurologic deficit with a vascular distribution of the left middle cerebral artery. Associated neuropsychiatric symptoms (NPS) are reviewed below.

Post-stroke depressive disorder (PSD) or depressive disorder due to another medical condition). Approximately 50% of stroke patients develop a depressive disorder (Robinson et al. 2008). PSD is difficult to diagnose because often a firm association between post-stroke depressive disorder, neuropathology, and brain location has not been established. Apathy, prosodic speech, abulia, sparse language, or flat affect often accompany stroke, but may not necessarily reflect features *specific* to PSD, the clues include:

- Refusal to participate in therapeutic interventions.
- Social withdrawal.
- Uncharacteristic behavior and mood, inconsistent with demeanor prior to stroke.

To rule out disorders other than post-CVA depressive disorder, consider the CVA Aphasic Depression Questionnaire-10 (SADQ-10), which has a sensitivity of 70% and specificity of 77%, using a cut-off score of ≥15 (Leeds et al. 2004).

Table 3.6 Screening for stroke *FAST* (Face Arm Speech Test)

If stroke is suspected act F.A.S.T. Note the time when symptoms first appear
F—face: ask the person to smile. Does one side of the face droop?
A—arms: ask the person to raise both arms. Does one arm drift downward?
S—speech: ask the person to repeat a simple phrase. Is the speech slurred or strange?
T—time: if you see any of these signs, call 9-1-1

Adapted from Powers et al. (2018)

PSD has a consistently negative effect on stroke outcomes (Kutlubaev and Hackett 2014); current and lifetime history of depressive disorder also impact functional outcomes post-stroke (Wulsin et al. 2012). When patients were matched for initial functional outcome, remission of prior depressive disorder was associated with a better functional outcome at 3 and 6 months compared to those who had continuation of a depressive disorder (Chemerinski et al. 2001).

The onset of a depressive disorder following a stroke has been reported to range from 33% at 1 year to 23% at 5 years after stroke (Hackett and Pickles 2014). Several *psychological* symptoms can help identify post-CVA depressive disorder: feeling discouraged/hopeless, thoughts of being punished, and being self-critical. *Physical* symptoms like fatigue are prevalent in geriatric patients but not as helpful in confirming a diagnosis of post-CVA depressive disorder (Tang et al. 2010).

A single question (*"Do you often feel sad or depressed?"*) from the Montgomery-Asberg depression rating scale (MADRS) demonstrated a specificity of 78% and sensitivity 86%, respectively, to screen for post-stroke depressive disorder (Watkins et al. 2001). The following risk factors and predictors are associated with PSD (Ayerbe et al. 2013; De Ryck et al. 2014; Hackett et al. 2014; Towfighi et al. 2017):

- Lack of family/social support
- Anxiety
- Physical disability
- Severity of stroke
- Cognitive impairment

PSD: Psychotherapeutic treatment. A Cochrane review and meta-analysis of three trials ($N = 445$) reported benefit from brief psychosocial therapies for established PSD and for prevention of depression (Hackett et al. 2008). A Living Well with Stroke Study derived from the Cochrane review included 101 stroke survivors. Subjects were randomized to either a brief psychosocial intervention of 9 counseling sessions or usual care. Remission or greater reduction in depression symptoms was achieved more often in the intervention group than usual care at all time points (9 weeks, 6 months, and 1 year). Antidepressants were recommended for all participants. By 12 months after the intervention, both modes of delivery were able to achieve a 40% reduction in Hamilton Depression Rating Scale scores, indicating equal efficacy (Mitchell et al. 2009). Psychotherapeutic telephone interventions have also been reported as beneficial (Kirkness et al. 2015).

PSD: Neuromodulation interventions and ECT. Several modalities have been used with some success to treat refractory post-stroke depressive disorders (Hackett et al. 2008). ECT is contraindicated in post-stroke patients if there is evidence of or significant risk of hemorrhage.

- *Repetitive Transcranial Magnetic Stimulation (rTMS)*: A 2016 systematic review of rTMS for depressive disorders associated with cerebrovascular disease (McIntyre et al. 2016) included five studies (three RCTs and two uncontrolled pre-post studies), with 186 participants overall, all diagnosed with either PSD or vascular depressive disorder (mean age: 51.9–67.9 years). For participants receiving active rTMS (as opposed to sham), three studies reported Hamilton Depression Rating Scale (HDRS) scores decreased by 33.1–42.4% (weighted average 38.8%) immediately posttreatment. One study reported a HDRS decrease of 38.5% at 2 weeks posttreatment, and 40.2% 4 weeks posttreatment. Remission rates ranged from 10.0 to 34.4% (weighted average 25.6%).
- A systematic review and meta-analysis reviewed RCTs of rTMS for PSD. Severity of

depressive disorder rated with the HDRS suggested that rTMS has beneficial effects on PSD. Change in HDRS scores from baseline to the end of treatment and a meta-analysis of the mean changes in scores of the experimental group and control group showed a mean difference: HDRS score was decreased by 6 points (95% CI −7.74 to −4.45, $P < 0.001$) favoring rTMS (Shen et al. 2022). Another systematic review of seven studies involving rTMS in PSD reported very low risk of adverse effects. The review concluded that rTMS was effective, although sample size was small and there was a lack of uniform diagnostic criteria for depressive disorders (Bucur and Papagno 2018). The long-term efficacy of these methods, alone and in combination with pharmacological treatment, awaits more study.
- Another extensive metanalysis reported that rTMS and tDCS were effective and safe treatment techniques for PSD (Shen et al. 2022). For further discussion, see Chap. 14: *Neuromodulation Therapies*.

PSD: Pharmacologic treatment. A review of seven trials compared SSRIs to placebo, two trials compared TCAs to placebo, and four trials, including combined flupentixol + melitracen, aniracetam, reboxetine, and trazodone, reported a small but significant improvement in depressive symptoms on illness remission (pooled odds ratio of 0.47 with 95% CI 0.22–0.98). However, a significant increase in adverse events was noted (Hackett et al. 2008).

A Cochrane review of seven trials involving 239 participants with stroke found that several trials showed antidepressant-related improvements in emotionalism, tearfulness, lability, and improved scores on the Pathologic Laughing and Crying Scale. This effect was not specific to a particular class of medications, and methodological deficiencies in the studies were noted (Hackett et al. 2010).

PSD: Prevention and management. A Cochrane review of 14 trials with 1515 participants found a small but significant effect of psychotherapy on improving mood and preventing depressive disorders following stroke. The review did not find evidence that prophylactic antidepressants *prevented* depressive disorders in the post-stroke period (Hackett et al. 2008).

A multisite prevention study looked at pharmacological and psychosocial treatment for 176 stroke survivors without depressive disorder who were enrolled within 3 months of stroke. Participants were randomized to 1 year of treatment with: (a) escitalopram ($n = 59$) (10 mg/day in the morning for patients <65 years and 5 mg/day for patients ≥65 years), (b) placebo ($n = 58$), or (c), a non-blinded arm with a problem-solving therapy group ($n = 59$). Those on placebo were *more likely* to report depressive disorder (HR, 4.5; 95% CI, 2.4–8.2) than those who participated in the therapy group (HR, 2.2; 95% CI, 1.4–3.5) or those taking escitalopram (Robinson et al. 2008).

While there is some evidence that prophylactic pharmacotherapy can prevent post-stroke depressive symptoms, its impact on function is less clear. The risk–benefit ratio in favor of prophylactic antidepressants has not been clearly established.

Post-stroke anxiety disorder (anxiety disorder due to another medical condition). In a 2017 meta-analysis of 13 studies, 2408 patients showed an association between post-stroke depressive and anxiety disorders (Wright et al. 2017). A structured or semi-structured interview is recommended during assessment (Schöttke and Giabbiconi 2015). A study of 73 participants with primary diagnosis of stroke was assessed with the Beck Anxiety Inventory. The most reported symptoms were *fearing the worst* (63%), *feeling scared* (60%), *fear of dying* (59%), and *unsteady gait* (53%); both emotional and somatic items were endorsed (Barker-Collo 2007).

Post-stroke anxiety disorder: non-pharmacological treatment. Standardized relaxation techniques have shown benefit for anxiety which is associated with neurological damage. A virtual reality system called Computer Assisted Rehabilitation Environment (CAREN) was combined with relaxation techniques and showed significantly superior results compared to relaxation techniques alone (De Luca et al. 2019).

Post-stroke anxiety disorder: pharmacological treatment. Consensus guidelines for medication treatment of post-stroke anxiety are sparse. Risks from benzodiazepines and Z-drugs, especially for the oldest-old, have been reported. In an open label, controlled clinical trial, 60 patients with post-stroke depressive disorder who received duloxetine, citalopram, or sertraline were studied. Duloxetine was substantially more effective than the other two medications for *anxiety* symptoms ($p < 0.01$) and well-tolerated (Karaiskos et al. 2012). For further discussion, see Chap. 2 *Geriatric Pharmacology Overview* and Chap. 10 *Anxiety Disorders*.

Post-stroke psychotic disorder (psychotic disorder due to another medical condition).

Psychosis has been estimated to occur in approximately 4% of post-stroke patients (Joyce 2018), and delusional disorder has been described as the most common psychotic disorder post-stroke. It is often localized to a right hemisphere lesion of the frontal, temporal, and/or parietal lobes (Stangeland and Vasiliki 2018). Visual hallucinations have been associated with the occipital lobe, and auditory hallucinations associated with subcortical strokes or cortical strokes (Hackett et al. 2014).

Post-stroke psychotic disorder: pharmacologic treatment. Standard antipsychotic (AP) treatment is appropriate (Ferreira et al. 2017). APs have been used with some success in treatment-resistant cases. For further discussion, see Chap. 9 *Psychotic Symptoms and Syndromes*.

Post-stroke apathy: description. A reduction in goal directed behavior and motivation, in the setting of normal cognitive abilities, mood, and level of consciousness is characteristic of apathy (Marin and Wilkosz 2005). Apathy can be present *without* the depressive constellation of depressed mood, morbid thoughts, self-blame, and low energy. A meta-analysis of 24 studies (2706 patients) showed a 35% prevalence of apathy, at a median of 120 days after stroke (van Dalen et al. 2013). Apathy can negatively impact functional recovery (Hama et al. 2011), rehabilitation participation, physical health, and health perception (Mayo et al. 2009). A study of 237 stroke patients identified 19.2% with apathy using the Neuropsychiatric Inventory (NPI). Compared with depressive disorder, apathy may be more often associated with diminished functional abilities and is more likely to impinge on recovery post-stroke (Sama et al. 2007).

Post-stroke apathy: pharmacologic treatment. A systematic review of double-blind RCTs of dopaminergic agents for various neuropsychiatric syndromes following stroke did not find studies which focused directly on apathy, or which demonstrated conclusive benefit (Sami and Faruqui 2015). One study compared combined dopaminergic treatment (methylphenidate and levodopa) to placebo at 90 and 180 days and reported considerable improvement on Geriatric Depression Scale scores (Delbari et al. 2011). Another study of apathy after a prefrontal cortex stroke reported that a dopamine receptor agonist had benefit (Kohno et al. 2010). A small, controlled trial of high dose nefiracetam showed a positive effect on apathy in a group of post-stroke depressive disorder patients (Robinson et al. 2008).

One RCT studied apathy in patients within 3 months of stroke. For 1 year, patients were treated with escitalopram, problem-solving therapy (PST), or placebo and assessed at 3, 6, 9, and 12 months; the apathy syndrome was 3.47 times more likely among patients given placebo than escitalopram, and 1.84 times more likely among patients given placebo than PST. Escitalopram and PST both prolonged the time to onset of post-stroke apathy even when patients with comorbid apathy and depression were excluded (Mikami et al. 2013). For further discussion, see Chap. 5 *NPS and Neurocognitive Disorder*, and Chap. 15 *Psychotherapeutic Interventions*.

Sleep-wake disturbances following stroke. Sleep-related breathing disorders are often evident within 24 h after stroke; if the patient get stroke while the patient was asleep, the breathing disorders tend to be more severe (Iranzo et al. 2002). Apparent cognitive impairment may be reversible in the context of sleep problems, especially when accompanied by sleep apnea, with daytime sleepiness, morning headaches, and poor energy (Janssens et al. 2000). Pre-existing sleep-related breathing disorders, common in patients with stroke, may be responsible [e.g., obstructive sleep apnea (OSA), central sleep apnea (CSA), and Cheyne-Stokes breathing].

Environmental factors such as poor lighting, excessive noise, and adjustment of surroundings can be corrected to minimize risk of injury or misinterpreting objects. Delirium should be ruled out, and sleep hygiene techniques emphasized (Lerner and Riley 2012). For further discussion, see Chap. 5 *NPS* and Chap. 8 *Sleep*.

Post-stroke mania (Bipolar and related disorder due to another medical condition). A systematic review of 32 studies described 49 cases of mania following a stroke, the majority (92%) of whom had elevated mood as the first symptom. Approximately 53% showed manic symptoms immediately after stroke, 23% during the first month after stroke and 23% *after the first month*. Frequent symptoms included an increased rate or amount of speech (71%), decreased sleep (69%), and agitation (63%). Clinical presentation was therefore like primary mania in the general population (Ferro et al. 2009).

Manic symptoms following a stroke may also be due to delirium (Santos et al. 2011). A search to rule out delirium and identify or correct any possible etiologies would be a first step. Treatment with mood stabilizers and antipsychotics, similar to treatment of primary mania, would be considered if harmful behavioral and psychiatric symptoms could not be otherwise managed. (See Chap. 6 *Delirium* and Chap. 12 *Bipolar and Related Disorders*).

Language and communication deficits following stroke. Neuropsychological testing as well as speech therapy consultation can help identify post-stroke disorders of language and speech. These conditions impact mood, functioning, and communication, leading to alienation, frustration, and agitation.

- *Apraxia* is an impairment of motor *programming*, rather than weakness or paralysis of the muscles needed for speech.
- *Speech apraxia is* the result of a neurological event which disrupts neural pathways involved in language production. The patient shows no apparent *effortful* struggle, but may have trouble expressing substitutions of phenomes, or difficulty in repeating multisyllabic words.
- *Verbal apraxia,* or *apraxia of speech*, results in no difficulty in producing automatic, or spontaneous speech, but impairment in *novel* verbal output. Misarticulations can escalate behavioral disruption and impact the relationship with others.
- *Aphasia* is loss of ability to produce and/or understand language, due to any insult or pathologic process in neural circuits which disrupt the language network.
- A*lexia* (inability to read), *acalculia* (poor understanding of written numbers), and *agraphia* (inability to write) are more specific language deficits.
- *Dysarthria* results when neuromuscular impairment of muscles involved in speech cannot function. A struggle to produce correct sounds can follow. Behavior described as "articulatory groping" results from attempts to compensate for communication deficits with different facial and oral maneuvers (such as grimacing).

The inability to clearly express one's needs or to follow exact instructions can contribute to strained interpersonal interactions; others may interpret that the patient as uncooperative by choice. These characteristics of non-fluent speech suggest a language deficit:

- Sparse output (decreased number of words per minute).
- Shortened phrases (5 words or less).
- Agrammatism: omission or substitution of words (prepositions, conjunctions, or suffixes).
- Effortful speech: hesitations and disruption of normal melodic rhythm.
- Breakdown of speech praxis: poor ability to coordinate the articulatory movements required for comprehensible speech.

For further discussion, see Chap. 4: *Laboratory, Neuroimaging, and Neuropsychological Testing*.

Transient Ischemic Attack (TIA)

An acute neurological event, indicating injury to the brain, that resolves within 24 h (World Health Organization 2004), is considered a *transient ischemic attack*. Most TIAs resolve within few hours. The ABCD2 score can help stratify the risk of subsequent stroke (see Table 3.7) (Johnston et al. 2007; Josephson et al. 2008).

When TIA is suspected in any setting (regardless of ABCD2 score), immediate transfer (within 24 h) to an ED or stroke center is recommended. Even patients who wake up with an acute neurological change with *unknown* time of onset (most likely greater than 4.5 h), should be transferred immediately because thrombectomy, can be of benefit only up to 24 h after the stroke onset (Nogueira et al. 2018).

Patients with a suspected TIA or minor ischemic stroke without a known cardioembolic source should be started on antiplatelet therapy even while waiting for neurology consultation and/or Emergency Department (ED) transfer. Exceptions are patients who are already on oral anticoagulation or have a clear new indication for anticoagulation.

Medication recommendations:

- For patients with high-risk TIA, defined as an ABCD^2 score of $\geq$4 dual antiplatelet therapy (DAPT) with aspirin (160–325 mg loading dose, followed by 50–100 mg daily) plus clopidogrel (300–600 mg loading dose, followed by 75 mg daily) should be considered.
- For patients with a low-risk TIA defined by an ABCD^2 score <4, aspirin monotherapy is started 162–325 mg/daily alone.

Table 3.7 ABCD2 Score

A	Age $\geq$60 years	No = 0	Yes = +1
B	Blood pressure $\geq$140/99 mmHg	No = 0	Yes = +1
C	Clinical features of TIA	• Unilateral weakness = +2 • Speech disturbances without weakness = +1 • Other symptoms = 0	
D1	Duration of symptoms	• <10 min = 0 • 10–59 min = +1 • $\geq$60 min = +2	
D2	History of diabetes mellitus	No = 0	Yes = +1

Adapted from Johnston et al. (2007) and Josephson et al. (2008)

Seizures

The possibility of seizure activity should be considered if untoward events include a loss of consciousness or altered consciousness, such as:

- Delirium.
- Sudden fall without warning or a clear orthopedic, gait, or neurological dysfunction, or another explanation.
- Recurrence of similar incidents under similar conditions.
- Arousal from sleep with confusion or disorientation.

The incidence of seizure is bimodal, with the first peak in early childhood and a second and higher peak in people over the age of 65 years (Sirven 2001). Seizures are approximately three to four times more common in aging adults than in younger adults, yet are more easily missed, because seizures in the elderly are *more* likely to:

- Lack an aura or prodrome.
- Lack observable motor phenomena.
- Occur in the context of major neurocognitive disorder.
- Be misidentified as delirium.

A delay in appropriate treatment can lead to continuation of seizures and complications, as well as unnecessary and contraindicated interventions (Shih and Schachter 2022). A thorough history from the patient, family, an eyewitness to the seizure (if available), neurological examination, laboratory work-up, including CBC, electrolytes, renal and liver-associated enzymes, neuroimaging, ECG, and electroencephalography (EEG) can help identify causes. These might include metabolic abnormalities (e.g. hypoglycemia, hyponatremia, uremia, hypocalcemia), stroke, CNS infection, trauma, and drug withdrawal) (Sirven 2001). A review of medications such as bupropion or tramadol, which can lower seizure threshold, is indicated (Thundiyil et al. 2007).

Status epilepticus. Almost one-third of aging adults with a first acute seizure present in *status epilepticus*, twice the rate in the general population (Sirven 2001) (see Table 3.8).

Table 3.8 Management of convulsive status epilepticus

Intervention	Recommendation
Airway protection	Turn the patient on the side and consider using oropharyngeal or nasopharyngeal airway
Oxygenation	Administer oxygen via nasal cannula or facemask (consider intubation if patient cannot turn, protect their airway or maintain oxygenation)
Check blood glucose	Check blood glucose and treat of the level is less than 60 mg/dL with intravenous thiamine followed by dextrose supplementation
Attempt IV access and collect blood for work-up (CBC, electrolytes, toxicology screen). If the seizure continues beyond the initial phase (longer than 5 min), patient is considered to have status epilepticus. At this point, transfer to the emergency department (ED), and/or contact rapid response team depending on availability	
Medication	First line: one of the following 3 equivalents: (a) Intravenous lorazepam (0.1 mg/kg/dose, maximum 4 kg/dose, maximum two doses) (b) Intramuscular midazolam (10 mg for >40 kg, 5 mg for 13–40 kg, single dose) (c) Intravenous diazepam (0.15–0.2 mg/kg/dose, maximum 10 mg/dose, maximum two doses) If none of above 3 options available, choose: • Intravenous phenobarbital (15 mg/kg/dose, single dose), or (d) Rectal diazepam (0.2–0.5 mg/kg, maximum 20 mg/dose, single dose) (e) Buccal or intranasal midazolam

Adapted from Drislane et al. (2022) and Glauser et al. (2016)

Acute Cardiac Events

Coronary heart disease (CAD) is the most common type of heart disease, killing 365,914 people in the US in 2017; 80% of these deaths were in ages greater than 65 (Centers for Disease Control and Prevention 2020b; Kochanek et al. 2019). Hypertension, hypercholesterolemia, diabetes mellitus, and smoking are key risk factors and are prevalent among aging adults (Seitz et al. 2012). Acute coronary syndrome (ACS) describes a range of conditions associated with sudden reduced blood flow to the heart (American Heart Association 2015), which can lead to myocardial infarction (MI). ACS and severe coronary spasm, a sudden contraction of a coronary artery, are common etiologies of MI (Centers for Disease Control and Prevention 2020a). See Six Common Symptoms of MI Table 3.9 (Centers for Disease Control and Prevention 2020a).

If the patient is unresponsive, hypotensive, tachycardic, bradycardic, and hypoxic, a rapid response team should be activated. If the patient is unresponsive and pulseless, code blue is indicated and basic life support (BLS) algorithm started (Kleinman et al. 2015).

The initial assessment and management depend on the availability of resources in the facility (Table 3.9). A 12-lead ECG should be obtained, and transfer to emergency department is indicated. An ECG can help triage the patient, depending upon whether ST elevation or new left bundle branch block (LBBB) is present. Emergency responders can transmit the results to the receiving hospital so that the cardiac catheterization laboratory can be notified prior to the patient's arrival.

Time is essential: if the onset of chest pain occurs in less than 12 h, the patient is a candidate for reperfusion therapy. A key performance quality metric in the treatment of ST-elevated myocardial infarction (STEMI) includes a door-to-balloon inflation goal of less than 90 min (for percutaneous intervention therapy) and a door-to-needle goal of less than 30 min (for fibrinolysis therapy) (Table 3.10)

Table 3.9 Six symptoms of myocardial infarction

Chest pain or discomfort; most heart attacks involve chest discomfort in the center or left side of the chest that lasts for more than a few minutes or that goes away and comes back. Patients usually describe as squeezing, fullness, or pain. Patients with history of diabetes may exhibit less chest symptoms due to impairment of sensation in the peripheral nerves. This phenomenon is called "silent" myocardial infarction
Weakness, lightheadedness, or syncope
Pain or discomfort in the jaw, left neck area or back. If the chest pain radiates to the back, aortic dissection is also on the differential diagnosis
Pain or discomfort in one or both arms or the shoulder, mostly on the left side
Shortness of breath
Nausea

Adapted from Reeder et al. (2022)

Skin Ulcers, Skin Breakdown, and Contributing Factors

Pressure to the skin for as little as 2 h, due to prolonged immobility, can result in reduced skin perfusion and soft tissue injury sufficient to cause damage. Neurologic conditions such as motor neurone disease and peripheral neuropathy can interfere with mobility and sensory perception. Vulnerabilities for reduced skin perfusion include volume depletion, hypotension, vasomotor failure, vasoconstriction, and underlying peripheral artery disease. If kidneys and the gastrointestinal tract are not adequately perfused, blood flow to the skin is reduced, which increases the risk of pressure-induced injuries.

Although absolute bedrest is medically necessary sometimes, most systemic medical conditions do not require it. Greater mobility can reduce risk of death at 2 years. These markers identify patients at risk for skin and soft tissue breakdown (Jansen et al. 2020).

- Reduction of sensory perception and/or ability to respond to discomfort of pressure.
- Exposure of skin to moisture.
- Reduction in motor activity and ability to change position.
- Poor nutrition and poor quality of food intake.
- Amount of skin friction and shear.
- Skin color.

Table 3.10 Emergency management of acute coronary syndrome (ACS)

Intervention	Recommendation
Obtain vital signs	Vital signs should be taken to determine the clinical stability of the patient into different categories: • If the patient is unresponsive, hypotensive, tachycardic, bradycardic, hypoxia, a rapid response team should be activated • If the patient is unresponsive and pulseless, code blue should be activated. The inpatient team should initiate the basic life support (BLS) algorithm in the meantime • If the patient is stable, the initial assessment and management depend on the availability of resource. An initial 12-lead ECG should be obtained if this can be performed to determine any concerning abnormality. Emergent transfer to emergency room is required if this cannot be done at the psychiatric facility to prevent the delay
Oxygenation	Correct hypoxia with oxygen therapy in acutely breathless patients or if oxygen saturation (SpO_2) is <94% (aiming for 94–100%, but caution in patients with history of COPD as they may be dependent on their hypoxic drive for respiration—aiming for SpO_2 88–92% instead)
Medication	If ACS is suspected, high-dose aspirin (325 mg) needs to be administered without delay, if there is no contraindication (e.g., bleeding or suspected aortic dissection) Consider sublingual nitroglycerin. Nitrates must be avoided in patient with hypotension, or recently have taken a phosphodiesterase inhibitor (e.g., sildenafil) in the previous 24 h
Reperfusion therapy	Transfer patient to nearest hospital that can provide reperfusion therapy (either percutaneous intervention therapy or fibrinolysis therapy)

Adapted from Bhatt et al. (2022)

- Variability in skin temperature.
- Level of dryness of skin.
- Decreased skin turgor.
- Location of wound and description.
- Current or prior skin ulcers and location.

Decubitus ulcers cannot heal if there is poor skin perfusion. Once risk is ascertained, interventions include redistribution of pressure with repositioning at least every 2 h, to minimize shear forces, keeping skin clean and dry, and the use of pressure-reducing products. Treatment can include treating and stabilizing hypotension, improving cardiac contractility, limiting vasoconstrictive agents, or revascularization for those patients who have severe peripheral artery disease (Jansen et al. 2020).

Constipation and Acute Bowel Obstruction

About one-third of adults 60 years or older report at least occasional constipation, and in nursing home residents, the prevalence is at 50% (Bouras and Tangalos 2009). Complaints include bowel movements fewer than 2–3 times/week, straining at defecation, hard feces, and/or feeling of incomplete evacuation. Aging adults are at risk for constipation due to

- Medications (e.g., opioids, calcium supplement, anticholinergic agents, certain antidepressants, antipsychotics, diuretics, and iron).
- Acute and chronic systemic medical conditions (e.g., colon tumor, dehydration, depressive disorder, hypothyroidism, immobility, Parkinson's disease, spinal cord injury, uremia, and stroke).
- Reduced mobility, lethargy, bedridden status.

On physical examination, including digital palpation, a large amount of feces can be palpated. Colonic fecal loading can be discerned on abdominal radiographs. If symptoms of bloating, abdominal pain, nausea, vomiting, cramping abdominal pain, inability to pass flatus or stool (obstipation) emerge, *small* bowel obstruction needs to be ruled out. These symptoms can overlap with symptoms of *large* bowel obstruction, which include bloating, abdominal pain, and obstipation. Prompt diagnosis and treatment are crucial since stercoral colitis can lead to a life-threatening condition and colonic perforation (35% mortality) (Naseer et al. 2017).

Age-adjusted preventive interventions can include lifestyle modifications (regular bowel movements), dietary changes (fiber), osmotic laxatives, stimulant laxatives, stool softeners, and suppositories, as well as enemas. All can be helpful in an appropriate sequence depending upon severity of constipation and response. In the context of opioid-induced constipation or paralytic ileus, peripherally acting mu opioid receptor antagonists, (e.g., alvimopan, methylnaltrexone, naloxegol, and naldemedine), may be considered. RCTs have demonstrated that biofeedback therapy for dyssynergic defecation can be superior to laxatives, standard therapy, sham therapy, placebo, and diazepam. Management of constipation for non-opioid related constipation and opioid-induced constipation is shown in Table 3.11.

Cancer

Cancer is the second leading cause of death in the geriatric population. According to the American Cancer Society, 77% of all cancers are diagnosed in people over the age of 55 (National Cancer Institute 2015). By age 85, the death rate from cancer begins to fall with slow-growing tumors being more common (Kochanek et al. 2019; National Cancer Institute 2015). Many cancer screenings may not be warranted in aging adults due to insufficient evidence of benefit. For example, screening is not recommended for breast cancer after age 75. Colon cancer screening for adults over age 75 in the US is only recommended in cases where there is a long-predicted life expectancy and a perceived strong capacity to tolerate cancer treatment. Screening for prostate cancer is not recommended due to frequent false positives and identification of slow-growing tumors. Caveat: Guidelines may change in the future as people continue to live longer. Table 3.2 (above) lists United States Preventive Services Task Force (USPSTF) recommendations for secondary prevention (US Preventive Services Task Force 2023).

Table 3.11 Management of non-opioid-related and opioid-induced constipation

Steps	Non-opioid related constipation	Opioid-induced constipation
Step 1	Stop all constipating medications, when possible	Avoid bulk-forming laxatives (e.g., methyl cellulose, psyllium) if sufficient oral fluid intake
Step 2	Increase dietary fiber, increase fluid intake to >1500 mL/day, and increase physical activity. If fiber exacerbates constipation (usually due to insufficient oral fluid intake), go to step 3	Start stimulants (e.g., bisacodyl, senna) and osmotic agents (e.g., polyethylene glycol). We recommend starting senna and polyethylene glycol (once or twice daily) when initiating patient on opioid
Step 3	Add an osmotic (e.g., polyethylene glycol)	Titrate medication in step 2
Step 4	Add stimulant laxative (e.g., senna, bisacodyl)	Suppository (e.g., bisacodyl)
Step 5	Suppository (e.g., bisacodyl)	Enema (tap water or oil-retention)
Step 6	Enema (tap water or oil-retention)	Consider lubiprostone, linaclotide, or plecanatide if idiopathic constipation Alvimopan, methylnaltrexone, naldemedine, or naloxegol if opioid-induced constipation Note: Consider gastroenterology consultation

Patients with prolonged constipation may need to start with Step 5 or Step 6

Infectious Disease

Long-term care facilities are populated with the oldest-old and frail patients who have compromised immune status, underlying health conditions, obesity, poor nutrition status, dementia, and terminal illnesses, among other vulnerabilities. All individuals in contact pose a high risk for transmission of pathogens. Common hospital-acquired (or nosocomial) infections and contributors include:

Clostridium difficile is a gram-positive anaerobic bacterium that causes antibiotic-associated colitis, is a significant cause of morbidity and mortality and the most frequent cause of nosocomial diarrhea. It often follows antibiotic therapy and colonizes the human intestinal tract after the normal flora has been altered (24). Strict precautions against contact, and isolation measures can help prevent the spread of *Clostridium difficile* spores.

Hospital-acquired pneumonia (HAP) occurs 48 h or more after admission. Patients with major neurocognitive disorder, Parkinson's disease, or other neurologic conditions are at high risk for aspiration pneumonia. Patients who develop swallowing dysfunction while on first-generation antipsychotics (FGAs), possibly due to laryngeal dystonia, are also at risk. Early signs include coughing when eating or drinking should be identified so measures can be instituted to prevent aspiration. These include avoidance of acid-blocking medications, attention to oral hygiene, and feeding only when the patient is alert and able to sit upright. Modifying consistency of foods, formal swallowing assessment, and assistance with feeding may be warranted.

Secondary nosocomial bacteremia and urinary tract infections (UTI) are often precipitated by use of Foley catheters; avoidance of unnecessary catheterization and removal of catheters when no longer indicated are best practices.

Airborne infection: A total of 8 out of 10 COVID-19 deaths reported in the US were in adults 65 years old and older. Lessons from COVID-19 pandemic suggest that vigilance for risk factors, prompt isolation and related precautions can minimize contagion from acute respiratory infections. Individuals age 85 or older have shown the greatest risk for severe illness (Centers for Disease Control and Prevention 2020c). Medical comorbidities associated with severity of illness and mortality included cardiovascular disease, diabetes mellitus, obesity, hypertension, chronic lung disease, cancer, chronic kidney disease, and smoking (CDC COVID-19 Response Team 2020 from https://www.cdc.gov/globalhealth/healthprotection/errb/global-rrt.htm accessed 08 May 2024; Liang et al. 2020).

Conclusions

At admission and during stay in a psychiatric, long-term care, or similar facility, scrutiny of the geriatric patient for under-treated acute and chronic medical events (such as stroke, chronic pain, or unrecognized seizures) is crucial. Psychiatric and behavioral symptoms often accompany or follow a medical condition. Prompt diagnosis and medical treatment can minimize medical complications, morbidity, and chronicity, and ameliorate associated neuropsychiatric symptoms (such as post-stroke depressive disorder—PSD).

Age-Adjusted Recommendations

1. Ensure a Comprehensive Geriatric Assessment (CGA) with laboratory studies for any geriatric patient admitted to long-term care, a psychiatric unit, or similar facility.

    - Rule out systemic medical etiologies when signs emerge of:
        - Cognitive impairment.
        - Psychotic symptoms.
        - Depressive symptoms or changes in mood.
        - Altered level of attention, consciousness, or arousal.
    - Determine whether medical treatment is within the capabilities of any receiving facility.
    - Gather history of medical co-morbidities, medications, seizure activity from reliable observers, family, and caregivers.
    - Assess for falls and their risk factors.
    - Assess and treat chronic pain with non-pharmacological modalities as well as pharmacotherapy.
    - Search for seizure activity and etiolog(ies) if there are alterations of consciousness.
    - Ensure availability of emergency medical resources and subspecialty consultation, and plan for emergency referral and transportation.

References

American Diabetes Association. Older adults: standards of medical care in diabetes—2020. Diabetes Care. 2020;43(Supplement 1):s152–62.

American Heart Association. Acute coronary syndrome. 2015.

Anderson AS, Loeser RF. Why is osteoarthritis an age-related disease? Best practice and research. Clin Rheumatol. 2010;24(1):15–26.

Armstrong C, Joint National Committee. JNC8 guidelines for the management of hypertension in adults. Am Fam Physician. 2014;90(7):503–4.

Ayerbe L, Ayis S, Wolfe CD, Rudd AG. Natural history, predictors and outcomes of depression after stroke: systematic review and meta-analysis. Br J Psychiatry. 2013;202:14–21. https://doi.org/10.1192/bjp.bp.111.107664.

Barker-Collo SL. Depression and anxiety 3 months post stroke: prevalence and correlates. Arch Clin Neuropsychol. 2007;22(4):519–31. https://doi.org/10.1016/j.acn.2007.03.002.

Beckett NS, Peters R, Fletcher AE, et al. Treatment of hypertension in patients 80 years of age or older. N Engl J Med. 2018;358(18):1887–98.

Benjamin EJ, Blaha MJ, Chiuve SE, et al. Heart disease and stroke statistics-2017 update: a report from the American Heart Association. Circulation. 2017;135(10):e146–603.

Benjamin EJ, Muntner P, Alonso A, et al. Heart disease and stroke statistics-2019 update: a report from the American Heart Association. Circulation. 2019;139(10):e56–528.

Bhatt DL, Lopes RD, Harrington RA. Diagnosis and treatment of acute coronary syndromes: a review. JAMA. 2022;327(7):662–75.

Blair E, Gruman C. Falls in an inpatient geriatric psychiatric population. J Am Psychiatr Nurses Assoc. 2005;11(6):351–4.

Bouras EP, Tangalos EG. Chronic constipation in the elderly. Gastroenterol Clin N Am. 2009;38(3):463–80.

Bucur M, Papagno C. A systematic review of noninvasive brain stimulation for post-stroke depression. J Affect Disord. 2018;238:69–78.

Centers for Disease Control and Prevention. Assessment timed Up&Go (TUG). 2017.

Centers for Disease Control and Prevention. Heart attack symptoms, risk, and recovery. 2020a. https://www.cdc.gov/heartdisease/heart_attack.htm.

Centers for Disease Control and Prevention. STEADI stopping elderly accidents, deaths and injuries materials for your older patients. 2020b.

Centers for Disease Control and Prevention. Stroke facts. 2020c.

Centers for Disease Control and Prevention. Stroke signs and symptoms. 2020d.

Chemerinski E, Robinson RG, Kosier JT. Improved recovery in activities of daily living associated

with remission of poststroke depression. Stroke. 2001;32:113.
Collerton J, Davies K, Jagger C, et al. Health and disease in 85-year-olds: baseline findings from the Newcastle 85+ cohort study. Br Med J. 2009;339:b4904.
De Luca R, Manuli A, De Domenico C, et al. Improving neuropsychiatric symptoms following stroke using virtual reality. Medicine. 2019;98(19):e15236.
De Ryck A, Brouns R, Geurden M, et al. Risk factors for poststroke depression: identification of inconsistencies based on a systematic review. J Geriatr Psychiatry Neurol. 2014;27:147–58. https://doi.org/10.1177/0891988714527514.
Delbari A, Salman-Roghani R, Lokk J. Effect of methylphenidate and/or levodopa combined with physiotherapy on mood and cognition after stroke: a randomized, double-blind, placebo-controlled trial. Eur Neurol. 2011;66:7–13.
Drislane FW, Garcia P, Edlow JA, et al. Convulsive status epilepticus in adults: management. UpToDate; 2022.
Edelstein BA, Brown SA. Falls among psychogeriatric patients. Clin Gerontol. 2000;21:17–3.
Ellis G, Whitehead MA, Robinson D, et al. Comprehensive geriatric assessment for older adults admitted to hospital. Cochrane Database Syst Rev. 2011;7:CD006211.
Elsawy B, Higgins KE. The geriatric assessment. Am Fam Physician. 2011;83(1):48–56.
Emberton M, Anson K. Acute urinary retention in men: an age old problem. Br Med J. 1999;318(7188):921–5.
Federal Interagency Forum on Aging-Related Statistics. Older Americans 2016: key indicators of well-being, 2016.
Ferreira MDC, Machado C, Santos B, Machado Á. Poststroke psychosis: how long should we treat? Trends Psychiatry Psychother. 2017;39:144–6.
Ferro JM, Caeiro L, Figueira ML. Neuropsychiatric sequelae of stroke. Nat Rev Neurol. 2016;12:269–80. https://doi.org/10.1038/nrneurol.2016.46.
Ferro JM, Caeiro L, Santos C. Poststroke emotional and behavior impairment: a narrative review. Cerebrovasc Dis. 2009;27(1):197–203. https://doi.org/10.1159/000200460. Epub 2009 Apr 3. PMID: 19342852.
Gangavati A, Hajjar I, Quach L, et al. Hypertension, orthostatic hypotension, and the risk of falls in a community-dwelling elderly population: the maintenance of balance, independent living, intellect, and zest in the elderly of Boston study. J Am Geriatr Soc. 2011;59(3):383–9.
Ganz DA, Latham NK. Prevention of falls in community-dwelling older adults. N Engl J Med. 2020;382(8):734–43.
Glauser T, Shinnar S, Gloss D, Alldredge B, Arya R, Bainbridge J, Bare M, Bleck T, Dodson WE, Garrity L, Jagoda A, Lowenstein D, Pellock J, Riviello J, Sloan E, Treiman DM. Evidence-based guideline: treatment of convulsive status epilepticus in children and adults: report of the guideline committee of the American Epilepsy Society. Epilepsy Curr. 2016;16(1):48–61. https://doi.org/10.5698/1535-7597-16.1.48. PMID: 26900382; PMCID: PMC4749120.
Guirguis-Blake JM, Michael YL, Perdue LA, et al. Interventions to prevent falls in community-dwelling older adults: a systematic review for the U.S. preventive services task force, vol. 319. Rockville: Agency for Healthcare Research and Quality (US); 2018. p. 1705.
Hackett ML, Pickles K. Part I: Frequency of depression after stroke: an updated systematic review and meta-analysis of observational studies. Int J Stroke. 2014;9:1017–25. https://doi.org/10.1111/ijs.12357.
Hackett ML, Anderson CS, House A, Xia J. Interventions for treating depression after stroke. Cochrane Database Syst Rev. 2008;4:CD003437.
Hackett ML, Yang M, Anderson CS, et al. Pharmaceutical interventions for emotionalism after stroke. Stroke. 2010;41(7):e460–1.
Hackett ML, Köhler S, O'Brien JT, Mead GE. Neuropsychiatric outcomes of stroke. Lancet Neurol. 2014;13:525–34.
Hama S, Yamashita H, Yamawaki S, Kurisu K. Poststroke depression and apathy: Interactions between functional recovery, lesion location, and emotional response. Psychogeriatrics. 2011;11(1):68–76. https://doi.org/10.1111/j.1479-8301.2011.00358.x. PMID: 21447112.
Hu YN, Chung YJ, Yu HK, et al. Effect of Tai Chi exercise on fall prevention in older adults: systematic review and meta-analysis of randomized controlled trials. Int J Gerontol. 2016;10:131.
Iranzo A, Santamaría J, Berenguer J, et al. Prevalence and clinical importance of sleep apnea in the first night after cerebral infarction. Neurology. 2002;58:911.
Izzo JL, Levy D, Black HR. Clinical advisory statement: importance of systolic blood pressure in older Americans. Hypertension. 2000;35(5):1021–4.
Jansen RCS, Silva KBA, Moura MES. Braden Scale in pressure ulcer risk assessment. Rev Bras Enferm. 2020;73(6):e20190413.
Janssens JP, Pautex S, Hilleret H, Michel JP. Sleep disordered breathing in the elderly. Aging. 2000;12:417–29.
Johnston SC, Rothwell PM, Nguyen-Huynh MN, et al. Validation and refinement of scores to predict very early stroke risk after transient ischaemic attack. Lancet (London, England). 2007;369(9558):283–92.
Josephson AS, Sidney S, Pham TN, et al. Higher ABCD2 score predicts patients most likely to have true transient ischemic attack. Stroke. 2008;39(11):3096–8.
Joyce EM. Organic psychosis: the pathobiology and treatment of delusions. CNS Neurosci Ther. 2018;24:598–603.
Karaiskos D, Tzavellas E, Spengos K, et al. Duloxetine versus citalopram and sertraline in the treatment of poststroke depression, anxiety, and fatigue. J Neuropsychiatry Clin Neurosci. 2012;24(3):349–53.
Kirkness CJ, Becker KJ, Cain KC, et al. Telephone versus in-person psychosocial behavioral treatment in poststroke depression. Stroke. 2015;46(suppl 1):AWP125.
Kleinman ME, Brennan EE, Goldberger ZD, et al. Adult basic life support and cardiopulmonary resuscitation quality: 2015 American Heart Association guidelines update for cardiopulmonary resuscitation and emer-

gency cardiovascular care. Circulation. 2015;132(18 Suppl 2):S414–35.
Kochanek KD, Murphy SL, Xu J, Arias E. Deaths: final data for 2017. National Vital Statistics Reports: from the Centers for Disease Control and Prevention, National Center for Health Statistics, National Vital Statistics System. Natl Vital Stat Rep. 2019;68(9):1–77.
Kohno N, Abe S, Toyoda G, et al. Successful treatment of post-stroke apathy by the dopamine receptor agonist ropinirole. J Clin Neurosci. 2010;17(6):804–6.
Kutlubaev MA, Hackett ML. Part II: predictors of depression after stroke and impact of depression on stroke outcome: an updated systematic review of observational studies. Int J Stroke. 2014;9:1026–36. https://doi.org/10.1111/ijs.12356.
Leeds L, Meara RJ, Hobson JP. The utility of the stroke aphasia depression questionnaire (SADQ) in a stroke rehabilitation unit. Clin Rehabil. 2004;18(2):228–31.
Lerner AJ, Riley D. Dementias associated with motor dysfunction. In: Yudofsky SC, Hales RE, editors. Clinical manual of neuropsychiatry. Washington, DC: American Psychiatric Publishing; 2012. p. 287–310.
Liang W, Liang H, Ou L, Chen B, Chen A, Li C, Li Y, Guan W, Sang L, Lu J, Xu Y, Chen G, Guo H, Guo J, Chen Z, Zhao Y, Li S, Zhang N, Zhong N, He J; China medical treatment expert group for COVID-19. Development and validation of a clinical risk score to predict the occurrence of critical illness in hospitalized patients with COVID-19. JAMA Intern Med. 2020;180(8):1081–9. https://doi.org/10.1001/jamainternmed.2020.2033. PMID: 32396163; PMCID: PMC7218676..
Marin RS, Wilkosz PA. Disorders of diminished motivation. J Head Trauma Rehabil. 2005;20:377–88.
Mayo NE, Fellows LK, Scott SC, et al. A longitudinal view of apathy and its impact after stroke. Stroke. 2009;40:3299–307.
McIntyre A, Thompson S, Burhan A, et al. Repetitive transcranial magnetic stimulation for depression due to cerebrovascular disease: a systematic review. J Stroke Cerebrovasc Dis. 2016;25(12):2792–800. https://doi.org/10.1016/j.jstrokecerebrovasdis.2016.08.043.
Mikami K, Jorge RE, Moser DJ, Arndt S, Jang M, Solodkin A, Small SL, Fonzetti P, Hegel MT, Robinson RG. Prevention of poststroke apathy using escitalopram or problem-solving therapy. Am J Geriatr Psychiatry. 2013;21(9):855–62. https://doi.org/10.1016/j.jagp.2012.07.003. Epub 2013 Feb 6. PMID: 23930743.
Mitchell PH, Veith RC, Becker KJ, et al. Brief psychosocial-behavioral intervention with antidepressant reduces poststroke depression significantly more than usual care with antidepressant: living well with stroke: randomized, controlled trial. Stroke. 2009;40:3073–8. https://doi.org/10.1161/STROKEAHA.109.549808.
Morley JE, Vellas B, van Kan GA, et al. Frailty consensus: a call to action. J Am Med Dir Assoc. 2013;14(6):392–7.
Naseer M, Gandhi J, Chams N, Kulairi Z. Stercoral colitis complicated with ischemic colitis: a double-edge sword. BMC Gastroenterol. 2017;17(1):1–6.
National Cancer Institute. Age and cancer risk. 2015.
National Center for Health Statistics. Percent of U.S. adults 55 and over with chronic conditions. 2015.
National Osteoporosis Foundation. Osteoporosis fast facts. 2015. https://cdn.nof.org/wp-content/uploads/2015/12/Osteoporosis-Fast-Facts.pdf.
National Osteoporosis Foundation. What women need to know. 2020. https://www.nof.org/preventing-fractures/general-facts/what-women-need-to-know/.
Nikolaus T, Bach M. Preventing falls in community-dwelling frail older people using a home intervention team (HIT): results from the randomized falls-HIT trial. J Am Geriatr Soc. 2003;51(3):300–5.
Nogueira RG, Jadhav AP, Haussen DC, et al. Thrombectomy 6–24 h after stroke with a mismatch between deficit and infarct. N Engl J Med. 2018;378(1):11–21.
Powers WJ, Rabinstein AA, Ackerson T, et al. Guidelines for the early management of patients with acute ischemic stroke: a guideline for healthcare professionals from the American Heart Association/American Stroke Association. Stroke. 2018;49:e49–99.
Reeder GS, Kennedy HL, Hoekstra J, Jaffe AS. Diagnosis of acute myocardial infarction. UpToDate; 2022.
Reuben DB, Herr K, Pacala JT, et al. Geriatrics at your fingertips. American Geriatrics Society; 2019.
Robinson RG, Jorge RE, Moser DJ, et al. Escitalopram and problem-solving therapy for prevention of post-stroke depression: a randomized controlled trial. JAMA. 2008;299(20):2391–400.
Ross AC, Taylor CL, Yaktine AL, Del Valle HB, editors. Institute of Medicine (US) Committee to review dietary reference intakes for vitamin D and calcium: dietary reference intakes for calcium and vitamin D. Washington (DC): National Academies Press (US); 2011.
Sama S, Yamashita H, Shigenobu M, et al. Depression or apathy and functional recovery after stroke. Int J Geriatr Psychiatry. 2007;22:1046–51.
Sami MB, Faruqui R. The effectiveness of dopamine agonists for treatment. Of neuropsychiatric symptoms post brain injury and stroke. Acta Neuropsychiatr. 2015;27(6):317–26.
Samuelsson E, Odeberg J, Stenzelius K, et al. Effect of pharmacological treatment for urinary incontinence in the elderly and frail elderly: a systematic review. Geriatr Gerontol Int. 2015;15(5):521–34.
Santos CO, Caeiro L, Ferro JM, Figueira ML. Mania and stroke: a systematic review. Cerebrovasc Dis. 2011;32(1):11–21. https://doi.org/10.1159/000327032. Epub 2011 May 11. PMID: 21576938.
Schöttke H, Giabbiconi CM. Post-stroke depression and post-stroke anxiety: prevalence and predictors. Int Psychogeriatr. 2015;27(11):1805–12.
Seitz DP, Vigod SN, Lin E, et al. Characteristics of older adults hospitalized in acute psychiatric units in

Ontario: a population-based study. Can J Psychiatr. 2012;57(9):554–63.
Shannon J, Shannon J, Modelevsky S, Grippo AA. Bisphosphonates and osteonecrosis of the jaw. J Am Geriatr Soc. 2011;59(12):2350–5.
Shen Y, Cai Z, Liu F, et al. Repetitive transcranial magnetic stimulation and transcranial direct current stimulation as treatment of poststroke depression: a systematic review and meta-analysis. Neurologist. 2022;27(4):177–82.
Sherrington C, Fairhall NJ, Wallbank GK, et al. Exercise for preventing falls in older people living in the community. Cochrane Database Syst Rev. 2019;1:CD012424.
Shih T, Schachter KE. Seizures and epilepsy in older adults: etiology, clinical presentation, and diagnosis. UpToDate; 2022.
Sirven JI. Acute and chronic seizures in patients older than 60 years. Mayo Clin Proc. 2001;76(2):175–83.
Smith NK, Albazzaz MK. A prospective study of urinary retention and risk of death after proximal femoral fracture. Age Ageing. 1996;25(2):150–4.
Social Security Administration. Life expectancy for social security. Social Security History. 2023. https://www.ssa.gov/history/lifeexpect.html.
SPRINT Research Group, Wright JT, Williamson JD, Whelton PK, et al. A randomized trial of intensive versus standard blood-pressure control. N Engl J Med. 2015;373(22):2103–016.
Stangeland H, Vasiliki OV. Review: Poststroke psychosis: a systematic review. J Neurol Neurosurg Psychiatry. 2018;89(8):879.
Tang WK, Chen YK, Mok V, et al. Acute basal ganglia infarcts in poststroke fatigue: an MRI study. J Neurol. 2010;257:178–82.
Thundiyil JG, Kearney TE, Olson KR. Evolving epidemiology of drug-induced seizures reported to a poison control center system. J Med Toxicol. 2007;3(1):15–9.
Towfighi A, Ovbiagele B, El Husseini N, et al. Poststroke depression: a scientific statement for healthcare professionals from the American Heart Association/American Stroke Association. Stroke. 2017;48(2):30–43.
US Preventive Services Task Force. A and b recommendations. 2023. https://www.uspreventiveservicestaskforce.org/uspstf/recommendation-topics/uspstf-and-b-recommendations.
US Preventive Services Task Force, Curry SJ, Krist AH, Owens DK, et al. Screening for osteoporosis to prevent fractures: US preventive services task force recommendation statement. JAMA. 2018;319(24):2521–31.
van Dalen JW, Moll van Charante EP, Nederkoorn PJ, van Gool WA, Richard E. Poststroke apathy. Stroke. 2013;44(3):851–60. https://doi.org/10.1161/STROKEAHA.112.674614. Epub 2013 Jan 29. PMID: 23362076.
van Hensbroek PB, van Dijk N, van Breda GF, et al. The CAREFALL triage instrument identifying risk factors for recurrent falls in elderly patients. Am J Emerg Med. 2009;27(1):23–36.
Watkins C, Daniels L, Jack C, van Den Broek M. Accuracy of a single question in screening for depression in a cohort of patients after stroke: comparative study. BMJ. 2001;323:1159.
Whelton PK, Carey RM, Aronow WS, et al. 2017 ACC/AHA/AAPA/ABC/ACPM/AGS/APhA/ASH/ASPC/NMA/PCNA guideline for the prevention, detection, evaluation, and management of high blood pressure in adults: a report of the American College of Cardiology/American Heart Association task force on clinical practice guidelines [Erratum: *Hypertension* 71(6): e13–115, 2018]. J Am Coll Cardiol. 2018;71(19):e127–248.
Wilson MP, Nordstrom K, Anderson EL, et al. American Association for Emergency Psychiatry Task Force on medical clearance of adult psychiatric patients. Part II: controversies over medical assessment, and consensus recommendations. West J Emerg Med. 2017;18(4):640–6.
World Health Organization. The atlas of heart disease and stroke. Geneva: World Health Organization; 2004.
Wright F, Wu S, Chun HY, Mead G. Factors associated with poststroke anxiety: a systematic review and meta-analysis. Stroke Res Treat. 2017;2017:2124743. https://doi.org/10.1155/2017/2124743. Epub 2017 Feb 22. PMID: 28321357; PMCID: PMC5340955.
Wulsin L, Alwell K, Moomaw CJ, et al. Comparison of two depression measures for predicting stroke outcomes. J Psychosom Res. 2012;72:175–9. https://doi.org/10.1016/j.jpsychores.2011.11.015.

Laboratory Studies, Neuroimaging, and Neuropsychological Testing

4

Andreea L. Seritan, Elizabeth B. Bruns, Ian O. Bledsoe, and Caroline A. Racine

Abstract

Laboratory studies, neuroimaging, and neuropsychological testing enhance physical examination findings. A systemic medical workup is even more important when patients present with atypical symptom profiles, new psychiatric manifestations occurring later than the typical onset ages in the general population, or treatment-resistant symptoms. In this chapter, we review common laboratory tests, with reference intervals and corresponding medical correlates, selected neuroimaging studies, and neuropsychological evaluation approaches that are helpful when caring for older adults. We propose a novel framework, by classifying laboratory tests and neuroimaging studies into three categories: *must-do* (necessary to confirm diagnosis), *supporting* (optional but not necessary, will only corroborate clinical diagnosis), and *not helpful* (will not provide additional relevant information, increase costs, and may cause patient anxiety and discomfort).

A. L. Seritan (✉) · E. B. Bruns
Department of Psychiatry and Behavioral Sciences, University of California, San Francisco, San Francisco, CA, USA

UCSF Weill Institute for Neurosciences, San Francisco, CA, USA
e-mail: Andreea.Seritan@ucsf.edu

I. O. Bledsoe
Department of Neurology, University of California, San Francisco, San Francisco, CA, USA

UCSF Weill Institute for Neurosciences, San Francisco, CA, USA
e-mail: ian.bledsoe@ucsf.edu

C. A. Racine
Department of Neurological Surgery, University of California, San Francisco, San Francisco, CA, USA

UCSF Weill Institute for Neurosciences, San Francisco, CA, USA
e-mail: caroline.racine@ucsf.edu

Case Vignette

A 70-year-old man presented with stiffness in his left arm and leg and worsening balance for several years. He fell approximately once a month. He had no tremor or micrographia. He reported a history of depression, for which he had received psychotherapy but no medications. Laboratory testing was nonrevealing, except for low vitamin B12 levels. He started taking cyanocobalamin 1000 mcg daily. A brain MRI was read as normal for age. The neurologist also ordered an I-123 ioflupane dopamine transporter single photon emission computerized tomography (DaT-SPECT) scan, which revealed asymmetric, slightly diminished radiotracer uptake in the right putamen, consistent with a presynaptic dopaminergic deficit.

The patient was diagnosed with Parkinson's disease (PD) and started on carbidopa-levodopa

H. H. Fenn et al. (eds.), *Age-Adjusted Psychiatric Treatment for the Older Patient*,
https://doi.org/10.1007/978-3-031-53976-3_4

25–100 mg, titrated to two tablets three times a day. He was also prescribed duloxetine, titrated to 60 mg daily, for depression. Over the next year, there was modest improvement in stiffness but increasing difficulty walking, and almost weekly falls. Spasticity and weakness, predominantly in the lower limbs, were noted on follow-up exam. An electromyogram and nerve conduction studies discovered acute and chronic denervation, consistent with motor neuron disease. The diagnosis was changed to amyotrophic lateral sclerosis (ALS).

This vignette illustrates a situation in which neuroimaging confounded, instead of clarifying, the diagnosis. A positive DaTscan may be nonspecific. The diagnosis of PD is ultimately a clinical one, particularly as DaTscans can be abnormal in atypical parkinsonism, such as multiple system atrophy (MSA) or progressive supranuclear palsy (PSP) and have been reported to be abnormal in some patients with motor neuron disease as well (D'Ascenzo 2012; Banks 2019).

Overview

Laboratory studies, neuroimaging, and neuropsychological testing are the foundation upon which accurate diagnoses and best treatment plans for geriatric patients are built. New psychiatric symptoms which emerge in late life often need further investigations to uncover other systemic medical illnesses. Older adults with a known psychiatric condition and those with new onset of psychiatric symptoms in late life can both benefit because systemic medical conditions may precipitate new symptoms. A systemic medical workup is also appropriate for atypical symptom profiles, new psychiatric symptoms with later onset than the typical age in the general population, or for treatment-resistant syndromes (Seritan et al. 2019).

Older individuals are more sensitive to medication side effects due to reduced glomerular filtration rate and slower hepatic metabolism, leading to accumulation of pharmacological agents with increased serum concentrations (Hommos et al. 2017; Klotz 2009). Additionally, the density of neurotransmitter receptors and transporters decreases with aging (Karrer et al. 2017). This dictates caution in titrating psychotropic agents and deciding treatment duration. Psychiatric disease increases the morbidity and mortality associated with systemic medical illness; clinicians should be vigilant and regularly screen for comorbidities (Khambaty et al. 2017).

Results of laboratory, neuroimaging, and/or neuropsychological testing should always be interpreted in the larger clinical context. High-yield neuroimaging and neuropsychological tests, including basic cognitive tests that can be performed in the office or hospital, can help guide the next diagnostic steps. In general, diagnostic tests should be ordered only if they change the treatment plan or uncover etiologies that would otherwise remain elusive. Results can help counsel patients and families about genetic risks, potentially modifiable risk factors, and other prevention strategies.

We propose a new framework that classifies laboratory tests and neuroimaging studies into three categories:

- **Must-do**: Necessary in order to confirm a diagnosis.
- **Supporting**: Optional but not necessary, i.e., clinical diagnosis is sufficiently accurate, and tests will only corroborate it.
- **Not helpful**: Increase costs, do not provide additional relevant diagnostic information, and/or may increase anxiety or discomfort, for example, brain magnetic resonance imaging (MRI) study in a patient with focal neurological findings and a chronic cerebrovascular accident (CVA) visible on a computerized tomography (CT) scan, assuming appropriate vessel imaging and other aspects of stroke workup have already been completed.

The focus here is on selected laboratory tests, neuroimaging studies, and neuropsychological testing which aid the differential diagnosis of psychiatric conditions in older adults. See Chap. 1 for medication monitoring guidelines.

Laboratory Tests and Procedures

In this section, we will describe the uses and interpretation of laboratory tests for older adults. Laboratory reference intervals (RIs) show concomitant variations with physiological aging. Most RIs used in medical practice are based on studies of adult populations under 60 years of age (Plebani and Lackner 2010). For the aged, test results may fall outside established RIs and still be within physiological norms. In some cases, RIs for older adults can be significantly higher than those for younger individuals.

Several prospective studies have established age-specific RIs, including for 75-year-old individuals, although few RIs have been published for the oldest-old (>85 years) (Huber et al. 2006; Risch et al. 2017). A cross-sectional study of over 15,000 adults in China reported that the 2.5th–97.5th percentile ranges for TSH in adults ≥65 years old were significantly higher (0.75–8.86, median 2.58 mIU/L) compared to younger adults (0.76–6.57, median 2.38 mIU/L) (Zhai et al. 2018). Another study of approximately 33,000 individuals showed that both lower and upper range limits for parathyroid hormone were higher by 63% in adults ≥80 years old, compared to those aged 18–29 (Farrell et al. 2018).

RIs should be distinguished from clinical decision limits (CDLs). RIs describe the typical distribution of results found in a healthy reference population, whereas CDLs are associated with a significantly higher risk for or indicate the presence of a particular condition (Ozarda et al. 2018). For example, hemoglobin A1c (HbA1c) values of 4.0–5.6% are considered normal (RI). A CDL of 5.7%–6.4% indicates higher risk of developing diabetes mellitus (DM), and levels ≥6.5% are consistent with DM (Ozarda et al. 2018).

Recommended Workup for Specific Psychiatric Syndromes

There are a few standardized diagnostic algorithms for older adults presenting with specific symptom clusters. Table 4.1 helps clinicians stratify the laboratory tests, procedures, and neuroimaging studies that can elucidate the etiology of common late-life syndromes.

For patients presenting with cognitive deficits, additional workup should be weighed carefully. Only 5% of adults with onset of major neurocog-

Table 4.1 Laboratory workup of psychiatric syndromes

Syndrome	Must-do tests	Supporting tests	Other tests
Alcohol use	LFTs	CBC (MCV), B_{12}, CDT, GGT, homocysteine, MMA; RBC-folate; UTox	B_1, electrolytes; neuroimaging
Anxiety	CBC, glucose, TSH	UTox; chest X-ray; ECG	24-h urine VMA
Cognitive deficits	B_{12}, BUN/Cr, CBC, electrolytes, glucose, LFTs, TSH; urinalysis	Vitamin D, ESR, HIV, homocysteine, MMA, RBC-folate, RPR, T4; UTox; neuroimaging	B_1, heavy metals; CSF; EEG
Delirium	BUN/Cr, CBC, electrolytes, glucose, LFTs; urinalysis	ESR, TSH, SARS-CoV-2 test; vitamin D; urine culture, UTox	Ammonia, B_1; CSF; EEG; neuroimaging
Depression	B_{12}, CBC, glucose, TSH	ESR; homocysteine, MMA (if low B_{12}); neuroimaging	CSF; EEG
Mania	B_{12}, calcium, glucose, TSH	ESR; homocysteine, MMA (if low B_{12}); UTox; neuroimaging	CSF; EEG
Psychosis	BUN/Cr, CBC, glucose, TSH, UTox	B_{12}, calcium, RBC-folate, RPR; SARS-CoV-2 test; neuroimaging	*C9orf72*; heavy metals; CSF; EEG

BUN Blood urea nitrogen, *CBC* Complete blood count, *CDT* Carbohydrate-deficient transferrin, *Cr* Creatinine, *CSF* Cerebrospinal fluid, *C9orf72 Chromosome 9 open reading frame 72*, *ECG* Electrocardiogram, *EEG* Electroencephalogram, *ESR* Erythrocyte sedimentation rate, *GGT* Gamma-glutamyl transferase, *HIV* Human immunodeficiency virus, *LFTs* Liver function tests, *MCV* Mean corpuscular volume, *MMA* Methylmalonic acid, *RBC* Red blood cell, *RPR* Rapid plasma reagin, *SARS-CoV-2* Severe acute respiratory syndrome coronavirus-2, *TSH* Thyroid-stimulating hormone, *UTox* Urine toxicology, *VMA* Vanillylmandelic acid

Sources: Hathaway and Wang (2023), Ford et al. (2013), Kaufman et al. (2017a), Levenson (2006), Seritan et al. (2009a)

nitive disorders (MNCDs) between the ages of 70 and 99 were found to have reversible causes of cognitive impairment (Knopman et al. 2006).

Common Laboratory Tests Used with Older Adults

The following section describes laboratory tests used in the workup of older adults and common medical conditions with neuropsychiatric correlates where these tests should be ordered. Table 4.2 summarizes common laboratory tests with RIs for geriatric patients and psychiatric symptoms that may be associated with abnormal results.

Complete Blood Count (CBC)

Although the CBC is useful in many clinical scenarios, it is not recommended in asymptomatic

Table 4.2 Common laboratory tests for older adults, with reference intervals

Laboratory Test	Reference interval	Psychiatric correlates of abnormal test results	Category	Other information
Complete blood count				
White blood cells	4500–11,000/μL	↑: infection (most common cause of delirium), stress, anxiety, seizures	Must do	Psychiatric medications can cause leukocytosis, neutropenia, or agranulocytosis (see Table 4.3)
Hemoglobin	Men: 13.5–17.5 g/dL Men >60 years old: >13.2 g/dL Women: 12–15.5 g/dL[a]	↓: cognitive deficits, depression ↑: cognitive deficits, depression, mania, psychosis	Must do	Psychiatric medications can cause anemia (see Table 4.3)
Mean corpuscular volume	80–100 μm^3	↑: excessive alcohol use, B_{12} or folate deficiency	Must do	↑: with ethanol intake >60 g/day Use in conjunction with other biomarkers
Platelets	150,000–450,000/μL	↓: valproic acid side effect ↑: mood changes	Must do	Thrombocytosis can increase risk of stroke.
Basic metabolic panel				
Sodium	136–145 mEq/L	↓: cognitive impairment, delirium, falls, seizures	Must do	Psychiatric medications can cause hyponatremia
Potassium	3.5–5.0 mEq/L	↓: anxiety, irritability	Must do	Hyperkalemia can be fatal
Blood urea nitrogen	8–20 mg/dL	↑: cognitive deficits, delirium, irritability, psychosis	Must do	Psychiatric symptoms are most severe with rapid development of uremia. Monitor when lithium is prescribed
Creatinine	Men: 0.70–1.30 mg/dL Women: 0.50–1.10 mg/dL			
Glucose, fasting	70–110 mg/dL	↓: anxiety, cognitive deficits, delirium ↑: delirium, depression, psychosis	Must do	Bidirectional correlation of diabetes mellitus with depression and cognitive deficits

Table 4.2 (continued)

Laboratory Test	Reference interval	Psychiatric correlates of abnormal test results	Category	Other information
Calcium, total	8.6–10.2 mg/dL	↓: anxiety, irritability, mania, psychosis 12–16 mg/dL: anxiety, depression, irritability >16 mg/dL: catatonia, delirium, psychosis, coma	If suspicion exists	Need to correct for total albumin: Corrected Calcium = Measured Calcium + 0.8 × (4 − albumin)
Liver function tests[b]				
Protein, total	5.5–9.0 g/dL	↓: cognitive deficits, depression	If suspicion exists	Hypoproteinemia may occur with inflammation, malnutrition and liver or renal disease
Albumin	3.5–5.5 g/dL	↓: cognitive deficits, depression	If suspicion exists	Hypoalbuminemia increases mortality risk
Aspartate aminotransferase	Men: 14–20 U/L Women: 9–32 U/L	↑ with excessive alcohol use	If suspicion exists	A >40% increase has >90% sensitivity and specificity for alcohol use disorder relapse
Alanine aminotransferase	Men: 10–40 U/L Women: 7–35 U/L	↑ with excessive alcohol use	If suspicion exists	A >20% increase has >80% sensitivity and specificity for alcohol use disorder relapse
Gamma-glutamyl transferase	Men: <50 IU/L Women: <30 IU/L	↑ with excessive alcohol use	If suspicion exists	Values >50 IU/L have 56–100% sensitivity, 100% specificity for excessive alcohol use
Ammonia	40–70 μg/dL	↑: anxiety, delirium, stupor	If suspicion exists	47% sensitivity, 78% specificity for hepatic encephalopathy
Other tests				
Folate	Serum: 1.8–9.0 ng/mL RBC: 150–450 ng/mL packed cells	↓: cognitive deficits, delirium, depression, psychosis	If suspicion exists	Measure RBC-folate (better correlated with cognitive scores than serum folate)
Thyroid-stimulating hormone	0.45–4.12 mU/L 51–70 years old: 0.5–4.5 mU/L 71–90 years old: 0.4–5.2 mU/L	↑: cognitive deficits, depression, psychosis ↓: anxiety, delirium, mania, psychosis, apathy/lethargy	Must do	Levels increase with age. Monitor with lithium treatment

(continued)

Table 4.2 (continued)

Laboratory Test	Reference interval	Psychiatric correlates of abnormal test results	Category	Other information
Thyroxine (T_4), serum	Total: 5–12 μg/dL Free: 0.8–1.8 ng/dL	↓: cognitive deficits, depression, psychosis	If suspicion exists	Levels remain unchanged or slightly increase with age
Vitamin B_{12}	200–800 pg/mL[c]	↓: cognitive deficits, delirium, depression, mania, psychosis	If suspicion exists	Check methylmalonic acid if vitamin B_{12} levels are borderline low (200–400 pg/mL)
Vitamin D: 25-hydroxyvitamin D	20–50 ng/mL[d]	↓: cognitive deficits, delirium, depression, psychosis, sleep disturbance	If suspicion exists	Vitamin D insufficiency: <20 ng/mL Vitamin D deficiency: ≤12 ng/mL

dL Deciliter, *g* Gram, *IU* International unit, *L* Liter, *mL* Milliliter, *mU* Milliunit, *ng* Nanogram, *pg* Picogram, *RBC* Red blood cell, *U* Unit, *μg* Microgram

Sources: Addolorato et al. (2013), American Board of Internal Medicine (2023), Dixit and Singh (2015), Evidence-Based Medicine Consult (2020), Gundling et al. (2013), Jewell (2020), Kaferle and Strzoda (2009), Lanier et al. (2018), Levenson (2006), Mendez and Cummings (2003)

[a]No age-specific reference interval for women

[b]Reference intervals may vary, depending on assay used

[c]Patients with values of 200–400 pg/mL may experience neuropsychiatric symptoms

[d]Values of 20–30 ng/mL can indicate insufficiency in patients with disorders of bone and mineral metabolism

Table 4.3 Hematologic adverse effects of common psychotropic agents SSRIs selective serotonin reuptake inhibitors

Side effect	Medications
Anemia	*Anticonvulsants* Carbamazepine, lamotrigine, valproic acid *Antidepressants* SSRIs, mirtazapine, nefazodone, trazodone, venlafaxine *Antipsychotics* Chlorpromazine, clozapine, risperidone *Benzodiazepines* Chlordiazepoxide, clonazepam, diazepam
Neutropenia/Agranulocytosis	*Anticonvulsants* Carbamazepine *Antidepressants* Mirtazapine *Antipsychotics* Haloperidol, phenothiazines, clozapine, olanzapine, quetiapine, risperidone, ziprasidone
Leukocytosis	Lithium
Thrombocytopenia	*Anticonvulsants* Carbamazepine, lamotrigine, valproic acid *Antidepressants* Mirtazapine, SSRIs, tranylcypromine, tricyclic antidepressants *Antipsychotics* First- and second-generation agents
Thrombocytosis	Lithium

Sources: Buoli et al. 2018; Flanagan and Dunk 2008; Rettenbacher et al. 2010l; Gitlin 2016 adults. In a systematic review, 11% of CBCs revealed abnormalities, yet only 1% of these led to a treatment plan change (Allan and Young 2017).

White Blood Cell (WBC) Count

Subtle signs of delirium in older individuals may emerge even in the absence of fluctuating levels of attention or hallucinations; any abrupt change from baseline in patients with cognitive impairment, especially those who cannot easily verbalize complaints, should prompt a delirium workup, including CBC and urinalysis. A reversed sleep-wake cycle (sleeping during the day and staying up at night, perhaps wandering from room to room) and/or new behavioral disturbances (e.g., aberrant motor behavior, agitation, or appetite changes) are examples. Delirium may persist for weeks after the underlying cause is treated; thus, the WBC and urinalysis may normalize well before delirium completely clears.

The WBC count is an important indicator for underlying systemic medical pathology which may be linked to psychiatric symptoms. Leukocytosis (WBC count >11,000/μL) indicates a proliferation of immune cells, which can be due to infection, inflammation, allergic reaction, or malignancy (Abramson and Melton 2000). Infections, particularly pneumonia and urinary tract infections (UTI), are the most common medical conditions associated with delirium (Oh et al. 2017). Treatment of underlying infections, if any, will help avoid costlier workups and result in symptomatic improvement.

Stressors—whether emotional or physical (e.g., seizure, anesthesia, overexertion)—can also lead to leukocytosis, as can certain medications, including beta-adrenergic agonists, lithium, and corticosteroids (Abramson and Melton 2000). Psychotropic agents can cause leukopenia (WBC count <4000/μL). Agranulocytosis is defined as absence of circulating granular WBCs (neutrophils, basophils, and eosinophils), consistent with a neutrophil count <500/μL (Flanagan and Dunk 2008). Clozapine carries an agranulocytosis risk of 0.8%, especially in the first year of treatment, while carbamazepine has a 0.5% risk of neutropenia (Flanagan and Dunk 2008).

Hemoglobin (Hgb)

Hgb should be checked for new or unexplained psychiatric manifestations, especially if these are accompanied by physical symptoms such as fatigue, lightheadedness, shortness of breath, or in populations at higher risk for nutritional deficiencies: institutionalized adults, recent immigrants, and refugees (Lanier et al. 2018).

Anemia is currently defined by the World Health Organization (WHO) as Hgb <13 g/dL in men and <12 g/dL in women. In practice, clinicians use lower reference values in older adults (Lanier et al. 2018). Causes include iron deficiency, hematological disorders, chronic renal or other disease, and less commonly vitamin B_{12} and folate deficiency, discussed below (Shah et al. 2009; Sharma et al. 2019). Anemia is common in the aged; 17% of participants in the Rush Memory and Aging Project (mean age, 81 years) had low Hgb (Shah et al. 2009). Anemia can present with anxiety, cognitive deficits, and depressive symptoms (Shah et al. 2009; Stewart and Hirani 2012).

Polycythemia (Hgb >18.5 g/dL in men and >16 g/dL in women) can be associated with a variety of physical (headache, dizziness, blurred vision) and neuropsychiatric symptoms such as agoraphobia, cognitive deficits, delirium, depression, mania, and psychosis, likely due to increased blood viscosity slowing transport of oxygen to essential organs, including the brain (Alkemade and Willems 2008; Shah et al. 2009).

Mean Corpuscular Volume (MCV)

MCV is a measure of the average red blood cell (RBC) volume and is helpful in identifying microcytosis (MCV <80 μm^3), often associated with iron deficiency, or macrocytosis (MCV >100 μm^3) (Kaferle and Strzoda 2009). Two salient neuropsychiatric conditions can be associated with high MCV: alcohol use disorder and vitamin B_{12} or folate deficiency. Vitamin B_{12} is a cofactor for folate metabolism, and folate is essential for nucleotide synthesis; deficiencies of either or both vitamins lead to inefficient erythropoiesis, with dyssynchrony between cytoplasm and nucleus maturation, resulting in immature, large nuclei, and macrocytosis (Fishman et al.

2000; Stabler 2013). Alcohol can cause macrocytosis through direct toxic effects on the marrow and/or B_{12} or folate nutritional deficiency (Kaferle and Strzoda 2009). A high MCV by itself does not imply a diagnosis of one of the aforementioned conditions and should be corroborated with other biomarkers.

Platelet Count

Thrombocytopenia, defined as low platelet count (<150,000 per μL) can occur during infection, autoimmune disease, or as a side effect of psychiatric medications. Among these, valproic acid (VPA) has the highest rate (12–18%) of thrombocytopenia; advanced age, female sex, and high doses increase the risk (Buoli et al. 2018). The severity of VPA-induced thrombocytopenia is dose-dependent; higher risk occurred with VPA plasma levels >100 μg/mL for women and >130 μg/mL for men (Nasreddine and Beydoun 2008). Recommendations on the management of this side effect are lacking; reducing the VPA dose often helps reverse the laboratory abnormality (Buoli et al. 2018).

Thrombocytosis can occur in the setting of infection, trauma, or myeloproliferative disease. Mood changes may be associated (Steardo et al. 2019). Thrombocytosis can also increase the risk of CVAs, in turn leading to cognitive, mood, or personality changes. Table 4.3 presents the hematological adverse effects of psychotropic agents.

Serum Electrolytes

A basic metabolic panel typically includes electrolytes (sodium, potassium, chloride), carbon dioxide, blood urea nitrogen (BUN), creatinine, glucose, and sometimes calcium.

*Hypo*natremia (<135 mEq/L) can be associated with confusion, delirium, dizziness, gait impairments, falls, and seizures (Mendez and Cummings 2003; Leth-Møller et al. 2016). Sodium levels should be monitored when prescribing medications known to cause hyponatremia, including anticonvulsants (carbamazepine, oxcarbazepine) and antidepressants, particularly serotonergic agents (Ozdemir 2013). The prevalence of hyponatremia due to SSRIs and SNRIs can reach 32%, with citalopram and clomipramine having the highest risk, while duloxetine, venlafaxine, and mirtazapine have the lowest risk (Ozdemir 2013; Leth-Møller et al. 2016). Medication-induced hyponatremia is usually caused by a syndrome of inappropriate secretion of antidiuretic hormone (SIADH), characterized by low serum osmolality and high urine osmolality, although the pathophysiological mechanism is not fully understood (Leth-Møller et al. 2016). Other causes of hyponatremia include primary polydipsia and adrenal insufficiency.

Chronic *hyper*natremia is better tolerated by the brain than chronic hyponatremia, although cognitive changes can occur (Mendez and Cummings 2003).

*Hyper*kalemia and *hypo*kalemia can both present as weakness or paralysis. Hyperkalemia can cause a fatal arrhythmia, whereas hypokalemia can be associated with anxiety and mood changes (Mazza et al. 2016). Hypokalemia, along with hypertension, hirsutism, and metabolic alkalosis, can indicate Cushing's syndrome, which is rare in older adults, but can present with anxiety, cognitive impairment, depression, and psychosis (Damanti et al. 2018).

Mild *hypo*calcemia can present with anxiety, irritability, and mood lability, while severe hypocalcemia can manifest with mania and psychosis (Levenson 2006). Mild to moderate *hyper*calcemia (serum calcium levels of 12–16 mg/dL) can be associated with apathy, depression, and irritability, whereas severe hypercalcemia (>16 mg/dL) can lead to delirium, psychosis, catatonia, lethargy, and may progress to coma (Levenson 2006; Mendez and Cummings 2003).

Blood Urea Nitrogen (BUN) and Creatinine

Renal function (BUN and creatinine) should be tested in patients with delirium and MNCDs and checked regularly in patients taking lithium (Kaufman et al. 2017a; Seritan et al. 2009b). Renal insufficiency is characterized by elevated BUN and creatinine levels, electrolyte abnormalities (hyponatremia, hyperkalemia, hypermagnesemia, hypocalcemia), and metabolic acidosis. Neuropsychiatric symptoms include poor concentration and memory, irritability, and psychosis, which are most pronounced with the rapid development of uremia (Mendez and Cummings 2003).

Erythrocyte Sedimentation Rate (ESR)

ESR is an inflammatory marker which can be elevated in rheumatoid arthritis, polymyalgia rheumatica, systemic lupus erythematosus, temporal (giant cell) arteritis, and other vasculitides.

ESR is a *must-do* test when inflammatory processes of the central nervous system are suspected, which can be associated with a range of neuropsychiatric symptoms: anxiety, mood disorders, psychosis, delirium, or MNCD (Isaac and Larson 2014).

Glucose and Hemoglobin A1c (HbA1c)

DM, hyperlipidemia, and hypertension constitute a triad of cerebrovascular disease risk factors, which can cause microvascular ischemic changes or strokes, resulting in cognitive dysfunction and/or mood disturbances (Mendez and Cummings 2003; Sharma et al. 2020). Eighteen percent of individuals with DM type II have depressive disorders, more common in women than men (Ali et al. 2006).

Cerebral glucose fluctuations can be associated with acute or chronic psychiatric features. *Hypo*glycemia may lead to fluctuating attention, cognitive slowing, or delirium, and a history of severe hypoglycemic episodes increases risk of MNCD (Levenson 2006; Whitmer et al. 2009). Hypoglycemia can also present with symptoms that mimic anxiety (dizziness, lightheadedness, nausea, sweating, tremor).

*Hyper*glycemia can be associated with delirium, depression, or psychosis (Mendez and Cummings 2003; Oh et al. 2017; Sharma et al. 2020). Depression increases the likelihood of hypo- and hyperglycemia due to inconsistent adherence to diet, exercise, blood sugar monitoring, and medication regimen; in turn, this can exacerbate cognitive deficits and depression, furthering the risk of poor glycemic control. HbA1c (glycated hemoglobin) measures the percentage of total hemoglobin bound to glucose and reflects the average blood sugar control over the previous 3 months.

Human Immunodeficiency Virus (HIV)

Effective antiretroviral therapies have reduced complications of HIV infection, including HIV-associated neurocognitive disorders (HAND). Testing for HIV is recommended for older adults with known risk factors and cognitive impairment (Valcour and Paul 2006). HAND is characterized by cognitive deficits, depression, and motor symptoms such as ataxia, bradykinesia, or tremor (Isaac and Larson 2014).

Liver Function Tests (LFTs)

LFTs consist of total protein, albumin, alkaline phosphatase, aspartate aminotransferase (AST), alanine aminotransferase (ALT), gamma-glutamyl transferase (GGT), and bilirubin. LFTs should be checked in older adults with a history of alcohol use, hepatic or metabolic disorders, and cognitive deficits, including delirium, as well as prior to starting medications that can cause liver damage.

Hypoalbuminemia is common in older adults and has been linked to increased morbidity and mortality (Hannan et al. 2012). Low albumin levels can indicate inflammation, reduced hepatic synthesis, such as in liver disease, or increased clearance (e.g., nephrotic syndrome) and have been correlated with cognitive loss and depressive symptoms (Pascoe et al. 2015).

Elevated transaminases can indicate acute hepatitis (of infectious or toxic etiology, including medication-induced) or alcohol intake. In men with alcohol use disorder, elevations in AST of >40% and ALT of >20% suggested alcohol use disorder relapse with a sensitivity and specificity higher than 90% for AST and 80% for ALT, even when transaminase values stayed within RIs (Addolorato et al. 2013). An AST/ALT ratio >2 is consistent with excessive alcohol use, but it may also indicate liver cirrhosis (Addolorato et al. 2013).

GGT values >50 IU/L have a 100% specificity and 56–100% sensitivity for excessive alcohol use although levels can also be affected by liver disease and medications such as antiepileptic agents and anticoagulants (Dixit and Singh 2015).

Serial ammonia levels can track severity of hepatic encephalopathy and response to treatment, but evidence shows this is not a valid tool. Levels ≥70 μg/dL have only a 47% sensitivity and 78% specificity for a diagnosis of hepatic encephalopathy; conversely, 60% of patients with advanced hepatic encephalopathy had normal ammonia levels (Gundling et al. 2013).

Thyroid Function Tests (TFTs)

Thyroid stimulating hormone (TSH, also known as thyrotropin) is the primary screening test for thyroid dysfunction and one of the most widely used laboratory tests in psychiatry. Thyroid disease affects between 3 and 21% of the population and is more common in women and older adults. The prevalence of overt hypothyroidism in the elderly ranges from 0.2 to 5.7% across studies (Leng and Razvi 2019). Thyroid disease should be distinguished from physiological changes that occur with aging. TSH levels rise with age, while free triiodothyronine (T_3) values decline and free T_4 levels increase or remain relatively unchanged (Papaleontiou and Haymart 2012; Zhai et al. 2018). Other factors that confound interpretation of TFT results include chronic illness (which may lead to low free T_3 levels), variable dietary iodine intake, autoimmune thyroid disease, and concurrent use of medications that interact with thyroid hormones, such as lithium or amiodarone (Papaleontiou and Haymart 2012; Gitlin 2016). If TSH is abnormal, serial tests over 3–6 months should be performed, with follow-up testing of free thyroxine (T_4) levels if abnormal TSH values persist. This can differentiate between subclinical (normal T_4 levels) and "overt" (abnormal T_4 levels) thyroid dysfunction (US Preventive Services Task Force 2015).

*Hypo*thyroidism is a common cause of depression and cognitive impairment in the aged although cognitive changes may not be fully reversible with thyroid replacement therapy (Isaac and Larson 2014; Knopman et al. 2006). Between 5% and 15% of patients with hypothyroidism can develop psychosis ("myxedema madness"); Capgras syndrome and catatonia have also been reported (Heinrich and Grahm 2003; Hines et al. 2015).

Although *hyper*thyroidism occurs most commonly in the second and third decade of life, 10–15% of patients are older than 60 years (Ajish and Jayakumar 2012). Hyperthyroidism can be accompanied by anxiety (as well as physical symptoms that mimic it: palpitations, tachycardia, tremor), delirium, depression, insomnia, irritability, mania, and psychosis (Isaac and Larson 2014; Levenson 2006). Paradoxically, severe hyperthyroidism may result in an "apathetic thyrotoxicosis" picture in older adults, with apathy, lethargy, psychomotor retardation, and weight loss (Ajish and Jayakumar 2012; Mendez and Cummings 2003).

Urinalysis

Urinalysis can detect diabetes insipidus, which may be an adverse effect of lithium (low specific gravity, indicating difficulty concentrating urine), glucosuria (presence of glucose in the urine, such as in DM), SIADH, or UTIs. As mentioned above, UTIs are the most frequent cause of delirium.

UTIs are the most common cause of bacterial infection in older adults, particularly women, accounting for almost a quarter of all infections (Lody and Juthani-Mehta 2014; Nicolle 2016). Symptomatic UTI is defined as both the presence of 10^5 colony-forming units (CFU)/mL of bacteria and pyuria (≥10 WBCs/high-powered field), alongside at least two UTI symptoms, including acute dysuria, urinary frequency, urgency or incontinence, gross hematuria, and suprapubic or costovertebral angle tenderness (Lody and Juthani-Mehta 2014; Nicolle 2016). A midstream clean-catch urinalysis should be obtained for all patients presenting with acute mental status changes, followed by urine cultures, if indicated.

Vitamin B_{12} and Folate

Vitamin B_{12} deficiency can be associated with cognitive impairment including MNCD (also delirium, infrequently), anxiety, depression, mania, and psychosis, as well as peripheral neuropathy (Isaac and Larson 2014; Mendez and Cummings 2003). Current B_{12} assays have low sensitivity and specificity and can yield up to

50% false-negative or false-positive results, making true vitamin B_{12} deficiency difficult to detect (Stabler 2013).

Levels of methylmalonic acid (MMA), homocysteine, or both, are recommended in patients with borderline low B_{12} levels (200–400 pg/mL) who have not yet received vitamin replacement (Kaferle and Strzoda 2009). Homocysteine and MMA levels are markedly elevated in vitamin B_{12} insufficiency and decrease immediately after treatment, so they are useful in guiding replacement therapy (Stabler 2013). Elevated MMA levels are more sensitive and specific for vitamin B_{12} deficiency than homocysteine, which can also increase with folate deficiency and renal failure (Stabler 2013).

Folate deficiency mimics B_{12} deficiency and can manifest as delirium with psychosis (in case reports), MNCD, or depression (Barnhardt et al. 2016; Mendez and Cummings 2003; Ramos et al. 2005). In folate deficiency, MMA level is normal, but homocysteine is elevated. Serum folate levels are not cost effective and fluctuate depending on dietary intake. If folate deficiency is suspected, RBC-folate should be measured since this marker correlates more accurately with folate deposits as well as with cognitive scores (Kaferle and Strzoda 2009; Ramos et al. 2005).

Other Laboratory Tests

Several additional laboratory tests can be considered when clinical suspicion exists.

Carbohydrate-deficient transferrin

CDT is a biomarker for chronic alcohol intake of more than 60 g ethanol/day which has been reported to be superior to GGT and MCV (Golka and Wiese 2004). The transferrin molecule has 3–5 carbohydrate side chains; because alcohol affects the enzymes that add or remove these, CDT has only 0–2 side chains (Sherwood 2008). %CDT is the percentage of total transferrin that is carbohydrate-deficient; values of <1.6% can be found in non-drinkers and 3–10% in individuals who misuse alcohol (Sherwood 2008). CDT has a 95% specificity but low sensitivity, and values can also be elevated in end-stage liver or cholestatic disease, iron deficiency (which raises transferrin levels), other chronic medical conditions such as rheumatoid arthritis, or with genetic transferrin variants (Fleming et al. 2004; Sherwood 2008). For this reason, CDT should be used in conjunction or with GGT and MCV.

Fluorescent Treponemal Antibody (FTA-ABS) Test

Neurosyphilis can present with agitation, depression, mania, personality changes, psychosis, or cognitive deficits (Crozatti et al. 2015; Friedrich et al. 2014). In patients with MNCD, screening for syphilis is recommended only if there is clinical suspicion (Knopman et al. 2001). FTA-ABS is a treponemal test which detects the presence of antibodies to *Treponema pallidum* and is usually performed to confirm a positive nontreponemal test result. FTA-ABS remains positive for the rest of life in individuals who had syphilis, so it cannot be used as a marker of active infection, in contrast to nontreponemal tests (discussed below).

Genetic Testing

Several genetic mutations can cause or increase the risk for neurodegenerative diseases, particularly movement disorders. Routine genetic testing of patients with MNCD is not common in clinical practice, nor are guidelines available (Knopman et al. 2001).

Heavy Metals

Heavy metal intoxication causes peripheral neuropathy and neuropsychiatric symptoms in adults. Lead exposure is often occupational or due to ingestion of lead-contaminated alcohol ("moonshine") and can be associated with agitation, poor attention and concentration, sleep difficulties, and psychosis (Mendez and Cummings 2003). Chronic mercury intoxication ("mad hatter disease") manifests with cognitive deficits, erethism (irritability in response to stimulation), neuropathy, ataxia, dysarthria, tremor, and the pathognomonic dark blue or black line along the gums (Kaufman et al. 2017a; Mendez and Cummings 2003). Although infrequent, manganese toxicity can cause cognitive deficits and parkinsonism. Manganese accumulates in the globus pallidus with a typical MRI appearance of bilateral symmetric hyperintensities on T1-weighted images (Mendez and Cummings 2003).

Lipid Panel

Cholesterol, triglycerides, high-density lipoprotein (HDL), and low-density lipoprotein (LDL)—direct and calculated—comprise the lipid panel. This can help ascertain risk of cerebrovascular disease and related vascular MNCD.

Parathyroid Hormone (PTH)

Hyperparathyroidism and the resulting hypercalcemia can be associated with anxiety, cognitive deficits, depression, insomnia, irritability, anger, psychosis, and suicidal ideation (Parks et al. 2017; Weber et al. 2013) (see Electrolytes, above). Lithium can cause hyperparathyroidism although symptoms are milder than in primary hyperparathyroidism (Gitlin 2016).

Rapid Plasma Reagin (RPR)

Nontreponemal tests such as the RPR and Venereal Disease Research Laboratory (VDRL) have a high false positive (up to 60%) and false negative (30%) rate; positive results should always be confirmed using treponemal tests (Geusau et al. 2015). Factors that can cause false-positive results include age >60 years, concurrent HIV infection, intravenous drug use, and autoimmune disease (Geusau et al. 2015). Latent syphilis, tertiary syphilis, treatment failure, and concurrent HIV infection should prompt a CSF examination (see below, Lumbar puncture) (CDC 2021).

Severe Acute Respiratory Syndrome-Coronavirus-2 (SARS-Cov-2) Test

SARS-CoV-2 infection can cause a variety of neuropsychiatric manifestations in aging adults, including cognitive deficits, delirium, mood changes, psychosis, and sleep disturbance (Helms et al. 2020; Rogers et al. 2020). A screening test should be ordered in patients with known or high likelihood of exposure, who present with suggestive symptoms (cough, shortness of breath, fever, fatigue, chills, anosmia, ageusia/dysgeusia, myalgias, sore throat, rash, or diarrhea), or who are otherwise at risk (e.g., living in long-term care facilities or other settings with high viral transmission). Viral tests include antigen and nucleic acid amplification tests (NAATs) such as the polymerase chain reaction (PCR), which detect the presence of viral genetic material (CDC 2023). Highly sensitive PCR tests can remain positive for up to 12 weeks after the infection, whereas antigen tests only detect an active infection.

Testosterone

Male hypogonadism can be associated with several nonspecific manifestations which overlap with depressive symptoms, (e.g., low energy, depressed mood, poor sleep, and poor concentration or memory) (Smith et al. 2018). Testosterone levels below RI can also be associated with low energy and depressed mood in women; however, testosterone replacement in women is controversial (Levenson 2006).

Urine Toxicology

Urine toxicology (UTox), or urine drug screen, can be helpful especially in emergency settings, for older adults presenting with first-onset psychosis, delirium, or signs and symptoms consistent with illicit drug intoxication such as pupillary changes, seizures, agitation, violent behavior, or those with known substance use disorders. Urine drug screens can detect alcohol metabolites (ethyl glucuronide and ethyl sulfate) for 12–24 h (up to 72 h with more sophisticated tests) after ingestion, as well as amphetamines, barbiturates, benzodiazepines, cocaine, marijuana, opioids, and phencyclidine. According to the National Epidemiologic Survey on Alcohol and Related Conditions—Wave 2, the prevalence of substance use disorders in those aged 65 years and older was 4.45%, with the oldest-old having very low rates (0.15%) (Reynolds et al. 2015). However, this is estimated to increase, particularly for cannabis and prescription medications (Reynolds et al. 2015; Kuerbis 2020). As such, a low threshold for ordering a UTox is advisable.

Vanillylmandelic Acid (VMA)

Vanillylmandelic acid (VMA) is measured in 24-h urine samples and is typically elevated in patients with pheochromocytoma. Plasma-free metanephrine levels (metanephrine, normetanephrine, and methoxytyramine) are more specific for pheochromocytoma and can help estimate the size and location (adrenal or extra-adrenal) of the tumor although they are not always measured correctly, making VMA the preferred test (Eisenhofer and Peitzsch 2014). Pheochromocytomas can manifest with anxiety, palpitations, paroxysmal hypertension, sweating, and tachycardia, mimicking panic attacks (Levenson 2006).

Vitamin B_1 (Thiamine)

Thiamine deficiency is often present in patients with chronic alcohol use disorder and concomitant malnutrition and can also be due to malabsorption, persistent vomiting, hypermetabolic states such as thyrotoxicosis, or dialysis (Arts et al. 2017; Isenberg-Grzeda et al. 2012). The biologically active form of thiamine, thiamine pyrophosphate, is essential for multiple biochemical pathways involved in carbohydrate metabolism.

Wernicke's encephalopathy (WE) is an acute syndrome that may occur in 12.5% of patients with chronic alcohol use, characterized by ataxia, delirium, and ophthalmoplegia although only 16% of patients have all three signs (Chandrakumar et al. 2019). WE is a medical emergency and can be fatal in 20% of cases; thiamine should be replaced without delay (Chandrakumar et al. 2019). Korsakoff's syndrome (alcohol-induced amnestic confabulatory mild NCD or MNCD in DSM-5-TR) is a late complication of WE which consists of anterograde and retrograde amnesia, executive dysfunction, confabulation, apathy, and mood lability (Arts et al. 2017; Chandrakumar et al. 2019).

Vitamin D

Vitamin D deficiency has been correlated with cognitive deficits, delirium, depressive disorders, psychosis, and sleep disorders (Ford et al. 2013; Mulcahy et al. 2016). Vitamin D is produced in the skin from 7-dehydrocholesterol (this step needs ultraviolet B light from the sun) or absorbed from the diet and converted into the 25-hydroxy D and then the active form, 1,25-dihydroxy D in the kidneys (Bikle 2014). Older adults are more susceptible to hypovitaminosis D than other groups because their skin doesn't produce vitamin D as efficiently when exposed to sun and the kidneys have a lower capacity to convert it into the active form. The prevalence of hypovitaminosis D can vary widely, ranging from 28% to 66% depending on the population studied (Rolizola et al. 2022). Institutionalized patients, tobacco smokers, obese individuals, people with dark skin, and those with hyperparathyroidism are at higher risk. Low sun exposure and a vegan diet predispose, whereas physical activity and a balanced diet reduce the risk of vitamin D deficiency (Mulcahy et al. 2016; Rolizola et al. 2022). The Endocrine Society recommends screening only patients at risk for deficiency; the preferred method is measuring the serum 25-hydroxy form (Holick et al. 2011).

Other Tests and Procedures

Chest Radiograph (Chest X-Ray)

The chest X-ray can help distinguish infections, such as pneumonia, a common cause of delirium, or pulmonary embolism, which may mimic panic attacks. Chest X-ray is a *must-do* test in older adults presenting with shortness of breath, confusion, or disorientation.

Electrocardiography (ECG)

The ECG is useful in diagnosing underlying cardiac conditions that can be associated with or resemble symptoms of anxiety (e.g., atrial fibrillation, tachycardia, thyrotoxicosis) or depression (bradycardia, adverse effects of beta-blockers). Serial ECGs should be obtained at baseline, prior to initiating treatment and during therapy with lithium (which can cause sinoatrial block or sick sinus syndrome) and medications that can prolong the QTc interval, including antidepressants (citalopram, TCAs), antipsychotics (haloperidol—especially with IV administration, pimozide, pimavanserin, quetiapine, ziprasidone), and cholinesterase inhibitors (donepezil) (Funk et al. 2020).

ECG monitoring is particularly important for older adults, women, individuals with congenital long-QT syndrome, structural heart disease, prior history of acquired QTc prolongation, concurrent treatment with multiple agents known to prolong QTc, hepatic and/or renal failure, hypomagnesemia, hypokalemia, or family history of sudden cardiac death (Funk et al. 2020).

Electroencephalography (EEG)

EEGs are not indicated in the routine psychiatric evaluation but should be ordered for patients with myoclonus, seizures, and rapidly progressive cognitive decline (Geschwind 2015; Kaufman et al. 2017a). Comorbid mood or psychotic symptoms in patients who have difficulty recalling certain time intervals ("lose time" or "drift away") should also prompt consideration of an EEG. Ambulatory EEG with a portable device is superior to routine EEG for capturing interictal epileptiform discharges (Seneviratne and D'Souza 2019). An inpatient 3–7 day hospitalization for video EEG monitoring (synchronized real-time continuous EEG recording and video recording) may be necessary to clarify the seizure type or aid in the pre-surgical evaluation of treatment-resistant epilepsy (Shih et al. 2018).

The EEG can confirm a diagnosis of herpes simplex viral (HSV) encephalitis, which typically affects the medial temporal lobes and is characterized by complex partial seizures with temporal lobe discharges, amnestic deficits, fever, and delirium. Periodic sharp wave complexes (1–3 s bursts of electrical discharges, followed by minimal activity, which clinically correlate with myoclonus) in one or both temporal lobes are diagnostic for sporadic Creutzfeldt-Jakob disease (CJD) but not present in variant CJD ("mad cow disease") (Kaufman et al. 2017a). Patients with focal or diffuse cognitive deficits, including delirium, often show commensurate slowing of EEG activity; psychotropic medications also cause EEG slowing (Racine-Belkoura and Geschwind 2016).

Electromyography (EMG)

EMG and nerve conduction studies can clarify the diagnosis of motor neuron disease such as ALS or other neuromuscular disorders. EMG can also aid in the differential diagnosis of frontotemporal dementia (FTD) with motor neuron disease (Racine-Belkoura and Geschwind 2016).

Lumbar Puncture (LP)

Lumbar puncture should be considered when trying to rule out meningitis or encephalitis in patients presenting with fever, headache, neck tenderness, rash, or who live or recently traveled to an area where they could have been exposed to endemic infectious agents (Oh et al. 2017). Infectious diseases to be considered include Lyme disease, neurosyphilis, viral encephalitis (e.g., HSV, West Nile virus), and CJD. Lyme disease diagnosis is based on history, clinical examination, CSF analysis, and *Borrelia burgdorferi* antibody testing, which should only be performed if there is high clinical suspicion (Koedel et al. 2015).

CSF testing can support a diagnosis of neurosyphilis, with elevated cell count or protein and a reactive VDRL test, in addition to reactive serologic tests CDC (2021). The CSF HSV polymerase chain reaction has a 94% sensitivity and 98% specificity although it can be negative when obtained within 72 h of symptom onset (Tüzün and Dalmau 2007). In patients with HIV disease, a positive CSF test for JC virus confirms the diagnosis of progressive multifocal leukoencephalopathy (Kaufman et al. 2017b).

CSF examination reveals higher levels of tau protein and reduced levels of β-amyloid and Aβ42 peptide in Alzheimer's disease (AD). The presence of oligoclonal bands and myelin basic protein in CSF confirms a multiple sclerosis diagnosis (Kaufman et al. 2017b). The utility of CSF biomarkers such as 14-3-3 protein, neuron-specific enolase, and total tau for sporadic CJD is unclear (Geschwind 2015).

If normal pressure hydrocephalus (NPH) is suspected, a large volume tap ($\geq$ 30 cc) is recommended, with pre- and post-gait and/or balance evaluation (Racine-Belkoura and Geschwind 2016).

Neuroimaging Studies

Neuroimaging is particularly important in older adults when assessing gradual cognitive changes, acute confusional states including delirium, or behavioral or personality changes. It is also a critical part of workup if clinical evidence suggests intracranial hemorrhage, ischemic stroke, or mass lesions, or for elucidating autoimmune or paraneoplastic processes that affect the central nervous system. In neurodegenerative conditions, neuroimaging is generally corroborative (*supporting*) because ultimately the diagnosis will rely on a broader set of clinical evaluations and testing, including a progressive course of behavioral, mood, cognitive, and/or personality changes. The distinctive cortical, subcortical, or brainstem atrophy pattern may be informative. If there is concern for a mimic of a neurodegenerative condition, such as vascular MNCD, or an acute or subacute time course, suggesting an infectious or paraneoplastic/autoimmune cause, neuroimaging is a *must-do*, because the treatment approach would differ significantly.

This section describes standard, clinically available neuroimaging techniques that are part of routine care and can highlight brain structure (CT and MRI) or neuronal function (SPECT and positron emission tomography—PET). Of note, functional imaging studies are not available in all centers.

Computed Tomography (CT)

CT scans of the head are of particular value in evaluating for intracranial hemorrhage or for bony abnormalities such as skull fractures, with excellent sensitivity for both (Heit et al. 2017; Rincon et al. 2016). When clinical suspicion is high for an intracranial hemorrhage, CT head is a *must-do* evaluation, such as after a fall, to rule out a subdural hematoma. The need for CT head relies on clinical judgment, guided by details of the fall or subsequent clinical changes (e.g., whether the head struck any surface, or presence of uncharacteristic confusion).

CT of the head is also part of emergency and hospital protocols for acute stroke, ruling out intracranial hemorrhage and (if CT angiography and CT perfusion imaging are available), evaluation for vessel cutoffs caused by a clot. CT perfusion studies are also helpful in determining the degree of tissue with reduced vascular perfusion that is at risk of additional injury and which might be salvaged with tissue plasminogen activator (tPA) or endovascular intervention, such as clot retrieval.

Signs of infarct on non-contrast CT are typically subtle and detected with low sensitivity within the first 6 h; associated hypodensities are often not apparent until the subacute or chronic phase (Caldwell et al. 2017). Significant limitations to CT exist in posterior and infratentorial regions given prominent bony artifact which may obscure small infarcts or mass lesions (Vilela and Rowley 2017). Normal CT study in the setting of clinical findings that might suggest a posterior circulation infarct or other brainstem abnormality may be falsely negative and, if clinical suspicion is high, MRI should follow.

Magnetic Resonance Imaging (MRI)

Compared to head CT, MRI of the brain generally has superior sensitivity for detecting intraparenchymal processes such as mass lesions, infarcts, demyelinating lesions, or infectious changes. MRI is the investigation of choice when evaluating for ischemic stroke, particularly in the acute phase or in posterior brain regions (Caldwell et al. 2017). Its use is limited in patients unable to lie still for a prolonged period of time or who have other contraindications such as MRI-incompatible implanted hardware. MRI findings in specific neuropsychiatric syndromes follow.

Delirium/Acute Confusional States

If symptoms suggest Wernicke's encephalopathy, MRI can detect changes in the medial thalami, mammillary bodies, periaqueductal region, and the tectum of the midbrain with 93% specificity but with a sensitivity of only 53% (Isenberg-Grzeda et al. 2012). MRI findings in Wernicke's encephalopathy may vary based on duration of alcohol use; individuals with chronic alcohol use show contrast enhancement in mamillary bodies and thalami more frequently than those without such a history (Zuccoli et al. 2009).

Infectious encephalitis may present with acute confusional states or delirium and feature MRI changes. HSV encephalitis shows changes on brain MRI in 80–100% of cases (Bertrand et al. 2017), typically with T2 or diffusion-weighted imaging (DWI) lesions in frontal and temporal regions, but also in the basal ganglia or thalami. Sensitivity for HSV-related changes is much higher acutely with MRI as compared to CT (Granerod et al. 2016). Varicella-zoster virus encephalitis may cause vasculopathy with unifocal or multifocal ischemic infarcts visible as DWI or fluid-attenuated inversion recovery (FLAIR) changes depending on acuity. In immunocompromised patients, cytomegalovirus encephalitis may show abnormal enhancement and T2 signal changes in the ventricular walls (Bertrand et al. 2017).

Neurodegenerative Diseases

In Alzheimer's disease (AD), cortical atrophy tends to be most prominent in the medial temporal lobes, temporoparietal regions, the precuneus, and posterior cingulate (Blamire 2018). In contrast, dementia with Lewy bodies (DLB) typically features relative preservation of medial temporal lobe structures, with atrophy in the temporal and frontal lobes, particularly the insula (Burton et al. 2002). Behavioral variant frontotemporal dementia (bvFTD) will characteristically demonstrate medial frontal, anterior temporal, and orbital-insular atrophy with relative sparing of more posterior cortical regions (Filippi and Agosta 2018).

Structural MRI is relatively unremarkable in PD. Patients with Richardson's syndrome, the originally described clinical phenotype of PSP (PSP-RS), typically have marked midbrain and superior cerebellar peduncle atrophy with relative sparing of the pons (Whitwell et al. 2017). Reduced midbrain-pons ratio on structural MRI (labeled the "hummingbird sign" in qualitatively obvious cases) was predictive of the development of PSP-RS within 15 months in patients with unclassifiable parkinsonism at baseline (Owens et al. 2016).

In multi-system atrophy (MSA), MRI may show pontine and cerebellar atrophy, particularly in the cerebellar subtype (MSA-C). The "hot cross buns" sign, with T2 hyperintensity in a slit-like configuration in the pons and middle cerebellar peduncles, results from selective atrophy in the lower basis-pontis, medulla, cerebellar hemispheres, and middle cerebellar peduncles with relative sparing of superior cerebellar peduncles and corticospinal tracts (Broski et al. 2014).

Vascular Disease

The diagnosis of chronic cerebrovascular disease, for example, subcortical ischemic vascular dementia (SIVD) or cerebral amyloid angiopathy (CAA) can be supported by neuroimaging. SIVD shows extensive subcortical white matter hyperintensities on T2 or FLAIR sequences and typically presents with executive dysfunction but may feature impairment in other cognitive domains, apathy, and depression (Risacher and Saykin 2019). CAA, related to amyloid deposition in the walls of small cerebral vessels, features numerous microhemorrhages in a cortical distribution which appear as areas of hypointensity on T2*-gradient echo or susceptibility weighted imaging—MRI sequences which are sensitive to hemoglobin breakdown products (Haacke et al. 2007). There may also be acute or subacute cortical or subcortical infarcts seen as areas of hyperintensity on DWI or T2 sequences (Risacher and Saykin 2019).

Autoimmune/Paraneoplastic Encephalitis

Autoimmune and paraneoplastic encephalitis can present with acute to subacute neuropsychiatric symptoms. Although more common in younger adults, limbic encephalitis can present with seizures, rapidly progressive memory changes, anxiety, mood, and psychotic symptoms (Tüzün and Dalmau 2007). MRI changes have been included as diagnostic criteria for paraneoplastic limbic encephalitis, in which 70-80% of patients have uni- or bilateral medial temporal lobe hyperintensities visible on MRI FLAIR or T2 sequences (Tüzün and Dalmau 2007). MRI is often normal in anti-N-methyl-D-aspartate (NMDA) receptor encephalitis although 44% of patients may have highly variable T2 and FLAIR signal changes throughout the brain (Kelley et al. 2017). Anti-Hu encephalitis, the most common of autoimmune paraneoplastic encephalitides, may feature T2 or FLAIR hyperintensities in medial temporal lobes in addition to brainstem and cerebellar regions (Kelley et al. 2017).

Dopamine Transporter Imaging (DaT-SPECT)

^{123}I-Ioflupane dopamine transporter SPECT scans were approved in 2011 by the U.S. Food and Drug Administration to help differentiate essential tremor from tremor occurring in parkinsonian syndromes and are marketed by GE Healthcare with the trade name DaTscan. An abnormal pattern of striatal uptake of the marker has a fairly high sensitivity for a neurodegenerative presynaptic dopaminergic deficit, indicative of PD. However, this does not distinguish PD from atypical parkinsonism syndromes such as MSA, PSP or DLB, all of which DLB), all of which can show abnormal findings with this technique (Ba and Martin 2015; Banks et al. 2019).

Drug-induced parkinsonism, on the other hand, typically features normal DaTscan findings (Ba and Martin 2015). Discontinuation of dopamine blocking agents (antipsychotics, etc.) in the setting of parkinsonism might be the first intervention considered. If the symptoms are purely drug-induced, parkinsonism should resolve within 6 months of the causative drug's removal although recovery may take up to 18 months.

Positron Emission Tomography (PET)

^{18}F-fluoro-2-deoxy-D-glucose positron emission tomography (^{18}F-FDG PET) highlights areas of reduced neuronal metabolism and may be used in the differential diagnosis of MNCDs and other neurodegenerative processes. Evaluation is typically qualitative though various semiquantitative methods have been introduced. ^{18}F-FDG PET can distinguish patients with AD from healthy controls with 99% sensitivity and 98% specificity (Mosconi et al. 2008). A meta-analysis of 24 studies demonstrated an 88% sensitivity and 84% specificity of ^{18}F-FDG PET in predicting conversion to AD in patients with mild cognitive impairment (MCI) (Yuan et al. 2009).

Amyloidβ PET (using β-amyloid tracers such as florbetapir and flutemetamol) and tau PET are newer modalities that can *support* the diagnosis of AD and help distinguish AD from other neurodegenerative diseases. These studies are used particularly in research settings; clinical benefit has yet to be established (Rice and Bisdas 2017). Amyloidβ PET was both sensitive (89%) and specific (83%) in discriminating AD from FTD, which can be helpful early in the disease course (Rabinovici et al. 2011). In 2020, the FDA-approved ^{18}F-flortaucipir, the first agent used to image tau pathology in patients being evaluated for AD (FDA 2020). Medicare covers FDG-PET scans for either the differential diagnosis of AD or FTD, under specific requirements. As of July 2023, Medicare was not covering amyloidβ PET although the Center for Medicare & Medicaid Services was reconsidering this limitation (CMS 2023).

Neuropsychological and Cognitive Testing

Neuropsychological testing is essential in the evaluation of older individuals with new cognitive complaints and/or co-occurring anxiety, mood, and cognitive disturbances. Selected tests can help differentiate depression from MNCD, cortical from subcortical impairments, and/or frontal from hippocampal deficit patterns. This section will cover commonly used cognitive tests and their diagnostic relevance. These tests are typically corroborative (*supporting*). Results should be interpreted in the clinical context, in conjunction with laboratory and neuroimaging studies.

Cognitive Screening Tests

The Mini-Mental State Exam (MMSE) and Montreal Cognitive Assessment (MoCA) can be performed in the office or at bedside to monitor cognitive function over time (Folstein et al. 1975; Nasreddine et al. 2005). The MMSE is the most widely used test although it focuses on cortical functions and may miss subcortical deficits (a score of ≤23 had only a 42% sensitivity to detect subcortical vascular MNCD) (Raimondi et al. 2012). A systematic review of 14 studies (totaling 10,185 patients) revealed an 88% sensitivity and 86% specificity for a cutoff score of 23/24 or 24/25 to detect MNCDs (Lin et al. 2013).

The MoCA is more sensitive to executive dysfunction and *frontal lobe deficits*. A score of <26 had a 90% sensitivity and 87% specificity for the presence of MCI (Nasreddine et al. 2005). A study conducted in a geriatric outpatient psychiatry clinic (Dautzenberg et al. 2020) found that the MoCA was useful to confirm normal cognition (score ≥26; 95% sensitivity), exclude MCI (score ≥26; negative predictive value [NPV] 94%), and exclude mild MNCD (score ≥21; NPV 98%). The MoCA was not as helpful for diagnosing MCI (score <26; positive predictive value [PPV] 33%) or mild MNCD (score <21; PPV 31%) (Dautzenberg et al. 2020). Several MoCA short forms have been developed and reported to have a median sensitivity of 88% (62–98%) and median specificity of 87% (7–98%); their use should be informed by the patient population examined (McDicken et al. 2019). The MoCA has been translated in 50 languages.

Other rating scales assess cognitive impairment in specific patient populations, such as the HIV Dementia Scale, which has several time-dependent subscales to quantify the significant psychomotor slowing; a score of ≤10 (out of 16) indicates the presence of HIV-associated MNCD (Power et al. 1995). This scale has also been validated in older adults with cognitive impairment due to subcortical vascular ischemic disease and NPH (van Harten et al. 2004). However, a systematic review found it to have low screening accuracy (Haddow et al. 2013).

Tables 4.4 and 4.5 list common neuropsychological tests conducted at bedside or office to detect deficits in cognitive domains, including attention, executive function, language, memory, and visuospatial skills.

Patterns and Constellations of Deficits

One of the most important clinical questions that can be answered by a neuropsychological evaluation is to identify the pattern of deficits (*frontal* vs. *hippocampal*) exhibited by patients, which in turn can help narrow down the localization of affected neural networks.

A *frontal pattern* of deficits consists of a combination of executive dysfunction, progressive learning (e.g., patients can learn lists, stories over consecutive trials), reduced spontaneous recall (which improves with cues), and generally intact recognition, along with intrusions or false-positive errors. It is important to note that both frontal cortical processes and subcortical pathology that involves the frontal-subcortical neural networks can result in a frontal deficit pattern (Bonelli and Cummings 2008). Disorders manifesting with a frontal deficit pattern include the behavioral/dysexecutive (also known as frontal) variant of AD (which tends to be more common among patients with early onset AD, before age 65), FTD, strokes, and mass lesions involving frontal lobes, as well as multifocal white matter diseases or even metabolic encephalopathy (Mendez et al. 2012; Mesulam 2000).

Fronto-subcortical MNCDs also reflect a frontal deficit pattern and can be due to HIV, multiple

Table 4.4 Attention and executive function tests

Test	Domains tested	Responses indicating dysfunction
Attention/concentration		
A-test[a]	Sustained attention	Errors of omission (missing A's) Errors of commission (responding to other letters)
Serial 7s[a,b]	Attention, working memory, calculation skills	Forgetting what is being subtracted; perseveration on other numbers
Digit span forward[a]	Simple attention	<7 digits (±2) <5 digits for adults >65 years old
Continuous performance tests (CPTs)	Sustained attention	Errors of omission (missing target) Errors of commission (responding to stimuli other than the target)
Executive function		
Clock drawing[a]	Planning, attention, language comprehension, visuospatial skills, numerical knowledge, motor skills	Poor spatial planning, hemineglect, poor number alignment, poor hand placement, stimulus bound behavior (placing clock hands at 10 and 11) Age-specific norms exist up to 85 years old
Digit span backward[a]	Working memory	<Digit span forward score—2 <4 digits for adults >65 years old
Three-step command[b]	Attention, memory, sequencing, language comprehension	Poor sequencing, motor perseveration (continuing to fold paper multiple times), inability to maintain all three steps in mind
Peaks and plateaus Tri-loops (spirals) 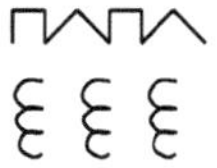	Motor programming	Motor perseveration (repeating the same element, adding loops to the spirals)
Luria hand sequence (fist-palm-side)	Sequencing, response inhibition	Motor perseveration, inability to maintain set
Verbal fluency[a] (FAS test or COWAT)	Self-initiation, fluency, perseverance, mental retrieval	<11–12 words/minute; errors (repetitions, rule violations for disallowed words), loss of task set (switching letters)
Stroop Interference Test	Susceptibility to interference, response inhibition	Errors of commission (inability to inhibit automatic responses)
Tower of Hanoi	Planning, sequencing	Difficulty with planning, rule maintenance, response inhibition, perseveration
Trail-Making Part B[a]	Set maintenance, response inhibition, susceptibility to interference (if timed)	Perseveration, inability to shift set (connecting only numbers or only letters)
Wisconsin Card Sorting Test (WCST)	Abstraction, hypothesis testing, mental flexibility	Perseveration, inability to shift set (in the 64-card version, cognitively intact adults should be able to switch categories at least 4 of the 6 possible times)

COWAT Controlled Oral Word Association Test
Sources: Racine-Belkoura and Geschwind (2016), Seritan et al. (2009b), Spreen and Benton (1977), Weintraub (2000)
[a]Included in the Montreal Cognitive Assessment
[b]Included in the Mini-Mental State Exam

Table 4.5 Language, memory, and visuospatial skills tests

Test	Domains tested	Responses indicating dysfunction
Language		
Boston Naming Test	Confrontational naming	<55/60 words (±5) <65 years old <50/60 words (±5) >75 years old
Repetition[a,b]	Word or sentence repetition	Difficulties with long sentences due to poor attention, grammatical errors, omission of particle words
Semantic fluency (e.g., animals)	Perseverance, fluency, mental retrieval	<18 (±5) per minute; errors (repetitions, rule violations for disallowed words), loss of task set (switching categories, returning to letter prompt)
Memory		
3-word 5–10 min recall[a,b]	Learning, recall	Encoding deficit (difficulties learning the words initially; suggests poor attention or hippocampal dysfunction) Retrieval deficit (difficulties recalling words spontaneously but improves with cues and recognition is intact; suggests frontal pattern) Rapid forgetting (no benefit from cues, reduced recognition; suggests hippocampal dysfunction)
California Verbal Learning Test	Word list learning, recall	Age-specific norms exist Short form (9-word list) usually more appropriate for older adults with known cognitive difficulties; long form (16-word) better for highly functioning older adults
Hopkins Verbal Learning Test—Revised	Word list learning, recall	Age-specific norms exist May be better for older adults given lack of interference trial and 12-word list
Wechsler Memory Scale—4th ed. Logical Memory	Story learning, recall	Age-specific norms exist Stories/information in context usually better preserved vs. list learning
Visuospatial skills		
Cube drawing[a,b]	Planning, organization	Poor planning, hemineglect, micrographia
Rey-Osterrieth Complex Figure	Visual attention, planning, organization	Poor planning, overlooking "large picture," omitting details Age-specific norms exist up to 89 years old

Sources: Brandt and Benedict (2001), Delis et al. (2000), Meyers and Meyers (1995), Racine-Belkoura and Geschwind (2016), Seritan et al. (2009b), Wechsler (2009), Weintraub (2000)
[a]Included in the Montreal Cognitive Assessment
[b]Included in the Mini-Mental State Exam

sclerosis, NPH, neurodegenerative movement disorders (e.g., Huntington's disease, PD, PSP, spinocerebellar ataxias), subcortical vascular ischemic disease, or vasculitides involving small- and medium-sized cerebral vessels. These patients present with bradykinesia and bradyphrenia (slowed thinking), difficulties with complex attention, executive dysfunction, and retrieval deficits, along with characteristic neurological signs and symptoms and prominent mood changes (apathy, depression, or irritability) (Bonelli and Cummings 2008).

A *hippocampal pattern* consists of a flat learning curve, poor recall (which does not improve with cues), and poor recognition. Neuropsychiatric disorders with a hippocampal pattern of deficits include AD, HSV encephalitis, alcohol-induced amnestic confabulatory (Korsakoff's) syndrome, limbic encephalitis, temporal lobe epilepsy, and strokes, tumors or infectious processes that affect the mesial temporal lobes.

The *dementia syndrome of depression* (formerly termed "pseudodementia") refers to the cognitive deficits that can occur in people with depression. Not uncommonly, patients with late-life depression display reduced processing speed, executive dysfunction, and impaired short-term memory (Wilkins et al. 2009). Patients with the dementia syndrome of depression typically score in the moderately impaired

(15–22) range on the MMSE (Spar and La Rue 2006). Poor effort and impaired performance on measures of attention, learning, and free recall can occur (Mendez and Cummings 2003). Older adults with depression often perform better on cognitive testing than people with AD and demonstrate a frontal, rather than hippocampal pattern (Masse et al. 2021).

Teleneuropsychological Assessment

The COVID-19 pandemic has made video visits/telemedicine common as the primary method of clinical evaluation. Prior research on teleneuropsychology suggests that for many verbally administered tasks (i.e., MMSE, digit span, naming, verbal fluency) results were highly similar across both in-person and video-based assessments in healthy controls and those with cognitive impairment (Cullum et al. 2014; Wadsworth et al. 2018). The MoCA has a "blind" version, which can be administered by video or phone without the written items; the written items can also be completed using a piece of paper at the examinee's home, allowing for full scoring.

Following the expansion of telemedicine visits, a new MoCA version for audio-visual meetings was released (https://mocacognition.com/). Studies conducted during the pandemic have further demonstrated the validity and reliability of many tests when performed via telehealth and high levels of satisfaction for both patients and clinicians (Hunter et al. 2021; Parsons et al. 2022). However, other authors have pointed out ongoing limitations including assessments of processing speed and executive function requiring written output (Salvadori and Pantoni 2023). Other limitations include access to technology, slow internet speed, and reduced ability to observe gait and behavior. Further development of validated, sensitive neuropsychological tests that can be administered via video visit is needed.

Conclusions

Laboratory, neuroimaging, and neuropsychological testing support a thorough history, physical, and neurological examination with evidence to diagnose and treat specific neuropsychiatric or neurocognitive symptoms. Routine laboratory tests are crucial (*must-do*) in many clinical situations. Additional workup should be considered, weighing benefits, risks, cost, and patient comfort. Age-specific laboratory RIs have yet to be widely used.

Neuroimaging studies are often *supporting* although they can be necessary (*must-do*) in certain clinical scenarios. Several, but not all, neuropsychological tests have norms for patients over age 65, and very few are normed for the oldest-old.

In summary, laboratory tests, neuropsychological evaluation, and imaging studies can confirm clinical diagnoses and help delineate neuropsychiatric diagnoses. This can guide specific treatment, which can minimize excessive or unnecessary interventions.

Age-Adjusted Recommendations

- We propose a practical framework for diagnostic test stratification: must-do (necessary), supporting (corroborative), and not helpful.
- Laboratory tests, neuroimaging studies, and neuropsychological evaluation results should always be interpreted within clinical context.
- Few age-specific reference intervals are available for laboratory tests.
- Neuroimaging studies can aid in the differential diagnosis of neurodegenerative diseases.
- Neuropsychological testing can identify patterns of cognitive decline and differentiate the cognitive deficits that occur in depressive disorders from major neurocognitive disorders.

References

Abramson N, Melton B. Leukocytosis: basics of clinical assessment. Am Fam Physician. 2000;62:2053–60.

Addolorato G, Mirijello A, Leggio L, et al. Management of alcohol dependence in patients with liver disease. CNS Drugs. 2013;27:287–99.

Ajish TP, Jayakumar RV. Geriatric thyroidology: an update. Indian J Endocrinol Metab. 2012;16:542–7.

Ali S, Stone MA, Peters JL, et al. The prevalence of comorbid depression in adults with type 2 diabetes: a systematic review and meta-analysis. Diabet Med. 2006;23:1165–73.

Alkemade GM, Willems JM. Polycythaemia presenting as sudden onset cognitive impairment. J Am Geriatr Soc. 2008;56:2362–3.

Allan GM, Young J. Complete blood count for screening? Can Fam Physician. 2017;63:772.

American Board of Internal Medicine: ABIM Laboratory Test Reference Ranges—July 2023. https://www.abim.org/~/media/ABIM%20Public/Files/pdf/exam/laboratory-reference-ranges.pdf. Accessed 8 Oct 2023.

Arts NJ, Walvoort SJ, Kessels RP. Korsakoff's syndrome: a critical review. Neuropsychiatr Dis Treat. 2017;13:2875–90.

Ba F, Martin WR. Dopamine transporter imaging as a diagnostic tool for parkinsonism and related disorders in clinical practice. Parkinsonism Relat Disord. 2015;21:87–94.

Banks KP, Peacock JG, Clemenshaw MN, et al. Optimizing the diagnosis of parkinsonian syndromes with (123)I-Ioflupane brain SPECT. AJR Am J Roentgenol. 2019;213:243–53.

Barnhardt EW, Jacque M, Sharma TR. Brief reversible psychosis and altered mental status in a patient with folate deficiency: a case report. Prim Care Companion CNS Disord. 2016;18 https://doi.org/10.4088/PCC.15l01839.

Bertrand A, Leclercq D, Martinez-Almoyna L, et al. MR imaging of adult acute infectious encephalitis. Med Mal Infect. 2017;47:195–205.

Bikle DD. Vitamin D metabolism, mechanism of action, and clinical applications. Chem Biol. 2014;21:319–29.

Blamire AM. MR approaches in neurodegenerative disorders. Prog Nucl Magn Reson Spectrosc. 2018;108:1–16.

Bonelli RM, Cummings JL. Frontal-subcortical dementias. Neurologist. 2008;14:100–7.

Brandt J, Benedict RHB. Hopkins verbal learning test-revised: professional manual. Psychological Assessment Resources (PAR); 2001.

Broski SM, Hunt CH, Johnson GB, et al. Structural and functional imaging in parkinsonian syndromes. Radiographics. 2014;34:1273–92.

Buoli M, Serati M, Botturi A, Altamura AC. The risk of thrombocytopenia during valproic acid therapy: a critical summary of available clinical data. Drug R D. 2018;18:1–5.

Burton EJ, Karas G, Paling SM, et al. Patterns of cerebral atrophy in dementia with Lewy bodies using voxel-based morphometry. NeuroImage. 2002;17:618–30.

Caldwell J, Heran MKS, McGuinness B, et al. Imaging in acute ischaemic stroke: pearls and pitfalls. Pract Neurol. 2017;17:349–58.

Center for Medicare & Medicaid Services. Beta amyloid positron emission tomography in dementia and neurodegenerative disease. July 18 2023. https://www.cms.gov/medicare-coverage-database/view/ncacal-decision-memo.aspx?proposed=Y&ncaid=308&ncacaldoctype=all&status=all&sortBy=status&bc=17. Accessed 4 Aug 2023.

Centers for Disease Control and Prevention: Sexually Transmitted Diseases Treatment Guidelines; 2021. https://www.cdc.gov/std/treatment-guidelines/hiv.htm. Accessed March 8, 2024

Centers for Disease Control and Prevention: COVID-19. Nucleic acid amplification tests (NAATs). Updated May 12, 2023. https://www.cdc.gov/coronavirus/2019-ncov/lab/naats.html. Accessed 12 Oct 2023.

Chandrakumar A, Bhardwaj A, 't Jong GW. Review of thiamine deficiency disorders: Wernicke encephalopathy and Korsakoff psychosis. J Basic Clin Physiol Pharmacol. 2019;30:153–62.

Crozatti LL, de Brito MH, Lopes BN, de Campos FP. Atypical behavioral and psychiatric symptoms: Neurosyphilis should always be considered. Autops Case Rep. 2015;5:43–7.

Cullum CM, Hynan LS, Grosch M, et al. Teleneuropsychology: evidence for video teleconference-based neuropsychological assessment. J Int Neuropsychol Soc. 2014;20:1028–33.

D'Ascenzo C, Cecchin D, Santelli L, et al. Parkinson-like features in ALS with predominant upper motor neuron involvement. Amyotroph Lateral Scler. 2012;13:137–43.

Damanti S, Abbate C, Chiodini I, et al. Behaviour disorder caused by Cushing's syndrome in an older person. Age Ageing. 2018;47:905–6.

Dautzenberg G, Lijmer J, Beekman A. Diagnostic accuracy of the Montreal Cognitive Assessment (MoCA) for cognitive screening in old age psychiatry: determining cutoff scores in clinical practice. Avoiding spectrum bias caused by healthy controls. Int J Geriatr Psychiatry. 2020;35:261–9.

Delis DC, Kramer JH, Kaplan E, et al. California verbal learning test. 2nd ed. San Antonio, TX: The Psychological Corporation; 2000.

Dixit S, Singh P. Usefulness of gamma glutamyl transferase as reliable biological marker in objective corroboration of relapse in alcohol dependent patients. J Clin Diagn Res. 2015;9:VC01–4.

Eisenhofer G, Peitzsch M. Laboratory evaluation of pheochromocytoma and paraganglioma. Clin Chem. 2014;60:1486–99.

Evidence-Based Medicine Consult 2020. https://www.ebmconsult.com/app/medical-calculators/calcium-correction-albumin-calculator. Accessed 1 Oct 2023.

Farrell CL, Nguyen L, Carter AC. Parathyroid hormone: data mining for age-related reference intervals in adults. Clin Endocrinol. 2018;88:311–7.

Filippi M, Agosta F. MRI of non-Alzheimer's dementia: current and emerging knowledge. Curr Opin Neurol. 2018;31:405–14.

Fishman SM, Christian P, West KP. The role of vitamins in the prevention and control of anaemia. Public Health Nutr. 2000;3:125–50.
Flanagan RJ, Dunk L. Haematological toxicity of drugs used in psychiatry. Hum Psychopharmacol Clin Exp. 2008;23(Suppl 1):27–S41.
Fleming MF, Anton RF, Spies CD. A review of genetic, biological, pharmacological, and clinical factors that affect carbohydrate-deficient transferrin levels. Alcohol Clin Exp Res. 2004;28:1347–55.
Folstein M, Folstein S, McHugh P. "Mini-Mental State": a practical method for grading the cognitive state of patients for the clinician. J Psychiatr Res. 1975;12:189–98.
Ford J, Hategan A, Bourgeois JA, et al. Hypovitaminosis D in delirium: a retrospective cross-sectional study. Can Geriatr J. 2013;16:186–91.
Friedrich F, Aigner M, Fearns N, et al. Psychosis in neurosyphilis—clinical aspects and implications. Psychopathology. 2014;47:3–9.
Funk MC, Beach SR, Bostwick JR, et al. QTc prolongation and psychotropic medications. Am J Psychiatry. 2020;177:273–4.
Geschwind MD. Prion diseases. Continuum (Minneap Minn). 2015;21:1612–38.
Geusau A, Kittler H, Hein U, et al. Biological false-positive tests comprise a high proportion of venereal disease research laboratory reactions in an analysis of 300,000 sera. Int J STD AIDS. 2015;16:722–6.
Gitlin M. Lithium side effects and toxicity: prevalence and management strategies. Int J Bipolar Disord. 2016;4:27.
Golka K, Wiese A. Carbohydrate-deficient transferrin (CDT)—a biomarker for long-term alcohol consumption. J Toxicol Environ Health B Crit Rev. 2004;7:319–37.
Granerod J, Davies NW, Mukonoweshuro W, et al. Neuroimaging in encephalitis: analysis of imaging findings and interobserver agreement. Clin Radiol. 2016;71:1050–8.
Gundling F, Zelihic E, Seidl H, et al. How to diagnose hepatic encephalopathy in the emergency department. Ann Hepatol. 2013;12:108–14.
Haacke EM, DelProposto ZS, Chaturvedi S, et al. Imaging cerebral amyloid angiopathy with susceptibility-weighted imaging. AJNR Am J Neuroradiol. 2007;28:316–7.
Haddow LJ, Floyd S, Copas A, Gilson RJ. A systematic review of the screening accuracy of the HIV Dementia Scale and International HIV Dementia Scale. PLoS One. 2013;8:e61826.
Hannan JL, Radwany SM, Albanese T. In-hospital mortality in patients older than 60 years with very low albumin levels. J Pain Symptom Manag. 2012;43:631–7.
van Harten B, Courant MN, Scheltens P, Weinstein HC. Validation of the HIV Dementia Scale in an elderly cohort of patients with subcortical cognitive impairment caused by subcortical ischaemic vascular disease or a normal pressure hydrocephalus. Dement Geriatr Cogn Disord. 2004;18:109–14.
Hathaway E, Wang S. Use of the laboratory in the diagnostic workup of older adults. In: Steffens DC, Zdanys KS, editors. The American Psychiatric Association publishing textbook of geriatric psychiatry. 6th ed. Washington, DC: American Psychiatric Association Publishing; 2023. p. 95–118.
Heinrich TW, Grahm G. Hypothyroidism presenting as psychosis: myxedema madness revisited. Prim Care Companion J Clin Psychiatry. 2003;5:260–6.
Heit JJ, Iv M, Wintermark M. Imaging of intracranial hemorrhage. J. Stroke. 2017;19:11–27.
Helms J, Kremer S, Merdji H, et al. Delirium and encephalopathy in severe COVID-19: a cohort analysis of ICU patients. Crit Care. 2020;24:491.
Hines A, Stewart J, Catalano G. A case of Capgras syndrome related to hypothyroidism. J Psychiatr Pract. 2015;21:445–8.
Holick MH, Binkley NC, Bischoff-Ferrari HA, et al. Evaluation, treatment and prevention of vitamin D deficiency: an Endocrine Society Clinical Practice Guideline. J Clin Endocrinol Metab. 2011;96:1911–30.
Hommos MS, Glassock RJ, Rule AD. Structural and functional changes in human kidneys with healthy aging. J Am Soc Nephrol. 2017;28:2838–44.
Huber KR, Mostafaie N, Stangl G, et al. Clinical chemistry reference values for 75-year-old apparently healthy persons. Clin Chem Lab Med. 2006;44:1355–60.
Hunter MB, Jenkins N, Dolan C, et al. Reliability of telephone and videoconference methods and cognitive assessment in older adults with and without dementia. J Alzheimers Dis. 2021;81:1625–47.
Isaac ML, Larson EB. Medical conditions with neuropsychiatric manifestations. Med Clin North Am. 2014;98:1193–208.
Isenberg-Grzeda E, Kutner HE, Nicolson SE. Wernicke-Korsakoff-syndrome: under-recognized and under-treated. Psychosomatics. 2012;53:507–16.
Jewell T. All about standard TSH ranges by age and life stage. January 8, 2020. https://www.healthline.com/health/tsh-normal-range-by-age. Accessed 6 Oct 2023.
Kaferle J, Strzoda CE. Evaluation of macrocytosis. Am Fam Physician. 2009;79:203–8.
Karrer TM, Josef KA, Mata R, et al. Reduced dopamine receptors and transporters but not synthesis capacity in normal aging adults: a meta-analysis. Neurobiol Aging. 2017;57:36–46.
Kaufman DM, Geyer HL, Milstein MJ. Dementia. In: Kaufman DM, et al., editors. Kaufman's clinical neurology for psychiatrists. 8th ed. Philadelphia, PA: Elsevier; 2017a. p. 105–49.
Kaufman DM, Geyer HL, Milstein MJ. Lumbar puncture and imaging studies. In: Kaufman DM, et al., editors. Kaufman's clinical neurology for psychiatrists. 8th ed. Philadelphia: PA, Elsevier; 2017b. p. 471–94.
Kelley BP, Patel SC, Marin HL, et al. Autoimmune encephalitis: pathophysiology and imaging review of an overlooked diagnosis. AJNR Am J Neuroradiol. 2017;38:1070–8.
Khambaty T, Callahan CM, Perkins AJ, et al. Depression and anxiety screens as simultaneous predictors of

10-year incidence of diabetes mellitus in older adults in primary care. J Am Geriatr Soc. 2017;65:294–300.

Klotz U. Pharmacokinetics and drug metabolism in the elderly. Drug Metab Rev. 2009;41:67–76.

Knopman DS, DeKosky ST, Cummings JL, et al. Practice parameter: diagnosis of dementia (an evidence-based review). Neurology. 2001;56:1143–53.

Knopman DS, Petersen RC, Cha RH, et al. Incidence and causes of nondegenerative nonvascular dementia: a population-based study. Arch Neurol. 2006;63:218–21.

Koedel U, Fingerle V, Pfister W. Lyme neuroborreliosis-epidemiology, diagnosis and management. Nat Rev Neurol. 2015;11:446–56.

Kuerbis A. Substance use among older adults: an update on prevalence, etiology, assessment, and intervention. Gerontology. 2020;66:249–58.

Lanier JB, Park JJ, Callahan RC. Anemia in older adults. Am Fam Physician. 2018;98:437–42.

Leng O, Razvi S. Hypothyroidism in the older population. Thyroid Res. 2019;12:2.

Leth-Møller KB, Hansen AH, Torstensson M, et al. Antidepressants and the risk of hyponatremia: a Danish register-based population study. BMJ Open. 2016;6:e011200.

Levenson JL. Psychiatric issues in endocrinology. Prim Psychiatry. 2006;13:27–30.

Lin JS, O'Connor E, Rossom RC, et al. Screening for cognitive impairment in older adults: an evidence update for the U.S. Preventive Services Task Force [Internet]. Rockville, MD: Agency for Healthcare Research and Quality (US); Report No.: 14-05198-EF-1.; 2013.

Lody M, Juthani-Mehta M. Urinary tract infections in older women: a clinical review. JAMA. 2014;311:844–54.

Masse C, Vandel P, Sylvestre G, et al. Cognitive impairment in late-life depression: a comparative study of healthy older people, late-life depression, and mild Alzheimer's disease using multivariate base rates of low scores. Front Psychol. 2021;12:724731.

Mazza A, Ravenni R, Armigliato M, et al. Mood disorders in uncontrolled hypertension despite multiple anti-hypertensive medications: searching for a link. High Blood Press Cardiovasc Prev. 2016;23:41–6.

McDicken JA, Elliott E, Blayney G, et al. Accuracy of the short-form Montreal cognitive assessment: systematic review and validation. Int J Geriatr Psychiatry. 2019;34:1515–25.

Mendez MF, Cummings JL. Toxic-metabolic causes of dementia and psychiatric dementias associated with psychiatric disorders, in dementia: a clinical approach. 3rd ed. Philadelphia, PA: Butterworth Heinemann; 2003. p. 421–502.

Mendez MF, Lee AS, Joshi A, Shapira JS. Nonamnestic presentations of early-onset Alzheimer's disease. Am J Alzheimers Dis Other Dement. 2012;27:413–20.

Mesulam M-M. Behavioral neuroanatomy. In: Mesulam MM, editor. Principles of behavioral and cognitive neurology. 2nd ed. New York: Oxford University Press; 2000. p. 1–120.

Meyers J, Meyers K. Rey complex figure test and recognition trial. San Antonio, TX: The Psychological Corporation; 1995.

Mosconi L, Tsui W, Herholz K, et al. Multicenter standardized 18F-FDG PET diagnosis of mild cognitive impairment, Alzheimer's disease, and other dementias. J Nucl Med. 2008;49:390–8.

Mulcahy KB, Trigoboff E, Oper L, Demmler TL. Physician prescribing practices of vitamin D in a psychiatric hospital. Innov Clin Neurosci. 2016;13:21–7.

Nasreddine W, Beydoun A. Valproate-induced thrombocytopenia: a prospective monotherapy study. Epilepsia. 2008;49:438–45.

Nasreddine ZS, Phillips NA, Bédirian V, et al. The Montreal Cognitive Assessment, MoCA: a brief screening tool for mild cognitive impairment. J Am Geriatr Soc. 2005;53:695–9.

Nicolle LE. Urinary tract infections in the older adult. Clin Geriatr Med. 2016;32:523–38.

Oh ES, Fong TG, Hshieh TT, Inouye SK. Delirium in older persons: advances in diagnosis and treatment. JAMA. 2017;318:1161–74.

Owens E, Krecke K, Ahlskog JE, et al. Highly specific radiographic marker predates clinical diagnosis in progressive supranuclear palsy. Parkinsonism Relat Disord. 2016;28:107–11.

Ozarda Y, Sikaris K, Streichert T, et al. Distinguishing reference intervals and clinical decision limits—a review by the IFCC Committee on Reference Intervals and Decision Limits. Crit Rev Clin Lab Sci. 2018;55:420–31.

Ozdemir O. Sodium and depression: hypothetical associations. Bull Clin Psychopharmacol. 2013;23:107–12.

Papaleontiou M, Haymart MR. Approach to and treatment of thyroid disease in the elderly. Med Clin North Am. 2012;96:297–310.

Parks KA, Parks CG, Onwuameze OE, Shrestha S. Psychiatric complications of primary hyperparathyroidism and mild hypercalcemia. Am J Psych. 2017;174:620–2.

Parsons MW, Gardner MM, Sherman JC, et al. Feasibility and acceptance of direct-to-home tele-neuropsychology services during the COVID-19 pandemic. J Int Neuropsychol Soc. 2022;28:210–5.

Pascoe MC, Skoog I, Blomstrand C, Linden T. Albumin and depression in elderly stroke survivors: an observational cohort study. Psychiatry Res. 2015;230:658–63.

Plebani M, Lackner K. Reference values: still a critical issue in laboratory medicine. Clin Chem Lab Med. 2010;48:577–8.

Power C, Selnes OA, Grim JA, McArthur JC. HIV dementia scale: a rapid screening test. J Acquir Immune Defic Syndr Hum Retrovirol. 1995;8:273–8.

Rabinovici G, Rosen H, Alkalay A, et al. Amyloid vs FDG-PET in the differential diagnosis of AD and FTLD. Neurology. 2011;77:2034–42.

Racine-Belkoura C, Geschwind M. The multidisciplinary evaluation of the atypical dementia patient. In: Geschwind M, Racine-Belkoura C, editors. Non-Alzheimer's and atypical dementia. Oxford, UK: Wiley Publishing; 2016. p. 6–16.

Raimondi C, Gleichgerrcht E, Richly P, et al. The Spanish version of the Addenbrooke's Cognitive

Examination—Revised (ACE-R) in subcortical ischemic vascular dementia. J Neurol Sci. 2012;322:228–31.
Ramos MI, Allen LH, Mungas DM, et al. Low folate status is associated with impaired cognitive function and dementia in the Sacramento Area Latino Study on Aging. Am J Clin Nutr. 2005;82:1346–52.
Rettenbacher MA, Hofer A, Kemmler G, Fleischhacker WW. Neutropenia induced by second generation antipsychotics: a prospective investigation. Pharmacopsychiatry. 2010;43:41–4.
Reynolds K, Pietrzak RH, El-Gabalawy R, Mackenzie CS, Sareen J. Prevalence of psychiatric disorders in U.S. older adults: findings from a nationally representative survey. World Psychiatry. 2015;14:74–81.
Rice L, Bisdas S. The diagnostic value of FDG and amyloid PET in Alzheimer's disease—a systematic review. Eur J Radiol. 2017;94:16–24.
Rincon S, Gupta R, Ptak T. Imaging of head trauma. Handb Clin Neurol. 2016;135:447–77.
Risacher SL, Saykin AJ. Neuroimaging in aging and neurologic diseases. Handb Clin Neurol. 2019;167:191–227.
Risch M, Nydegger U, Risch L. SENIORLAB: a prospective observational study investigating laboratory parameters and their reference intervals in the elderly. Medicine (Baltimore). 2017;96:e5726.
Rogers JP, Chesney E, Oliver D, et al. Psychiatric and neuropsychiatric presentations associated with severe coronavirus infections: a systematic review and meta-analysis with comparison to the COVID-19 pandemic. Lancet Psychiatry. 2020;7:611–27.
Rolizola PMD, Freiria CN, Silva GMD, et al. Vitamin D insufficiency and factors associated: a study with older adults people from primary health care network. Ciênc Saúde Colet. 2022;27:653–63.
Salvadori E, Pantoni L. Società Italiana di NeuroGeriatria (SINEG): Teleneuropsychology for vascular cognitive impairment: which tools do we have? Cereb Circ Cogn Behav. 2023;5:100173.
Seneviratne U, D'Souza DJ. Ambulatory EEG. Handb Clin Neurol. 2019;160:161–70.
Seritan AL, McCloud MK, Hinton L. Geriatric depression—review for primary care. Curr Psychiatr Rev. 2009a;5:137–42.
Seritan AL, McCloud MK, Hinton L. Dementias. In: McCarron R, Xiong G, Bourgeois JA, editors. Primary care psychiatry. Philadelphia, PA: Lippincott Williams & Wilkins; 2009b. p. 187–200.
Seritan AL, Rienas C, Duong T, et al. Ages of onset of anxiety and depressive disorders in Parkinson's disease. J Neuropsychiatry Clin Neurosci. 2019;31:346–52.
Shah RC, Wilson RS, Tang Y, et al. Relation of hemoglobin to cognitive function in older persons. Neuroepidemiology. 2009;32:40–6.
Sharma D, Suri V, Pannu AK, et al. Patterns of geriatric anemia: a hospital-based observational study in North India. J Family Med Prim Care. 2019;8:976–80.
Sharma G, Parihar A, Talaiya T, et al. Cognitive impairments in type 2 diabetes, risk factors and prevention strategies. J Basic Clin Physiol Pharmacol. 2020;31:2.
Sherwood R. Carbohydrate deficient transferrin (CDT). May 2008. http://www.viapath.co.uk/sites/default/files/upload/BloodSciences/cdt%20report2.pdf. Accessed 26 Oct 2023.
Shih JJ, Fountain NB, Herman ST, et al. Indications and methodology for video-electroencephalographic studies in the epilepsy monitoring unit. Epilepsia. 2018;59:27–36.
Smith JB, Rosen J, Colbert A. Low serum testosterone in outpatient psychiatry clinics: addressing challenges to the screening and treatment of hypogonadism. Sex Med Rev. 2018;6:69–76.
Spar JE, La Rue A. Mood disorders—introduction, in clinical manual of geriatric psychiatry. Washington, DC: American Psychiatric Publishing; 2006. p. 67–110.
Spreen O, Benton AL. Neurosensory center comprehensive examination for aphasia. Revised edition. Victoria, BC: University of Victoria Neuropsychology Laboratory; 1977.
Stabler SP. Vitamin B12 deficiency. N Engl J Med. 2013;368:149–60.
Steardo L, Staltari F, Segura-Garcia C, et al. Thrombocytosis in bipolar disorder: a case report. Bipolar Disord. 2019;21:800–2.
Stewart R, Hirani V. Relationship between depressive symptoms, anemia, and iron status in older residents from a national survey population. Psychosom Med. 2012;74:208–13.
Tüzün E, Dalmau J. Limbic encephalitis and variants: classification, diagnosis and treatment. Neurologist. 2007;13:261–71.
U.S. Food and Drug Administration. FDA approves first drug to image tau pathology in patients being evaluated for Alzheimer's disease. May 28, 2020. https://www.fda.gov/news-events/press-announcements/fda-approves-first-drug-image-tau-pathology-patients-being-evaluated-alzheimers-disease. Accessed 8 Oct 2023.
US Preventive Services Task Force. Screening for thyroid dysfunction: recommendation statement. Am Fam Physician. 2015:91. https://www.aafp.org/afp/2015/0601/od1.html. Accessed 8 Oct 2023.
Valcour V, Paul R. HIV infection and dementia in older adults. Clin Infect Dis. 2006;42:1449–54.
Vilela P, Rowley HA. Brain ischemia: CT and MRI techniques in acute ischemic stroke. Eur J Radiol. 2017;96:162–72.
Wadsworth HE, Dhimas K, Womack KB, et al. Validity of teleneuropsychological assessment in older patients with cognitive disorders. Arch Clin Neuropsych. 2018;33:1040–5.
Weber T, Eberle J, Messelhäuser U, et al. Parathyroidectomy, elevated depression scores, and suicidal ideation in patients with primary hyperparathyroidism: results of a prospective multicenter study. JAMA Surg. 2013;148:109–15.
Wechsler D. Wechsler memory scale. 4th ed. San Antonio, TX: The Psychological Corporation; 2009.
Weintraub S. Neuropsychological assessment of mental state. In: Mesulam MM, editor. principles of behavioral and cognitive neurology. 2nd ed. New York: Oxford University Press; 2000. p. 121–73.

Whitmer RA, Karter AJ, Yaffe K, et al. Hypoglycemic episodes and risk of dementia in older patients with type 2 diabetes mellitus. JAMA. 2009;301:1565–72.
Whitwell JL, Hoglinger GU, Antonini A, et al. Radiological biomarkers for diagnosis in PSP: where are we and where do we need to be? Mov Disord. 2017;32:955–71.
Wilkins CH, Mathews J, Sheline YI. Late life depression with cognitive impairment: evaluation and treatment. Clin Interv Aging. 2009;4:51–7.
Yuan Y, Gu ZX, Wei WS. Fluorodeoxyglucose-positron-emission tomography, single-photon emission tomography, and structural MR imaging for prediction of rapid conversion to Alzheimer disease in patients with mild cognitive impairment: a meta-analysis. AJNR Am J Neuroradiol. 2009;30:404–10.
Zhai X, Zhang L, Chen L, et al. An age-specific serum thyrotropin reference range for the diagnosis of thyroid diseases in older adults: a cross-sectional survey in China. Thyroid. 2018;28:1571–9.
Zuccoli G, Santa Cruz D, Bertolini M, et al. MR imaging findings in 56 patients with Wernicke encephalopathy: nonalcoholics may differ from alcoholics. AJNR Am J Neuroradiol. 2009;30:171–6.

Part II

Neurocognitive Disorders

5 Neuropsychiatric Symptoms (NPS) and Neurocognitive Disorders

Zainab Bhojani, Sheena Ghodasara, James Patience, Elyse Ross, Rita Hitching, Howard H. Fenn, and Amer M. Burhan

Abstract

Nearly all patients with major neurocognitive disorder (MNCD, formerly dementia) or mild neurocognitive disorder (mNCD) will develop *non-cognitive* neuropsychiatric symptoms (NPS) at some point in the course of their disease. Clinicians of any discipline or medical specialty who treat geriatric patients will inevitably see patients with MNCDs and associated behavioral and psychological symptoms of dementia (BPSD). NPS may present in the prodromal phase of Alzheimer's disease (AD) and other neurodegenerative disorders, and they often increase in frequency throughout the course of the illness. Comorbid depressive and psychotic disorders, among NPS, are associated with more rapid cognitive decline in AD. Given their enormous impact on quality of life, safety, function, caregiver burden, and cost of care, BPSD become the primary

Z. Bhojani
Ontario Shores Centre for Mental Health Sciences, Whitby, ON, Canada

Schulich School of Medicine and Dentistry, London, ON, Canada

Geriatric Psychiatry, London Health Sciences Centre, London, ON, Canada
e-mail: zainab.bhojani@lhsc.on.ca

S. Ghodasara
Geriatric Psychiatry, Halton Health, Halton, ON, Canada

J. Patience
Parkwood Institute, London, ON, Canada

E. Ross
Division of Geriatric Psychiatry, Department of Psychiatry, Western University and London Health Sciences Centre, London, ON, Canada

Division of Geriatric Psychiatry, Department of Psychiatry, Dalhousie University, Halifax, Nova Scotia, Canada
e-mail: elysec.ross@nshealth.ca

R. Hitching
University of Newcastle, Newcastle, Australia

H. H. Fenn
Department of Psychiatry and Behavioral Sciences, Stanford University, Stanford, CA, USA

VA Health Care System, Palo Alto, CA, USA

e-mail: hhfenn@aol.com, howard.fenn@va.gov

A. M. Burhan (✉)
Ontario Shores Centre for Mental Health Sciences, Whitby, ON, Canada

Department of Psychiatry, Temerty School of Medicine, University of Toronto, Whitby, ON, Canada
e-mail: burhana@ontarioshores.ca

H. H. Fenn et al. (eds.), *Age-Adjusted Psychiatric Treatment for the Older Patient*,
https://doi.org/10.1007/978-3-031-53976-3_5

concern of family and caregivers. The demand for treatment of BPSD is significant: a cross-sectional analysis of Medicare claims in the United States in 2018 found that 13.9% of older individuals with MNCD filled prescriptions for CNS-active polypharmacy (Maust et al. JAMA 325:952–61, 2021).

This chapter discusses an *age-adjusted* approach to NPS: ruling out modifiable contributors to MNCDs, treating systemic medical comorbidities, correcting environmental factors, and instituting non-pharmacological interventions as first-line interventions. A *minimalist* ethic endorses pharmacological treatment when it is needed for the management of disruptive or dangerous psychiatric symptoms but always with the goal of limiting risk of adverse effects.

Case Example: BPSD in a Patient with Alzheimer's Disease

A 67-year-old physician complained that she had trouble recognizing staff members and could not find the way to her office, which she had occupied for 20 years. There was no history of head trauma, substance abuse, seizure disorder, stroke, TIAs, cardiovascular disease, or an amnestic disorder. The patient's mother had developed Alzheimer's disease in her 60s and died at 73.

At the primary care visit for these symptoms, she scored 25/30 on a Mini-Mental State Exam (MMSE). A thorough systemic medical work-up did not reveal any treatable condition that could have contributed to the cognitive deficits. The only chronic systemic medical condition was osteoarthritis of the knees.Over the following year, the patient misplaced objects and accused others of stealing them. She became lost walking in the neighborhood where she had lived for 30 years and was convinced that strangers were following her. She insisted that her husband was her brother who was raping her, and that he was having an affair with her daughter. She wandered out of the house at night.

One year later, the MMSE scored 19/30. The patient now could not perform digit span backwards, remember three words after 5 min, follow a three-step command, or retain any new memory items. A diagnosis of probable Alzheimer's disease with behavioral disturbance was offered and she was started on donepezil 5 mg BID. Memantine 10 mg daily was added but without benefit for either cognition or behavior.

Over the next year, the patient had three involuntary psychiatric hospitalizations of 2 weeks each for self-harmful and dangerous behaviors (wandering and threatening neighbors). Once hospitalized the patient paced the units aimlessly, tried to open doors, and was easily agitated. She did not participate in psychotherapy and walked out of recreational and dance therapy groups within 5 min.

During the first hospitalization, a dose of citalopram 10 mg daily was started, increased to 20 mg daily, but discontinued after 8 weeks without benefit. Risperidone 2 mg at bedtime was added but caused restlessness and was discontinued. Intramuscular olanzapine 2.5 mg as needed every 4 h was used for episodes of severe agitation.

Carbamazepine at a dose of 200 mg TID was prescribed for the agitation, a dose chosen in anticipation of the tendency of CBZ to auto-induce its own metabolism. CBZ reached a steady state serum level of 0.9 mg/L after 10 days, and ECG did not demonstrate any conduction abnormalities. This medication regimen was continued as an outpatient over the next 3 months, but paranoid delusions, episodes of agitation, or wandering continued unchanged.

A second hospitalization came 3 months later after the patient threw a glass jar at her husband. During this hospitalization she fell twice, possibly due to a hypotensive episode, bradycardia, dehydration, and two doses of 1 mg lorazepam. The bradycardia was attributed to carbamazepine and/or donepezil. Both carbamazepine and donepezil were discontinued and quetiapine 100 mg at bedtime was started.

A third hospitalization, 2 months later, was in response to wandering; once the patient was lost near a freeway. She no longer recognized her husband or children and her MMSE was untestable. A conservatorship for person and estate was instituted during hospitalization, and the patient was placed in a secure memory care unit. Quetiapine 100 mg at bedtime was continued. The agitated behaviors improved on 50 mg of quetiapine at noon, 50 mg at

6 PM, and 100 mg at bedtime. Olanzapine 2.5 mg intramuscular every 4 h PRN helped reduce the severity of screaming and threatening.

(a) *Discussion:* This patient met DSM-5-TR criteria for major neurocognitive disorder due to Alzheimer's disease, based upon: A decline in memory and learning, and a severe deficit in at least one other cognitive domain, in this case, executive functioning.
(b) Steadily progressive, gradual decline in cognition, without extended plateaus.
(c) No signs of mixed etiology.

Efforts to treat BPSD with interpersonal interventions were not possible, and medications were only partially effective. Carbamazepine and donepezil may have contributed to the onset of bradycardia. The patient's family concluded that placement in a secure facility was needed prevent the dangerous behaviors.

Diagnosis, Search for Etiology, and Assessment

When psychological and behavioral symptoms emerge in late life:

1. Diagnose or rule out major neurocognitive disorder (MNCD). The DSM-5-TR criteria for probable MNCD are listed in Table 5.1; evidence from neuroimaging and neuropsychological testing are corroborative.
2. Identify etiologies, medical comorbidities, or treatable causes of cognitive decline.
3. Rule out, treat, or correct systemic medical disorders, delirium, environmental stressors, or other factors which contribute to the psychological and behavioral symptoms.

Table 5.1 DSM-5-TR diagnostic criteria for Major Neurocognitive Disorder (MNCD)

Criterion A. Evidence of significant cognitive decline from a prior level of performance in one or more cognitive domains: • complex attention • executive function • learning and memory • language • perceptual-motor • social cognition	Evidence for criterion A cognitive decline based upon: 1. Concern of the individual, knowledgeable informant, or clinician that there has been a significant decline and 2. A substantial impairment in cognitive performance preferably documented by standardized testing or another quantified neurocognitive clinical assessment[a]
Criterion B. The cognitive deficits interfere with independence in everyday activities, indicated by needing assistance **Criterion C.** The cognitive deficits do not occur exclusively in the context of a delirium **Criterion D.** The cognitive deficits are not better explained by another mental disorder such as major depressive disorder or schizophrenia	

Notes. Diagnostic Criteria from DSM-5-TR American Psychiatric Association 2022

[a]Neurocognitive or neuropsychological (NP) testing is not required as evidence to support the MNCD diagnosis though it is corroborative and can help track the course of specific cognitive domains. Executive function deficits and memory impairments can provide insight into the MNCD etiology (Sivasathiaseelan et al. 2019)

Step 1: Diagnosis

Cognitive changes noticed by the patient or reliable observers should prompt a search for:

- The chronology of the cognitive decline and the onset of behavioral/psychiatric symptoms
- Changes in systemic medical conditions, medications, or other factors
- History of brain trauma, neurodegenerative disease, environmental insults, substance abuse, alcohol abuse, or psychosocial stressors
- Symptomatology of pre-existing major mental disorder (MMD) or psychiatric symptomatology

- A cognitive rating scale, such as the Mini-Mental State Examination (MMSE) or Montreal Cognitive Assessment (MoCA), should be used to quantify and track the course of any cognitive decline (Lees et al. 2014).

Neuropsychological testing, though not required to diagnose MNCD, can be helpful:

- To identify cognitive impairments which reflect patterns specific to certain MNCD subtypes.
- To identify the *dementia syndrome of depression (DSD),* a pattern of potentially reversible cognitive deficits found in a major depressive disorder. Aging adults with cognitive impairment *and* depressive disorder have been shown to be at greater risk for progressing to MNCD than those who have depression *without* prominent cognitive difficulties. (Ganguli et al. 2006).
- To differentiate DSD from early AD. Although deficits in memory, attention, confrontation naming, verbal fluency, visuospatial ability, processing speed, and executive functioning are seen in depressive disorder, these deficits are usually less severe than those seen in early AD. Individuals with depressive disorders tend to perform more poorly than controls relative to the amount of effort required to complete a task (Wright and Perad 2007). AD patients have also shown greater false-positive errors during recognition memory tasks, whereas depressed patients tend to show more false-negative errors, suggesting less motivation by depressed patients to produce the correct answer (Ganguli et al. 2006). Individuals with early AD present often with impairments in temporal orientation, praxis, and gnosis functions, such as measured through tasks of visual recognition and visuo-construction.
- To identify cognitive impairments which may respond to non-pharmacological interventions for depressive symptoms (Watt et al. 2019).

Step 2. Search for Etiology of MNCD or Cognitive Impairment

Neuroimaging and laboratory evaluations can help:

- Determine the pathophysiology and patterns of deficits underlying the MNCD.
- Support the clinical diagnosis of MNCD; the final diagnosis of a specific neurodegenerative disorder may depend upon the progression of cognitive deficits.
- Rule out intracranial hemorrhage, ischemic stroke, mass lesions, autoimmune or paraneoplastic processes. MRI diagnostic algorithms have been shown to identify the etiology about 70% of the time (Tong et al. 2017) and can help differentiate specific subtypes of MNCD. Neuroimaging can identify neuropathological characteristics with distinctive cortical, subcortical, or brainstem atrophy patterns.
- Rule out brain neuropathology. Executive function deficits and memory impairments can provide insight into the MNCD etiology (Sivasathiaseelan et al. 2019).
- Differentiate vascular MNCD from other neurodegenerative pathophysiology.
- Rule out an infectious or paraneoplastic/autoimmune causes.
- Rule out treatable central nervous system (CNS) diseases such as CNS tumor, subdural hematoma, neuroinflammatory illnesses, or normal pressure hydrocephalus (NPH).

Although a CT scan can rule out most acute CNS injuries or relatively large lesions, an MRI provides more information about smaller lesions, subcortical structures, white matter abnormalities, vascular structures, microbleeds, and patterns of regional atrophy or reduced perfusion. Genetic testing can identify known genes associated with MNCD, and genetic testing can identify risk in other family members. Biomarkers are not generally used in the clinical diagnosis of MNCD (Isaacs and Boenink 2020; Ahmed et al. 2014). For further discussion, see Chap. 4.

Step 3: Search for Contributing Factors

BPSD is a diagnosis of exclusion, and factors which can contribute to its onset, severity, and continuation need to be ruled out. Identification and treatment of the following symptoms and conditions can improve management.

Other Major Mental Disorders. NPS in the aging adult can be manifestations of another, pre-existing, major mental disorder (MMD) *unrelated* to an MNCD. The prevalence of schizophrenia, for example, has been reported to be rising in nursing homes from 7.3% to 8.7% from 2011 to 2015.

Schizophrenia and bipolar disorder are associated with cognitive deficits also confer a higher risk of developing MNCD. Neuropsychiatric symptoms of MNCD overlap or mimic symptoms of other major mental disorders. The historical information listed in Fig. 5.1 can help identify MMDs in the aging adult. If suspected, a pre-existing major mental disorder (MMD) may suggest different treatment approaches:

- Symptoms of MMD with onset earlier in life may have a different trajectory than NPS of MNCD. Patients with MNCDs who have other major mental illnesses have shown a faster cognitive decline compared with those with MNCD *without* comorbid mental illness. Patients with bipolar disorder and MNCD showed greater decline when compared with patients with *only* MNCD. Treatment of bipolar disorder patients should therefore include interventions to minimize factors which impact cognition (Bendayan et al. 2021).
- Major mental disorders which began earlier in life may be associated with cognitive deficits which occur primarily *during an active psychotic episode*, and which may improve when psychotic symptoms diminish.
- MMD symptoms in late life raise the question as to whether the patient is adherent to their regimen of antipsychotic or mood-stabilizing medications (Bowie et al. 2018).
- mNCD: If MNCD is *not* diagnosed, the patient may meet DSM-5-TR criteria for a mild neurocognitive disorder (mNCD), but little high-quality evidence has been found to support effective pharmacological treatments for mNCD (Petersen et al. 2018). Serial cognitive assessments can help identify when mNCD devolves to MNCD. See Table 5.2.

Delirium. The onset of behavioral and psychiatric symptoms in an aging patient should raise the possibility of delirium, which is associated with prolonged inpatient length of stay, discharge to a higher level of care, readmission within 30 days (Zenilman 2017), and increased incidence of future MNCD (Fong et al. 2017). To distinguish delirium from BPSD:

- Administer the Confusion Assessment Method (CAM), a validated instrument to screen for delirium and/or predict its future emergence (Fong et al. 2017; Marcantonio 2017; Marcantonio 2011). Inattention and disorganized thinking have been found to *precede* 92.7% of the episodes of full syndrome delirium by several weeks; these symptoms identify 90.2% of the episodes, and the symptoms may persist *after* the apparent resolution of delirium (Cole et al. 2012; Maust et al. 2019). A positive CAM result for delirium necessitates a full psychiatric assessment for delirium, including use of standardized cognitive rating scales.
- Review laboratory findings for metabolic disturbances such as hyponatremia, urinary tract infections, or systemic infections which can support a diagnosis of delirium.
- Review medications which have high anticholinergic burden (AB) and those with sedative-hypnotic properties.

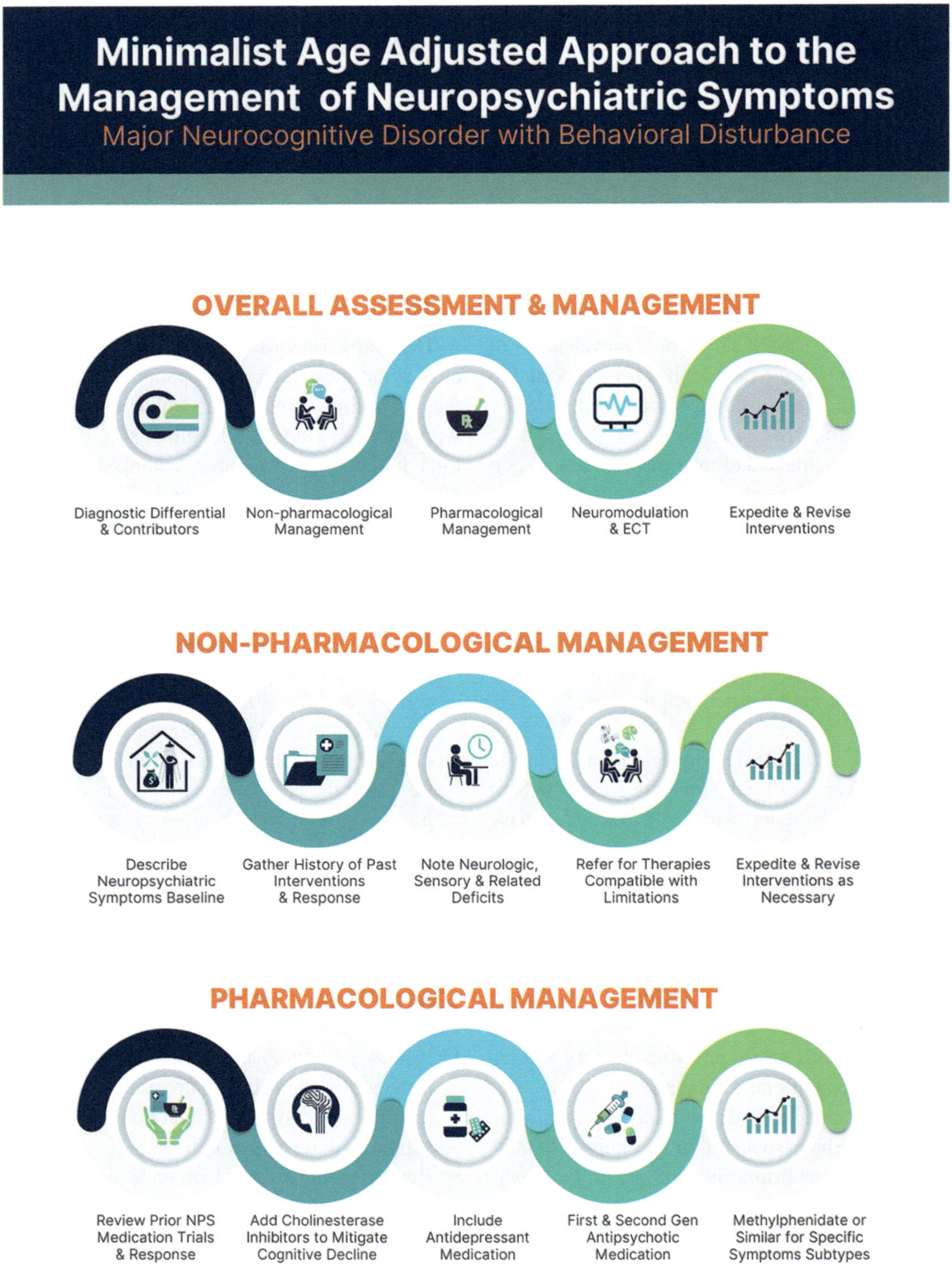

Fig. 5.1 Minimalist approach to management of NCS in MNCD (Rita Hitching, MSc)

Table 5.2 Features of pre-existing Major Mental Disorders (MMDs)

Mental disorders pre-dating neurocognitive disorders			
	Bipolar I & II	Depressive spectrum	Schizophrenia spectrum
Episodic Presentations Course of Illness	Depressive episodes—morbid thoughts, motivation or reduced energy Manic episodes—intense, elevated, irritable mood, or pressured speech	Reduced interest, joy & motivation worthlessness, hopelessness, self-blame & suicidality	Thought disorder often between episodes Paranoid or bizarre delusions prominent during episodes Auditory hallucinations
Medications Treatment Response	Mood—stabilizing medications improve acute symptoms	Antidepressant medication trials response at adequate doses & duration	Antipsychotic medications at adequate dose & duration ameliorate acute psychotic symptoms
Medications Treatment Response	Hospitalizations & emergency visits during acute mood episodes	Hospitalizations or other psychiatric interventions during depressive & suicidal episodes	Hospitalizations & psychiatric interventions often associated with medication non-compliance
Relationships Family & Partners	Relationships disrupted during mood disorder episodes	Isolation, withdrawal, detachment during acute depressive episodes	Disconnected from others or persistent dependence on others
Age of Symptom Onset Diagnosed Disorder	Onset before age 30 chronic & relapsing course recurrent episodes	Onset any time in life, may be spontaneous or associated with loss or stressors	Onset of psychotic symptoms before age 30
Developmental Landmarks Anticipated Milestones	Incomplete due to mood disorder episodes & impaired functioning	Interrupted during depressive episodes Functioning below potential	Incomplete or disrupted educational, military, social, marital, occupational

(Rita Hitching, MSc)
Neurocognitive or neuropsychological (NP) testing is not required as evidence to support the MNCD diagnosis though it is corroborative and can help track the course of specific cognitive domains. Executive function deficits and memory impairments can provide insight into the MNCD etiology (Sivasathiaseelan et al. 2019)

- Assess for recent discontinuation from benzodiazepines and other factors associated with onset of delirium. (Marcantonio 2017)
- Consider the risk of delirium or exacerbation of BPSD following general anesthesia. A retrospective study of 152 patients (mean age 86.5 for men, 83.1 for women) who had surgery under general anesthesia for fracture of the proximal femur reported three risk factors with the highest incidence of delirium or exacerbation of BPSD: presence of dementia, serum albumin level ≤3.7 g/dL, and peripheral lymphocyte count ≤1200/μL (Tanaka 2015). For further discussion, see Chap. 6 Delirium.

Pain. In-person interviews with a nationally representative sample of community-dwelling U.S. Medicare beneficiaries aged 65 and older with MNCD found that 670 (63.5%) of participants with MNCD experienced bothersome pain, and 347 (43.3%) had pain that limited activity (Hunt et al. 2015). Of 2822 nursing home residents (mean age 84.1), 538 (19.1%) were found to have pain which was significantly and positively associated with disruptive behaviors, abnormal thought processes, and/or resistance to care (Tosato et al. 2012). Wandering behavior, was *inversely* associated with pain (Husebo et al. 2011), perhaps because movement exacerbates pain (see Fig. 5.2).

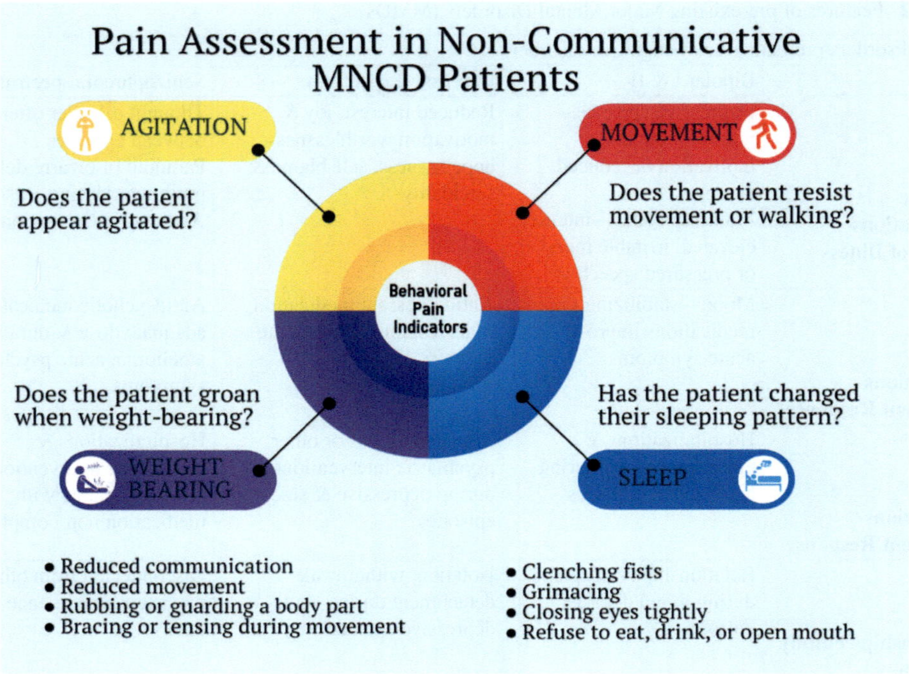

(Rita Hitching, MSc)

Sources: Makris et al. 2014; Husebo et al. 2016)

Fig. 5.2 Pain assessment in non-communicative patients (Rita Hitching, MSc). Sources: Makris et al. (2014), Husebo et al. (2016)

Pain in those with impaired communication skills can be assessed with validated, reliable pain rating scales such as the Pain Assessment in Elderly Adults with Dementia (PAINAD) (Ammaturo et al. 2017; Chibnall and Tait 2001; Hadjistavropoulos et al. 2014), and the Mobilization-Observation-Behavior-Intensity-Dementia Scales (MOBID and MOBID-2) (Makris et al. 2014; Husebo et al. 2016).

Treatment for pain has been shown to mitigate the severity of BPSD. One RCT studied 352 patients over age 65 with MNCD and NPS who either received stepwise treatment of pain or usual management. The intervention group had an average reduction of agitation on the Cohen-Mansfield Agitation Inventory (CMAI) at weeks 2, 4, and 8, and a reduction of overall severity of behavioral disturbances. When analgesic treatment was *withdrawn* at week 8 in the intervention group, CMAI agitation scores worsened (Husebo et al. 2011).

Sleep Disorders. Insomnia disorder affects 30% to 50% of aging adults (Suzuki et al. 2017), and compared with age-matched controls, is present in an even higher proportion of adults with MNCD. Sleep loss prevents protein clearance in the brain and may hasten the progression from mild cognitive impairment (MCI) to Alzheimer's dementia (AD)/MNCD (Romanella et al. 2020). History of sleep disturbance from a credible observer (Grimes et al. 2019) should include the quality and duration of sleep, environmental factors, behavior during the night, sleep hygiene, as well as substance and medication use. These observations can help differentiate between sleep-related behaviors, parasomnias, and agitation due to BPSD. These assessment scales can determine the severity of sleep disordered symptoms:

- PD sleep scale (PDSS)
- Epworth sleepiness scale (ESS) for daytime sleepiness to screen and to measure severity
- Inappropriate sleep composite score (ISCS) for severe daytime sleepiness or sleep attacks to screen and to measure severity
- Stanford sleepiness scale (SSS): rates sleepiness and measure severity at a specific moment

First-line interventions for disrupted sleep and insomnia disorders include:

- Minimize activating medications which affect sleep or alertness
- Assess pain and stiffness, enhance pain management (e.g., adding a non-opioid analgesic before bedtime)
- Light therapy: increasing bright-light exposure in the mornings
- In Parkinson's disease (PD), optimize dopaminergic medications which may cause sleep-interfering distress

Medication interventions for insomnia include:

- Doxepin: A small pilot RCT of doxepin 10 mg bedtime in PD improved subjective sleep measures with no evidence of worsening cognition (Rios-Romenets et al. 2013)
- Melatonin 3–5 mg at bedtime
- Quetiapine 12.5–25 mg at bedtime (Ferreira et al. 2013)
- Mirtazapine 7.5 mg at bedtime
- Trazodone 25–50 mg at bedtime

Rapid Eye Movement Sleep Behavior Disorder (RBD) is a progressive disorder often associated with alpha-synucleinopathies (e.g., Parkinson's disease dementia (PDD), multiple system atrophy (MSA), and dementia with Lewy bodies (DLB)). It is characterized by involuntary episodes of arousal often accompanied by complex motor behaviors and vocalizations during REM sleep (American Psychiatric Association 2013). The vocalizations and movements are secondary to lack of motor inhibition (atonia) during this sleep phase. It is more common in men and often predates DLB diagnosis.

Motor behaviors can pose a risk of injury to the patient and bed partner. In suspected RBD, safety precautions include sleeping on a mattress on the floor, securing sharp or dangerous objects, installing padding on furniture edges, and a separate bedroom for the bed partner (Romanella et al. 2020). Small nighttime doses of melatonin, clonazepam, or both, may be helpful.

Restless Legs Syndrome (RLS). An urge to move the lower extremities, often in response to uncomfortable physical sensations, characterizes this syndrome. The urge typically occurs during periods of rest, is relieved by movement, and is worse during evening/night hours (American Psychiatric Association 2013). Severity may worsen with antidepressants, antipsychotics, and long-term treatment with dopaminergic medications. RLS is associated with PD, iron deficiency, renal failure, rheumatoid arthritis, diabetes, peripheral nerve dysfunction, and thyroid disease. RLS may improve with reduction of dopamine agonist treatment or treatment with pregabalin (Grimes et al. 2019). Strategies for treatment of milder cases of RLS include avoidance of alcohol, caffeine, and tobacco; stretching; massage; and good sleep hygiene (Neikrug and Ancoli-Israel 2021). For further discussion, see Sleep Chap. 8.

Sedative, Hypnotic, Opioid, Anxiolytic, or Alcohol Abuse, Misuse, and/or Dependence. Aging individuals who take benzodiazepines or opioids regularly for as little as 3 months duration may be at risk of physiologic dependence. Misuse of these medications or symptoms of withdrawal from these medications, such as rebound anxiety, can disrupt sleep. The DSM-5-TR criteria for Sedative, Hypnotic, or Anxiolytic Withdrawal consist of:

(a) Cessation of (or reduction in) the substance after prolonged use, and physiologic symptoms of withdrawal (such as autonomic hyperactivity, insomnia, anxiety, agitation) within a few days of cessation of the substance (Brett and Murnion 2015). Of note: NPS in the context of dementia are not confined to, or necessarily associated with, either criteria A or B.

Inappropriate medication use is suspected when there are multiple prescribers, changes in clinicians, hospitalizations, psychosocial isolation, patient-driven pro re nata (p.r.n.) use of benzodiazepines and hypnotics (e.g., Z-drugs), and impaired cognition. For further discussion, see Chap. 2 Geriatric Pharmacology Overview and and Chap. 7 Substance Use Disorders.

Major Neurocognitive Disorders (MNCDs)

Alzheimer's Disease (AD) and All-Cause Dementia

The National Institute of Aging-Alzheimer's Association (NIA-AA) recommends that the diagnosis of MNCD start with a designation of *all-cause dementia*, categorized as DSM-5-TR *Major Neurocognitive disorder* (McKhann et al. 2011). The diagnosis of etiologies and subtypes of MNCD follows. The NIA-AA defines Alzheimer's disease as a dementia syndrome with insidious onset, gradual worsening, and either an amnestic or a non-amnestic presentation. Criteria include "changes in personality, behavior, or comportment" as one of two clinical features leading to a diagnosis of dementia. Alzheimer's disease (AD), as the most prevalent MNCD, is responsible for a significant proportion of neuropsychiatric symptoms (NPS) of MNCD, such as apathy and sundowning.

AD is often seen in combination with another MNCD, in which case the diagnosis is *mixed* dementia. Either AD+VaD or AD+DLB is the second most common cause of MNCD in the United States. One study reported that in persons with MNCD, over 50% had multiple diagnoses (AD, PD/LBD, or infarcts). After controlling for age, persons with multiple diagnoses were almost three times (OR = 2.8; 95% CI = 1.2, 6.7) more likely to exhibit dementia compared to those with one pathologic diagnosis. Mixed brain pathologies account for most dementia cases in community-dwelling older persons (Schneider et al. 2007).

Risk of Alzheimer's disease (AD) and vascular dementia (VaD) increases with age, especially for the oldest-old (>80), while the prevalence of frontotemporal dementia (FTD) peaks among young-old adults (~65). Less common MNCD causes, like HIV and prion diseases, have their onset typically at younger ages.

Any combination of behavioral and psychiatric symptoms listed in Table 5.3 can be found in any patient with MNCD. Many patients have two or more MNCD neuropathological findings and a mixture of NPS detailed below. *Apathy,* for example, is characterized as reduced interest,

Table 5.3 Behavioral and Psychiatric Symptoms of Dementia (BPSD)

Neuropsychiatric symptoms	Typical presentation
Anxiety	Apprehensive, tense, nervousness out of proportion to situation, rapid heart rate, sighing, short of breath
Delusions	Believes and/or accuses others of stealing, harming, or betraying
Dysphoria	Sad mood, tearfulness, loss of sense of pleasure or joy
Disinhibition	Impulsive, socially, and sexually inappropriate behavior (e.g., indiscreet comments and non-consensual sexual behavior—often under-reported)
Hallucinations	Auditory/visual/sensory perceptions not based in reality. Responds to people, objects, animals, or other stimuli not present
Sleep Disorders	When awakening from sleep and arising from bed
Elation and Euphoria	Elevated mood out of proportion to the situation
Motor Disturbances	Repetitive activities, wandering, pacing, and meaningless actions
Irritability and Lability	Easily angered, impatient, sudden, or frequent change of moods, poor coping with waiting
Apathy and Indifference	Reduced interest in activities, plans, or the future
Agitation and Aggression	Increased motor activity, fidgeting, gesturing, clenching fists, shaking, hitting, holding, scratching, gouging, and kicking, wandering
Appetite and Eating Disturbance	Craving odd foods, sweets, and gorging

Note. Adapted from Cummings et al. (1994)

lack of initiative, and diminished activity and affects 20–70% of Alzheimer's disease (AD) patients. Its presentation can overlap with psychomotor retardation of depressive disorders, hypoactive delirium, lethargy, or sedation, which makes apathy challenging to recognize (See Table 5.1 above). *Sundowning*, another condition, is marked by motor agitation, confusion, or aggressive behavior, often occurring near bedtime, which interferes with restful sleep.

Dementia with Lewy Bodies (DLB) and Parkinson's Disease Dementia (PDD)

These two neurodegenerative diseases, known under the general category of Lewy body diseases, overlap in neuropathology and clinical symptoms. Parkinson's disease dementia (PDD) and Dementia with Lewy bodies (DLB) together account for 15%–20% of the global cases of dementia. Both are marked by the presence of Lewy bodies (protein aggregates of alpha-synuclein that cause neuronal atrophy), parkinsonian motor symptoms, and cognitive decline.

Cognitive deficits in the DLB and PDD spectrum can be exacerbated by anticholinergic burden (AB) of medications (Jaïdi et al. 2018; Kröger et al. 2015).

DLB is considered by some authorities a distinct MNCD, differentiated from PDD by early onset of dementia, preceeding motor symptoms, and more rapid progression. DLB by itself has been reported as the third most common dementia (5% of cases) with a prevalence that peaks around 75 years of age (Vann Jones and O'Brien 2014). In DLB, the pattern of atrophy is characterized by relative sparing of medial temporal lobe structures compared to AD and more involvement of occipital areas (Banerjee et al. 2020). It shows a significant deficit in acetylcholine neurotransmission compared to other dementing illnesses.

Fluctuation in levels of arousal and psychotic symptoms, lasting seconds to hours, are seen in 60% to 80% of DLB patients, highlighting the need to rule out delirium. Vivid, well-formed, recurrent, and complex visual hallucinations (e.g., people, animals) occur in about one third of patients with Dementia of Lewy Bodies (DLB). Hallucinations in other sensory modalities are less frequent, and patients may have insight into their hallucinations.

The cognitive symptoms of DLB *precede* its motor symptoms. Conversely, the duration of motor symptoms of parkinsonism in PDD *prior* to the development of MNCD is longer than in DLB. PDD patients exhibit more frequent cardiovascular and autonomic dysfunction compared to DLB, vascular dementia, and AD (Lenka et al. 2015). Nonetheless, in its most progressed state, DLB is clinically indistinguishable from PDD.

DLB may have a poorer prognosis than PDD; its average duration is 5 to 8 years from symptom onset. Vascular risk factors are less associated with DLB than with AD (Jellinger and Korczyn 2018). DLB and PDD can sometimes be differentiated by cerebral amyloid angiopathy and the neuropathology in Alzheimer's disease, which are usually more frequent and severe in DLB versus PDD (Sezgin et al. 2019; McFarland et al. 2021).

Parkinson's Disease Dementia (PDD)

Approximately 1% of the population over 60 years of age are affected by Parkinson's disease (PD). The *motor features* of Parkinson's disease (PD) include resting tremor, bradykinesia, muscle rigidity, and postural instability; its *non-motor* symptoms include depressed mood, apathy, sleep problems, and cognitive decline (Borek et al. 2006). Among patients who experience Parkinson's disease for 20 years, 83% will develop Parkinson's disease dementia (PDD) (Sezgin et al. 2019). PDD,visual impairment and advancing age are risk factors for the development of psychotic symptoms. (Lerner and Riley 2012)

Psychosis has been reported in 40% of Parkinson's disease (PD) patients, anxiety in 60%, and depressed mood in 35% (Armstrong and Okun 2020). The long-term cumulative prevalence of psychosis in PD is 60% (Forsaa et al. 2010a) and is associated with increased mortality

(Forsaa et al. 2010b), reduced quality of life (Alvarado-Bolaños et al. 2015), and worse prognosis (Friedman 2013).

Neuropsychiatric symptoms (NPS) are also prevalent in Parkinson's disease (PD) *prior* to the onset of MNCD. Some of the NPS in PD are direct physiologic effects of PD and some are attributable to psychological reactions to PD (Ismail et al. 2016).

Generally, hallucinations are seen in later-stage PD, with visual hallucinations being most common. Auditory, tactile, and olfactory hallucinations may also occur (Fénelon et al. 2010). In patients of advancing age and/or those with cognitive impairment, hallucinations may manifest earlier in the disease course and can be associated with PD medication (Connolly and Lang 2014). Delusions are typically paranoid in nature (Borek et al. 2006). The "phantom boarder" delusion, a belief that other people are living in the patient's home, and a feeling of "presence" are common.

Dopamine agonists such as pramipexole which are used as alternatives to L-DOPA carry an acceptable risk (Seppi et al. 2019). However, dopamine agonists, levodopa (L-DOPA), MAO-B or COMT inhibitors, or amantadine, used to treat parkinsonian symptoms, can precipitate or exacerbate psychosis, and increase the risk of visual hallucinations compared to placebo (Ffytche et al. 2017). In situations where psychotic symptoms are harmful, doses may need to be reduced or medications discontinued (Grimes et al. 2019). Therefore, treatment with dopamine agonists and L-DOPA for optimal control of motor symptoms of PD must be balanced against the need to minimize neuropsychiatric symptoms (Connolly and Lang 2014). Clinical judgment may also direct psychotic symptoms to be left untreated in PD if they are well tolerated by the patient and caregivers (NICE 2017).

Depressive symptoms such as psychomotor retardation and anhedonia in the context of Parkinson's disease (PD) and Dementia of Lewy Bodies (DLB) are challenging to distinguish from the apathy, flat or unresponsive facial expression, loss of motivation, and inertia, all of which are manifestations of PD. These clinical observations can help differentiate depressive symptoms, apathy, and negative symptoms of PD:

- *Non-motor* aspects of PD, PDD, or DLB, such as apathy do not change significantly with antidepressant treatment (Borek et al. 2006). SSRIs and SNRIs may improve the depressive symptoms in PD patients but apathy will likely not respond (Takahashi et al. 2019).
- Motor slowing during "off" periods in PD and PDD can present like depressive symptoms when dopaminergic medications wear off (Aarsland et al. 2012). If depressive symptoms are confined to "off" periods when dopaminergic effect is low, adjusting dopaminergic therapy may reduce the apparent depressive symptoms, which are related to PD motor symptoms (Connolly and Lang 2014). (Seppi et al. 2019).
- Predisposing risk factors for depression include female sex, worse cognitive status, worse functioning on daily activities, family and/or personal history of depressive or anxiety disorder (Leentjens et al. 2013). See Table 5.4.

Vascular MNCD (VaD)

The core features of vascular MNCD/dementia (VaMNCD/VaD) are cognitive impairments, inattention, slow information processing, and poor executive function, in the context of systemic vascular disease (Stebbins et al. 2008). Impairment of frontostriatal circuits in VaMNCD/VaD may underly an association with depressive disorders and impaired gait speed (Patience et al. 2019), A review of patients with VaD showed 92% had NPS, of whom 65% showed apathy, 45% depressive symptoms, 42% irritability, and 40% agitation/aggression (Cruz-Jentoft et al. 2005). The finding of executive dysfunction *without* memory impairment suggests a diagnosis of VaD over AD (Reed et al. 2007). For cognitive screening, the MoCA is preferred over the MMSE for the assessment of executive dysfunction in VaD due to its higher sensitivity (Lees et al. 2014). VaD patients with small-ves-

Table 5.4 Parkinson's disease distinctions: depressive disorder, apathy, major depressive disorder

Features	Depressive disorder in PD	Apathy in PD	Major depressive disorder
Mood	Anxiety and irritability common On-off depressive and anxiety symptoms which may correlate with dopaminergic treatment Lower rates of self-blame and guilt	Absence of hopelessness or depressed mood Absence of discernable mood Dulled/disinterested emotional tone Absence of depressive thoughts, such as self-blame	Depressed mood, hopelessness, morbid thoughts, self-blame, and absence of joy every day and throughout each day Anxiety and irritability less common Higher rates of guilt, self-blame, self-punishment
Behavior	More brooding	Lack of concern over anything	Brooding
Anhedonia	Prevalent	Indifference, lack of motivation, interest, initiative	Less prevalent than depression in PD
Cognitive processes	Greater cognitive deficits	Variable cognitive deficits and poor effort on testing	Fewer cognitive deficits
Motor symptoms and function	Parkinsonian features Psychomotor retardation more frequent	Diminished goal-directed physical activity, inertia	Psychomotor retardation Depressed geriatric individuals *without* PD may also have motor signs (bradykinesia, tremor, rigidity)
Other distinctive characteristics	Suicidal ideation more common Fatigue frequent	Suicidal ideation not typical Sparse goal-directed speech	Suicidal ideation less common Fatigue less frequent (than depression in PD)

References: Alves et al. (2004), Leentjens et al. (2003), Oguru et al. (2010), Marsh (2013)

sel findings on neuroimaging display more apathy, aberrant motor behavior, and hallucinations than those with large-vessel disease. Cholinesterase inhibitors or memantine in VaD have *not* proven effective treatment for global functioning, activities of daily living (ADLs), or NPS (Rabins et al. 2014).

Reduction of blood pressure has failed to show efficacy in limiting cognitive decline in VaD, likely due to the limited intervention duration and given that vascular damage is accrued over decades (O'Brien and Thomas 2015). A high proportion of cases of late-life dementia can be attributed to cardiovascular risk factors (e.g., hypertension, diabetes, and obesity) and psychosocial factors (e.g., education, entertainment, social engagement, and leisure activities). Cardiovascular health and MNCD were studied in two large longitudinal cohort studies, which compared midlife high cardiovascular health to *low* cardiovascular health and found that better cardiovascular health at midlife and improvement of cardiovascular health within midlife were associated with lower dementia risk.

The Perindopril Protection Against Recurrent Stroke Study (PROGRESS) studied the effect of lowering blood pressure on the risk of dementia and cognitive decline among individuals with CVD; no clear effect of treatment on the overall risk of dementia was found. However, the study reported that the risk of the composite outcome of "dementia with recurrent stroke" was reduced by one-third, suggesting that the benefits of treatment are primarily the consequences of stroke prevention rather than a direct effect on MNCD or cognitive decline (Tzourio 2003). Another study of diet, exercise, cognitive training, and vascular risk monitoring reported that these interventions could improve or maintain cognitive functioning in those at risk of vascular dementia (Ngandu et al. 2015). Stroke, post-stroke depressive disorder, other post-stroke psychiatric sequelae, and NPS are discussed in Chap. 3.

Frontotemporal Dementia (FTD)

FTD, a neurodegenerative disorder whose prevalence peaks around age 65, in general has an earlier onset than AD or PDD. It accounts for 42% of MNCD in middle aged adults (Snowden et al. 2011a, b). Atrophy of the frontal and/or temporal lobes is the primary etiology. The gross neuropathology, although heterogeneous, is characterized as frontotemporal lobar degeneration (FTLD) (Warren et al. 2013).

FTLD pathology encompasses three clinical presentations of MNCD: behavioral variant FTD (bvFTD), and two types of primary progressive aphasia (PPA). The bvFTD subtype, the most prevalent variant, has been reported as the third most common MNCD, following Alzheimer's disease (AD) and dementia with Lewy bodies (DLB). The two aphasia variants are semantic variant primary progressive aphasia (svPPA), and non-fluent variant primary progressive aphasia (nfvPPA) (Woollacott and Rohrer 2016). Symptoms of FTD variants have significant overlap, especially in late-stage FTD (Murley et al. 2020).

Accurate diagnosis of FTD can direct better treatment. Language deficits, prominent in FTD spectrum of MNCD (Woollacott and Rohrer 2016), can look like thought disorders and other psychotic symptoms, leading to unsuccessful antipsychotic (AP) interventions accompanied by a risk of adverse effects. The onset of apathy, disinhibition, loss of empathy, new compulsive behaviors, hyperorality, and executive dysfunction which are uncharacteristic of the patient can be misdiagnosed as psychiatric disorders. Flat affect and inappropriate behavior can approximate schizophrenia; disinhibition and intrusiveness can appear like mania. Conversely, those with a major mental disorder (MMD) are sometimes inaccurately diagnosed with bvFTD.

bvFTD often presents with behavioral disinhibition, apathy or inertia, loss of sympathy or empathy; perseverative, stereotyped, or compulsive/ritualistic behavior; or hyperorality and dietary changes. Symptoms of bvFTD which overlap with symptoms of psychiatric disorders:

- *Manic-spectrum symptoms* misidentified as bipolar disorder.
- *Apathy and/or reduced empathy* misidentified as symptoms of a major depressive disorder. Non-pharmacological treatment, such as *simulated presence*—a personalized audiotape which simulates a person, has been reported to improve apathy and withdrawn behavior associated with bvFTD (Theleritis et al. 2018).
- *Disinhibition* may appear as anti-social behavior and includes inappropriate touching, taking items from others, offensive language, socially inappropriate behavior, and uninvited intrusions, including sexual advances.
- *Sexually Inappropriate Behaviors (SIB)* have been associated with bvFTD (Sachdev 2017; Cipriani et al. 2016). Behavioral interventions such as redirection and distraction are first-line treatments; but to date no well-conducted studies of behavioral are available.
- *Hyperorality* can manifest as a change in food preferences (e.g., excessive desire for sweets), binge eating, gorging, and even trying to eat inedible objects.
- *Excessive craving* for sweet foods is common (95%) in bvFTD (compared to 29% in AD). Musicophilia or music aversion and altered pain/temperature sensation is rare in nfvPPA and AD but moderately common in other variants (Fletcher et al. 2015; Marshall et al. 2017).

Episodic memory and set-shifting are spared in FTD, relative to AD, while lexical fluency, emotion naming, and error sensitivity are impaired (Ranasinghe et al. 2016). AD aphasia tends to be logopenic, including anomia and word finding pauses, unlike FTD (Marshall et al. 2018).

FTD also presents with changes in sensory perception. A pathological preference for eating sweet foods is common (95%) in bvFTD (compared to 29% in AD) while musicophilia or music aversion and altered pain/temperature sensation is rare in nfvPPA and AD but moderately common in other variants (Fletcher et al. 2015). One study found that those with svPPA have poor

Table 5.5 Key clinical features across FTD variants

FTD variants	Key clinical features (Murley et al. 2020)
All Variants	Behavioral impairment, especially toward later stages of the illness
bvFTD	Apathy, inertia, impulsivity, loss of empathy, loss of social interest, and executive dysfunction each found in 60–70% of patients Impaired language, not as severe as svPPA (Hardy et al. 2016)
svPPA	Surface dyslexia, circumlocution, impaired single word, and object recognition
nfvPPA	Speech apraxia, agrammatism, and impaired syntactic comprehension

heartbeat counting accuracy, indicating impaired interoceptive accuracy (Marshall et al. 2017).

Roughly one-third of patients with FTD have a family history of the illness and 15% have a relevant genetic mutation like progranulin, MAPT, or *C9orf72* (Coyle-Gilchrist et al. 2016). Genetic factors are most strongly associated with bvFTD then nfvPPA and have little association with svPPA (Mishra et al. 2017) (Table 5.5).

While biomarkers are increasingly available to assess for Alzheimer's disease pathology, no specific biomarker is available for bvFTD. Diagnosis depends primarily upon clinical assessment. While current diagnostic criteria for bvFTD perform reasonably well in distinguishing underlying Alzheimer's pathology from frontotemporal lobar degeneration, these criteria are less helpful for distinguishing FTD, an incurable progressive neurodegenerative disease, from primary psychiatric disorders whose treatment differs.

Diagnostic Tools. Neuroimaging is useful for verifying suspected FTD. Please consult Table 5.6 for common patterns of neuronal atrophy observed in FTD variants.

Non-Pharmacological Treatment for bvFTD. Behavioral interventions are first-line treatments for FTD although well-conducted studies are lacking. The younger age of onset in FTD may direct changing employment/financial decisions to accommodate the disorder.

Pharmacological Treatment for bvFTD. Treatment recommendations for bvFTD are sparse. Among the SSRIs, findings from well-controlled studies suggest that trazodone (Lebert et al. 2004), citalopram (Herrmann et al. 2012), and sertraline (Mendez et al. 2005) may be effective with a 40% reduction in behavior symptoms. There is evidence for the efficacy of paroxetine but there are reports that it also may impair cognitive function (Deakin et al. 2004). Antipsychotic use in patients with FTD has not been widely endorsed due to vulnerability to extrapyramidal side effects (Pijnenburg et al. 2003).

Table 5.6 Key features of neurodegeneration across FTD variants

FTD variant	Key features of neurodegeneration
All variants	Structural abnormalities in the insula and temporal lobes (5–10 years before onset in those with genetic risk) (Rohrer et al. 2010). Greater orbitofrontal/temporal polar cortex and frontostriatal circuit atrophy has been implicated in greater FTD behavioral impairment (Lansdall et al. 2017)
bvFTD	Atrophy primarily in the anterior right temporal lobe and throughout the frontal lobes with some parietal atrophy (Whitwell et al. 2009)
svPPA	Predominantly left hemisphere atrophy in the anteromedial/inferior temporal lobes, amygdala, hippocampus, and fusiform gyrus with a characteristic "knife-blade" appearance of the temporal pole (Sivasathiaseelan et al. 2019)
nfvPPA	Left inferior frontal, insular, and anterior superior temporal gyral atrophy (Sivasathiaseelan et al. 2019)

There is little evidence for cholinergic loss in bvFTD. Cholinesterase inhibitors and memantine have been found ineffective (Tsai and Boxer 2016; Noufi et al. 2019); rather *worsening* of behavioral symptoms or cognition with cholinesterase inhibitors has been reported (Woolley et al. 2007). Apathy in FTD has been treated with stimulants, but screening for potential cardiac effects and regular monitoring is recommended.

Prion Diseases

These rare conditions affect 0.0001% of people/year worldwide (Chen and Dong 2016). Cases can be sporadic (80–95%), genetic (10–15%), or acquired (2–5%) in etiology and are caused by a change in the prion protein structure from alpha-helical to beta-pleated, inducing a chain reaction of misfolding that leads to the protein aggregate responsible for brain atrophy in prion disease (Geschwind 2015). Symptoms vary among Creutzfeldt-Jakob disease, Gerstmann-Sträussler-Scheinker syndrome, and fatal familial insomnia, but can include rapidly progressive MNCD, behavioral abnormalities, and motor disorders with age of onset between 50 and 60 (Brown and Mastrianni 2010). Genetic testing, electroencephalography (detection of biphasic and triphasic 1 Hz sharp-wave complexes), cerebrospinal fluid analysis (14-3-3 proteins and tau biomarkers), and neuroimaging (DWI and FLAIR) have high sensitivity and specificity for detecting prion diseases, with variation among types (Green 2019; Steinhoff et al. 2004; Vitali et al. 2011). No successful treatments of prion diseases have been found.

HIV-Associated Neurocognitive Disorders (HAND)

Symptoms typically include executive dysfunction and impaired information processing. Different presentations are possible, but recall and language impairment are uncommon. For further discussion, see Chap. 4.

Neurocognitive Disorder Due to Substance Use and Alcohol

Substance-induced MNCD manifests as impairments in executive function, memory, and learning domains beyond the period of intoxication and withdrawal. Large cohort studies tend to report that light-moderate alcohol consumption has little impact on MNCD risk (Handing et al. 2014) while high alcohol consumption (>14 drinks/week) is linked to increased MNCD risk (Wiegmann et al. 2020).

Neurocognitive Effects of Coronavirus Disease 2019 (COVID-19)

Neuroinflammatory and neurovascular effects, including an attenuated delirium syndrome, have been reported in patients with COVID-19 infection (Butler et al. 2020). One study compared cognitive performance on the MoCA in asymptomatic COVID-19 with healthy controls. The COVID-19 group reported significantly lower performance on visuoperceptual, fluency, and naming items (Amalakanti et al. 2021).

Non-pharmacological Treatment

MNCD can present with a range of behavioral and psychiatric symptoms which are not specific to any one MNCD subtype or variant. Neuropathological findings overlap between MNCD subtypes and combinations, such as AD+CVD and AD+LBD. Non-pharmacological/behavioral approaches therefore can apply across to MNCDs of many different etiologies, tailored primarily to the individual's cognitive capacity and behavior.

One meta-analysis of 148 RCTs of treatment for aggression or agitation in 21,686 MNCD patients reported that *non-pharmacological* interventions and structured therapies, were equal to, or more effective than, usual care pharmacology for aggressive and agitated behaviors. Recreation therapy, multidisciplinary care, massage, touch therapy, and music combined with massage and touch therapy were found to perform better than the usual care for agitation and aggression (Watt et al. 2019). However, 46% of studies were noted to be at high risk of bias because of missing outcome data. In addition, the harms and costs of therapies were not evaluated, and the studies did not address or rule out delirium (Watt et al. 2019).

One process for first-line non-pharmacological interventions is D-I-C-E (Kales et al. 2014):

- ***Describe*** in detail the problematic behaviors, including antecedents, precipitants, and social context. Rating scales like the Cohen-Mansfield Agitation Inventory (CMAI) help quantify maladaptive behavior its precipitants, severity, frequency, quality, duration, precipitants, and response to treatment.
- ***Investigate*** NPS to discover underlying causes and exclude treatable conditions.
- ***Create*** a realistic and non-pharmacological treatment plan.
- ***Evaluate*** the effect of the treatment plan on the problematic behavior.

The **D-I-C-E** model incorporates the following behavioral interventions into an individualized treatment plan.

Interpersonal Interactions

Patients with MNCD may become distressed and disruptive during administration of medications, ADL care, toileting, washing, and feeding (Gitlin et al. 2012). Anticipating these situations can help prepare the patient with calm reminders, soothing tone of voice, and clear, simple explanations can help ameliorate anxiety and minimize agitated behavior (Nelson et al. 2013; Thakur and Gwyther 2015). Prevention of dehydration, constipation, and pain (as noted above) and correction of environmental factors such as poor lighting and excessive noise can also alleviate some behavioral symptoms. See Table 5.7.

Table 5.7 Interpersonal factors which impact disturbed behavior

Factors which impact disturbed behavior in MNCD patients	
 Family & Others	Interpersonal interactions which coincide with agitation, anxiety, resistance in patient & others (e.g., toileting).
 Environment situation	Timing, frequency, duration, severity of interactions which appear to contribute to distress of patient & others.
 Daily routine	Changes in routine, schedule, activities, locations, time of day which coincide with NPS. (e.g. change of shift or staff).
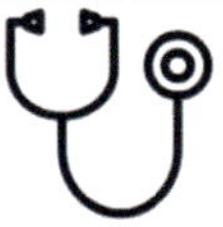 Physical & Medical Considerations	Symptoms & discomfort that coincide with disturbances of behavior (e.g., incontinence, constipation, thirst, need to urinate, pain, infection, fatigue).

(Rita Hitching, MSc)

Psychotherapeutic Interventions

- *Cognitive Behavioral Therapy* (CBT) may offer relief for caregivers and help them manage the demands imposed by disturbing behaviors (Cheng et al. 2019; Fortinsky et al. 2020; Gerlach and Kales 2018; Newkirk et al. 2020).
- *Functional analysis* (FA): A meta-analysis reviewed 18 RCTs of this strategy to manage difficult behaviors in MNCD populations. The intervention appeared to result in benefit shortly after each session, but its efficacy could not be determined from the studies reviewed (Cook et al. 2012).
- *Aromatherapy* with lemon balm or lavender oil can be delivered by either inhalation or skin application and has yielded mixed results (Forrester et al. 2014).
- *Massage and touch therapy* have been described as potentially beneficial.
- *Exercise training* and caregiver education may improve outcomes in patients with Alzheimer's disease (AD). A randomized trial in 153 community-dwelling AD patients found that, compared with routine medical care, those on exercise (goal minimum of 30 min per day), and whose caregivers received training in managing behavioral problems, had improved physical functioning and less depression measured on the GDS (Geriatric Depression Scale) (Jacquart et al. 2014).
- *Music therapy, crafts, and pet therapy* have shown evidence of efficacy (van der Steen et al. 2018).

- *Body-based therapies, for example, yoga, tai-chi, and mind-body techniques* can increase mindfulness and physical fitness, thereby improving health outcomes.
- *Art therapy* such as expressive art encourages the development of a narrative though this may challenge those with severe cognitive impairment.

Other Psychotherapy Models

Loss of social roles and role transition may be addressed by counseling for patients who have adequate cognitive functioning. Techniques such as Interpersonal Therapy IPT, CBT, Dialectic Behavioral Therapy (DBT), and Acceptance and Commitment Therapy (ACT) have not been studied extensively in MNCD/dementia patients.

Correction of Communication Barriers. Perceptual, sensory, speech, and language deficits can impair communication and exacerbate NPS in patients with MNCD. Aphasias, dysphasias, dysarthria, and simple auditory deficits, for example, can result in the misidentification of stimuli and deficits in processing and expressing language. Miscommunication and frustration can escalate to disruptive behaviors. Thorough evaluation of sensory limitations and providing hearing, speech, and vision assistance can help avoid untoward behavior (Potkins et al. 2003).

Planning for Loss of Functioning. Diagnosis of MNCD as early as possible allows for the development of ways to compensate for functional deficits. Transportation, financial management, decision-making, and food preparation can be anticipated and assisted. Often simplification (using a model of "safe/calm/consistent"), routine implementation, calm interactions/reassurance, redirection to pleasurable activities, and communication of only *necessary* information can bolster functioning. For further discussion, see Chap. 15

Neuromodulation Modalities and ECT

Several studies have found that ECT can be effective for BPSD. One retrospective study of 60 subjects with ultra-brief right unilateral pulse ECT demonstrated a decrease in agitation after 3 sessions (Hermida et al. 2020). An uncontrolled study found resolution of agitation and aggressive behavior for BPSD in 72% of cases, and the response to maintenance ECT was 87% (Isserles et al. 2017). Research is not conclusive as to the benefit of neuromodulation modalities for BPSD in the elderly. For further discussion, see Chap. 14 *Neuromodulation modalities.*

Pharmacological Treatment

When non-pharmacological or behavioral approaches fail to sufficiently manage harmful NPS or BPSD, pharmacological interventions can help. Although neuropathology, neurobiological processes, and neural pathways of NPS are active areas of research, the etiology of NPS has not been delineated definitively (Lanctôt et al. 2017).

RCTs have reported that antipsychotic (AP) medications and other medications can reduce the relapse of neuropsychiatric symptoms (NPS) (Ballard et al. 2015a, b). To date, only brexpiprazole has been FDA-approved for the treatment of any psychiatric indication in dementia, specifically, agitation. Categories of medications used for BPSD and treatment recommendations are reviewed below.

The avoidance of medication adverse effects and recognition of the risks of medications is paramount, and guidance can be found in QUM-D and Beers Criteria (Maust et al. 2021). The Quality Use of Medications in Dementia (QUM-D) identifies 10 prescribing practices to avoid (Peisah et al. 2015) and the Beers Criteria AGS lists potentially inappropriate medications (PIM) to avoid in older adults (American Geriatrics Society 2019).

Many algorithms offer steps in behavioral approaches and medication treatment for BPSD though each algorithm differs slightly. The Algorithm Project from Harvard, for example, suggests that treatment for *non-emergent* BPSD starts with decreasing anticholinergic load, optimizing pain control and sleep, followed by a sequence of donepezil, then escitalopram and sertraline. For *emergent* BPSD, it suggests intramuscular olanzapine as first line, followed by intramuscular haloperidol, and then intramuscular benzodiazepines (Chen et al. 2021). The Sequential Drug Treatment Algorithm suggests first to use risperidone, followed by quetiapine or aripiprazole, then carbamazepine (Davies et al. 2018). Several other evidence-based guidelines are available (McDermott and Gruenewald 2019; Delfino et al. 2019).

Prescribing practices differ across individual practitioners, institutions, and nursing homes (Cioltan et al. 2017) (Silwanowicz et al. 2017).

Antidepressants (ADs)

Serotonin-Specific Reuptake Inhibitors (SSRIs). Conclusive studies and recommendations are sparse, yet citalopram for NPS has been most studied in RCTs and shows the most evidence of benefit (Aga 2019). The CitAD study of citalopram 20 mg per day versus a placebo followed outpatients with AD for over 9 weeks (Porsteinsson et al. 2014). Citalopram 20 mg per day showed a statistically significant improvement in agitation on validated behavioral scales and was associated with decreased delusions, hallucinations, anxiety, and irritability/lability at 9 weeks (Leonpacher et al. 2016). A review of 692 patients in 9 trials reported that sertraline and citalopram of varying doses were well tolerated and improved agitation and psychosis compared to placebo (Seitz et al. 2011). Citalopram has not shown evidence of benefit for NPS of DLB.

Class I evidence of effectiveness was found for paroxetine (HAM-D score reduction of 6.2 points; $p < 0.0007$) and venlafaxine ER (Ham-D score reduction of 4.2 points ($p < 0.02$)) without worsening of motor function, in an RCT (Richard et al. 2012). However, paroxetine CR has been reported to be not efficacious (Menza et al. 2009). Some well-controlled studies have also suggested that trazodone 150 mg/day (Lebert et al. 2004), citalopram 40 mg/day (Herrmann et al. 2012), and sertraline 25 mg/day (Mendez et al. 2005) may be effective with a 40% reduction in behavioral symptoms. There is evidence for the efficacy of paroxetine 30 mg/day but also reports that it may impair cognitive function (Deakin et al. 2004).

Tricyclic Antidepressants (TCAs) are not currently recommended for the treatment of BPSD due to their anticholinergic burden. For example, amitriptyline shows increased risk of falls (Seppala et al. 2018). A small pilot RCT of doxepin 10 mg bedtime in PD demonstrated improvement in subjective sleep measures with no evidence of worsening cognition (Rios-Romenets et al. 2013).

Serotonin-Norepinephrine Reuptake Inhibitors (SNRIs), such as duloxetine, venlafaxine, and levomilnacipran for BPSD have not been studied sufficiently in the aging population to provide recommendations (Asnis and Henderson 2015). One RCT of 59 patients with moderate AD and MDD observed improvement with venlafaxine in the first 4–8 weeks but benefit then waned (Mokhber et al. 2014).

Monoamine Oxidase B Inhibitors are not recommended in combination with SSRI/SNRI/TCA (serotonin syndrome risk potential). (NICE 2009).

Trazodone. In an open-label, retrospective study of trazodone (50–100 mg QHS) in 178 MNCD patients (64% with Alzheimer type), 65.7% of patients on trazodone reported evidence of improvement in sleep maintenance, as assessed on NPI (Camargos et al. 2011). One RCT of trazodone (50–300 mg daily) vs. placebo for agitation in MNCD showed no statistically significant benefits (Lebert et al. 2004).

Mirtazapine has been used successfully at a dose of 7.5 mg for sleep initiation in patients with dementia. In a randomized, double-blind, placebo-controlled trial it has not been found beneficial for agitation in dementia (Banerjee et al. 2021). Mirtazapine has been reported to exacerbate REM Behavior Disorder (RBD (Gomperts 2016) although its sedative and appetite stimulating properties may be beneficial in some cases.

Cholinesterase Inhibitors (ChEIs)

A Cochrane meta-analysis review reported moderate- to high-certainty evidence that donepezil 5 mg/day, donepezil 10 mg/day, and galantamine 16–24 mg/day have a slight beneficial effect on cognition in people with mild neurocognitive impairment (MCI) but advised that the size of the change was not clinically important. Donepezil 10 mg/day and galantamine 16–24 mg/day were likely associated with more adverse events than placebo, but evidence of this for rivastigmine was less certain. The data suggest that donepezil 10 mg/day has the greatest effect on cognition, but at the cost of adverse effects. Further research into rivastigmine is needed, including the use of transdermal patches.

ChEIs have been shown to delay BPSD onset (McDermott and Gruenewald 2019), but no evidence that they have improved quality of life. A systematic literature search of RCTs found no conclusive benefit from ChEIs for AD or BPSD in patients with significant functional impairments (Seibert et al. 2021). In one study, participants on rivastigmine were noted to be less anxious and to have fewer hallucinations (McKeith et al. 2000). Donepezil and rivastigmine have demonstrated effectiveness for the treatment of cognitive impairment in PDD (Rolinski et al. 2012). Another Cochrane review concluded that acetylcholinesterase inhibitors like donepezil and rivastigmine are efficacious for the treatment of cognitive impairment in PDD (Rolinski et al. 2012). In one study, participants on rivastigmine were also found to be less anxious and to have fewer hallucinations (McKeith et al. 2000). Sudden withdrawal of ChEIs, it should be noted, may cause deterioration in cognition.

Rivastigmine, Donepezil, and Galantamine were compared to placebo in a systematic review of 14 RCTs for NPS in possible/probable Alzheimer's disease with little evidence supported the effectiveness of rivastigmine for NPS of MNCD (Rodda et al. 2009).

Donepezil 10 mg daily vs. placebo demonstrated *no* statistically significant improvement in a 12-week RCT of 272 patients with AD and NPS (Howard et al. 2007). An RCT of AD-related agitation compared aromatherapy (massaged into hands or arms twice daily) to donepezil started at 5 mg daily, increased to 10 mg daily after 1 month, to placebo at 4 and 12 weeks. No differences in outcome were found between the donepezil group versus the two groups *without* donepezil, but 37% improved on the NPI across all groups. This suggested a therapeutic benefit of hand massage and touch (Burns et al. 2011).

In VaD, cholinesterase inhibitors or memantine have not proven effective for global functioning, activities of daily living (ADLs), or NPS (O'Brien and Thomas 2015). Another study reported moderate to high-certainty evidence that donepezil 5 mg/day, donepezil 10 mg/day, and galantamine had a slight beneficial effect on cognition in people with vascular cognitive impairment (VCI) although the size of the change was not thought to be clinically important. However, both donepezil 10 mg and galantamine 16–24 mg were found to be associated with more adverse events than placebo. Donepezil 10 mg has appeared to benefit cognition, but with adverse effects, but without other treatments, the use of this intervention should be considered (Battle et al. 2021).

Adverse effects of ChEIs can be significant and dose-related, especially for individuals over age 85 who are vulnerable to stimulation of muscarinic and nicotinic receptors (Kröger et al. 2015). Gastrointestinal symptoms are most common, and the risk of bradycardia is also important to consider; these medications are discontinued if they lead to symptomatic bradycardia.

Memantine is a partial NMDA receptor antagonist thought to limit damaging glutamatergic excitation, thus protecting neurons. A 2006 Cochrane review concluded that memantine provides a small but statistically significant benefit at 6 months in those with moderate to severe MNCD, but not MCI (McShane et al. 2006). Memantine has been reported as ineffective and may worsen cognition or behavior (Tsai and Boxer 2016). Another meta-analysis concluded that memantine does not improve function in LBD (Matsunaga et al. 2015a, b). A post hoc analysis of three RCTs of moderate to severe AD patients with baseline agitation/aggression or psychosis found that memantine demonstrated significant improvement at all time points in NPS scores compared to placebo, especially in agitation/aggression (55.3% vs. 43.1% at week 12, $p = 0.011$; 61.0% vs. 45.0% at week 24/28, $p < 0.001$) (Wilcock et al. 2008; Wang et al. 2015; McShane et al. 2006; Maidment et al. 2008). Memantine or ChEIs may improve RBD in some cases (Gomperts 2016).

For DLB, rivastigmine (6–12 mg/day) and donepezil (5–10 mg/day) have been tested in randomized, placebo-controlled trials; both agents demonstrated beneficial effects on cognitive and behavioral symptoms *in DLB* patients. However, ChEIs also may increase vivid dreaming; daytime dosing is recommended (Boot et al. 2013).

There is evidence that the combination of cholinesterase inhibitors and memantine together may have superior efficacy to ChEIs alone across cognitive scores, ADLs, and behavioral scores (Dysken et al. 2014). However, this improvement also had small clinical significance. A post hoc analysis reported that the *addition* of memantine to ongoing treatment with donepezil reduced agitation/aggression, irritability, and appetite/eating disturbances on the NPI, compared to the addition of *placebo* to donepezil (Howard et al. 2007; Cummings et al. 2006). A meta-analysis of 17 RCTs ($n = 1798$) of ChEIs vs. controls in subjects with Lewy body disorders (PD, PDD, and DLB) reported no significant improvements in cognitive dysfunction, behavioral disturbances, activities of daily living, and global impairment. This same meta-analysis found no beneficial effect of memantine for cognition in DLB patients (Matsunaga et al. 2015a, b).

One systematic meta-analysis reviewed RCTs with several pharmacological agents (including ChEIs) vs. placebo for AD patients, with NPI as an outcome measure (Wang et al. 2015). A subgroup analysis, excluding trials with estimated SDs, demonstrated that only galantamine (−0.13, 95% CI: −0.22 to −0.03) had a modest but significant improvement in NPI scores, while donepezil did not (−0.09, 95% CI: −0.27 to 0.08). All groups taking ChEIs were at increased risk for adverse effect-related dropouts (2.25 95% CI: 1.53–3.26) (Wang et al. 2015).

Antipsychotic Medications (APs)

Antipsychotics (APs) are often necessary when non-pharmacological or behavioral approaches fail to manage NPS which are harmful or interfere with medical care or daily health needs. The choice of medication, dosing, and sequence is guided by balancing the risk from the psychiatric/behavioral symptoms with the risk of adverse effects. Older patients are sensitive to adverse effects of APs (both FGAs and SGAs) which can worsened parkinsonism and cognition, or a syndrome such as neuroleptic malignant syndrome (NMS), with profound autonomic instability. See Table 5.8.

First-Generation Antipsychotics (FGAs). For geriatric patients, risks from FGAs have been reported as higher than SGAs (American Psychiatric Association 2016; Maust et al. 2015; Reus et al. 2016). High potency D2 antagonist APs especially may precipitate parkinsonian motor symptoms or neuroleptic malignant syndrome (NMS), with delirium, rigidity, and autonomic instability. Other adverse effects for APs (Wang et al. 2005; Narang et al. 2010; Porsteinsson and Antonsdottir 2017) include community-acquired pneumonia (Trifirò et al. 2010), falls/fractures (Fraser et al. 2015), and worsening cognition (Steinberg and Lyketsos 2012; Vigen et al. 2011). Long-acting injectable APs should be used when non-compliance leads to relapse and dangerous behaviors (American Psychiatric Association 2016).

Second-Generation Antipsychotics (SGA). SGAs may be needed to manage harmful behavioral symptoms which cannot otherwise be controlled. An FDA black box warning for SGAs

Table 5.8 American Psychiatric Association (APA) recommendations for antipsychotic use in MNCD

Symptom	Recommendation
Agitation and Psychosis	Used for agitation or psychosis only when symptoms are severe, dangerous, or cause significant distress to the patient
Non-pharmacological Treatment Fail	A clinical response to non-pharmacological interventions should be reviewed before any non-emergency use
Lowest Effective Dose	Treatment should be started at a low dose and titrated up to the minimum effective dose tolerated
No Response Discontinue after 4 Weeks	If no clinically significant response is evident after a 4-week trial of an adequate dose taper and withdraw treatment
Effective Response Taper within 4 Months	If treatment is effective, an attempt to taper should made within 4 months unless a prior attempt resulted in recurrence of target symptoms
Reassess Monthly During Taper	After medication discontinuation reassess symptoms at least monthly, for 4 months minimum, lookout for any sign of symptom recurrence; recommend risk-benefit analysis to restart treatment
Delirium Haloperidol Acceptable	In the absence of delirium, and if non-emergency treatment is needed, haloperidol should not be used as first-line treatment

Note. Adapted from Rues (2016) and Yohanna and Cifu 2017

cautions against increased of cerebrovascular events and sudden death in geriatric patients with MNCD (Steinberg and Lyketsos 2012). SGAs can also contribute to exacerbation of parkinsonian motor symptoms, cognitive decline, drowsiness, confusion, orthostatic hypotension, urinary incontinence, and falls. A retrospective case-control study of 90,786 veterans ≥65 years with MNCD reported differences between FGAs and SGAs in odds ratios of increased mortality and number-needed-to-harm (NNH): haloperidol (OR = 3.8%, NNH 26), risperidone (OR = 3.7%, NNH 27), olanzapine (OR = 2.5%, NNH 40), quetiapine (OR = 2.0%, NNH 50) after controlling for relevant risk factors (Maust et al. 2015). SGAs such as risperidone, aripiprazole, quetiapine are used for NPS in VaD with caution and informed consent. *Olanzapine* may cause motor deterioration (Miyasaki et al. 2006). *Risperidone* and *aripiprazole* may worsen parkinsonian symptoms (Ferreira et al. 2013). Antipsychotics for symptoms of bvFTD has not been widely endorsed due vulnerability to extrapyramidal side effects (Pijnenburg et al. 2003). Low D2 antagonist APs, such as clozapine and quetiapine may be used, but also with caution.

Quetiapine may be less likely than other SGAs to exacerbate parkinsonian motor features in DLB and PDD (Stinton et al. 2015). It is often prescribed for NPS, but there is inconclusive evidence of its efficacy. A systematic review of 7 RCTs (n = 241) (mean dose of 103.0 mg/day) reported no statistically significant benefit (Desmarais et al. 2016). Another RCT reported that quetiapine, 100 mg twice a day, was *more effective* than placebo for agitation, while doses of 100 mg/day were not (Zhong et al. 2007). Quetiapine has also been associated with the lowest mortality risk among APs (Gerhard et al. 2014).

Clozapine has a low dopamine-2 antagonist activity and thus has much less risk of exacerbating Parkinsonian symptoms than other SGAs or FGAs; it can be used as an alternative to quetiapine for PDD or DLB (NICE 2017) although few RCTs have studied clozapine in DLB (Gatt et al. 2017; Stinton et al. 2015). Adverse effects include delirium, cardiomyopathy, neutropenia, seizures, constipation, and bowel obstruction, some due to the high anticholinergic burden (AB), for which geriatric individuals are at risk. Clozapine therefore requires frequent (at least monthly) monitoring of serum levels and WBCs; agranulocytosis may occur in 0.38% of treated patients. Echocardiography is needed if concern for cardiomyopathy is high.

Aripiprazole: A meta-analyses that included 17 trials of SGAs compared to placebo found aripiprazole decreased agitation and was safer than olanzapine, risperidone, and quetiapine (Yunusa et al. 2019). *Brexpiprazole* is an SGA pharmacologically and structurally similar to aripiprazole. Two RCTs for agitation in over 700

AD subjects reported that brexpiprazole 2 mg/day reduced agitation compared with age-matched patients receiving placebo (Grossberg et al. 2020).

Third-Generation Antipsychotics (TGAs). Some authors have categorized *pimavanserin* as a TGA, in part because of its profile as a 5-HT2A inverse agonist and to a lesser extent 5HT-2C (Fox 2014), with minimal dopamine (D2) receptor antagonism. It has been approved by FDA (US) for the treatment of Parkinson's disease (PD) psychosis and is well tolerated (Bozymski et al. 2017). Pimavanserin demonstrated efficacy in patients with hallucinations and delusions associated with Parkinson's disease. In a trial of patients with PD, 61% had moderate-to-severe dementia. The double-blind phase was planned for 26 weeks of follow-up of each subject but was stopped early for efficacy; the median duration of exposure during this phase was approximately 18 weeks in the pimavanserin group and 11 weeks in the placebo group (Tariot et al. 2021).

Because Lewy body diseases share similar neuropathology, pimavanserin may improve psychosis in patients with DLB and PDD as well as PD with psychosis. It has been tried in Alzheimer's disease-related psychosis (Yunusa, et al. 2020), but does not appear to show benefit over time; an RCT of pimavanserin vs. placebo in AD patients showed initial improvement on the NPI-nursing home (NPI-NH) psychosis scores at week 6, but by week 12 the benefit was not significant (Ballard et al. 2018).

A randomized discontinuation trial of pimavanserin was conducted in patients with psychosis and several types of neurodegenerative diseases. The study examined sustained response to pimavanserin treatment and relapse of psychosis after discontinuation of pimavanserin. Approximately 15% of the patients in the trial had Parkinson's disease. Among those who continued to receive pimavanserin the percentage of patients who had a relapse of psychosis was 13% (either delusions or hallucinations) versus 28% among those who were switched to placebo. The trial was stopped early because the active pimavanserin was found to be clearly effective; subjects who had previously responded to the drug had a higher risk of relapse of psychosis than those who continued to receive pimavanserin.

Adverse events which occurred more frequently with pimavanserin than with placebo were headache, constipation, and urinary tract infection. The mean change in QTc in patients exposed to pimavanserin in the open label phase was 5.4 ms, consistent with the current labeling of the medication, and five adverse events involving asymptomatic prolongation of the QTc interval were reported (Tariot et al. 2021). For further discussion, see Ch 01 *Overview of Geriatric Pharmacology* and Ch 08 *Psychotic Symptoms.*

Mood Stabilizers

Carbamazepine (CBZ) at a mean dose 300 mg/day has demonstrated modest, but statistically significant improvement in NPS ratings compared to placebo (Seitz et al. 2013). However, its adverse effects, such as agranulocytosis, hyponatremia, and liver toxicity, can have an impact on the aging individual (McDermott and Gruenewald 2019). Special attention should be paid to drug–drug interactions in which CBZ can enhance metabolism of itself and other medications, resulting in lower serum levels. Regular serum monitoring and gradual upward titration is recommended, with starting dose at 50 mg daily for the oldest-old and frail patients (Davies et al. 2018).

Valproic Acid (VPA) has not shown RCT evidence of benefit for NPS (Tariot 2011). A multicenter, RCT of flexible dose of VPA (target dose of 10–12 mg/kg/day) in 313 moderate AD patients did not prevent agitation/aggression or psychosis. Somnolence due to hyperammonemic encephalopathy in patients with urea cycle disorders and hepatic failure has been reported.

Gabapentin has shown benefit for NPS in small case reports.

Topiramate and Lamotrigine have not shown conclusive RCT evidence of benefit for BPSD (Liu et al. 2016).

Lithium has not demonstrated sustained effectiveness for NPS of MNCD; its CNS risks such as toxicity, ataxia, and delirium may overwhelm any potential benefits for the oldest-old and/or those with renal insufficiency (Boecker et al. 2011). One case series of 6 MNCD patients (3 AD, 3 FTD), reported that lithium improved agitation/aggression at doses of 300–600 mg daily (Devanand et al. 2017).

Hormonal Agents. Leuprolide acetate, a Luteinizing Hormone-Releasing Hormone (LHRH) agonist has been employed for SIB in bvFTD. It can limit the production of luteinizing hormone, which stimulates testicles to release testosterone, and thereby diminishes libido; but ethical concerns have been raised (DeGiorgi and Series 2016).

Buspirone. Evidence of benefit for NPS is limited. A retrospective observational study of buspirone for NPS in 179 patients, *without a comparator arm*, (average daily dose of 25.7 mg ± 12.50 mg) reported 68% had improved scores on the Clinical Global Impression scale (McDermott and Gruenewald 2019).

Melatonin (3–12 mg at bedtime) has demonstrated effectiveness for insomnia and REM Behavior Disorder (RBD), based upon observations (Almeida et al. 2017).

Methylphenidate (Stimulant) and Modafinil (Wakefulness Promoter). Methylphenidate has been found beneficial for apathy (van Dyck et al. 2021), but the evidence is not conclusive. It may also contribute to appetite suppression, weight loss, insomnia (if given close to bedtime), and arrhythmias. Modafinil, thought to increase adrenergic, histaminergic, glutamatergic, and hypocretin brain activity, is FDA-approved for narcolepsy, shift-work sleep disorder, obstructive sleep apnea (OSA) (Frakey et al. 2012). Evidence is insufficient to suggest that modafinil reduces risk posed by somnolence during activities such as driving (Zesiewicz et al. 2010; NICE 2017). Hypersomnia observed in PDD may be treated with modafinil, though few, if any, RCTs are available.

Adrenergics: Prazosin, Clonidine, and Propranolol. The possibility of noradrenergic dysfunction in Alzheimer's disease (Gannon et al. 2015) prompted the study of medications that modulate the adrenergic system, such as propranolol (beta 1,2-antagonist), prazosin (alpha-1 antagonist) (Seitz et al. 2013), and clonidine (alpha-2 agonist). A small RCT with propranolol (mean dose 106 mg/d ±38 mg/d) versus placebo in patients with probable or possible Alzheimer's disease showed statistically significant reductions in agitation/aggression and anxiety on the NPI (Peskind et al. 2005). Asthmatic/reactive airway disease, low heart rate, and those at risk of syncope, or orthostatic hypotension are contraindications. Prazosin (mean dose 5.7 mg/day ±0.9 mg/day) compared to placebo, improved agitation/aggression in Alzheimer's disease patients for 8 weeks and was well tolerated (outcome measures NPI, BPRS, and CGI-Change scales) (Wang et al. 2009).

Monoclonal antibodies. *Lecanemab* and *Aducanumab* have been approved by the US-FDA only for the treatment of cognitive decline in AD. They are discussed here because they may also be prescribed for patients with BPSD.

Aducanumab. This monoclonal antibody was approved by FDA for the treatment of Alzheimer's disease on June 7, 2021. It targets aggregated beta-amyloid, a core molecular feature of the disease's pathophysiology but its efficacy in preventing cognitive decline has not been conclusively demonstrated. Vasogenic edema and cortical microhemorrhages (together called amyloid-related imaging abnormalities [ARIA]) occurred in about 40% of participants in two RCT high-dose aducanumab groups, compared with 10% of those received placebo (Rabinovici 2021). Further efficacy and safety trials can hopefully find evidence of consistent, longer-term benefit.

Lecanemab. The US Food and Drug Administration (FDA) in early 2023 approved lecanemab (Leqembi) for the treatment of Alzheimer's disease based on phase 2 trial data that showed a reduction in amyloid β (Aβ) plaques in patients at an early stage. Similar efficacy and safety concerns to *Aducanumab* have been raised. The FDA recommended that lecanemab should be initiated only in patients with mild cognitive impairment or in those in the mild dementia stage of disease (Mahase 2023).

Cannabinoids and Dronabinol. Dronabinol, a synthetic cannabinoid, has been approved by

FDA for nausea and vomiting related to chemotherapy or AIDS-associated anorexia. A retrospective chart review of MNCD patients treated with dronabinol for agitation/aggression or resistance to care showed improvement from baseline based upon outcomes on the Pittsburgh Agitation Scale (Woodward et al. 2014).

Benzodiazepines. As of October 2020, the FDA has required a warning for benzodiazepine use due to physiological dependence and risks of withdrawal syndromes. A review of RCTs found little evidence to support a favorable risk-benefit ratio for benzodiazepines in NPS (Defrancesco et al. 2015). While short-term use may be safe, the risks of longer term benzodiazepine use (weeks to months) include ataxia, falls, fractures, as well as delirium, confusion, impairment of immediate recall, and rebound anxiety upon abrupt discontinuation (Aspinall et al. 2019). Benzodiazepines are also among the list of Potentially Inappropriate Medications (PIM) (American Geriatrics Society 2019 Updated AGS Beers Criteria® 2019). However, clonazepam has been found effective for REM Behavior Disorder (RBD) although evidence is primarily observational (Almeida et al. 2017). For insomnia, clonazepam (0.5–2.0 mg at bedtime) has shown benefit although evidence is also based upon observations (Almeida et al. 2017). In frail elderly patients, caution is advised with clonazepam due to sedation and risk of falls.

Zopiclone, Eszopiclone, Zaleplon, And Zolpidem. These "Z-drugs" are US FDA-approved for insomnia and have been used for agitation in MNCD. However, they also pose risks to cognitively impaired individuals due to increased cognitive impairment, withdrawal seizures, and rebound anxiety.

Dextromethorphan and Quinidine. The US FDA has approved this combination for the treatment of the pseudobulbar affect (PBA). A multicenter RCT has compared dextromethorphan + quinidine to placebo, over 10 weeks and demonstrated statistically significant reductions in NPI scores for agitation in Alzheimer's disease. Stable dosages of antidepressants, antipsychotics, hypnotics, and cognitive enhancers were allowed in the trial. There was no apparent cognitive impairment, sedation, nor clinically significant QTc prolongation (Ballard et al. 2015a, b).

Conclusions

An *age-adjusted* approach to neuropsychiatric symptoms (NPS) or behavioral and psychological symptoms of dementia (BPSD) in the geriatric patient should include a comprehensive evaluation to:

1. Diagnose—or rule out—MNCD and other cognitive impairments.
2. Determine the etiology(ies) of the MNCD.

   Evaluate and treat systemic medical comorbidities and other factors which could contribute to, exacerbate, or precipitate neuropsychiatric symptoms (NPS).

First-line interventions for BPSD consist of non-pharmacological therapies and behavioral interventions. When harmful NPS cannot be otherwise managed, medications are recommended, age-adjusted with doses that accommodate pharmacokinetics, pharmacodynamics, medical comorbidities, tolerance, and frailty. While pharmacotherapy algorithms and guidelines may differ in terms of choice and sequence of medications, there is consensus about which medications to avoid or minimize, based both upon neuropathology and physiology (Arvanitakis et al. 2019).

Age-Adjusted Recommendations

- Establish baseline NPS with the Neuropsychiatric Inventory (NPI) or similar instrument.
- Identify and treat contributors to NPS such as pain, disrupted sleep, sensory deficits, systemic medical comorbidities, medication effects, and delirium.
- Search for psychosocial and environmental factors which may be associated with NPS.
- Diagnose/treat pre-existing or co-morbid major mental disorders whose onset was earlier in life.

- Determine prior treatment and their impact on NPS.
- Recommend behavioral/environmental/psychotherapeutic interventions as first-line.
- If medications are indicated, observe for potential adverse effects.
- Follow established treatment algorithms.
- Collaborate with family and credible observers for accurate information about symptoms, adherence to and response to medications, and adverse effects.
- Attend to Beers Criteria to minimize Potentially Inappropriate Medications (PIMs), anticholinergic burden (AB), risk of parkinsonian symptoms and of other adverse effects.
- Follow APA prescribing recommendations for antipsychotics.

References

Aarsland D, Ballard C, Rongve A, et al. Clinical trials of dementia with Lewy bodies and Parkinson's disease dementia. Curr Neurol Neurosci Rep. 2012;12(5):492–501.

Aga VM. When and how to treat agitation in Alzheimer's disease dementia with citalopram and escitalopram. Am J Geriatr Psychiatry. 2019;27(10):1099–107.

Ahmed RM, Paterson RW, Warren JD, et al. Biomarkers in dementia: clinical utility and new directions. J Neurol Neurosurg Psychiatry. 2014;85(12):1426–34.

Almeida L, Ahmed B, Walz R, et al. Depressive symptoms are frequent in atypical parkinsonian disorders. Mov Disord Clin Pract. 2017;4(2):191–7.

Alves G, Wentzel-Larsen T, Larsen JP. Is fatigue an independent and persistent symptom in patients with Parkinson disease? Neurology. 2004;63(10):1908–11.

Alvarado-Bolaños A, Cervantes-Arriaga A, Rodríguez-Violante M, et al. Impact of neuropsychiatric symptoms on the quality of life of subjects with Parkinson's disease. J Parkinsons Dis. 2015;5(3):541–8.

Amalakanti S, Arepalli KVR, Jillela JP. Cognitive assessment in asymptomatic COVID-19 subjects. Virus disease. 2021;32(1):146–9.

American Geriatrics Society Beers Criteria® Update Expert Panel. American Geriatrics Society 2019 updated AGS Beers Criteria® for potentially inappropriate medication use in older adults. J Am Geriatr Soc. 2019;67(4):674–94.

American Psychiatric Association. The American Psychiatric Association practice guideline on the use of antipsychotics to treat agitation or psychosis in patients with dementia. American Psychiatric Pub; 2016.

Ammaturo DA, Hadjistavropoulos T, Williams J. Pain in dementia: use of observational pain assessment tools by people who are not health professionals. Pain Med. 2017;18(10):1895–907.

Armstrong MJ, Okun MS. Diagnosis and treatment of Parkinson disease: a review. JAMA. 2020;323(6):548–60.

American Psychiatric Association. Diagnostic and statistical manual of mental disorders (DSM-5®). American Psychiatric Pub; 2013.

Asnis GM, Henderson MA. Levomilnacipran for the treatment of major depressive disorder: a review. Neuropsychiatr Dis Treat. 2015;11:125–35.

Aspinall SL, Springer SP, Zhao X, et al. Central nervous system medication burden and risk of recurrent serious falls and hip fractures in veterans affairs nursing home residents. JAGS. 2019;67(1):74–80.

Arvanitakis Z, Shah RC, Bennett DA. Diagnosis and management of dementia: review. JAMA. 2019;322(16):1589–99.

Ballard C, Sharp S, Corbett A. Dextromethorphan and quinidine for treating agitation in patients with Alzheimer's disease dementia. JAMA. 2015a;314(12):1233–5.

Ballard C, Banister C, Khan Z, et al. Evaluation of the safety, tolerability, and efficacy of pimavanserin versus placebo in patients with Alzheimer's disease psychosis: a phase 2, randomised, placebo-controlled, double-blind study. Lancet Neurol. 2018;17(3):213–22.

Ballard C, Thomas A, Gerry S, et al. A double-blind randomized placebo-controlled withdrawal trial comparing memantine and antipsychotics for the long-term treatment of function and neuropsychiatric symptoms in people with Alzheimer's disease (MAIN-AD). J Am Med Dir Assoc. 2015b;16(4):316–22.

Banerjee D, Muralidharan A, Hakim Mohammed AR, et al. Neuroimaging in dementia: a brief review. Cureus. 2020;12(6):e8682.

Banerjee S, High J, Stirling S, et al. Study of mirtazapine for agitated behaviours in dementia (SYMBAD): a randomised, double-blind, placebo-controlled trial. Lancet. 2021;398:1487–97.

Boeker H, Seidl A, Schopper C. Neurotoxicitiy related to combined treatment with lithium, antidepressants and atpyical neuroleptics: a series of cases. Schweizer Archiv für Neurologie und Psychiatrie. 2011;162(2):72–6.

Boot BP, McDade EM, McGinnis SM, Boeve BF. Treatment of dementia with lewy bodies. Curr Treat Options Neurol. 2013 Dec;15(6):738-64. https://doi.org/10.1007/s11940-013-0261-6. PMID: 24222315; PMCID: PMC3913181.

Bowie CR, Best MW, Depp C, et al. Cognitive and functional deficits in bipolar disorder and schizophrenia as a function of the presence and history of psychosis. Bipolar Disord. 2018;20(7):604–13.

Bozymski, Kevin M., Denise K. Lowe, Kiersten M. Pasternak, Travis L. Gatesman, and Ericka L. Crouse.

"Pimavanserin: A Novel Antipsychotic for Parkinson's Disease Psychosis." The Annals of Pharmacotherapy 51, no. 6 (June 2017): 479–87. https://doi.org/10.1177/1060028017693029.

Brett J, Murnion B. Management of benzodiazepine misuse and dependence. Aust Prescr. 2015;38(5):152–5.

Brown K, Mastrianni JA. The prion diseases. J Geriatr Psychiatry Neurol. 2010;23:277–98.

Burns A, Perry E, Holmes C, et al. A double-blind placebo-controlled randomized trial of Melissa officinalis oil and donepezil for the treatment of agitation in Alzheimer's disease. Dement Geriatr Cogn Disord. 2011;31(2):158–64.

Butler M, Pollak TA, Rooney AG, et al. Neuropsychiatric complications of covid-19. Br Med J. 2020;371

Camargos EF, Pandolfi MB, Freitas MPD, et al. Trazodone for the treatment of sleep disorders in dementia: an open-label, observational and review study. Arq Neuropsiquiatr. 2011;69(1):44–9.

Chen C, Dong XP. Epidemiological characteristics of human prion diseases. Infect Dis Poverty. 2016;5:47.

Chen A, Copeli F, Metzger E, et al. The Psychopharmacology Algorithm Project at the Harvard South Shore Program: an update on management of behavioral and psychological symptoms in dementia. Psychiatry Res. 2021;295:13364.

Cheng ST, Au A, Losada A, et al. Psychological interventions for dementia caregivers: what we have achieved, what we have learned. Curr Psychiatry Rep. 2019;21(7):59.

Borek LL, Amick MM, Friedman JH: Non-motor aspects of Parkinson's disease. CNS Spectr. 11(7):541–54, 2006.

Battle CE, Abdul-Rahim AH, Shenkin SD, Hewitt J, et al. Cholinesterase inhibitors for vascular dementia and other vascular cognitive impairments: a network meta-analysis. Cochrane Database Syst Rev. 2021;2(2):CD013306: 1–68.

Chibnall JT, Tait RC. Pain assessment in cognitively impaired and unimpaired older adults: a comparison of four scales. Pain. 2001;92(1–2):173–86.

Cioltan H, Alshehri S, Howe C, et al. Variation in use of antipsychotic medications in nursing homes in the United States: a systematic review. BMC Geriatr. 2017;17(1):32.

Cipriani G, Ulivi M, Danti S, et al. Sexual disinhibition and dementia. Psychogeriatr. 2016;16(2):145–53.

Cohen JM, Blustein J, Weinstein BE, et al. Studies of physician-patient communication with older patients: how often is hearing loss considered? A systematic literature review. JAGS. 2017;65(8):1642–9.

Cole, Martin G., Jane McCusker, Philippe Voyer, Johanne Monette, Nathalie Champoux, Antonio Ciampi, Minh Vu, Alina Dyachenko, and Eric Belzile. "Symptoms of Delirium Occurring before and after Episodes of Delirium in Older Long-Term Care Residents." Journal of the American Geriatrics Society 60, no. 12 (December 2012): 2302–7. https://doi.org/10.1111/j.1532-5415.2012.04237.x.

Connolly BS, Lang AE. Pharmacological treatment of Parkinson disease: a review. JAMA. 2014;311(16):1670–83.

Cook ED, Swift K, James I, et al. Functional analysis-based interventions for challenging behaviour in dementia. Cochrane Database Syst Rev. 2012;2

Coyle-Gilchrist ITS, Dick KM, Patterson K, et al. Prevalence, characteristics, and survival of frontotemporal lobar degeneration syndromes. Neurology. 2016;86(18):1736–43.

Cruz-Jentoft AJ, Burón JA, Diago JI, et al. Risperidone in the treatment of behavioural and psychological symptoms of dementia in patients diagnosed with vascular or mixed-type dementia. Int J Psychiatry Clin Pract. 2005;9(1):45–51.

Cummings JL, Schneider E, Tariot PN, et al. Behavioral effects of memantine in Alzheimer disease patients receiving donepezil treatment. Neurology. 2006;67(1):57–63.

Cummings JL, Mega M, Gray K, et al. The neuropsychiatric inventory: comprehensive assessment of psychopathology in dementia. Neurology. 1994;44(12):2308–14.

Davies SJ, Burhan AM, Kim D, et al. Sequential drug treatment algorithm for agitation and aggression in Alzheimer's and mixed dementia. J Psychopharmacol. 2018;32(5):509–23.

Deakin JB, Rahman S, Nestor PJ, et al. Paroxetine does not improve symptoms and impairs cognition in frontotemporal dementia: a double-blind randomized controlled trial. Psychopharmacol. 2004;172(4):400–8.

Defrancesco M, Marksteiner J, Fleischhacker WW, Blasko I. Use of benzodiazepines in Alzheimer's disease: a systematic review of literature. Int J Neuropsychopharmacol. 2015;18(10):pyv055.

Delfino LL, Komatsu RS, Komatsu C, et al. Dementia management strategies associated with neuropsychiatric symptoms of elderly people with Alzheimer's disease. Dementia. 2019;18(7–8):2747–59.

Desmarais P, Massoud F, Filion J, et al. Quetiapine for psychosis in Parkinson disease and neurodegenerative parkinsonian disorders: a systematic review. J Geriatr Psychiatry Neurol. 2016;29(4):227–36.

DeGiorgi R, Series H. Treatment of inappropriate sexual behavior in dementia. Curr Treat Options Neurol. 2016;18(9):41.

Devanand DP, Pelton GH, D'Antonio K, et al. Low-dose lithium treatment for agitation and psychosis in Alzheimer disease and frontotemporal dementia: a case series. Alzheimer Dis Assoc Disord. 2017;31(1):73–5.

Dysken MW, Sano M, Asthana S, et al. Effect of vitamin E and memantine on functional decline in Alzheimer disease: the TEAM-AD VA cooperative randomized trial. JAMA. 2014;311(1):33–44.

Fénelon G, Soulas T, Zenasni F, et al. The changing face of Parkinson's disease-associated psychosis: a cross-sectional study based on the new NINDS-NIMH criteria. Mov Disord. 2010;25(6):763–6.

Ferreira JJ, Katzenschlager R, Bloem BR, et al. Summary of the recommendations of the EFNS/MDS-ES review on therapeutic management of Parkinson's disease. Eur J Neurol. 2013;20(1):5–15.
Ffytche DH, Creese B, Politis M, et al. The psychosis spectrum in Parkinson disease. Nat Rev Neurol. 2017;13(2):81–95.
Fletcher PD, Downey LE, Golden HL, et al. Auditory hedonic phenotypes in dementia: a behavioural and neuroanatomical analysis. Cortex. 2015;67:95–105.
Fong TG, Inouye SK, Jones RN. Delirium, dementia, and decline. JAMA Psychiatry. 2017;74(3):212–3.
Forrester LT, Maayan N, Orrell M, et al. Aromatherapy for dementia. Cochrane Database Syst Rev. 2014;2:CD003150.
Forsaa E, Larsen J, Wentzel-Larsen T, et al. A 12-year population based study of psychosis in Parkinson disease. Arch Neurol. 2010a;67:996–1001.
Forsaa E, Larsen J, Wentzel-Larsen T, Alves G. What predicts mortality in Parkinson disease? A prospective population-based long-term study. Neurology. 2010b;75:1270–6.
Fortinsky RH, Kuchel GA, David C, et al. Clinical trial testing in-home multidisciplinary care management for older adults with cognitive vulnerability: rationale and study design. Contemp Clin Trials. 2020;92:105992.
Fox SH. Pimavanserin as treatment for Parkinson's disease psychosis. Lancet. 2014;383(9916):494–6.
Frakey LL, Salloway S, Buelow M, Malloy P. A randomized, double-blind, placebo-controlled trial of modafinil for the treatment of apathy in individuals with mild-to-moderate Alzheimer's disease. JCP. 2012;73(6):796–801.
Fraser LA, Liu K, Naylor KL, et al. Falls and fractures with atypical antipsychotic medication use: a population-based cohort study. JAMA Intern Med. 2015;175(3):450–2.
Friedman JH. Parkinson disease psychosis: update. Behav Neurol. 2013;27(4):469–77.
Ganguli M, Du Y, Dodge HH, et al. Depressive symptoms and cognitive decline in late life. Arch Gen Psychiatry. 2006;63:153–60.
Gannon M, Che P, Chen Y, et al. Noradrenergic dysfunction in Alzheimer's disease. Front Neurosci. 2015;9
Gatt A, Ekonomou A, Somani A, et al. Importance of proactive treatment of depression in Lewy body dementias: the impact on hippocampal neurogenesis and cognition in a post-mortem study. Dement Geriatr Cogn Disord. 2017;44(5–6):283–93.
Gerhard T, Huybrechts K, Olfson M, et al. Comparative mortality risks of antipsychotic medications in community-dwelling older adults. Br J Psych. 2014;205(1):44–51.
Gerlach LB, Kales HC. Managing behavioral and psychological symptoms of dementia. Psychiatr Clin North Am. 2018;41(1):127–39.
Geschwind MD. Prion diseases. Continuum. 2015;21:1612–38.
Gitlin LN, Kales HC, Lyketsos CG. Managing behavioral symptoms in dementia using nonpharmacologic approaches: an overview. JAMA. 2012;308(19):2020–9.
Gomperts SN. Lewy body dementias: dementia with Lewy bodies and Parkinson disease dementia. Continuum (Minneap Minn). 2016;22:435–63.
Green AJE. RT-QuIC: a new test for sporadic CJD. Pract Neurol. 2019;19(1):49–55.
Grimes D, Fitzpatrick M, Gordon J, et al. Canadian guideline for Parkinson disease. CMAJ. 2019;191:E989.
Grossberg GT, Kohegyi E, Mergel V, et al. Efficacy and safety of brexpiprazole for the treatment of agitation in Alzheimer's dementia: two 12-week, randomized, double-blind, placebo-controlled trials. Am J Geriatr Psychiatry. 2020;28(4):383–400.
Hadjistavropoulos T, Herr K, Prkachin KM, et al. Pain assessment in elderly adults with dementia. Lancet Neurol. 2014;13(12):1216–27.
Handing EP, Andel R, Kadlecova P, et al. Midlife alcohol consumption and risk of dementia over 43 years of follow-up: a population-based study from the Swedish twin registry. J Gerontol A Biol Sci Med Sci. 2014;70(10):1248–54.
Hardy CJD, Buckley AH, Downey LE, Lehmann M, Zimmerer VC, Varley RA, Warren JD. The language profile of behavioral variant frontotemporal dementia. Journal of Alzheimer's Disease. 2016;50(2):359–71. https://doi.org/10.3233/JAD-150806.
Herrmann N, Black SE, Chow T, et al. Serotonergic function and treatment of behavioral and psychological symptoms of frontotemporal dementia. Am J Geriatr Psychiatry. 2012;20(9):789–97.
Hermida AP, Tang YI, Glass O, et al. Efficacy and safety of ECT for behavioral and psychological symptoms of dementia (BPSD): a retrospective chart review. Am J Periatr Psychiatry. 2020;28(2):157–63.
Howard RJ, Juszczak E, Ballard CG, et al. Donepezil for the treatment of agitation in Alzheimer's disease. NEJM. 2007;357(14):1382–92.
Hunt LJ, Covinsky KE, Yaffe K, et al. Pain in community-dwelling older adults with dementia: results from the National Health and Aging Trends Study. J Am Geriatr Soc. 2015;63(8):1503–11.
Husebo BS, Ballard C, Sandvik R, et al. Efficacy of treating pain to reduce behavioural disturbances in residents of nursing homes with dementia: cluster randomised clinical trial. BMJ. 2011;343:d4065.
Husebo BS, Achterberg W, Flo E. Identifying and managing pain in people with Alzheimer's disease and other types of dementia: a systematic review. CNS Drugs. 2016;30(6):481–97.
Ismail Z, Smith EE, Geda Y, et al. Neuropsychiatric symptoms as early manifestations of emergent dementia: provisional diagnostic criteria for mild behavioral impairment. Alzheimers Dement. 2016;12(2):195–202.
Isserles M, Daskalakis ZJ, Kumar S, et al. Clinical effectiveness and tolerability of electroconvulsive therapy in patients with neuropsychiatric symptoms of dementia. J Alzheimers Dis. 2017;57:45–51.
Isaacs JD, Boenink M. Biomarkers for dementia: too soon for routine clinical use. Lancet Neurol. 2020;19(11):884–5.
Jacquart SD, Marshak HH, Santos HD, et al. The effects of simultaneous exercise and psychotherapy on depres-

sive symptoms in inpatient, psychiatric older adults. Adv Mind-Body Med. 2014;28(4):8–17.

Jaïdi Y, Nonnonhou V, Kanagaratnam L, et al. Reduction of the anticholinergic burden makes it possible to decrease behavioral and psychological symptoms of dementia. Am J Geriatr Psychiatry. 2018;26(3):280–8.

Jellinger KA, Korcyzn AD. Are dementia with Lewy bodies and Parkinson's disease dementia the same disease? BMC Med. 2018;16(1):34.

Kales HC, Gitlin LN, Lyketsos CG. Management of neuropsychiatric symptoms of dementia in clinical settings: recommendations from a multidisciplinary expert panel. JAGS. 2014;62(4):762–9.

Kröger E, Mouls M, Wilensky M, et al. Adverse drug reactions reported with cholinesterase inhibitors: an analysis of 16 years of individual case safety reports from VigiBase. Ann Pharmacother. 2015;49(11):1197–206. https://doi.org/10.1177/1060028015602274.

Lansdall, C. J., Coyle-Gilchrist, I. T. S., Jones, P. S., Rodríguez, P. V., Wilcox, A., Wehmann, E., … Rowe, J. B. (2017). Apathy and impulsivity in frontotemporal lobar degeneration syndromes. Brain, 140(6), 1792–1807. https://doi.org/10.1093/brain/awx101.

Lanctôt K, Amatniek J, Ancoli-Israel S, et al. Neuropsychiatric signs and symptoms of Alzheimer's disease: new treatment paradigms. Alzheimers Dement Transl Res Clin Intervent. 2017;3(3):440–9.

Lebert F, Stekke W, Hasenbroekx C, et al. Frontotemporal dementia: a randomised, controlled trial with trazodone. Dement Geriatr Cogn Disord. 2004;17(4):355–9.

Leentjens AF, Marinus J, Van Hilten JJ, Lousberg R et al: The contribution of somatic symptoms to the diagnosis of depressive disorder in Parkinson's disease: a discriminant analytic approach. J Neuropsychiatry Clin Neurosci 15(1):74–77;2003.

Leentjens AF, Moonen AJ, Dujardin K, et al. Modeling depression in Parkinson disease: disease-specific and nonspecific risk factors. Neurology. 2013;81(12):1036–43.

Lees R, Selvarajah J, Fenton C, et al. Test accuracy of cognitive screening tests for diagnosis of dementia and multidomain cognitive impairment in stroke. Stroke. 2014;45(10):3008–18.

Lenka A, Jhunjhunwala KR, Saini J, Pal PK. Structural and functional neuroimaging in patients with Parkinson's disease and visual hallucinations: a critical review. Parkinsonism Relat Disord. 2015;21:683–91.

Lerner AJ, Riley D. Dementias associated with motor dysfunction. In: Yudofsky SC, Hales RE, editors. Clinical manual of neuropsychiatry. Washington DC: American Psychiatric Publishing; 2012. p. 287–310.

Leonpacher AK, Peters ME, Drye LT, et al. Effects of citalopram on neuropsychiatric symptoms in Alzheimer's dementia: evidence from the CitAD study. Am J Psychiatry. 2016;173(5):473–80.

Liu D, Myles H, Foley DL, et al. Risk factors for obstructive sleep apnea are prevalent in people with psychosis and correlate with impaired social functioning and poor physical health. Front Psych. 2016;7:139.

Mahase E. Alzheimer's disease: FDA approves lecanemab amid cost and safety concerns. BMJ. 2023;380:73.

Maidment ID, Fox CG, Boustani M, et al. Efficacy of memantine on behavioral and psychological symptoms related to dementia: a systematic meta-analysis. Ann Pharmacotherapy. 2008;42(1):32–8.

Makris UE, Abrams RC, Gurland B, Reid MC. Management of persistent pain in the older patient: a clinical review. JAMA. 2014;312(8):825.

Marcantonio ER. Delirium. Ann Internal Med. 2011;154(11):ITC6.

Marcantonio ER. Delirium in hospitalized older adults. NEJM. 2017;377(15):1456–66.

Marsh L. Depression and Parkinson's disease: current knowledge. Curr Neurol Neurosci Rep. 2013;13(12):409.

Marshall CR, Hardy CJD, Russell LL, et al. Impaired interoceptive accuracy in semantic variant primary progressive aphasia. Front Neurol. 2017;8

Marshall CR, Hardy CJD, Volkmer A, et al. Primary progressive aphasia: a clinical approach. J Neurol. 2018;265(6):1474–90.

Matsunaga S, Kishi T, Iwata N. Memantine for Lewy body disorders: systematic review and meta-analysis. Am J Geriatr Psychiatry. 2015a;23(4):373–83.

Matsunaga S, Kishi T, Iwata N. Memantine monotherapy for Alzheimer's disease: a systematic review and meta-analysis. PLoS One. 2015b;10(4):e0123289.

Maust DT, Kim HM, Seyfried LS, et al. Antipsychotics, other psychotropics, and the risk of death in patients with dementia: number needed to harm. JAMA Psychiatry. 2015;72(5):438–45.

Maust DT, Strominger J, Kim HM, et al. Prevalence of central nervous system–active polypharmacy among older adults with dementia in the US. JAMA. 2021;325(10):952–61.

McDermott CL, Gruenewald DA. Pharmacologic management of agitation in patients with dementia. Curr Geriatr Rep. 2019;8(1):1–11.

McFarland N, DeKosky ST, Tung GA. Clinical features and diagnosis of dementia with Lewy bodies, UpToDate Literature review current through: Sep 2022.| This topic last updated: Aug 30, 2021.

McKeith I, Del Ser T, Spano PF, et al. Efficacy of rivastigmine in dementia with Lewy bodies: a randomised, double-blind, placebo-controlled international study. Lancet. 2000;356(9247):2031–6.

McKhann GM, Knopman DS, Chertkow H, et al. The diagnosis of dementia due to Alzheimer's disease: recommendations from the National Institute on Aging-Alzheimer's association workgroups on diagnostic guidelines for Alzheimer's disease. Alzheimers Dement. 2011;7(3):263–9.

McShane R, Areosa Sastre A, Minakaran N. Memantine for dementia. Cochrane Database Syst Rev. 2006;2:CD003154.

Mendez MF, Shapira JS, Miller BL. Stereotypical movements and frontotemporal dementia. Mov Disord. 2005;20(6):742–5.

Menza M, Dobkin R, Marin H, et al. A controlled trial of antidepressants in patients with Parkinson's disease and depression. Neurology. 2009;72:886–92.

Mishra A, Ferrari R, Heutink P, et al. Gene-based association studies report genetic links for clini-

cal subtypes of frontotemporal dementia. Brain. 2017;140(5):1437–46.
Mokhber NE, Abdollahian A, Soltanifar R, et al. Comparison of sertraline, venlafaxine and desipramine effects on depression, cognition and the daily living activities in Alzheimer patients. Pharmacopsychiatry. 2014;47(04/05):131–40.
Miyasaki JM, Shannon K, Voon V, et al. Practice parameter: evaluation and treatment of depression, psychosis, and dementia in Parkinson disease (an evidence-based review). Report of the quality standards subcommittee of the American Academy of Neurology. Neurology. 2006;66(7):996–1002.
Murley A, Coyle-Gilchrist I, Rouse M, et al. Redefining the multidimensional clinical phenotypes of frontotemporal lobar degeneration syndromes. Brain. 2020;143(5):1555–71.
Narang, Puneet, Mostafa El-Refai, Roop Parlapalli, Lilia Danilov, Sainath Manda, Gagandeep Kaur, and Steven Lippmann. "Antipsychotic Drugs: Sudden Cardiac Death among Elderly Patients." Psychiatry (Edgmont (Pa.: Township)) 7, no. 10 (October 2010): 25–29.
National Institute for Health and Care Excellence: Depression in adults with a chronic physical health problem: recognition and management. Clinical Guideline CG91. Available at: https://www.nice.org.uk/guidance/cg91. Published date 28 October 2009. Accessed May 15, 2020
National Institute for Health and Care Excellence: Parkinson's disease in adults. NICE guideline NG71. Available at: www.nice.org.uk/guidance/ng71. Published date 19 July 2017. Accessed May 1, 2020
Neikrug AB, Ancoli-Israel S. Sleep-wake disturbances and sleep disorders in patients with dementia. UpToDate, Literature review current through: Aug 2022. | This topic last updated: Nov 12, 2021.
Nelson JC, Delucchi KL, Schneider LS. Moderators of outcome in late-life depression: a patient-level meta-analysis. Am J Psychiatry. 2013;170(6):651–9.
Newkirk LA, Dao VL, Jordan JT, et al. Factors associated with supportive care service use among California Alzheimer's disease patients and their caregivers. J Alzheimers Dis. 2020;73(1):77–86.
Ngandu T, Lehtisalo J, Solomon A, et al. A 2 year multidomain intervention of diet, exercise, cognitive training, and vascular risk monitoring versus control to prevent cognitive decline in at-risk elderly people (FINGER): a randomised controlled trial. Lancet. 2015;385(9984):2255–63.
Noufi P, Khoury R, Jeyakumara S, Grossberg GT. Use of cholinesterase inhibitors in non-Alzheimer's dementias. Drugs Aging. 2019;36(8):719–31.
O'Brien JT, Thomas A. Vascular dementia. Lancet. 2015;386:1698–706.
Oguru M, Tachibana H, Toda K, et al. Apathy and depression in Parkinson disease. J Geriatr Psychiatry Neurol. 2010;23(1):35–41.
Patience J, Lai KSP, Russel E, et al. Relationship between mood, thinking, and walking: a systematic review examining depressive symptoms, executive function, and gait. Am J Geriatr Psychiatry. 2019;27(12):1375–83.
Peisah C, Strukovski J-A, Wijeratne C, et al. The development and testing of the quality use of medications in dementia (QUM-D): a tool for quality prescribing for behavioral and psychological symptoms of dementia (BPSD). International Psychogeriatrics.27(8). Published online by Cambridge University Press: 02 February 2015.
Peskind ER, Tsuang DW, Bonner LT, et al. Propranolol for disruptive behaviors in nursing home residents with probable or possible Alzheimer disease: a placebo-controlled study. Alzheimer Dis Assoc Disord. 2005;19(1):23–8.
Petersen RC, Lopez O, Armstrong MJ, et al. Practice guideline update summary: mild cognitive impairment. Neurology. 2018;90:126–35.
Pijnenburg YAL, Sampson EL, Harvey RJ, et al. Vulnerability to neuroleptic side effects in frontotemporal lobar degeneration. Int J Geriatr Psychiatry. 2003;18(1):67–72.
Porsteinsson AP, Antonsdottir IM. An update on the advancements in the treatment of agitation in Alzheimer's disease. Expert Opin Pharmacother. 2017;18(6):611–20.
Porsteinsson AP, Drye LT, Pollock BG, et al. Effect of citalopram on agitation in Alzheimer disease: the CitAD randomized clinical trial. JAMA. 2014;311(7):682–91.
Potkins D, Myint P, Bannister C, et al. Language impairment in dementia: impact on symptoms and care needs in residential homes. Int J Geriatr Psychiatry. 2003;8(11):1002–6.
Rabins, Peter V., Barry W. Rovner, Teresa Rummans, Lon S. Schneider, and Pierre N. Tariot. "Guideline Watch (October 2014): Practice Guideline for the Treatment of Patients with Alzheimer's Disease and Other Dementias." FOCUS 15, no. 1 (January 2017): 110–28. https://doi.org/10.1176/appi.focus.15106.
Rabinovici GD. Controversy and progress in Alzheimer's disease—FDA approval of aducanumab. N Engl J Med. 2021;385:771–4.
Ranasinghe KG, Rankin KP, Lobach IV, et al. Cognition and neuropsychiatry in behavioral variant frontotemporal dementia by disease stage. Neurology. 2016;86(7):600–10.
Reed BR, Mungas DM, Kramer JH, et al. Profiles of neuropsychological impairment in autopsy-defined Alzheimer's disease and cerebrovascular disease. Brain. 2007;130(3):731–9.
Reus VI, Fochtmann LJ, Eyler AE, et al. The American Psychiatric Association practice guideline on the use of antipsychotics to treat agitation or psychosis in patients with dementia. Am J Psychiatry. 2016;173(5):543–6.
Richard IH, McDermott MP, Kurlan R, et al. A randomized, double-blind, placebo-controlled trial of antidepressants in Parkinson disease. Neurology. 2012;78(16):1229–36.
Rios-Romenets S, Creti L, Fichten C, et al. Doxepin and cognitive behavioural therapy for insomnia in patients

with Parkinson's disease—a randomized study. Parkinsonism Relat Disord. 2013;19(7):670–5.

Rodda J, Morgan S, Walker Z. Are cholinesterase inhibitors effective in the management of the behavioral and psychological symptoms of dementia in Alzheimer's disease? A systematic review of randomized, placebo-controlled trials of donepezil, rivastigmine and galantamine. Int Psychogeriatr. 2009;21(5):813.

Rohrer, Jonathan D., and Jason D. Warren. "Phenomenology and Anatomy of Abnormal Behaviours in Primary Progressive Aphasia." Journal of the Neurological Sciences 293, no. 1–2 (June 2010): 35–38. https://doi.org/10.1016/j.jns.2010.03.012

Rolinski M, Fox C, Maidment I, McShane R. Cholinesterase inhibitors for dementia with Lewy bodies, Parkinson's disease dementia and cognitive impairment in Parkinson's disease. Cochrane Database of Syst Rev. 2012;2014

Romanella SM, Roe D, Tatti E, et al. The sleep side of aging and Alzheimer's disease. Sleep Med. 2020;77:209–25.

Reus, Victor I., Laura J. Fochtmann, A. Evan Eyler, Donald M. Hilty, Marcela Horvitz-Lennon, Michael D. Jibson, Oscar L. Lopez, et al. "The American Psychiatric Association Practice Guideline on the Use of Antipsychotics to Treat Agitation or Psychosis in Patients with Dementia." The American Journal of Psychiatry 173, no. 5 (01 2016): 543–46. https://doi.org/10.1176/appi.ajp.2015.173501.

Sachdev PS. Inappropriate sexual behaviors in dementia. Am J Geriatr Psychiatry. 2017;25(4):372–3.

Schneider JA, Arvanitakis Z, Bang W, Bennett DA. Mixed brain pathologies account for most dementia cases in community-dwelling older persons. Neurology. 2007;69(24):2197–204.

Seibert M, Mühlbauer V, Holbrook J, et al. Efficacy and safety of pharmacotherapy for Alzheimer's disease and for behavioral and psychological symptoms of dementia in older patients with moderate and severe functional impairments: a systematic review of controlled trials. Alzheimers Res Ther. 2021;13(1):1–20.

Seitz DP, Adunuri N, Gill SS, et al. Antidepressants for agitation and psychosis in dementia. Edited by Cochrane Dementia and Cognitive Improvement Group. Cochrane Database Syst Rev. 2011;

Seitz DP, Gill SS, Herrmann N, et al. Pharmacological treatments for neuropsychiatric symptoms of dementia in long-term care: a systematic review. Int Psychogeriatr. 2013;25(2):185–203.

Seppala LJ, Wermelink AM, de Vries M, et al. Fall-risk-increasing drugs: a systematic review and meta-analysis: II Psychotropics. J Am Med Dir Assoc. 2018;19(4):371–e11.

Seppi K, Ray Chaudhuri K, Coelho M, et al. Update on treatments for nonmotor symptoms of Parkinson's disease-an evidence-based medicine review. Mov Disord. 2019;34(2):180–98.

Sezgin M, Bilgic B, Tinaz S, Emre M. Dementia and Lewy body disease. Semin Neurol. 2019;39:274–82.

Silwanowicz, Ryan M., Donovan T. Maust, Lisa S. Seyfried, Claire Chiang, Claire Stano, and Helen C. Kales. "Management of Older Adults with Dementia Who Present to Emergency Services with Neuropsychiatric Symptoms: Management of Older Adults with Dementia with NPS." International Journal of Geriatric Psychiatry 32, no. 12 (December 2017): 1233–40. https://doi.org/10.1002/gps.4599.

Sivasathiaseelan H, Marshall CR, Agustus JL, et al. Frontotemporal dementia: a clinical review. Semin Neurol. 2019;39(2):251–63.

Snowden JS, Hu Q, Rollinson S, et al. The most common type of FTLD-FUS (aFTLD-U) is associated with a distinct clinical form of frontotemporal dementia but is not related to mutations in the FUS gene. Acta Neuropathol. 2011a;122(1):99–110.

Snowden JS, Thompson JC, Stopford CL, et al. The clinical diagnosis of early-onset dementias: diagnostic accuracy and clinicopathological relationships. Brain. 2011b;134:2478–92.

Stebbins GT, Nyenhuis DL, Wang C, et al. Gray matter atrophy in patients with ischemic stroke with cognitive impairment. Stroke. 2008;39(3):785–93.

Steinberg M, Lyketsos CG. Atypical antipsychotic use in patients with dementia: managing safety concerns. Am J Psychiatry. 2012;169(9):900–6.

Steinhoff BJ, Zerr I, Glatting M, et al. Diagnostic value of periodic complexes in Creutzfeldt-Jakob disease. Ann Neurol. 2004;56(5):702–8.

Stinton C, McKeith I, Taylor JP, et al. Pharmacological management of Lewy body dementia: a systematic review and meta-analysis. Am J Psychiatry. 2015;172(8):731–42.

Suzuki K, Miyamoto M, Hirata K. Sleep disorders in the elderly: diagnosis and management. Gen Fam Med. 2017;18(2):61–71.

Takahashi M, Tabu H, Ozaki A, et al. Hamano Tfor the REBORN study group: antidepressants for depression, apathy, and gait instability in Parkinson's disease: a multicenter randomized study. Intern Med. 2019;58(3):361–8.

Tanaka T. Factors predicting perioperative delirium and acute exacerbation of behavioral and psychological symptoms of dementia based on admission data in elderly patients with proximal femoral fracture: a retrospective study. Geriatr Gerontol Int. 2015;16(7):821–8.

Tariot PN. Chronic divalproex sodium to attenuate agitation and clinical progression of Alzheimer disease. Arch Gen Psychiatry. 2011;68(8):853.

Tariot PN, Cummings JL, Soto-Martin ME, et al. Trial of Pimavanserin in dementia-related psychosis. N Engl J Med. 2021;385(4):309–13.

Thakur M, Gwyther L. Agitation in older adults. In: Steffens DC, Blazer DG, Thakur ME, editors. The American Psychiatric Publishing textbook of geriatric psychiatry. 5th ed. American Psychiatric Publishing; 2015. p. 507–23.

Theleritis C, Siarkos K, Politis AA, et al. A systematic review of non-pharmacological treatments for apathy in dementia. Int J Geriatr Psychiatry. 2018;33(2):e177–92.

Tong T, Ledig C, Guerrero R, et al. Five-class differential diagnostics of neurodegenerative diseases using random undersampling boosting. Neuroimage Clin. 2017;15:613–24.

Tosato M, Lukas A, van der Roest HG, et al. Association of pain with behavioral and psychiatric symptoms among nursing home residents with cognitive impairment: results from the SHELTER study. Pain. 2012;153(2):305–10.

Trifirò G, Gambassi G, Sen EF, et al. Association of community-acquired pneumonia with antipsychotic drug use in elderly patients: a nested case-control study. Ann Intern Med. 2010;152(7):418–25, W139–40.

Tsai RM, Boxer AL. Therapy and clinical trials in frontotemporal dementia: past, present, and future. J Neurochem. 2016;138:211–21.

Tzourio C. Vascular factors and cognition: toward a prevention of dementia? J Hypertens Suppl. 2003;21(5):S15–9.

Van der Steen JT, Smaling HJ, van der Wouden JC, et al. Music-based therapeutic interventions for people with dementia. Cochrane Database Syst Rev. 2018;7(7)

Van Dyck CH, Arnsten AFT, Padala PR, et al. Neurobiologic rationale for treatment of apathy in Alzheimer's disease with methylphenidate. Am J Geriatr Psychiatry. 2021;29(1):51–62.

Vann Jones SA, O'Brien JT. The prevalence and incidence of dementia with Lewy bodies: a systematic review of population and clinical studies. Psychol Med. 2014;44:673–83.

Vigen CL, Mack WJ, Keefe RS, et al. Cognitive effects of atypical antipsychotic medications in patients with Alzheimer's disease: outcomes from CATIE-AD. Am J Psychiatry. 2011;168(8):831–9.

Vitali P, MacCagnano E, Caverzasi E, et al. Diffusion-weighted MRI hyperintensity patterns differentiate CJD from other rapid dementias. Neurology. 2011;76(20):1711–9.

Wang PS, Schneeweiss S, Avorn J, et al. Risk of death in elderly users of conventional vs. atypical antipsychotic medications. NEJM. 2005;353(22):2335–41.

Wang LY, Shofer JB, Rohde K, et al. Prazosin for the treatment of behavioral symptoms in patients with Alzheimer's disease with agitation and aggression. Am J Geriatr Psychiatry. 2009;17(9):744–51.

Wang J, Yu JT, Wang HF, et al. Pharmacological treatment of neuropsychiatric symptoms in Alzheimer's disease: a systematic review and meta-analysis. JNNP. 2015;86(1):101–9.

Warren JD, Rohrer JD, Rossor MN. Frontotemporal dementia. Br Med J. 2013;347

Watt JA, Goodarzi Z, Veroniki AA, et al. Comparative efficacy of interventions for aggressive and agitated behaviors in dementia: a systematic review and network meta-analysis. Ann Intern Med. 2019;171(9):633.

Whitwell, J. L., Przybelski, S. A., Weigand, S. D., Ivnik, R. J., Vemuri, P., Gunter, J. L., ... Josephs, K. A. (2009). Distinct anatomical subtypes of the behavioural variant of frontotemporal dementia: A cluster analysis study. Brain, 132(11), 2932–2946. https://doi.org/10.1093/brain/awp232.

Wiegmann C, Mick I, Brandl EJ, et al. Alcohol and dementia—what is the link? A systematic review. Neuropsychiatr Dis Treat. 2020;16:87–99.

Wilcock GK, Ballard CG, Cooper JA, Henrik Loft H. Memantine for agitation/aggression and psychosis in moderately severe to severe Alzheimer's disease: a pooled analysis of 3 studies. JCP. 2008;69(3):341–8.

Woodward MR, Harper DG, Stolyar A, et al. Dronabinol for the treatment of agitation and aggressive behavior in acutely hospitalized severely demented patients with noncognitive behavioral symptoms. Am J Geriatr Psychiatry. 2014;22(4):415–9.

Woollacott IOC, Rohrer JD. The clinical spectrum of sporadic and familial forms of frontotemporal dementia. J Neurochem. 2016;138:6–31.

Woolley JD, Wilson MR, Hung E, et al. Frontotemporal dementia and mania. Am J Psychiatry. 2007;164(12):1811–6.

Wright S, Perad C. Distinguishing between depression and dementia in older persons: neuropsychological and neuropathological correlates. J Geriatr Psychiatry Neurol. 2007;20:189–98.

Yohanna D, Cifu AS. Antipsychotics to treat agitation or psychosis in patients with dementia. JAMA. 2017;318(11):1057–8.

Yunusa I, Alsumali A, Garba AE, et al. Assessment of reported comparative effectiveness and safety of atypical antipsychotics in the treatment of behavioral and psychological symptoms of dementia: a network meta-analysis. JAMA. 2019;2(3):e190828.

Yunusa I, El Helou ML, Alsahali S. Pimavanserin: a novel antipsychotic with potentials to address an unmet need of older adults with dementia-related psychosis. Front Pharmacol. 2020;11(87)

Zenilman, Michael E. "Delirium: An Important Postoperative Complication." JAMA 317, no. 1 (03 2017): 77–78. https://doi.org/10.1001/jama.2016.18174.

Zesiewicz TA, Sullivan KL, Arnulf I, et al. Practice parameter: treatment of nonmotor symptoms of Parkinson disease: report of the quality standards Subcommittee of the American Academy of neurology. Neurology. 2010;74(11):924–31.

Zhong, Kate, P. Tariot, J. Mintzer, M. Minkwitz, and N. Devine. "Quetiapine to Treat Agitation in Dementia: A Randomized, Double-Blind,Placebo-Controlled Study." Current Alzheimer Research 4, no. 1 (February 1, 2007): 81–93. https://doi.org/10.2174/156720507779939805.

Delirium

6

Boski Patel, Rita Hitching, and Yelizaveta Sher

Abstract

Delirium in aging adults correlates strongly with poor outcomes and inappropriate interventions (Bellelli et al. Front Aging Neurosci 13:1–13, 2021). Unfortunately, it is also often missed (Hercus and Hudaib BMC Health Serv Res 20:1–7, 2020). Rates of misdiagnosis have been estimated as high as 64% (de la Cruz et al. Supportive Care Cancer 23(8): 2427–2433, 2015). This chapter offers an overview of delirium to encourage its early identification, its non-pharmacological management, and, where needed, *age-adjusted* pharmacotherapy.

Accurate, timely diagnosis, and appropriate treatment of delirium has implications for the health delivery system at large. The fiscal impact of delirium is enormous; annual healthcare costs attributed to delirium in the United States are estimated at $164 billion due in part to longer hospitalizations, increased readmission rates, increased morbidity, functional decline, and increased rates of institutionalization and mortality (Maldonado, Crit Care Clin, 33:461–519, 2017).

B. Patel (✉)
Department of Psychiatry, The Permanente Medical Group, Kaiser Permanente, Northern California, Santa Clara, CA, USA
e-mail: bpatel@uchc.edu

R. Hitching
University of Newcastle, Newcastle, Australia

Y. Sher
Division of Medical Psychiatry, Psychiatric and Psychological Services, Adult Cystic Fibrosis Program, Stanford University and Medical Center, Stanford, USA
e-mail: ysher@stanford.edu

Case Example: Missed Delirium

A 73-year-old financial advisor with a history of diabetes mellitus and hypertension was hospitalized with acute respiratory distress syndrome (ARDS) due to COVID-19 infection. On hospital day #3, oxygenation by pulse oximeter was recorded as 89%. The patient required support with oxygen and intravenous fluids, and treatment with dexamethasone and remdesivir. Daily evaluation with the Confusion Assessment Method-ICU (CAM-ICU) through hospital day #6 demonstrated that she could write the date, time, location, and circumstances, and was able to spell WORLD backward. On the "A" test for vigilance, she had no positive or negative errors.

However, over the course of the next 5 days she became lethargic, withdrawn, and appeared dejected. Oxygenation fell to 85%. With worsening respiratory status, she was intubated on day #7. On hospital day #10 and #11, she wrote several notes that she wanted to die and asked for her breathing tube to be removed.

The patient's family members reported that her cognitive status before hospitalization was

H. H. Fenn et al. (eds.), *Age-Adjusted Psychiatric Treatment for the Older Patient*,
https://doi.org/10.1007/978-3-031-53976-3_6

not impaired, adequate for her fulltime work, and her mood was always upbeat and optimistic. They insisted that she was now depressed and that this contributed to passive suicidality. The medical team determined that the patient now lacked decision-making capacity over her medical treatment and ventilation. The patient's husband was the surrogate decision-makers and the treatment plan was continued.

The patient was not sleeping at night, expressed depressed mood, hopelessness, and did not engage with others. The primary team consulted psychiatry. Mirtazapine 15 mg was started for the depressive symptoms and insomnia. Neither the insomnia nor mood improved over the next 3 days, and on Hospital Day #13 the mirtazapine dose was increased to 30 mg QHS.

On hospital day #15, the Confusion Assessment Method (CAM) demonstrated that she did not know the date, time, location, or circumstances, and was unable to spell WORLD backwards. On the "A" test for vigilance, she had 3 positive errors and 2 negative errors. A second psychiatric consultant noted that the patient was inattentive, lethargic, and detached. She followed simple commands, such as opening her eyes, but could not perform more complex commands; her recall after 3 min was 0 out of 3 objects. Positive palmomental and grasp reflexes bilaterally were noted. No prior history of depressive symptoms, major depressive disorder, or major neurocognitive disorder (MNCD) could be found.

The diagnosis was changed to *hypoactive delirium*. Mirtazapine was discontinued over 2 days, and supportive oxygenation continued. Her eyeglasses and hearing aids were provided. Nighttime interruptions were minimized, and blinds were opened during the day. Family visits with masks began. As she became more aroused and attentive, her respiratory condition stabilized, she was extubated on day #16. By hospital days #18, the patient was able to concentrate and was less distractible. Mood, motor energy, and engagement with family improved. She affirmed that she did *not* want to die.

Discussion: The patient's dysphoria, suicidal statements, impaired decision-making capacity, social withdrawal, lethargy, and sleep disruption were manifestations of delirium. A corrected diagnosis of delirium, persistent, with *hypoactive* specifier, suggested the need for non-pharmacological interventions. Mirtazapine was not a good choice because isolated insomnia was not a target symptom and its weak anticholinergic properties may have exacerbated delirium.

Diagnosis and Phenomenology

Diagnostic criteria for delirium in the American Psychiatric Association's Diagnostic and Statistical Manual of Mental Disorders, Fifth Edition Text Revision (DSM-5-TR) comprise:

- Disturbance in attention and awareness.
- Develops acutely representing an acute change from baseline attention and awareness and tends to fluctuate in severity *represents an acute change from baseline attention and awareness* and tends to fluctuate in severity during the course of a day.
- An additional disturbance in cognition (e.g., memory deficit, disorientation, language, visuospatial ability, or perception).
- *The disturbances in Criteria A and C* are not better explained by a pre-existing, established, or evolving neurocognitive disorder and *do not occur in the context of a severely reduced level of arousal such as coma.*
- Evidence from the history, physical examination, or laboratory findings that the disturbance is *a direct* physiological consequence of another medical condition, *substance intoxication or withdrawal* (i.e., *due to a drug of abuse or to a medication), or exposure to a toxin, or is due to multiple etiologies.*

Delirium can be categorized into three subtypes, broadly defined by *motor* features:

- *Hyperactive*: Agitation, irritability, increased psychomotor activity, and restlessness, often with psychotic symptoms and paranoid ideation. Its rapid onset and potential danger to self and/or others due to motor agitation are hallmarks that make it easily recognizable.

- *Hypoactive*: The most prevalent subtype in geriatric patients (Oh et al. 2017) presents with lethargy, reduced psychomotor activity/withdrawal, and apathy. Severe forms can present with catatonia, marked by limited responsiveness to external stimuli. The vegetative symptoms associated with *hypoactive delirium* include low appetite, low motivation, reduced energy, which can be misdiagnosed as a depressive disorder, resulting in inappropriate treatment with antidepressants, undertreatment of underlying causes, and prolongation of delirium (Krishnan 2020; Maldonado 2017).
- *Mixed*: A combination of *hyperactive* and *hypoactive* features, which displays fluctuation between agitation and hypoactivity; the hypoactive phase can be precipitated by psychoactive medications.

Delirium has also been characterized by two symptom courses:

- A *subsyndromal* constellation of symptoms presents with cognitive impairment *without* meeting full DSM-5-TR criteria for delirium, which some experts term *acute brain failure* (Maldonado 2017). This can be considered a *prodromal* phase, presenting within hours to days with anxiety, irritability, changes in sleep, and increased sensitivity to light and sound. Its features may follow or *precede* delirium, and they may never meet full diagnostic criteria for delirium (Maldonado 2017).
- A *persistent* constellation of symptoms continues for weeks or months after the initial delirium episode despite correction and/or treatment of underlying pathology and risk factors and often shows features of the hypoactive subtype. *Persistent* delirium has been associated with worse outcomes, including progression to dementia, severe delirium, hypoxia, and other systemic medical conditions (Maldonado 2017).

Delirium can present with the following signs and symptoms (Inouye et al. 2014):

- *Reversal and fragmentation of sleep-wake cycle*: Early in its course, insomnia, midnight awakenings, daytime somnolence and sleeping, and nighttime wakefulness.
- *Perceptual disturbances*: Auditory and visual hallucinations, delusions, and illusions, such as paranoid ideation focused on caregivers, staff, or family
- *Emotional lability and dysregulation*: Agitation, irritability, dysphoria
- *Psychomotor disturbances:* Agitation, retardation, hypoactivity
- *Cognitive changes:* Impaired memory, poor executive functioning, disorientation, disorganization, poor language comprehension or expression
- *Alteration of arousal:* Impaired concentration and/or attention (e.g., inability to recite days of the week or months of the year backward)

Prevalence

Delirium is prevalent in treatment settings wherein aging individuals predominate. In palliative care, delirium has been reported in up to 85% of patients (Inouye et al. 2014), while in rehabilitation facilities, it has been identified in between 18% and 36.8% (Morichi et al. 2018). In nursing homes, the prevalence of delirium has been reported up to 40% (Inouye et al. 2014). In the intensive care unit (ICU), it has been found in 31% of patients (Krewulak et al. 2018), and up to 85% of mechanically intubated patients (Ely et al. 2004). Following elective surgical procedures, estimates of delirium range between 15 and 25% with up to 50% after high-risk procedures (Marcantonio 2017). A systematic review and meta-analysis of 33 studies using validated diagnostic criteria reported a prevalence rate of delirium at 23% (95% CI 19–26%) (Gibb et al. 2020).

Assessment

Biomarkers

The pathogenesis of delirium has not been conclusively determined, and a systematic review did not support the use of any one biomarker for the identification of delirium (Dunne et al. 2021). Although changes to levels of neurotransmitters and neuronal inflammation appear to play a central role in the pathogenesis of delirium, in the absence of validated diagnostic tests, the diagnosis of delirium rests often upon its course and presentation, with core disturbances in attention and awareness, memory deficits, disorientation, or perception, and sudden changes in behavior and cognition (see Fig. 6.1). For further discussion, see Chap. 4.

Historical information, neurological findings, and laboratory findings which may help explain the etiology and diagnosis are as follows:

- New prescriptions, adherence history, changes in dosing, abrupt medication discontinuation, and use of over-the-counter/herbal supplements along with a full list of medications and doses from all prescribers
- Medications with significant anticholinergic burden (AB) (Garpestad and Devlin 2017)
- Cognitive decline; or abrupt, unexplained changes in behavior and cognition
- Prior episodes of delirium
- Substance use, to include quantity, frequency, timing, and withdrawal from alcohol, nicotine, opioids, benzodiazepines, or stimulants
- Daily sleep, nutrition, physical activity
- Falls, head trauma, loss of consciousness episodes (warranting head CT scan)
- Recent illnesses, invasive medical procedures, surgeries
- Urinary tract infection (UTI) symptoms
- Recent flu or upper respiratory infection symptoms, including viral infections may warrant a chest-X-ray and pulse oximeter
- Reduced concentration and impaired vigilance following an infection
- Depressive symptoms.

Assessment Instruments

Standardized instruments have a high degree of sensitivity and specificity in detecting signs and symptoms of delirium. Apart from diagnosis, tests administered multiple times during the illness can measure severity, risk factors, agitation/sedation, and cognition.

The Confusion Assessment Method (CAM) or CAM-ICU takes less than 2 min each to administer. The CAM targets multiple cognitive domains: auditory and visual procession, motor execution, and language, posing some difficulties in the assessment of delirium in older patients with dementia (Duggan et al. 2021). The CAM assesses fluctuations in mental status as measured by (i) inattention, (ii) disorganized thinking, and (iii) altered level of consciousness baseline in acute presentations.

The CAM-ICU, developed for the Intensive Care Unit (ICU) or similar setting, has good inter-rater reliability and specificities. One study found that the CAM-ICU had the most supportive evidence to identify a delirium diagnosis in critically ill *older* adults with baseline dementia and has a sensitivity of 80% and specificity of 96% (Duggan et al. 2021).

However, the CAM and CAM-ICU have not shown good sensitivity in clinical settings with a predominance of *hypoactive* delirium, possibly because both instruments rely on patient's active cooperation. A prospective study of patients admitted to an inpatient geriatric unit noted that the sensitivity of CAM performed by bedside nurses was 66.7% (Lemiengre et al. 2006).

The Age-Friendly Health Systems Initiative of the Institution for Healthcare Improvement, the Coalition for Quality in Geriatric Surgery that sets hospital standards for surgical care of older adults, and the Pain, Agitation, Delirium, Immobility, and Sleep (PADIS) guidelines all recommend use of the CAM and CAM-ICU, ideally in tandem with the ABCDEF (A2F) bundle.

The ABCDEF bundle. This group of recommendations encourages assessment, prevention, and management of pain; a spontaneous awakening trial and spontaneous breathing trial; choice of sedation and analgesia; delirium assessment,

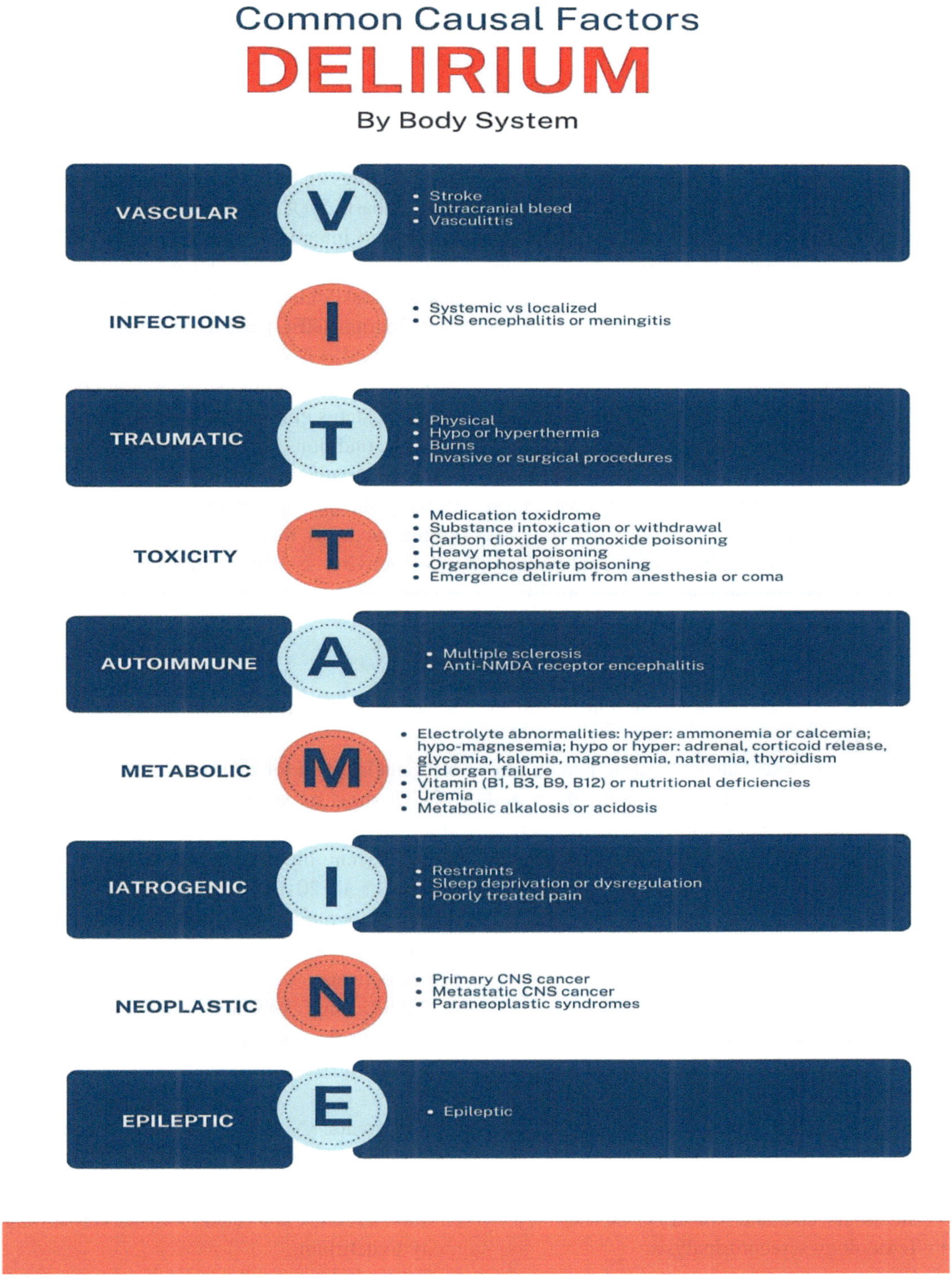

(Rita Hitching, MSc)

Fig. 6.1 Common causes of delirium by system (Rita Hitching, MSc) early mobility, and exercise; and family engagement (Duggan et al. 2021).

Stanford Proxy Tool for Delirium (S-PTD). This tool uses nursing assessment throughout the day, does not need direct patient participation, and is based on the ICD-10 and DSM-5-TR criteria for delirium. It has been shown to be robust even in the face of fluctuating symptoms of delirium and lack of patient cooperation (Alosaimi et al. 2018; Maldonado et al. 2020). The S-PTD has demonstrated a sensitivity of 80.72% and a specificity of 90.37% (Maldonado et al. 2020). See Table 6.1.

Focal Neurological Signs of Delirium

- Pupillary response: opioid (symmetric pupil constriction) or anticholinergic (symmetric pupil dilatation).
- Tremors: withdrawal from a CNS substance.
- Asterixis: hepatic or renal encephalopathy.
- Nystagmus or myoclonic jerks can point towards non-convulsive seizures.
- Lacrimation, piloerection, vital sign instability: substance intoxication or withdrawal or infection.
- Primitive reflexes such as palmomental, glabellar, grasp, snout, rooting, snout, grasp, and suck reflexes although not specific to an etiology suggest disease localized to the frontal cortex (Maldonado 2017).

Laboratory Studies

The following are the laboratory tests which can support the diagnosis of delirium (Marcantonio et al. 2006):

- Complete basic cell count (CBC)
- Comprehensive metabolic panel (CMP) including renal and liver function tests
- Toxicology screen/urinalysis
- C-reactive protein, a general marker for inflammation (Speciale et al. 2008)
- Potentially: serum melatonin, tryptophan, cortisol levels, genetic alleles like the *A9* allele of the dopamine transporter and Apolipoprotein *E4* allele (Dunne et al. 2021)

Imaging, Lumbar Puncture for CSF and EEG

The diagnostic yield of head imaging for patients with acute confusion on admission, without any focal findings on neuro exam, is low (Hufschmidt and Shabarin 2008). A lumbar puncture for CSF to rule out infection of the CNS or a subarachnoid hemorrhage has also been reported to have a low clinical yield (Cole 2005). The electroencephalogram (EEG) can help distinguish delirium from other CNS pathologies that can present with similar symptoms, such as non-convulsive seizures, status epilepticus, as well as other psychiatric conditions (Oh et al. 2017). Typical EEG findings in patients with delirium include diffuse slowing and disorganization of the cortical background activity, increased theta or delta slow-wave activity, as well as reduced reactivity to eye-opening and closing (Jacobson and Jerrier 2000).

Specific Risk Factors and Predictors

National Institute for Health and Care Excellence (NICE) suggests specific risk factors for delirium: age >65, MNCD or other cognitive impairment, current hip fracture, and severe illness (Young et al. 2010). Risk factors are additive; despite recognition and treatment of one risk factor, other factors may still lead to the continuation of delirium.

Predisposing (chronic) and precipitating (acute and/or potentially modifiable) risk factors (Maldonado 2017) include:

- Age greater than 75 years, male gender, with prior cognitive impairment or MNCD. Age-related damage to neurons and other parts of brain structure and function foster susceptibility to delirium.
- Frailty indicates reduced resilience to stressors and low functional reserve; it has an especially high prevalence in the geriatric population. One review found that frailty was an independent predictor for delirium development (Persico et al. 2018).

Table 6.1 Delirium assessment instruments

Measure type	Time to complete	Domains	Interpretation	
NEECHAM	10 min	• Attention • Orientation • Following commands	Delirium score 0–30, cut-offs • 0–20 moderate to severe • 20–24 mild	
DOS	5 min	Early recognition and assessment, with focus on effective treatment	Maximum score 46, • Severity scores 0–3 • Diagnostic items 0–2 or 0–3 • Score 0 indicates no delirium	
Nu-DESC	1 min	Disorientation Inappropriate behavior Inappropriate communication Hallucination, Psychomotor retardation	Each feature is scored by severity from 0 (absent) to 2 (severe)	
Diagnostic and symptom assessments				
SPTD	1 min	Only tool validated for DSM-5-TR and ICD-11	12 items	
CAM	5 min	Presence and severity Acute onset/varying course Inattention Disorganized thinking Disorientation Altered consciousness level Memory impairment Perceptual disturbances Agitation or retardation Altered sleep-wake cycle	Complete cognitive screen (e.g., MiniCog). Positive if patient cognitively impaired with acute onset or with varying course and inattention, plus any symptom 3–9	
CAM-ICU	1 min	Limited speech or non-verbal 1. Acuity of onset 2. Inattention 3. Altered level of consciousness 4. Disorganized thinking	Positive if patient manifests 1 and 2, and either feature 3 or 4	
Cognitive symptoms screening				
MMSE	8 min	Education can affect scores Orientation to time and place Word registration and recall Language Visual construction	Level of cognitive impairment 20–24 mild 13–20 moderate 0–12 severe	
Clock Drawing	HCP	5 min	Comprehension Visuospatial skills Motor execution and planning	Scores 0 or 1—correct or incorrect
Digit Span	HCP	5 min	Forward Backward Sequencing	Digit span of <5 considered atypical
Vigilance A	HCP	10 min	Attention Motivation Memory	Abnormal ≥2 errors

CAM Confusion Assessment Method, *CAM-ICU* Confusion Assessment Method Intensive Care Unit, *DOS* Delirium Observation Screening, *HCP* Health Care Professional Psychiatrist or Psychologist, *MMSE* Mini-Mental State Examination, *Nu-DESC* Nursing Delirium Screening scale, *NEECHAM* Neelon and Champagne Confusion Assessment, *SPTD* Stanford Proxy Test for Delirium

Sources: Grover and Kate (2012), Maldonado et al. (2020)

- Multiple systemic medical comorbidities, for example, stroke, renal or hepatic disease.
- Sensory impairments (auditory or visual) confer threefold risk in hospitalized patients.
- Malnutrition, dehydration, and indwelling catheters (Inouye 2000).
- Social isolation and reduced or low physical mobility.
- Polypharmacy, especially sedative/hypnotic or anticholinergic medications.
- Systemic metabolic or infectious disorder.
- Physical restraints and recent trauma or surgeries (Inouye et al. 2014).

In geriatric medical inpatients, the following five independent and modifiable variables were found to predict the onset of delirium (Otremba et al. 2016):

- Pre-existing diagnosis of MNCD
- Previous history of delirium
- Transfer between hospital wards
- Previous falls
- Use of proton-pump inhibitors

Differential Diagnosis (Table 6.2)

Missed Delirium

Delirium is often missed or under-reported in aging patients, especially in emergency departments. One prospective observational study used a pretest–post-test design for patients over the age of 70 seen in an academic emergency department. A diagnosis of delirium was derived from medical records in the pretest group ($N = 490$) and from the CAM-ICU in the post-test group ($N = 478$). By medical record review alone, only 14 patients (3%) were diagnosed with delirium, versus 48 patients (10%) diagnosed with delirium using the CAM-ICU (Van de Meeberg et al. 2017).

Several common assumptions can contribute to a missed delirium. See Table 6.3.

Depressive and Manic Symptoms vs. Delirium

Depressive symptoms and major depressive disorder symptoms can be prodromal to delirium and can overlap with delirium, resulting in misdiagnosis. For example, of 67 hospitalized patients older than 60 years of age referred to an inpatient psychiatric consultation service for "depression," 28 or 42% were later diagnosed with delirium by the psychiatry service (Farrell and Ganzini 1995). The patients with delirium often endorsed depressive symptoms, including depressed mood (60%), sense of worthlessness (68%), and frequent thoughts of death (52%). A presentation of depressive disorder will likely be more sub-

Table 6.2 Differential diagnosis for delirium

Neurological		Systemic Medical			Psychiatric
Structural	**Generalized**	**Organ Dysfunction**	**Metabolic Cause**	**Medication-Induced**	Major Neurocognitive disorder Depressive disorder
• Stroke • Tumors • TBI	• Non-convulsive status epilepticus • PRES • Catatonia • Limbic encephalitis • Infectious encephalitis/ meningitis	• Liver • Kidney • Heart • Lungs	• Wernicke's encephalopathy • Vitamin Deficiency • Thyroid	• Anticholinergic • Serotonin toxicity • NMS • Steroid-induced • CNS withdrawal[a]	• Psychotic disorder • Dissociative disorder • Personality disorder

TBI Traumatic brain injury, *PRES* Posterior reversible encephalopathy syndrome, *NMS* Neuroleptic malignant syndrome

[a]Alcohol, benzodiazepines, barbiturates

Table 6.3 Assumptions which can lead to missed delirium

Historical assumptions
• Cognitive deficits present are long-standing and are likely due to a major neurocognitive disorder (MNCD) responsible for *current* cognitive symptoms. (assumption)
• Depressive, mania, or related labile mood symptoms *fully explain* the current presentation
• The current altered cognitive status is the patient's baseline
• Substance abuse or substance/medication withdrawal has been ruled out
Screening assumptions
• Delirium is ruled out because no positive laboratory findings have been identified
• Delirium has resolved because of successful prior treatment of a urinary tract infection (UTI) or another infection
• Somnolence, lethargy, fatigue, detachment, and social withdrawal indicate depression rather than delirium
• Labile, irritable, intense moods reflect long-standing and pre-existing personality traits
Medication assumptions
• *Anticholinergic burden* from medications or OTC substances are not contributing to the presentation.
• The patient is taking medications as prescribed or as recommended.
• All medications, including over-the-counter, nutraceuticals, and other substances, have been identified.
• All prescribers have been identified.
• Adverse medication effects or interactions have been ruled out.

Sources: Cole (2005), Fick et al. (2002), Inouye (2006)

acute, and patients will likely lack primitive reflex signs seen in delirium. If delirium is treated successfully, a co-existing depressive disorder might become more apparent. (See Table 6.4). See Chap. 11.

According to DSM-5-TR, a manic episode is characterized as "a distinct period of abnormally and persistently elevated, expansive, or irritable mood … [often accompanied by] … inflated self-esteem or grandiosity … lasting at least 1 week …" This contrasts with *hyperactive* delirium, in which the onset of intense, fluctuating mood is abrupt and can fluctuate within minutes.

Table 6.4 Features of delirium vs. Major neurocognitive disorder (MNCD)

	Delirium	MNCD
Onset	Rapid onset hours—days-to weeks	Gradual onset: Years
Course and duration	Fluctuating and may return to baseline Duration: days to weeks; hypoactive delirium may prolong to months	Progressive decline Duration: indefinite
Fluctuating attention and impaired concentration	Yes	Varies with etiology
Level of arousal altered	Yes	Varies with etiology
Disorganized thought process	May be present	Typically absent unless a language or communication deficit present
Sleep-wake cycle disturbance	Present	Present
Perceptual disturbances: hallucinations, delusions	Visual hallucinations common Paranoid delusions	Visual hallucinations present in PDD, LBD Auditory hallucinations in all MNCD
Cognitive impairment course: can return to baseline functioning	Yes	No
Etiology discoverable	Yes	Varies with etiology

Notes: PDD Parkinson's disease dementia
DLB Dementia with Lewy bodies
Differentiation of delirium from dementia, especially end-stage MNCD, can be challenging because of many overlapping symptoms and signs
BPSD Behavioral and psychological symptoms of dementia

Substance or medication-induced/substance withdrawal symptoms can also mimic symptoms of delirium (Table 6.4).

Table 6.5 Features of delirium vs. depressive disorder

Features of delirium	Overlapping features	Major depressive disorder
• Acute or abrupt onset except hypoactive subtype • Underlying medical etiology • Fluctuating symptom severity • Altered arousal or consciousness • Inattentive to surroundings • Disorientation • Disorganization of thoughts • New comprehension deficits	• Mood dysphoric or low • Labile or inappropriate affect • Altered emotional expression • Apathy • Change in affect • Social withdrawal • Reduced motivation, activity, or lethargy • Impaired cognition and memory	• Identifiable stressors • Sustained low mood and energy • Anhedonia and loss of joy • Anxiety • Rumination • Morbid thoughts and preoccupation with loss • Self-doubt • Low self-esteem • Poor appetite

Major Neurocognitive Disorders (MNCD) vs. Delirium (Table 6.5)

MNCD has also been noted to increase the risk for developing delirium. In one study of 444 outpatients with dementia, assessed in a memory clinic, 85 had probable delirium (prevalence of 19%), and 10 had subsyndromal delirium (2%). The most common causes of delirium were infection (42%), drug-intoxication or withdrawal (22%), and metabolic/endocrine disturbance (12%). Age (OR 1.07, 95% CI 1.02–1.11) and prior delirium (OR 3.34, 95% CI 1.28–8.69) were independent nonmodifiable factors associated with an increased risk of delirium. The only independent *modifiable* risk factor was infection (OR 17.31, 95% CI 8.44–35.49) (Quispel-Aggenbach et al. 2021).

A study of hospitalized patients with AD (N = 263) followed for a median duration of 3.2 years found that 56% developed delirium during hospitalization. After controlling for MNCD severity, comorbidity, and demographic features, cognitive deterioration in patients who developed delirium in the year following hospitalization proceeded at twice the rate as those who had not developed delirium (Gross et al. 2012).

Behavioral and Psychological Symptoms of Dementia (BPSD) vs. Delirium

Correction of factors which contribute to delirium can help rule out delirium and differentiate it from BPSD.

Non-convulsive Status Epilepticus (NCSE) vs. Delirium

NCSE is defined as any alteration in mental status and corresponding changes on EEG indicative of seizures; its incidence is underestimated. Studies report the presence of NCSE in 5.2% of palliative care patients and 8.0% of comatose ICU patients (Lorenzl et al. 2010). Although no obvious outward motor signs are present; making this diagnosis is crucial. The oldest-old and critically ill patients with NCSE may present with confusion, personality change, dysphasia, subtle motor activity, and nystagmus (Beyenburg et al. 2007). If NCSE is suspected, at least 24–48 h of continuous EEG is needed for its diagnosis, as the spot EEG (usually 30–60 min) will miss approximately 50% of the cases. NCSE is treated by addressing contributing etiologies and initiating anticonvulsants (Beyenburg et al. 2007). For further discussion, see Chap. 3.

Posterior Reversible Encephalopathy Syndrome (PRES)

PRES can emerge in a hypertensive emergency, autoimmune disease, or concomitant with high dose immunosuppressants (e.g., after transplantation). Autonomic instability, headache, nausea/vomiting, seizures (which may be non-convulsive), and visual disturbances (e.g., hallucinations alterations in vision including cortical blindness) are often present. Brain imaging, especially magnetic resonance imaging (MRI), will typically demonstrate symmetric, posterior occipital/parietal/temporal predominantly white matter edema although atypical locations or asymmetric lesions can also occur (Schusse et al. 2013). Treatment includes supportive measures, discontinuation of offending agents, and control of high blood pressure and/or seizures.

Substance-Induced Mood Disorder vs. Hyperactive Delirium

A substance-induced state, or substance withdrawal syndrome, can be distinguished from delirium when exposure to a specific substance, which could cause the symptomatology, is identified and symptoms resolve when the substance is withdrawn.

Catatonia vs. Hypoactive Delirium

Catatonia is a neuropsychiatric syndrome with motor (rigidity), vocal, mood, and behavioral manifestations, including alterations in external (environmental) and internal (proprioceptive) awareness, which can overlap with, or mimic, delirium. Other medical factors (beyond antecedent psychiatric illnesses) account for greater than 50% of catatonia encountered in hospital; at least 80% of older adults are seen for catatonia by consult psychiatry or those who are critically ill have been found to have delirium (Oldham et al. 2018). If treated with antipsychotics, there is an increased risk for the neuroleptic malignant syndrome (NMS).

Autoimmune Encephalitis vs. Mixed Delirium

Autoimmune encephalitis, which may be associated with a malignancy, can occur without obvious comorbidity in geriatric patients with malignancy who present with neuropsychiatric symptoms. It is characterized by subacute onset of confusion, altered mental status, memory problems, or other psychiatric symptoms, associated with motor signs and/or characteristic findings on MRI and/or lumbar puncture (Graus et al. 2016).

Contagion

Aging individuals in specific settings are at high risk for contagion of any kind. In one study delirium was identified in 28% of 817 older adults with COVID-19 who were seen in the ED (Kennedy et al. 2020).

Pathophysiology

The *systems integration failure* hypothesis explains the etiology of delirium as a cascade of adverse neuronal events, in which neurotransmitter dysregulation and network dysconnectivity lead to what some authors have characterized as *acute brain failure* (Maldonado 2018). Neuronal aging, neuroinflammation, oxidative stress, neuroendocrine dysregulation, and circadian dysregulation are all affected by precipitating factors, such as underlying systemic medical illness. Neuronal aging, in turn, leads to increased vulnerability to stress and neuronal loss affecting how neurotransmitters are regulated. Peripheral inflammation from sources such as infection or invasive procedures (e.g., surgery) can incite inflammation that crosses the blood–brain barrier leading to neuronal and synaptic dysfunction. Oxidative stress to lipids that line the myelin sheaths damages neuronal structures and prevents normal neurotransmitter synthesis. Dysregulation of the hypothalamus-pituitary-adrenal axis leads to high basal glucocorticoid levels which impair neuronal activity and survivability. Poor sleep regulation, a risk factor for delirium, may be due to dysregulation of the melatonin-tryptophan metabolism leading to abnormal pineal gland melatonin secretion.

Delirium appears also to be correlated with changes to serum melatonin, tryptophan, cortisol levels, genetic alleles like the *A9* allele of the dopamine transporter, apolipoprotein *E4* allele (Dunne et al. 2021), and C-reactive protein—a general marker for inflammation (Speciale et al. 2008). The release of cerebral cytokines that alter neurotransmitter function have also been proposed as a possible mechanism for delirium onset (Hshieh et al. 2020). Studies of interleukins and C-reactive protein suggest that they may serve as biomarkers of delirium in the future (Hshieh et al. 2020). Chronic stress caused by trauma, severe illness, or surgery can activate the sympathetic and immune systems resulting in hypercortisolism, thyroid dysfunction, or modified permeability to the blood–brain barrier (Hshieh et al. 2020).

The aforementioned processes can result in abnormal neurotransmitter levels with *lower levels* of acetylcholine (i.e., high anticholinergic state) and *increased release and levels* of dopamine, norepinephrine, and glutamate. Depending upon the specific etiology of delirium, other neurotransmitters (i.e., serotonin, histamine, and gamma-aminobutyric acid [GABA]) are increased or decreased. Disturbance of functional neural networks can lead to failure to integrate complex information and process sensory and motor stimuli. The aged are especially vulnerable to impaired attention and other phenotypic delirium symptoms (Maldonado 2017).

Prevention and Treatment

Prevention

Prevention of delirium (Oh et al. 2017) often starts with a review of the medication regimen and tapering or discontinuing offending medications. Treatment of infection, re-hydration, correction of electrolyte abnormalities, and support of vital organ function (e.g., dialysis) are also crucial (Maldonado et al. 2017). Polypharmacy may require de-prescribing or switching medications that can contribute to delirium (Garpestad and Devlin 2017; Marcantonio 2017).

Structural brain events, such as a stroke, traumatic brain injury, or a tumor can precipitate delirium. A thorough history can elicit, for example, acute versus chronic presentation, history of trauma or falls, preceding factors, and risk factor. A neurological exam for focal neurological deficits and often neuroimaging are necessary to identify or rule out these processes.

Early mobilization (sitting up, walking) has been shown to be an effective preventative strategy. Frequent communication and education with clinical team members and caregivers can facilitate this (Inouye 2014). Home rehabilitation after acute hospitalization and an early geriatric consult have also been found to reduce delirium incidence and severity (Marcantonio 2017; Mittal et al. 2011).

Ongoing in-person or virtual connection with loved ones, supplemented by photographs, cognitive stimulation, and re-orientation, are all important. Eyeglasses and hearing aids, preservation of sleep-wake cycle, and prevention of dehydration, malnutrition, and pain are intuitive corrective measures which may be over-looked.

The ABCDEF bundle, also described under Assessment section, is a multidisciplinary intervention in the ICU to improve and/or preserve patients' function and neurocognitive status (Hshieh et al. 2018). It can decrease ICU delirium prevalence, mean number of days spent in delirium, duration of mechanical ventilation, patients' length of hospital stay, and costs associated with hospitalization (Hshieh et al. 2018).

Non-pharmacological Management

The Hospital Elder Life Program (HELP) is delivered by a multidisciplinary team consisting of caregivers, an elder life specialist, nurse specialist, geriatrician, and trained volunteers. The interventions provide orientation, therapeutic activities, sleep enhancement, early mobilization, vision and hearing adaptation, fluid repletion, feeding assistance, and pain management. A meta-analysis of 14 interventional studies demonstrated that multi-component approaches can lead to significant reductions in delirium incidence (Odds Ratio (OR) 0.47, 95% CI 0.38–0.58); decreased rate of falls (OR 0.38, 95% CI 0.25–0.60); trend towards decrease in length of stay decreased rate of institutionalization, and reduced costs of hospitalization (Hshieh et al. 2015).

Pharmacological Interventions

If preventive measures or non-pharmacological strategies cannot fully manage dangerous or self-harmful behavior due to delirium, medications should be considered.

Antipsychotics (APs). A review of 16 RCTs and 10 observational studies reported that the evidence does not support *routine* use of haloperidol or second-generation antipsychotics to treat delirium in adult inpatients. These results can be extrapolated to the geriatric population (Nikooie et al. 2019).

A meta-analysis reported that prophylactic antipsychotics (APs) in the perioperative period in aged patients at high risk for delirium *can* decrease the risk of delirium development by 50% (Teslyar et al. 2013). Several reviews and meta-analyses noted the effectiveness of APs in selected patient populations (Neufeld et al. 2016). *Dopamine antagonists* in perioperative patients have demonstrated a reduction in the development of delirium (Maldonado 2017).

Other reviews and meta-analyses have *not* demonstrated that APs alter the duration of delirium, length of hospital stay, discharge disposition, or health-related quality of life. No differences were reported in mortality or extrapyramidal side effects between individuals treated with APs as compared to those who were not (Burry et al. 2018; Nikooie et al. 2019). APs might be considered for treatment of symptoms on a case-by-case basis. Low doses of agents with minimal anticholinergic activity (e.g., risperidone) are preferred in aging patients. The *hypoactive* subtype might require especially small doses. A review of specific medications used for delirium follows below.

Haloperidol, a high potency first-generation antipsychotic (FGA) has the longest track record of being used for the treatment of delirium, and it is convenient due to its availability in (off label) intravenous form. Second-generation antipsychotics (SGAs) associated with less QTc prolongation (e.g., aripiprazole) have an advantage over haloperidol in patients where QTc is a concern. Quetiapine might be helpful in patients with symptoms of parkinsonism.

Alpha-2 agonists, in particular dexmedetomidine, have been shown to be effective for delirium prevention in patients at risk (Maldonado et al. 2009). A study of 700 patients who were 65 years of age or older admitted to the ICU for non-cardiac surgery demonstrated that delirium was significantly lower in the dexmedetomidine group compared to the placebo group (9% versus 23%; OR 0.35, 95% CI 0.22–0.54; $p < 0{\cdot}0001$) (Su et al. 2016).

Cholinesterase inhibitors. Current evidence does not support the efficacy of acetylcholinesterase inhibitors, such as rivastigmine, for delirium in aging adults.

Melatonin and its agonists have been reported as effective to prevent postoperative delirium, particularly in older patients (Campbell et al. 2019). It influences sleep-wake cycle regulation inherent in delirium symptomatology and has anti-inflammatory and antioxidant effects (Maldonado 2017). *Ramelteon*, a melatonin receptor agonist, has evidence to support its treatment of delirium (Maldonado 2017).

Suvorexant, a novel sleep agent and a selective dual orexin receptor antagonist, shows promise to prevent delirium in aging adults. A group of 72 patients (ages 65–89 years) admitted for emergency care, were randomly assigned to receive either suvorexant or placebo nightly for three nights. Delirium developed significantly *less often* among patients taking suvorexant than among those taking placebo (0% [$n/N = 0/36$] vs 17% [6/36], respectively, $P = 0.025$) (Hatta et al. 2017).

NMDA antagonists, wakefulness-promoting agents (e.g., *modafinil), and stimulants* (e.g., *methylphenidate)* have been advocated for delirium symptoms, especially for hypoactive delirium (Maldonado 2017; Sher et al. 2015a, b). A risk-benefit analysis for the frail and those with cardiac pathology such as arrythmias would be needed.

Valproate and divalproex. Multiple retrospective and prospective case series support its use in delirium, but RCTs have not conclusively established its benefit (Crowler et al. 2020; Gagnon et al. 2017; Sher et al. 2015a, b).

Delirium in Special Populations

Management of delirium in aging *ethnic* or *underserved* populations has not been thoroughly studied, and one must rely upon clinical judgment. Patients and families unfamiliar with Western conceptualization of brain failure and/or medical practice may view sudden changes or fluctuations in behavior/cognition seen in delirium as signs of mental illness. The clinician can help with explanations to prevent stigmatization or isolation of the patient.

Conclusions

When delirium is suspected, a thorough history, physical exam, and medical work-up can lead to correction and treatment of systemic medical and other etiologies. Extra vigilance is necessary to identify the *hypoactive* subtype, which is often misdiagnosed or missed entirely.

Prevention or recognition of delirium early in its course can reduce mortality, morbidity, healthcare costs, and excessive or unnecessary interventions. Prompt treatment can benefit outcome (O'Hanlon and Inouye 2020) and minimize hospitalization length; non-pharmacological interventions should be considered first. The identification of cognitive deficits following delirium in the ICU and elsewhere can facilitate rehabilitation of any residual cognitive deficits. (Tingey et al. 2022). Evaluation for impaired decision-making capacity due to delirium can avoid medical-legal complications.

A JAMA review of 127 articles, involving 11,616 treated patients, concluded that "... prevention of delirium using nonpharmacologic approaches is documented to be effective, while pharmacologic prevention and treatment of delirium remains controversial ...." (Oh et al. 2017). *Age-adjusted* medication use, however, may be necessary when non-pharmacological approaches do not ameliorate harmful symptoms and behaviors.

Age-Adjusted Recommendations

- Rule out delirium if neuropsychiatric/behavioral symptoms emerge in the geriatric patient who has no history of a major mental disorder.
- Suspect and rule out *hypoactive* delirium, when alteration of arousal, withdrawal, or lethargy emerges and is not accompanied by agitation or motor hyperactivity.
- Use screening tools such as the CAM, CAM-ICU, SPTD.
- Institute preventive measures for the aged patient at high risk for delirium.
- Employ non-pharmacological modalities as first-line interventions.
- Use medications second line to manage harmful behaviors/symptoms which cannot otherwise be managed.
- Institute pro-active preventive measures in settings at risk of delirium
  - Minimize nighttime awakenings.
  - Provide orientation, therapeutic activities, sleep enhancement, early mobilization, aids for poor vision and hearing, fluid repletion, feeding assistance, family visits, and pain management.

References

Beyenburg S, Elger CE, Reuber M. Acute confusion or altered mental state: consider nonconvulsive status epilepticus. Gerontology. 2007;53(6):388–96.

Burry L, Mehta S, Perreault MM, et al. Antipsychotics for treatment of delirium in hospitalised non-ICU patients. Cochrane Database Syst Rev. 2018;6

Campbell AM, Axon DR, Martin JR, et al. Melatonin for the prevention of postoperative delirium in older adults: a systematic review and meta-analysis. BMC Geriatr. 2019;19(1):272.

Cole MG. Delirium in elderly patients. Focus. 2005;12(2):7–332.

Crowler KE, Urben L, Hacobian G, Geiger KL. Valproic acid for the management of agitation and delirium in the intensive care setting: a retrospective analysis. Clin Ther. 2020;42(4):e65–73.

Duggan MC, Van J, Ely EW. Delirium assessment in critically ill older adults: considerations during the COVID-19 pandemic. Cri Care Clin. 2021;37(1):175–90.

Dunne SS, Coffey JC, Konje S, et al. Biomarkers in delirium: a systematic review. J Psychosom Res. 2021;147:110530.

Ely EW, Shintani A, Truman B, et al. Delirium as a predictor of mortality in mechanically ventilated patients in the intensive care unit. JAMA. 2004;291:1753–62.

Farrell KR, Ganzini L. Misdiagnosing delirium as depression in medically ill elderly patients. Arch Intern Med. 1995;155(22):2459–64.

Fick DM, Agostini JV, Inouye SK. Delirium superimposed on dementia: a systematic review. J Am Geriatr Soc. 2002;50(10):1723–32.

Gagnon DJ, Fontaine GV, Smith KE, et al. Valproate for agitation in critically ill patients: a retrospective study. J Crit Care. 2017;37:119–25.

Garpestad E, Devlin JW. Polypharmacy and delirium in critically ill older adults: recognition and prevention. Clin Geriatr Med. 2017;33(2):189–203.

Gibb K, Seeley A, Quinn T, et al. The consistent burden in published estimates of delirium occurrence in medical inpatients over four decades: a systematic review and meta-analysis study. Age Ageing. 2020;49(3):352–60.

Graus F, Titulaer MJ, Balu R, et al. A clinical approach to diagnosis of autoimmune encephalitis. Lancet Neurol. 2016;15(4):391–404.

Gross AL, Jones RN, Habtemariam DA, et al. Delirium and long-term cognitive trajectory among persons with dementia. Arch Intern Med. 2012;172(17):1324.

Grover S, Kate N. Assessment scales for delirium: a review. World J Psychiatry. 2012;2(4):58.

Hatta K, Kishi Y, Wada K, et al. Preventive effects of suvorexant on delirium: a randomized placebo-controlled trial. J Clin Psychiatry. 2017;78(8):970–9.

Hshieh TT, Yue J, Oh E, et al. Effectiveness of multicomponent nonpharmacological delirium interventions: a meta-analysis. JAMA Intern Med. 2015;175(4):512–20.

Hshieh TT, Yang T, Gartaganis SL, et al. Hospital elder life program: systematic review and meta-analysis of effectiveness. Am J Geriatr Psychiatry. 2018;26(10):1015–33.

Hshieh TT, Inouye SK, Oh ES. Delirium in the elderly. Clin Geriatr Med. 2020;36:183–99.

Hufschmidt A, Shabarin V. Diagnostic yield of cerebral imaging in patients with acute confusion. Acta Neurol Scand. 2008;118(4):245–50.

Inouye SK. Prevention of delirium in hospitalized older patients: risk factors and targeted intervention strategies. Ann Med. 2000;32(4):257–63.

Inouye SK. Delirium in older persons. N Engl J Med. 2006;354(11):1157–65.

Inouye SK, Westendorp RG, Saczynski JS. Delirium in elderly people. Lancet. 2014;383(9920):911–22.

Jacobson S, Jerrier HEEG. EEG in delirium. Semin Clin Neuropsychiatry. 2000;5(2):86–92.

Kennedy M, Helfand BKI, Gou RY, et al. Delirium in older patients with COVID-19 presenting to the emergency department. JAMA Netw Open. 2020;3(11):e2029540.

Krewulak KD, Stelfox HT, Leigh JP, et al. Incidence and prevalence of delirium subtypes in an adult ICU: a systematic review and meta-analysis. Crit Care Med. 2018;46(12):2029–35.

Krishnan V. Delirium in the elderly. BMH Med J. 2020;7(Suppl):2348–392X.

Lemiengre J, Nelis T, Joosten E, et al. Detection of delirium by bedside nurses using the confusion assessment method. J Am Geriatr Soc. 2006;54(4):685–9.

Lorenzl S, Mayer S, Feddersen B, et al. Nonconvulsive status epilepticus in palliative care patients. J Pain Manag. 2010;40(3):460–5.

Maldonado JR. Acute brain failure: pathophysiology, diagnosis, management, and sequelae of delirium. Crit Care Clin. 2017;33(3):461–519.

Maldonado JR. Delirium pathophysiology: an updated hypothesis of the etiology of acute brain failure. Int J Geriatr Psychiatry. 2018;33(11):1428–57.

Maldonado JR, Wysong A, Van Der Starre PJ, et al. Dexmedetomidine and the reduction of postoperative delirium after cardiac surgery. Psychosomatics. 2009;50(3):206–17.

Maldonado JR, Sher YI, Benitez-Lopez MA, et al. A study of the psychometric properties of the Stanford Proxy Test for Delirium (S-PTD): a new screening tool for the detection of delirium. Psychosomatics. 2020;61(2):116–26.

Marcantonio ER, Rudolph JL, Culley D, et al. Serum biomarkers for delirium. J Gerontol A Biol Sci. 2006;61(12):1281–6.

Mittal V, Muralee S, Williamson D, et al. Delirium in the elderly: a comprehensive review. Am J Alzheimers Dis Other Dement. 2011;26(2):97–109.

Morichi V, Fedecostante M, Morandi A, et al. A point prevalence study of delirium in Italian Nursing Homes. Italian Study Group on Delirium. Dement Geriatr Cogn Disord. 2018;46(1–2):27–41.

Neufeld KJ, Yue J, Robinson TN, et al. Antipsychotic medication for prevention and treatment of delirium in hospitalized adults: a systematic review and meta-analysis. J Am Geriatr Soc. 2016;64(4):705–14.

Nikooie R, Neufeld KJ, Oh ES, et al. Antipsychotics for treating delirium in hospitalized adults: a systematic review. Ann Intern Med. 2019;171(7):485–95.

O'Hanlon S, Inouye SK. Delirium: a missing piece in the COVID-19 pandemic puzzle. Age Ageing. 2020;49:497.

Oh ES, Fong TG, Hshieh TT, Inouye SK. Delirium in older persons: advances in diagnosis and treatment. JAMA. 2017;318(12):1161–74.

Oldham MA, Flaherty JH, Maldonado JR. Refining delirium: a transtheoretical model of delirium disorder with preliminary neurophysiologic subtypes. Am J Geriatr Psychiatry. 2018;26(9):913–24.

Otremba I, Wilczyński K, Szewieczek J. Delirium in the geriatric unit: proton-pump inhibitors and other risk factors. Clin Interv Aging. 2016;11:397.

Persico I, Cesari M, Morandi A, et al. Frailty and delirium in older adults: a systematic review and meta-analysis of the literature. J Am Geriatr Soc. 2018;66(10):2022–30.

Quispel-Aggenbach DW, Schep-de Ruiter EP, van Bergen W, et al. Prevalence and risk factors of delirium in psychogeriatric outpatients. Int J Geriatr Psychiatry. 2021;36(1):190–6.

Schusse CM, Peterson AL, Caplan JP. Posterior reversible encephalopathy syndrome. Psychosomatics. 2013;54(3):205–11.

Sher Y, Cramer ACM, Ament A, et al. Valproic acid for treatment of hyperactive or mixed delirium: rationale and literature review. Psychosomatics. 2015a;56(6):615–25.

Sher Y, Miller AC, Lolak S, et al. Adjunctive valproic acid in management-refractory hyperactive delirium: a case series and rationale. J Neuropsychiatry Clin Neurosci. 2015b;27(4):365–70.

Speciale S, Bellelli G, Guerini F, Trabucchi M. C-reactive protein levels and delirium in a rehabilitation ward. Age Ageing. 2008;37(1):122–3.

Su X, Meng ZT, Wu XH, et al. For prevention of delirium in elderly patients after non-cardiac surgery: a randomised, double-blind, placebo-controlled trial. Lancet. 2016;388(10054):1893–902.

Teslyar P, Stock VM, Wilk CM, et al. Prophylaxis with antipsychotic medication reduces the risk of post-operative delirium in elderly patients: a meta-analysis. Focus. 2013;11(4):544–51.

Tingey JL, Dasher NA, Bunnell AE, Starosta AJ. Intensive care-related cognitive impairment: a biopsychosocial overview. PM&R. 2022;14(2):259–72.

Van de Meeberg EK, Festen S, et al. Improved detection of delirium, implementation and validation of the CAM-ICU in elderly emergency department patients. Eur J Emerg Med. 2017;24(6):411–6.

Young J, Murthy L, Westby M, et al. Diagnosis, prevention, and management of delirium: summary of NICE guidance. BMJ. 2010;341:c3704.

Part III

Psychiatric Syndromes

Substance Use Disorders

7

Chinyere I. Ogbonna, Howard H. Fenn, and Rita Hitching

Abstract

The physiology of aging and systemic medical comorbidities exposes geriatric patients to increased risks from psychoactive substances, alcohol, stimulants, opioids, benzodiazepines, or hypnotics. Often the potential for adverse effects of these agents, even when appropriately prescribed, and the risk of abuse and/or misuse, are not explored sufficiently in aging adults. Abuse of illegal substances or prescribed medications can exacerbate age-related physical, cognitive decline, and impaired social and relationship changes. Impaired level of arousal, delayed reaction times, sedation, and imbalance all can contribute to falls, car accidents, burns, and head injuries, which accelerate loss of independence (Kuerbis et al. Clin Geriatr Med 30(3): 629–654, 2014; Markota et al. Mayo Clin Proc 91(11): 1632–1639, 2016; SAMHSA, Substance abuse among older adults. Treatment Improvement Protocol (TIP) Series, no 26. HHS Publication No. (SMA) 12–3918. Rockville, MD, Substance Abuse and Mental Health Services Administration, 2012).

This chapter reviews substance use disorders in the aging individual to encourage early recognition and appropriate interventions, which can avoid later, more severe psychiatric and systemic medical complications. We distinguish *early-onset* substance abuse which continues into older age, from *late-onset,* substance abuse, which is often associated with stressors of aging such as retirement, loss of a partner, financial strain, relocation, family conflict, social isolation, chronic pain, or health problems.

Case Example: Alcohol Use Disorder (AUD) and Anxiolytic Use Disorder

A 69-year-old corporate attorney presented to the emergency department (ED) with her daughter. The patient had slipped in the shower and fallen. X-rays showed no fractures. The patient's daughter revealed that the patient's performance at work lately had been unreliable, with many absences. An apparent decline in short-term

C. I. Ogbonna (✉)
Addiction Medicine and Recovery Services, Kaiser Permanente San Jose, San Jose, CA, USA
e-mail: cogbonna@stanford.edu; Chinyere.Ogbonna@kp.org

H. H. Fenn
VA Health Care System, Palo Alto, CA, USA

Department of Psychiatry and Behavioral Sciences, Stanford University, Stanford, CA, USA
e-mail: hhfenn@aol.com, howard.fenn@va.gov

R. Hitching
School of Medicine and Public Health, University of Newcastle, Newcastle, Australia

H. H. Fenn et al. (eds.), *Age-Adjusted Psychiatric Treatment for the Older Patient*,
https://doi.org/10.1007/978-3-031-53976-3_7

memory, general weakness, and depressed mood had been observed since the death of her husband of 45 years, 9 months earlier. Three days after the first ED visit, the patient was brought back to the ED by her daughter who now noticed her slurred speech and incoherence on the phone. The patient had been found on the floor at home next to an empty wine bottle. She was now confused, frail, diaphoretic, and tremulous. Her blood alcohol level (BAL) was noted to be 128 mg/dL. Her daughter reported that the patient lived alone, worked from home, and had been more isolated since the loss of her husband.

Over the prior 12 months, a primary care provider (PCP) had prescribed clonazepam 0.5 mg po daily as needed for anxiety, dysphoria, and insomnia following the loss of her husband; this was titrated up to 2 mg po daily as the patient reported that lower doses of clonazepam were not effective. The PCP had noticed that the patient requested early refills of clonazepam almost monthly for the past 6 months, suggesting that she had been taking more than prescribed. Appointments to review her use of clonazepam had been scheduled, but the patient did not show up.

Medical history included hypertension (blood pressure was 180/93 mm Hg in ED), poorly controlled type II diabetes mellitus, and peripheral neuropathy. Her adherence with metformin or the lisinopril was not confirmed. When finally seen in primary care, she acknowledged drinking "a glass of wine or two" every evening at dinner, after which she took clonazepam to help "calm my nerves" and initiate sleep. She did not know how much clonazepam she took daily and she noted she had become more forgetful but attributed this to aging. She also endorsed symptoms of depression, which were likely related to bereavement and/or substance-induced depressive disorder.

Discussion: Family provided a history of diminished nutrition, a 20 lb. weight loss, intermittent unsteady gait, falls, and judgment lapses along with abuse of clonazepam prescriptions, marked by early refills. The diagnosis was *anxiolytic use disorder*. Alcohol and benzodiazepine withdrawal were successful over the course of a 7-day inpatient stay without complications, using the Clinical Institute Withdrawal Assessment for Alcohol revised (CIWA-Ar) protocol. The patient was then referred to a specialized inpatient unit for treatment of depressive disorder, anxiolytic use disorder, and alcohol use disorder.

Diagnosis of SUD and Epidemiology

At least two of the following 11 DSM-5 criteria must be met within a 12-month period to fulfill SUD. Medications which have been appropriately prescribed can still fulfill SUD criteria for a substance use disorder if criteria are met (See Fig. 7.1).

Data from the National Surveys on Drug Use and Health (NSDUH) estimates past-year substance use disorder (SUD) rates among adults >50 years at 2.8 million in 2006–2016; this was expected to reach 5.7 million in 2020 (Han et al. 2009). Other studies report that excessive use of opioids among geriatric patients alone may also account for the increase in total substance use in the United States (Blow and Barry 2014; Kuerbis et al. 2014). SUD in aged individuals has also been associated with an increase in mortality. Drug overdose deaths in those >65 years, with both opioid analgesics and benzodiazepines, increased by 0.3 per 1,000,000 population between 2004 and 2011 (Jones and McAninch 2015). Risk factors for substance use in later life include the previous history of substance abuse, poor health status, chronic psychiatric and/or medical comorbidities, chronic pain, polypharmacy, gender (men: alcohol, women: prescription drugs), affluence, and limited coping skills (Kuerbis et al. 2014).

The National Ambulatory Care Survey from 2014 to 2016 reported that the rate of office visits with benzodiazepine and opioid prescriptions increased by age, with those 65 years old and older receiving more prescriptions than younger age cohorts. Well-intentioned prescribing practices to relieve pain, anxiety, and insomnia may be partially responsible. Women aged 65 and older have been the most prescribed age group (Santo et al. 2020).

The majority of adults aged 50 years and older with substance use disorders have been projected to be white (76%) and male (71%); Latino and

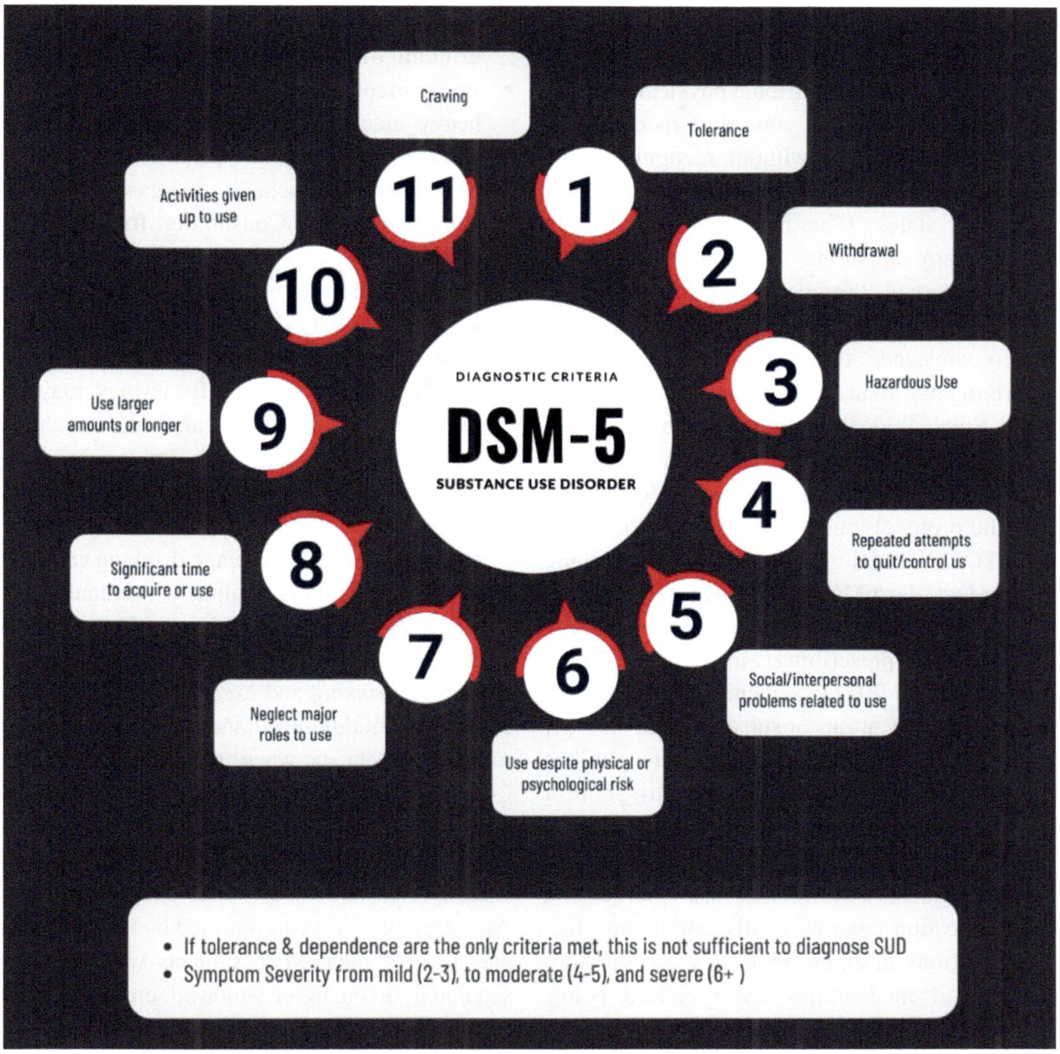

(Rita Hitching, MSc.)

Fig. 7.1 DSM-5 Substance Use Criteria

Black individuals 50 years and older were projected to have a similar prevalence of substance use disorders in 2020 (10% and 10.5%, respectively). However, these numbers were based upon self-report (Wu and Blazer 2011).

Assessment

Aging adults may present with complaints of changes in sleep patterns, recurrent falls, somatic symptoms, dizziness and lightheadedness, anxiety, and changes to mood or alertness, all of which may be attributed to aging and/or comorbid medical and psychiatric conditions. These concerns can obscure recognition of physical dependence, substance misuse, or substance use disorder (SUD). Dependence upon some medications, such as benzodiazepines, may become obvious with the onset of withdrawal symptoms (rebound anxiety and increased dysphoria) when the medication dose is lowered. These symptoms may be misinterpreted as evidence that the medication is effectively controlling an underlying anxiety disorder or depression, prompting a continuation or even increase in the dose.

Aging patients may attribute physical and psychological problems to comorbid medical and psychiatric conditions without recognizing the substance-induced impact to their cognitive or functional status (Kuerbis et al. 2013). In addition, any apparent alteration of cognitive functioning (e.g., "fogginess" or forgetfulness), or emergence of psychiatric symptoms can be due to substance intoxication rather than an underlying psychiatric condition (Han and Moore 2018). Suicidal ideation, intent, and attempts are more likely lethal when substance use is involved (Choi et al. 2015; Han and Moore 2018).

Some protocols such as the EU (7)-PIM List, the STOPP/START (https://www.ncbi.nlm.nih.gov/pmc/articles/pMC4339726/) and Beers criteria offer guidance on screening for potentially inappropriate prescribing in aging people (Perpétuo et al. 2021). Screening for misuse of *prescribed* medications or substance use disorder can also help identify psychosocial interventions that address stressors which may be triggers for continued medication misuse or substance abuse (Blow and Barry 2014).

The diagnosis of substance use disorder and safe medication tapering or discontinuation recommendations in aging adults for specific substances and medications are reviewed below (Bart et al. 2020; Maree et al. 2016).

Alcohol

Prevalence

At least 17% of Americans aged >60 years have an alcohol or prescription drug use disorder (National Institute on Alcohol Abuse and Alcoholism (NIAAA 2020)). The presence of alcohol use disorders in aging patients is reported at 30% in medical settings and 50% in psychiatric units. Substantial functional, medical, and psychiatric impairments are associated with alcohol abuse and aging (Jemberie et al. 2020).

Patterns of excessive alcohol use among older adults are as follows:

- Continuous: Ongoing, continuous pattern of drinking over the years.
- Intermittent drinking: A return to regular, heavy alcohol use after a period of stable abstinence of at least 3 years. The risk of intermittent drinking behavior increases with age.
- Binge drinking: Consuming four or more drinks per occasion; but can also be described as short periods of excessive alcohol use alternating, with periods of abstinence or reduced alcohol use (SAMHSA 2012). Binge drinkers can be difficult to identify as they may not experience the usual social, occupational, or legal consequences often experienced by younger drinkers.

Both intermittent and binge drinking can be as hazardous to the older adult as continuous drinking (SAMHSA 2012). A nationwide survey in the United States by Blazer and Wu (2009) concluded that *binge drinking* and *excessive* alcohol use are common in middle-aged and older adults and are more prevalent between the ages of 50 and 64 years. Tobacco and illicit drug use were associated with binge drinking across all age groups. For older age groups ≥65 years, binge drinking was reported in 3% of women and 14% of men. At-risk alcohol use was reported by 8% of women and 13% of men. Male subjects were typically separated, divorced, or widowed, employed, high income, and using prescription medications for non-medical purposes. In contrast, females were more likely to be African American and less educated (Blazer and Wu 2009). Based on surveys done in 2018, the rates of past-month binge alcohol use were 18.1% for adults 50 or older and 10.7% for adults 65 or older (SAMHSA 2019).

At-risk drinking (more than 3 drinks per occasion or more than 7 drinks per week) is more prevalent than alcohol use disorder for adults older than 65 years (Kuerbis et al. 2014).

Assessment

Most screening tools were created and validated in younger populations and may *under-identify* older adults with problematic alcohol use.

Table 7.1 Substance and alcohol use disorder screening tools

Assessment	Acronym	Clinical Usefulness	Limitations	Minutes
Alcohol use disorders identification test	AUDIT	First-line use validated in older adults for hazardous or problematic. Lower cut-off scores are recommended	Only half of the screen is sensitive and specific for older adults consequences of consumption less relevant to older adults	2
Michigan alcoholism screening test geriatric	MAST-G	Highly sensitive and specific, explores stressors and behaviors relevant to late-life use of alcohol	No information on quantity, frequency, and current problems with alcohol use	8
Cut-down annoyed guilty eye-opener	CAGE	First-line use and useful at identifying dependence	Poor at detecting heavy or binge use, and consequences of use	1
Brief drinker profile	BDP	Guidance on consumption, drinking patterns, and commensurate impairment	Limited normative data, lengthy to administer not ideal for screening	4
Quantity frequency	Q-F	Ideal to screen consumption	Limited at measuring dependence and consequences of use	1
Alcohol dependence scale	ADS	Screens for dependence and impact of use	High threshold and less suitable for older adults	5

Patients with a positive score on any screening tool should undergo further assessment.

The National Institute on Alcohol Abuse and Alcoholism (NIAAA) single-item screener is effective for problematic alcohol use (Smith et al. 2009). For patients that screen positive on the single-item screener, the Alcohol Use Disorders Identification Test (AUDIT-C) and the Michigan Alcoholism Screening Test (MAST-Geriatric or short version SMAST-G) are recommended as additional screening for unhealthy or at-risk alcohol use (Knightly et al. 2016). Nevertheless, alcohol-related harm among aging adults is possible even without meeting full criteria of AUD using DSM-5-TR criteria. Alcohol use screening tools for older individuals are summarized in Table 7.1.

Alcohol Intoxication

Excessive consumption of alcohol is characterized by behavioral and psychological changes correlated with severity of intoxication, such as impaired memory and attention, unsteady gait, loss of coordination, stupor, and coma, nystagmus, paired with a loss of social or sexual inhibition, increased aggression, and mood changes (Butt et al. 2020; Jemberie et al. 2020). Age-related changes, such as loss of lean body mass, decreased total body water, decreased liver metabolism of alcohol, increased permeability of the blood–brain barrier, and neuronal sensitivity to alcohol in the brain, make older individuals more susceptible to physical and cognitive impairment compared with younger adults (Kuerbis et al. 2014).

Alcohol Withdrawal

Management of withdrawal for the young-old and oldest-old is accomplished best in an inpatient setting. Symptoms include dysphoria, pupillary piloerection or dilation, aches and pains, yawning, lacrimation and rhinorrhea, insomnia, nausea and vomiting, autonomic hyperactivity (temperature, heart rate, blood pressure), psychomotor agitation, delusions and hallucinations, tremor, seizures, delirium, and coma. The Clinical Institute Withdrawal Assessment for Alcohol revised (CIWA-Ar) offers standard withdrawal protocols, adjusted individually for physical health, substance use history, prior withdrawal attempts, and complications (DiBartolo and Jarosinski 2017; Mulkey and Olson 2020). In chronic, severe alcohol abuse, the patient will likely have depleted nutritional reserves; multivitamins, thiamine, and folate may be recommended (Eloma et al. 2018). The CIWA-Ar guidelines provide dosing schedules for medications such as lorazepam or diazepam to facilitate uncomplicated alcohol and benzodiazepine withdrawal.

Management of alcohol withdrawal in geriatric adults also requires vigilance for concomitant neurological and medical complications. The young-old face fewer risks than older alcoholics, including a less extreme increase in blood pressure (BP), less pronounced alcoholic liver disease, and reduced risk of breast cancer in menopausal women. Aging adults who adhere to an alcohol discontinuation protocol show 20% abstinence rates after 4 years (Caputo et al. 2012).

Benzodiazepines and anti-epileptic drugs (AEDs) have the strongest evidence for the management of alcohol withdrawal (Hammond et al. 2015). An *age-adjusted* approach suggests dosages at one-third to one-half or less of the usual benzodiazepine dose, continual monitoring, and rapid tapering within 1–2 days (Sachdeva et al. 2015).

Alcohol Use Disorder Treatment: Psychosocial Interventions for Aging Patients

Aging individuals who have an extensive history of alcohol abuse or dependence may not be able to achieve the goal of absolute abstinence but can minimize *excessive* use (Han and Moore 2018). Community-based residential treatment and outpatient treatment programs have a role. An *age-adjusted* approach to AUD in aging adults emphasizes psychosocial interventions as first-line, before medications. Treatment outcomes have shown that aged patients who engage in residential treatment in age-integrated programs have good outcomes, at least as comparable to those experienced by middle-aged and younger patients, and better outcomes over a 5-year follow-up period, when compared to younger patients (Lemke and Moos 2003). Although aged patients tended to have similar patterns of alcohol use at initiation of treatment as younger patients, they experienced fewer negative consequences and fewer symptoms of psychological distress. Both aging and younger patients benefitted from longer treatment stays, more counseling sessions, and an emotionally supportive treatment environment. Yet all age groups had poor outcomes in programs with fewer activities and poorly defined treatment goals.

Age-integrated programs with varied therapeutic emphasis appear to work well for aging adults regardless of whether tailored for older patients or not (Lemke and Moos 2003). Variations in polysubstance use, medical comorbidities, and cognitive functioning were not related to positive outcomes and did not affect the participation of aged adults in informal support groups or in professional outpatient care (Lemke and Moos 2003). At discharge, personal functioning characteristics, specifically situational confidence, and approach-coping strategies, were the strongest outcome predictors. This suggests an important area of focus during treatment. After discharge from residential care programs, the duration of time in self-help group participation was also found to be important to maintain gains. Discharge planning should anticipate and reduce barriers to meeting attendance and strive to establish a relationship with a sponsor (Lemke and Moos 2003).

Alcohol Use Disorder (AUD) Treatment: Pharmacological Interventions for Aging Patients

There are three FDA-approved medications for AUD: disulfiram (Antabuse), acamprosate (Campral), and naltrexone (ReVia oral, Vivitrol IM), but their long-term efficacy in older adults has not been established. Medications can enhance motivation, strengthen adherence, improve coping skills, and reduce cravings or withdrawal symptoms that trigger relapse. Treatment plans are most effective when medications combine with behavioral interventions.

Disulfiram was the first medication approved by the FDA for the treatment of AUD in 1951. It is an alcohol-aversive or alcohol-sensitizing agent which results in a drug-ethanol reaction (DER) when mixed with alcohol. Disulfiram inhibits the enzyme aldehyde dehydrogenase, which interrupts the normal metabolism of alcohol and temporarily increases the concentration of acetaldehyde to 5 to 10 times the normal blood concentration. The DER is proportional to the amount of disulfiram and alcohol ingested but can be unpredictable in the onset and severity of symptoms.

DER consists of sweating, flushing of the upper chest and face, respiratory difficulty, blurred vision, headache, GI disturbance, chest palpitations, weakness, syncope, and confusion. Severe reactions may include arrhythmias, myocardial infarction, acute congestive heart failure, respiratory depression, seizures, and even death. Due to the potential for severe DER, disulfiram is contraindicated in patients with a history of severe cardiac disease or liver disease, or in the frail or oldest-old. Monitoring liver enzymes for signs of hepatotoxicity and checking for impulsivity or cognitive impairment are good practices (CSAT 2009).

Prescribing disulfiram requires assessment for capacity to consent since patients with mild cognitive deficits would be at risk of adverse effects or of unintentional alcohol use. No withdrawal symptoms are associated with disulfiram, but a DER can occur if alcohol is consumed within 14 days of the last dose (CSAT 2009), which also makes cognitive impairment an inherent risk (Ogbonna and Lembke 2019).

Acamprosate can reduce the post-acute symptoms of alcohol withdrawal by modulating brain excitability via interaction with glutamate although the exact mechanism of action is not well understood. Acamprosate has been found to decrease the number of drinking days and increase the number of abstinent days, lengthening the time to relapse (CSAT 2009). Its efficacy has not been well-studied among aging adults, but it is considered safe (Kuerbis et al. 2014). *Acamprosate* is typically started 5 days after the last drink but can be started during medically supervised withdrawal and can be continued in the event of relapse. The best outcomes are observed in individuals who are motivated to achieve complete abstinence. Contraindications include severe renal impairment although it can be prescribed to aged adults with renal insufficiency if renal function tests are done and medication is started at a reduced dose, with periodic monitoring. Intolerance of GI side effects and difficulty with three times daily schedule are common reasons for discontinuation. There are no known withdrawal symptoms associated with the discontinuation of acamprosate (CSAT 2009).

Naltrexone is an opioid antagonist that exerts its effect by blocking alcohol-induced dopamine release in the brain. It is contraindicated for anyone taking opioid agonists for chronic pain (Kuerbis et al. 2014). It has been studied among aging adults and shown effective when taken daily to reduce craving and the pleasurable feeling from drinking alcohol (Kuerbis et al. 2014). *Naltrexone* has a low incidence of adverse effects and few drug interactions (CSAT 2009). To avoid precipitating opioid withdrawal, especially in the aged individual, naltrexone should be started after at least 7–10 days from the last dose of opioids; conversely, opioids should not be initiated until at least 7 days after the *last dose* of naltrexone (CSAT 2009). In the United States, an X-waiver to prescribe Suboxone (trade name for buprenorphine/naloxone) should be considered for psychiatrists who treat geriatric patients.

In addition to abstinence, *naltrexone* can be effective in *reducing* the amount of alcohol intake. Most common side effects: headache, nausea, and fatigue. Strategies to minimize adverse effects include starting at a lower dose and increasing the dose gradually as tolerated to the FDA recommended treatment dose of 50 mg daily. Liver monitoring tests are performed before initiation of therapy and at regular intervals thereafter. Caution is advised if liver enzyme tests greater than five times the upper limit of normal or if there is a history of moderate to severe renal impairment. *Naltrexone* can be prescribed as an oral medication (ReVia) administered daily or as an intramuscular injection (Vivitrol) every 4 weeks in case of poor adherence (CSAT 2009). Patients with comorbid depression should also be monitored for worsening depressive symptoms (Kuerbis et al. 2014).

Benzodiazepines, Sedative-Hypnotics, Barbiturates, and Z-Drugs

Benzodiazepines are typically prescribed for anxiety and insomnia. For the aging adult, the loss of economic and social supports, and medical/mental health problems, all increase the risk for prescription misuse and abuse. Benzodiazepines with long half-lives, longer duration of action, and those with active metabolites may increase vulnerability for adverse events (SAMHSA 2012).

Poor physical health and female gender confer the greatest risk for psychoactive drug misuse. Other risk factors for psychoactive drug abuse include middle—and late-life divorces, widowhood, less education, lower income, more physical and psychiatric disorders, and chronic somatic problems (SAMHSA 2012).

The absence of a prior history of substance use is not enough to rule out substance misuse or abuse. Even without firm evidence, aberrant behaviors may offer clues: craving or a "need" to take psychoactive medication to function, requests for early prescriptions, multiple "lost" prescriptions, requests for increased dose (tolerance), or attempts to obtain prescription medications from other prescribers (Markota et al. 2016).

The US FDA issued a boxed warning for benzodiazepines in September of 2020 due to "serious risks of abuse, addiction, physical dependence, and withdrawal reactions" among this class of medications (Hirschtritt et al. 2021). In the United States, common benzodiazepines include alprazolam (Xanax), diazepam (Valium), lorazepam (Ativan), flurazepam (Dalmane), chlordiazepoxide (Librium); common barbiturates include clorazepate (Tranxene), secobarbital (Seconal), and pentobarbital (Nembutal).

Even if benzodiazepines are taken as prescribed at therapeutic doses for 2 months, patients will likely develop physiological dependence and/or experience uncomfortable withdrawal symptoms when tapered or discontinued (Conn et al. 2020). The diminished ability to metabolize substances over the age of 65 years paired with increased brain sensitivity, compounds the risk of withdrawal symptoms, irrespective of the level of abuse or dependence.

The need to taper off benzodiazepines is suggested by:

- Daily benzodiazepine use for longer than 1 month.
- Age > 65 years with increased risk of falls and cognitive adverse effects.
- Several benzodiazepines or concurrent opioids, sedatives, or stimulants (Guina and Merrill 2018; Markota et al. 2016).
- Supra-therapeutic doses of benzodiazepines.
- History of traumatic brain injury.
- Current or history of substance use disorder—especially alcohol or sedative-hypnotic use disorder (Ogbonna and Lembke 2017).
- The use of benzodiazepines at doses or schedules which are not recommended, as well as early refills, multiple prescribers, medications from non-prescribers.

Recommendations for Tapering Benzodiazepines

After 4–6 months of chronic benzodiazepine use, withdrawal symptoms are experienced by 40–80% of people regardless of abrupt discontinuation or gradual taper (SAMHSA 2012). The following are symptoms associated with benzodiazepine withdrawal are similar to alcohol withdrawal (SAMHSA 2012):

- Increased anxiety and agitation.
- Impaired concentration.
- Derealization and depersonalization.
- Insomnia.
- Tremor, poor coordination, dizziness.
- Loss of appetite.
- Lethargy.

If a benzodiazepine taper is done too quickly, the aforementioned withdrawal symptoms may not be tolerable; if so, consider maintaining a current dose before resuming the taper (SAMHSA 2012).

Dose *increases,* however, with the intent of relieving withdrawal symptoms can result in a gradual return of the *original symptoms* for which the benzodiazepines were prescribed, due to the development of tolerance. These original symptoms may be difficult to ameliorate despite resuming benzodiazepines or adding adjuvant medications (SAMHSA 2012). Withdrawal symptoms typically resolve within 3–5 weeks after discontinuation of the benzodiazepine but have been known to last as long as several months. The approach of avoiding dose increases can help distinguish withdrawal symptoms from the original symptoms.

Strategies for deprescribing benzodiazepine and other hypnotics include pharmacist and clinician-directed tapers, patient education, psychotherapy, and pharmacologic substitution (e.g., with SSRIs for anxiety, or melatonin for insomnia) (Reeve et al. 2017). For patients at risk of severe or life-threatening adverse effects, some authors recommend avoiding medications with narrow therapeutic indices (Fluyau et al. 2018). Few RCTs show clear evidence of the efficacy of medication substitution when tapering benzodiazepines (Fluyau et al. 2018), but anti-epileptics seem to offer modest improvement (Brett and Murnion 2015). Psychotherapeutic interventions can minimize avoidance behaviors, promote cognitive processing, and help extinguish fear upon exposure to stressors (Guina and Merrill 2018).

The following are strategies which support a clinician–patient alliance of tapering (Ogbonna and Lembke 2017):

- Establish rapport with a trial of dose reduction, to bolster the patient's confidence, sense of control, and to reduce anxiety prior to a full withdrawal protocol.
- Educate about the long-term benefits of discontinuation.
- Offer choices in the rate of dose reduction, dose increments, and the frequency of reduction; doses can be reduced gradually in tiny increments.
- Consider the dose, potency, duration of benzodiazepine use, timing of doses, and psychosocial stressors.
- Employ psychotherapy, such as cognitive-behavioral therapy (CBT) in the first few months of tapering although these effects diminish after 3 months (Darker et al. 2015).
- Emphasize a *uni-directional* taper; the dose will only be *reduced, never increased* (Guina and Merrill 2018).
- Allow flexibility in scheduling the taper during the last 10%–20% of dose reduction (Guina and Merrill 2018).

With successful withdrawal, other factors, including stressors and psychiatric symptoms, which contributed to the development of the SUD, can be identified and addressed.

Barbiturates are not prescribed widely in the United States, and there is little information about the need for their tapering. A Medicare Part D prescriptions database for 2019 (https://www.cms.gov/Research-Statistics-Data-and-Systems/Statistics-Trends-and-Reports/Information-on-Prescription-Drugs/MedicarePartD) did not list beneficiaries who had received secobarbital or pentobarbital.

Non-benzodiazepine receptor agonists or "Z-drugs," such as zolpidem (Ambien) and zaleplon (Sonata), chemically similar to benzodiazepines, are typically prescribed for insomnia, but may not be effective beyond short-term use. They are associated with increased risk for delirium, falls, fractures, and motor vehicle accidents (Markota et al. 2016). They also pose a risk of adverse effects and potential for addiction, particularly among the old-old over time (McHugh et al. 2020; National Institute of Drug Abuse (NIDA) 2020; Han and Moore 2018).

Polysubstance Misuse and Overdose

Hospital admissions for overdoses within geriatric populations has been reported as high as 38% in 2012 (Chhatre et al. 2017). Co-ingestion of multiple substances obscures which specific withdrawal symptom is associated with which substance (Chhatre et al. 2017). Polysubstance use, sudden discontinuation, or restarting medication after a period of abstinence increases the risks of overdose, drug–drug interactions, autonomic hyperactivity, or seizures. Use beyond the patient's typical daily dose can lead to disinhibition and motor impairment similar to excessive alcohol use (McHugh et al. 2020; Fluyau et al. 2018).

Alternative Medications for Insomnia

Sleep restriction and CBT show evidence of benefit among older adults (Markota et al. 2016). Non-benzodiazepine medications and melatonin receptor antagonists are the safest and most efficacious medications available for the treatment of insomnia. Prescribers should review both prescription and over-the-counter medications taken for chronic medical/psychiatric conditions to identify factors which may cause or exacerbate insomnia (Bloom et al. 2009). For further discussion, see Chap. 8.

Opioids

Prevalence of Misuse and Use Disorder

Opioid abuse in aging adults is a leading cause of emergency department visits, representing 34% of all opioid-related hospitalizations and a 74% increase between 2010 and 2015 (Weiss et al. 2018). According to the US Centers for Disease Control (CDC), 20% of Americans use analgesics multiple times per week and 18% of Americans diagnosed with chronic pain also met DSM-5 criteria for opioid abuse or dependence in 2018. A representative sample of middle-aged and older adults estimated 1.4% of aging adults reported nonprescription use of opioids during the previous year (Blazer and Wu 2009).

The CDC also reported that Americans aged ≥65 years demonstrated a 17% increase in opioid overdose deaths between 2016 and 2017 (Scholl et al. 2019). A global increase in opioid prescribing for chronic pain has emerged (Bedson et al. 2016) and appears greater in the United States, which consumes above 80% of the global opioid supply and up to 99% of the world's oxycodone and hydrocodone (Häuser and Tölle 2017). From 1999 to 2014 an increase in prescription opioid use by US adults rose from 4.1% in 1999 to 6.8% in 2014. This increase correlated with a history of heroin use, poor health, and concurrent benzodiazepine use (Mojtabai 2018). While some patients benefit from long-term opioid use, the risks of dependence, abuse, self-poisoning, and falls are high (Saunders et al. 2010).

Aging adults metabolize opioids slower due to decreased gastrointestinal absorption of orally ingested formulations, and they experience a longer duration of action due to age-related decreases in liver function. Age-related changes in opioid receptor sensitivity contribute to the rapid development of tolerance and dependence which raise the risk for adverse effects from chronic opioid use (SAMHSA 2012).

The prescribing data supports the recommendation that aging adults with acute chronic pain receive "the lowest effective dose of the least potent immediate-release opioid for ≤ 3 days and rarely > 7 days" (Rieb et al. 2020). For treatment of chronic non-cancer pain, non-opioid pain management modalities should be exhausted before starting chronic opioid therapy. Geriatric patients without a history of substance use disorder or active mental illness may be candidates for chronic low dose opioid therapy; treatment should be discontinued if there is no evidence of functional improvement or with the onset of adverse effects. Polypharmacy and co-prescribing of other CNS-depressant medications should be avoided (Rieb et al. 2020).

Assessment

Screening tools for opioid use disorder (OUD) include the Opioid Risk Tool (ORT), the National Institute of Drug Abuse Quick Screen (NMASSIT) for patients with pain, and the Screener and Opioid Assessment for Patients with Pain Revised (SOAPP-R). Positive screening results should be followed by a medication review, cognitive assessment, and a functional and physical exam, with attention to signs of intoxication, withdrawal, or other physical signs of substance abuse. A urine drug screen can be considered (Reib et al. 2002). Table 7.2 lists substance-abuse-specific presenting symptoms.

Opioid Intoxication

Symptoms of sedation, and impairment of psychomotor function, vision, attention, and motor coordination can present as dose-dependent manifestations (SAMHSA 2012). Visible behavioral and cognitive changes range from mild to severe, depending on the level of intoxication. Changes to mood and affect can result in apathy, even if the initial mood was euphoric or dysphoric. Psychomotor retardation or agitation, hallucinations, and pupil dilation or constriction may be caused by anoxia. Other symptoms of intoxication include cognitive impairment, judgment, memory, and attention, slurred speech; diminished arousal, drowsiness, or coma (Guina and Merrill 2018; Stitt and Kumar 2020).

Naloxone, a short-acting opioid antagonist, can be administered in emergency situations to treat opioid overdose (McQuade et al. 2021).

Table 7.2 Symptoms and features of substance use disorders[a]

	Alcohol and Benzodiazepines	Opioids	Hypnotics	Marijuana	Stimulants
Behavioral changes	• Impaired judgment • Mood changes • Sexual disinhibition • Aggressive behavior	• Psychomotor agitation or retardation • Tachycardia • Orthostatic hypertension • Impaired judgment • Euphoria, dysphoria, or apathy	• Drowsiness or coma • Confusion • Euphoria, dysphoria, or apathy • Dry mouth • Nausea	• Increased appetite • Mood changes and irritability • Reduced focus and attention • Nausea and diarrhea	• Mood swings • Euphoria and increased confidence • Reduced appetite • Sexual arousal. • Dehydration • Appetite changes
Symptoms Signs	• Impaired memory or attention • Nystagmus • Poor coordination • unsteady gait • Slurred speech • Stupor or coma	• Nystagmus • Ataxia or slurred speech • Memory or attention deficit • Respiratory changes • Drowsiness or coma • Pupillary changes • Hallucinations	• Poor short-term memory • Hallucinations • Headache • Rebound insomnia • Fatigue • Abnormal dreams	• Impaired coordination and dizziness • Slowed reaction time • Impaired memory • Lack of motivation • Hallucinations and delusions • Distorted perception • Drowsiness and relaxation	• Impaired memory • Lack of motivation • Aggression and paranoia • Anxiety and panic attacks • Distorted perception • Relaxed state or sleepiness • Tremor and seizure
Intoxication overdose management	• IV fluids • oxygen and airway protection • Vitamin infusion, thiamine, and folate	• Oxygen and airway protection • Administer naloxone (Narcan) for acute opioid overdose • Clonidine, gabapentin, hydroxyzine, trazodone for supportive management of opioid withdrawal • Buprenorphine or methadone for medication-assisted therapy (MAT)	• Monitor and manage aspiration, respiratory depression, hypoxia, hypotension, and cardiac arrhythmias • Consider ultrashort acting methohexital and thiopental • In severe cases flumazenil	• Oxygen and airway protection • Manage hypoglycemia if present • Pneumothorax or pneumomediastinum manage with oxygen if severe needle decompression or chest tube • Manage asthma with nebulizer and short-acting beta2 agonist	• Ensure airway and oxygen is clear • Benzodiazepine or low dose antipsychotic for anxiety and agitation in severe cases intramuscular droperidol or zuclopenthixol acetate • Monitor serotonin toxicity, delirium, and confusion

[a]Adapted from Kuerbis et al. 2014

Risk factors for opioid overdose include concomitant use of benzodiazepines, opioid doses of ≥50 morphine milligram equivalents (MME) per day, history of alcohol use disorder, and a previous history of opioid overdose (Luther et al. 2021). Although geriatric individuals are at-risk for overdose due to age-related physiologic changes that impact opioid pharmacokinetics, a national pharmacy study examining naloxone dispensing rates in 2018 showed fewer than 0.75% of adults older than 65 years of age filled a naloxone prescription. For aging adults with risk factors, clinicians should consider prescribing naloxone. To reduce hesitancy and uncertainty due to fear of offending patients, many health systems have implemented naloxone prescribing protocols (Luther et al. 2021). Where access to primary care providers and pharmacies are limited, provider-extenders and home health workers can give training on the use of naloxone to reverse opioid overdose to community-dwelling older adults. One such program is the SAFE—Home Opioid Management Education (SAFE-HOME) in aging adults, a naloxone awareness program for home health workers (McQuade et al. 2021).

Opioid Withdrawal Management

Opioid withdrawal is uncomfortable, but rarely life-threatening, unlike withdrawal syndromes for alcohol or benzodiazepines (SAMHSA 2012). Acute symptoms present within 8 to 24 h from last use for short-acting opioids and within 36 h from last use with long-acting opioids. The severity of opioid withdrawal symptoms is dose-dependent based on the level of physical dependence, duration of use, and specific opioids taken by the patient. Opioid withdrawal is often accompanied by gastroenteritis, severe influenza, anxiety, and dysphoria (SAMHSA 2020). Common symptoms of acute opioid withdrawal also include lacrimation, rhinorrhea, dilated pupils, yawning, tachycardia, nausea/vomiting, diarrhea, anorexia, piloerection, myalgias/arthralgias, GI distress, restlessness, and insomnia.

Acute withdrawal symptoms peak between 1 and 3 days from last use and last about 7–10 days for short-acting opioids, and peak between 3 and 4 days from last use and last about 14 days or more for long-acting opioids. Symptoms of dysphoria, craving, insomnia, and hyperalgesia can persist for weeks to months after last use. Clinical tools such as the Clinical Opiate Withdrawal Scale (COWS) and the Clinical Institute Narcotic Assessment (CINA) Scale for Withdrawal Symptoms provide objective and standardized data points to assess severity of withdrawal symptoms (SAMHSA 2022).

To taper aging adults off opioids, decrease the dose of opioids with a slowly, by 5% every 2 to 8 weeks with rest periods. Slower tapers minimize the risk of severe opioid withdrawal symptoms and are often better tolerated compared to more rapid tapers or abrupt discontinuation. Aging adults may benefit from time-limited use of adjuvant medication with the precaution to adjust dosing for age-related changes to metabolism, comorbid medical conditions, and tolerability of adverse effects (Rieb et al. 2020).

Low dose buprenorphine initiation can help avoid the more severe discomfort of opioid withdrawal. Its starting dose is low and gradually increased to therapeutic levels over a period of days. This results in slow displacement of full opioid agonist from mu-opioid receptors and can avoid more severe opioid withdrawal symptoms while minimizing the risk of precipitating opioid withdrawal. Evidence for low dose buprenorphine initiation in the geriatric population is limited. A contaminated opioid drug supply and high potency synthetic opioids, which contribute to overdose deaths should encourage further study of buprenorphine use in this population (Cohen et al. 2022).

Opioid Use Disorder (OUD) Treatment

Opioid agonist treatment, with buprenorphine/naloxone (Suboxone), is a first-line treatment for aged adults. Suboxone can be prescribed for both opioid withdrawal management and as long-term opioid agonist medication-assisted treatment (MAT), along with methadone maintenance. Methadone MAT can be considered as an alternative long-term opioid agonist treatment for aging patients who are not able to tolerate Suboxone or who have not been successful with previous Suboxone treatment trials (Rieb et al. 2020).

Both Suboxone and methadone maintenance treatment are proven safe and effective treatments for opioid use disorders in geriatric patients who do not have contraindications to long-term opioid agonist treatment. Initial doses may be lower and titrated at slower rates (25–50%, respectively) compared to younger adults. The goal is to find the lowest effective dose for improving symptoms of cravings and resolving symptoms of physical withdrawal. Patients should be monitored for adverse effects and cautioned about co-ingestion of alcohol, benzodiazepines, and other CNS depressants while on opioid agonist treatment.

For patients who cannot tolerate Suboxone and methadone, initiation of naltrexone, an opioid antagonist, can be a long-term treatment after a period of abstinence from opioids lasting at least 7–10 days (Reib et al. 2020). Suboxone can be prescribed for opioid use disorder by primary care providers who have an X-license as office-based opioid treatment (OBOT). Methadone for opioid use disorder is dispensed at US federally regulated opioid treatment programs (OTPs). Given the increasing prevalence of opioid use disorders in aging adults, access to OBOT treatment can be life-saving.

SAMHSA Practice Guidelines were updated in April 2021 in response to the COVID19 pandemic and to encourage providers to prescribe OBOT and reduce barriers to accessing treatment for OUD. The change allows for an alternative Notice of Intent (NOI) process for eligible providers (physicians, physician assistants, clinical nurse specialists, certified registered nurse anesthetists, certified nurse midwives) to forego the training requirement to obtain an X-license, with the stipulation to provide OBOT to no more than 30 patients at any one time. To treat more than 30 patients, providers will still need to complete the appropriate training and obtain a full DATA 2000 waiver. All providers caring for aging adults are encouraged to apply for an NOI and consider additional training DATA 2000 waiver (SAMHSA 2019)

Patients with mild to moderate OUD can be managed by experienced clinicians. For patients with more severe OUD, addiction specialist consultation can increase accessibility for opioid agonist treatment in primary care settings (Rieb et al. 2020).

Outcome studies of opioid use disorder treatment among geriatric individuals appears to show that older adults do *better* in treatment compared to their younger counterparts; older women 55 to 77 years old tend to have longer periods of abstinence and remain in treatment longer compared to men in the same age group (Carew and Comiskey 2018). Psychosocial interventions and medication management can be components of a comprehensive addiction treatment plan but should not be mandatory for accessing pharmacologic treatment. Aging adults may benefit from age-appropriate peer group support (Reib et al. 2020).

Cannabis

Prevalence of Cannabis Misuse and Use Disorder

After alcohol and tobacco, cannabis is the most common substance used in the United States. Geriatric individuals have reported that self-medication with cannabis is prompted primarily by pain, need to stimulate appetite, and wish to relieve stress rather than for pleasure (Yang et al. 2021). In a nationally representative sample of older adults in 2018, about 6% of adults aged 50 or older and 3.2% of adults aged 65 and older reported the use of cannabis within the past month (NSDUH 2019). Among 13 states and Washington, DC with medical cannabis statutes, most registered medical cannabis participants were male and aged 50 or older (Fairman 2016).

Delta-9-tetrahydrocannabinol (THC) is the main psychoactive component of cannabis that exerts its effect by binding primarily to the CB1 receptor found in the brain and spinal cord. There are several other cannabinoids found in the cannabis plant, some of which do not produce a psychoactive effect (cannabidiol [CBD], cannabidiol

[CBN]) (Mehmedic et al. 2010). Even after controlling for other potential risk factors comorbid medical, psychiatric, and substance use disorders may increase vulnerability to injury among older adults, cannabis use can lead to increased healthcare utilization (Fairman 2016).

The psychological, behavioral, and physiological effects of cannabis vary depending on the concentration of THC, the dose and route of administration, previous experience with the drug, expectations/attitudes, and social setting of drug use. The potency of available cannabis preparations has gradually risen over the years, with confiscated samples containing an average potency of 2.0% to 4.5% from 1980 to 1997 and 3.4% to 8.8% from 1993 to 2008 (Mehmedic et al. 2010). Aging adults using cannabis preparations with higher ratios of THC to CBD are unlikely to experience the potential off-setting effect of CBD, a non-psychoactive component of cannabis (McLaren et al. 2008).

Among aged individuals who use cannabis, there is a perception of lower risk of harm in users with a previous history of use, compared to those who reported *never* using cannabis. Older adults who met the criteria for cannabis use disorder reported moderate or great risk perception of cannabis use, likely due to the negative consequences experienced because of their use disorder (Choi et al. 2017).

Cannabis Intoxication

Cannabis intoxication causes euphoria, relaxation, and alterations in time and sensory perceptions. Delayed reaction time, motor impairment, and deficits in memory and concentration are common symptoms of intoxication, which can impair performance of skilled tasks. Cannabis with higher concentrations of THC has been associated with adverse effects of anxiety, panic, paranoia, derealization/depersonalization, and psychosis (visual > auditory hallucinations) (Wilkins et al. 2014). Cannabis-induced psychosis tends to be transient, but a predisposition of psychopathology (previous history of psychosis, family history of schizophrenia) may increase the risk of panic attacks and psychosis (Wilkins et al. 2014; Turner and Agrawal, 2020). Physiologic signs of acute cannabis intoxication include tremors, pupil constriction, conjunctival injection, vasodilation, tachycardia, arrhythmias, orthostatic hypotension, increased appetite, dry mouth, and urinary retention, all usually mild, self-limited, and do not require medication management (Wilkins et al. 2014).

Acute psychosis related to cannabis can be managed with low doses of benzodiazepines or antipsychotic medications (Wilkins et al. 2014). Further treatment of acute cannabis intoxication depends on factors like age and the amount of cannabis ingested. Inhaled doses of 2 to 3 mg of THC and ingested doses of 5 to 20 mg of THC (e.g., cannabis cookies, brownies, teas, gummy candies) are associated with symptoms of cognitive impairment, with inhaled doses higher than 7.5 mg/m^2 producing more severe central nervous system (CNS) depression. Accidental overdoses have been reported in geriatric patients, resulting in intensive care (ICU) admissions due to CNS depression, and raises suspicion of co-ingestion of alcohol or other substances (Turner and Agrawal 2020).

Aged individuals who use cannabis are at high risk for Major Depressive Disorder (MDD) and rapid progression of age-related cognitive decline (e.g., slowed reaction time and memory impairment). These effects add risk to activities of independent living (ADLs) such as driving (Turner and Agrawal 2020).

Cannabis Withdrawal

Little information about cannabis withdrawal in the aged population has been reported. Cannabis withdrawal syndrome (CWS) can be seen in up to 30–75% of regular cannabis users, typically within a week after abrupt discontinuation of the daily or almost daily pattern of use, which is also a predictor of cannabis dependence (Wilkins et al. 2014).

Management of Cannabis Abuse and Dependence

Older cannabis users, especially those who meet the criteria for cannabis use disorder, have higher rates of other psychiatric disorders (e.g., MDD, anxiety disorder, PTSD, bipolar disorder) and substance use (alcohol, nicotine, and/or other drugs) compared to non-users; they reported significantly more life stressors and lower perceived social support. Life stressors were primarily around interpersonal relationships, debt burden, legal problems, and crime victimhood. Perceived deficient social support were in the domains of appraisal, belonging, and tangible forms of support (Choi et al. 2016).

Stimulants

Prevalence

Between 1999 and 2012, stimulant prescribing to older adults ≥65 years old increased (Kantor et al. 2015). According to the National Surveys on Drug Use and Health (2019), there was also a significant increase in amphetamine use in males >50 years from 2019 to 2020.

Stimulant Intoxication

Cocaine, amphetamines, and derivatives exert effects through stimulating the release of catecholamine neurotransmitters, which result in the activation of the dopamine reward circuit and the psychological and behavioral effects (Wilkins et al. 2014). Increased energy, elevated mood, increased attention, decreased need for sleep, and appetite suppression are common. High dose and frequent stimulant use are associated with increased anxiety, irritability, stereotypical behaviors, and psychosis (e.g., hallucinations, paranoia, delusions). Stimulant-induced psychosis may present with symptoms similar to schizophrenia although cocaine-induced psychosis tends to present with fewer negative symptoms, less thought disorder, and fewer auditory or visual hallucinations (Wilkins et al. 2014). The physiological impact of acute stimulant intoxication affects multiple organ systems: HEENT (pupil dilation, bruxism); respiratory (hyperventilation, chest pain, hemoptysis); cardiovascular (palpitations, hypertension, arrhythmias, myocardial infarction); neurologic (ischemic and hemorrhagic, tremor, hyperreflexia, seizures); renal (diuresis, renal failure); gastrointestinal (nausea, vomiting, mesenteric ischemia); and alterations in body temperature regulation (fever, malignant hyperthermia) (Wilkins et. 2014).

Mild intoxication symptoms do not require hospitalization and may be managed by "ART": "**A**cceptance" of the patient's immediate needs, "**R**eassurance" that the effects of the substance are transient and will likely resolve within a few hours, and "**T**alking down" the patient to avoid agitation and reorient the patient to reality (Wilkins et al. 2014).

Management of *moderate to severe* intoxication should include a thorough drug history and drug toxicology to confirm stimulant intoxication and to assess for co-ingestion of other substances. Cocaine poses a health hazard for aging adults after immediate and long-term use, primarily from myocardial infarction, heatstroke, cerebrovascular accident, and delirium.

Symptom management of *severe* intoxication requires hospitalization and should focus on stabilization of vital signs, adequate hydration, and cardiorespiratory and neurological monitoring (Wilkins et al. 2014). Medical or neuropsychiatric conditions that may mimic acute stimulant intoxication should be ruled out. See Table 7.3.

Stimulant Withdrawal

The intensity of cue-induced cravings during the early withdrawal period contributes to an increased risk of relapse (Wilkins et al. 2014). Psychosocial interventions (cognitive-behavioral therapy-CBT and contingency management (CM) have shown the best evidence for the management of stimulant use disorder. No medications have US FDA approval for treating stimulant use disorders yet, and few have shown promise in

Table 7.3 Standard withdrawal protocols

Objective Measures of Withdrawal Symptoms	Alcohol CIWA-Ar[a]	Benzodiazepines BWSQ[b]	Opioids COWS[c]	Marijuana	Stimulants
Geriatric adaptations	• Discuss age-related risks: Decreased liver metabolism, increased permeability of the blood–brain barrier, and increased neuronal sensitivity • Remain vigilant for concomitant neurological and medical complications • Management of withdrawal for the young-old and oldest-old are best accomplished in an inpatient setting	• Discuss age-related risks: Changes to metabolism and increased brain sensitivity • Assess degree of motivation to taper and • Provide psychoeducation and anticipatory guidance about tapering and common withdrawal symptoms • For insomnia: Sleep restriction and CBT have evidence of benefit among older adults	• Discuss age-related risks: Decreased GI absorption, longer duration of action due to decreases in liver function, increased opioid receptor sensitivity • Provide psychoeducation and anticipatory guidance about tapering and common withdrawal symptoms • Buprenorphine or methadone preferred for management of opioid withdrawal symptoms over adjuvant medications alone	• Discuss age-related risks: Higher risk for depression, and rapid progression of age-related cognitive decline • Average cannabis potency has gradually risen over the years • Provide psychoeducation and anticipatory guidance about common withdrawal symptoms	• Discuss age-related risks: Increased risk of myocardial infarction, heatstroke, cerebrovascular accident, and delirium • Provide psychoeducation and anticipatory guidance about common withdrawal symptoms
Monitoring	• Monitor and assess vital signs regularly • Administer CIWA-Ar every 4 h to evaluate symptoms • Assess medication effects every hour • Monitor fall and sedation risk	• Monitor and assess vital signs regularly • Administer BWSQ to evaluate symptoms • monitor fall and sedation risk	• Monitor and assess vital signs regularly • Administer COWS to evaluate symptoms • Monitor fall and sedation risk	• Monitor for elevated blood pressure • Monitor for changes in mood, anxiety, sleep, appetite, and cravings	• Monitor and assess vital signs regularly • Monitor for changes in mood, anxiety, energy, sleep, appetite, and cravings • Monitor for severe depression and suicidal ideation

Minimizing adverse effects	• Prescribe benzodiazepines and anticonvulsants at dosages one-third to one-half or less the usual dose for younger adults	• Uni-directional, gradual taper • Consider switch to long-acting benzodiazepine at minimal viable dose • Review both prescription and over-the-counter medications taken by the patient to identify anything that may cause or exacerbate common withdrawal symptoms	• Uni-directional, gradual taper • Consider buprenorphine or methadone for managing opioid withdrawal symptoms • Can consider time-limited use of adjuvant medications if no contraindications • Advise of risks of co-ingestion of alcohol, benzodiazepine, and other prescription CNS depressants	• Symptomatic treatment of withdrawal symptoms • Address comorbid mental health and substance use disorders • Improve psychosocial support and coping skills for managing age-related life stressors	• Symptomatic management of withdrawal symptoms • Focus on self-management strategies of rest, exercise, and eating a healthy diet • Engagement in psychosocial interventions (e.g., CBT or CM)
Process of tapering	• Ideally, rapidly taper off medications within 1–2 days	• Gradual dose reduction over a 4 to 5-month timeline, with option to hold at a stable dose prior to resuming taper • Avoid up-dosing to manage withdrawal symptoms • Can offer non-benzodiazepine medications and melatonin receptor antagonist for treatment of insomnia	• Gradual reduction of opioid dose by 5% every 2 to 8 weeks with rest periods as appropriate • Lowest effective dose of buprenorphine or methadone as first-line for resolving cravings and physical withdrawal symptoms. • Offer psychosocial interventions—Older adults benefit from age-appropriate peer group support	• Discontinuation of use followed by symptomatic management of withdrawal • No evidence-based taper strategies	• Discontinuation of use followed by symptomatic management of withdrawal • No evidence-based taper strategies

[a] Clinical Institute Withdrawal Assessment Alcohol Revised
[b] Benzodiazepine Withdrawal Symptom Questionnaire
[c] Clinical Opiate Withdrawal Scale

addressing milder dependence or patients with comorbid depression, bipolar disorder, and schizophrenia when prescribed in combination with psychosocial interventions. Medications which have shown some benefit in managing symptoms of stimulant withdrawal include TCAs (desipramine, imipramine), anticonvulsants (topiramate), other antidepressants (bupropion, citalopram), and antipsychotics (quetiapine).

In general, stimulant withdrawal is associated with symptoms of depression, anhedonia, anergia, increased appetite, hypersomnia, and intense cravings. Treatment trials have typically excluded participants aged >65 years, in order to minimize any confounding variables such as chronic medical conditions and cognitive decline (Lam et al. 2019). The choice of medication management should consider the severity of dependence, withdrawal status, and psychiatric and other medical comorbidities (Gorelick 2014).

Withdrawal from stimulants can be mistaken for major depressive disorder; the intense "crash" can include depressed mood and suicidal ideation. However, most symptoms of stimulant withdrawal are mild, and resolve within 1–2 weeks *without* treatment. Self-management with rest, exercise, and eating a healthy diet can help the patient return to baseline moods and functioning (Wilkins et al. 2014).

ADHD and Stimulants in Geriatrics

Current FDA regulations approve the use of ADHD medication up to age 65. But there is a paucity of data about neuropsychiatric effects of long-term stimulant use in the aging ADHD population (Lakhan and Kirchgessner 2012). Cardiovascular issues commonly associated with aging may be responsible, rather than a result of any stimulant (Lakhan and Kirchgessner 2012). A review of 64 studies on the long-term use of stimulants highlighted a *reduced* incidence of depression and suicide in patients on methylphenidate for ADHD (Krinzinger et al. 2019).

Overview of Psychosocial and Behavioral Interventions

Psychosocial approaches (including self-help groups) and pharmacotherapy can aid relapse prevention (Blow and Barry 2014). Although substance abuse programs specifically for aging individuals are not always available, cognitive-behavioral therapy (CBT) and supportive therapy models (STM) can foster a culture of support, improve self-esteem, and encourage healthy coping skills (Kuerbis et al. 2014). Outpatient medical settings can provide normative feedback, education about the harms of substance use, and enhance motivation. The approach of FRAMES (Feedback of personal risk; personal Responsibility; Advice to change; offering a Menu of options; Empathetic counseling style; and enhancing patient Self-efficacy) facilitates brief outpatient interventions (SAMHSA 2012).

Conclusions

The prevalence of SUD and medication misuse is increasing in adults aged ≥65 years due in part to disproportional prescribing of opioids, benzodiazepines, and other controlled medications to this age group. An increase in rates of polysubstance use among geriatric individuals (Chhatre et al. 2017) underscores the need to screen for alcohol abuse, non-medical use of prescription drugs, and other illicit substance use (Choi et al. 2016; Han and Moore 2018). An *age-adjusted* approach to SUD and misuse starts with an accurate history, identification of risk factors, and scrutiny for clues of abuse or misuse. Unfortunately, although clinical time may limit a comprehensive evaluation of actual medication use, misuse, or substance abuse, all members of the clinical the clinical team can assist in screening.

Enlisting the entire healthcare team, including pharmacists and nursing staff can help. With patient's permission, family and caregivers should be included in gathering history, assessment of possible abuse, and implementing a treatment plan. Nonjudgmental explanations can help patients and family appreciate how age-related changes in metabolism and medication interactions can cause adverse systemic medical and psychiatric events (Han et al. 2009; Blow and Barry 2014).

Judicious prescribing and frank discussions solidify an alliance among patients, family, and the medical team to address medication misuse or substance abuse. Discuss these topics:

- The long-term effect on the patient's health.
- Physiologic changes in age which increase the risk of harm from problematic substance use.
- Drug–drug interactions due to reduced metabolism, pharmacokinetics, and pharmacodynamics of aging.
- Age-related cognitive decline, for example, slower reaction times, which contribute to misuse.
- The threat to independent living and risk to autonomy (e.g., driver's license).

Age-Adjusted Recommendations

- Search behavioral history for signs of excessive alcohol use, medication misuse, or substance abuse/misuse.
- Recognize that the impact of substance abuse on social and vocational life in the aged patient may not be obvious because social and vocational demands are reduced, and there is less incentive to avoid abuse.
- Recognize that the isolated aging adult may be able to obscure chronic substance abuse or misuse and/or alcohol abuse.
- Emphasize the adverse impact of substance use upon chronic medical and psychiatric problems (Blow and Barry 2014; Kuerbis et al. 2014).
- Question the assumption that a decline in functioning is due only to chronic medical conditions or aging rather than SUD or medication adverse effects.
- Attend to clues of substance use or misuse:
  - Obvious craving or a need to take a psychoactive medication to function.
  - Requests to increase the dose of a controlled substance without a clear indication.
  - Pattern of early refill requests for a controlled substance due to lost medications.
  - Use of medication for reasons other than prescribed.
  - Attempts to obtain prescriptions from different providers or sources.
  - Unexplained, abrupt changes in behavior.
  - New onset or unexplained exacerbation of psychiatric symptoms.
  - Unclear, vague, or inconsistent answers about substance or alcohol use.
  - Cognitive deficits in patients for whom medications are self-administered.

References

Bart GB, Saxon A, Fiellin DA, et al. Developing a clinical decision support for opioid use disorders: a NIDA center for the clinical trials network working group report. Addict Sci Clin Pract. 2020;15(1):4.

Bedson J, Chen Y, Hayward RA, et al. Trends in long-term opioid prescribing in primary care patients with musculoskeletal conditions: an observational database study. Pain. 2016;157(7):1525–31.

Blazer DG, Wu LT. Nonprescription use of pain relievers by middle-aged and elderly community-living adults: National Survey on drug use and health. J Am Geriatr Soc. 2009;57(7):1252–7.

Bloom HG, Ahmed I, Alessi CA, Ancoli-Israel S, Buysse DJ, Kryger MH, Phillips BA, Thorpy MJ, Vitiello MV, Zee PC. Evidence-based recommendations for the assessment and management of sleep disorders in older persons. J Am Geriatr Soc. 2009;57(5):761–89. https://doi.org/10.1111/j.1532-5415.2009.02220.x. PMID: 19484833; PMCID: PMC2748127

Blow FC, Barry KL. Treatment of older adults. In: Ries RK, Fiellin DA, Miller SC, Saitz R, editors. The ASAM principles of addiction medicine Philadelphia. PA: Wolters Kluver; 2014. p. 541–54.

Brett J, Murnion B: Management of benzodiazepine misuse and dependence. Australian prescriber 2015;38:152–55.

Butt PR, White-Campbell M, Canham S, et al. Canadian guidelines on alcohol use disorder among older adults. Can Geriatr J. 2020;23(1):143–8.

Caputo F, Vignoli T, Leggio L, et al. Alcohol use disorders in the elderly: a brief overview from epidemiology to treatment options. Exp Gerontol. 2012;47(6):411–6.

Carew AM, Comiskey C. Treatment for opioid use and outcomes in older adults: a systematic literature review. Drug Alcohol Depend. 2018;182:48–57.

Center for Substance Abuse Treatment. Incorporating Alcohol Pharmacotherapies Into Medical Practice: A Review of the Literature. Rockville (MD): Substance Abuse and Mental Health Services Administration (US); 2009. (Treatment Improvement Protocol (TIP) Series, No. 49s.) Available from: https://www.ncbi.nlm.nih.gov/books/NBK65180/

Chhatre S, Cook R, Mallik E, Jayadevappa R. Trends in substance use admissions among older adults. BMC Health Serv Res. 2017;17:584.

Choi NG, DiNitto DM, Marti CN. Middle-aged and older adults who had serious suicidal thoughts: who made suicide plans and nonfatal suicide attempts? Int Psychogeriatr. 2015;27(3):491–500.

Choi NG, DiNitto DM, Marti CN. Older marijuana users: life stressors and perceived social support. Drug Alcohol Depend. 2016;169:56–63.

Choi NG, DiNitto DM, & Marti CN. Older marijuana users' marijuana risk perceptions: associations with marijuana use patterns and marijuana and other substance use disorders. International Psychogeriatrics, 2017;30(9);1311–22

Cohen SM, Weimer MB, Levander XA, et al. Low dose initiation of buprenorphine: a narrative review and practical approach. J Addict Med. 2022;16(4):399–406.

Conn DK, Hogan DB, Amdam L, et al. Canadian guidelines on benzodiazepine receptor agonist use disorder among older adults. Can Geriatr J. 2020;23(1):116–22.

Darker CD, Sweeney BP, Barry JM, et al. Psychosocial interventions for benzodiazepine harmful use, abuse, or dependence. Cochrane Database Syst Rev. 2015;5:CD009652.

DiBartolo MC, Jarosinski JM. Alcohol use disorder in older adults: challenges in assessment and treatment. Issues Ment Health Nurs. 2017;38(1):25–32.

Eloma AS, Tucciarone JM, Hayes EM, Bronson BD. Evaluation of the appropriate use of a CIWA-Ar alcohol withdrawal protocol in the general hospital setting. Am J Drug Alcohol Abuse. 2018;44(4):418–25.

Fairman BJ. Trends in registered medical marijuana participation across 13 US states and District of Columbia. Drug Alcohol Depend. 2016;159:72–9.

Fluyau D, Revadigar N, Manobianco BE. Challenges of the pharmacological management of benzodiazepine withdrawal, dependence, and discontinuation. Ther Adv Psychopharmacol. 2018;8(5):147–68.

Gorelick DA. Pharmacologic interventions for cocaine, methamphetamine, and other stimulant addiction. In: Ries RK, Fiellin DA, Miller SC, Saitz R, editors. The ASAM principles of addiction medicine. Philadelphia, PA: Wolters Kluver; 2014. p. 796–810.

Guina J, Merrill B. Benzodiazepines I: upping the care on downers: the evidence of risks, benefits, and alternatives. J Clin Med. 2018;7(2):17.

Hammond CJ, Niciu MJ, Drew S, Arias AJ. Anticonvulsants for the treatment of alcohol withdrawal syndrome and alcohol use disorders. CNS Drugs. 2015;29(4):293–311.

Han B, Gfroerer JC, Colliver JD, Penne MA. Substance use disorder among older adults in the United States in 2020. Addiction. 2009;104(1):88–96.

Han BH, Moore AA. Prevention and screening of unhealthy substance use by older adults. Clin Geriatr Med. 2018;34(1):117–29.

Häuser W, Tölle T. Problematic use of prescribed opioids for chronic noncancer pain—no scarcity of data outside the United States. Pain. 2017;158(11):2277.

Hirschtritt ME, Olfson M, Kroenke K. Balancing the risks and benefits of benzodiazepines. JAMA. 2021;325(4):347–8.

Jemberie WB, Padyab M, Snellman F, Lundgren L. A multidimensional latent class analysis of harmful alcohol use among older adults: subtypes within the Swedish addiction severity index registry. J Addict Med. 2020;14:e89–99.

Jones CM, McAninch JK. Emergency department visits and overdose deaths from combined use of opioids and benzodiazepines. Am J Prev Med. 2015;49(4):493–501.

Kantor ED, Rehm CD, Haas JS, et al. Trends in prescription drug use among adults in the United States from 1999-2012. JAMA. 2015;314(17):1818–31.

Knightly R, Tadros G, Sharma J, et al. Alcohol screening for older adults in an acute general. Hospital: FAST v. MAST-G assessments. BJPsych Bull. 2016;40(2):72–6.

Krinzinger H, Hall CL, Madeleine J, et al. Neurological and psychiatric adverse effects of long-term methylphenidate treatment in ADHD: A map of the current evidence. Neurosci Biobehav Rev. 2019;107(2019):945–68.

Kuerbis AN, Hagman BT, Sacco P. Functioning of alcohol use disorders criteria among middle-aged and older adults: implications for DSM-5. Subst Use Misuse. 2013;48(4):309–22. https://doi.org/10.3109/10826084.2012.762527. Epub 2013 Feb 1. PMID: 23373632.

Kuerbis A, Sacco P, Blazer DG, Moore AA. Substance abuse among older adults. Clin Geriatr Med. 2014;30(3):629–54.

Lakhan SE, Kirchgessner A. Prescription stimulants in individuals with and without attention deficit hyperactivity disorder: misuse, cognitive impact, and adverse effects. Brain Behav. 2012;2(5):661–77.

Lam AP, Matthies S, Graf E, et al. Comparison of methylphenidate and psychotherapy in adult ADHD study (COMPAS) consortium. Long-term effects of multimodal treatment on adult attention-deficit/hyperactivity disorder symptoms: follow-up analysis of the COMPAS trial. JAMA Netw Open. 2019;2(5):e194980.

Lemke S, Moos RH. Outcomes at 1 and 5 years for older patients with alcohol use disorders. J Subst Abuse Treat. 2003;24(1):43–50.

Luther CD, Hughes TD, Ferreri SP. Naloxone prescribing to older adults in primary care. J Am Geriatr Soc. 2021;69(12):3681–3.

Maree RD, Marcum ZA, Saghafi E, et al. A systematic review of opioid and benzodiazepine misuse in older adults. Am J Geriatr Psychiatry. 2016;24(11):949–63.

Markota M, Rummans TA, Bostwick JM, Lapid MI. Benzodiazepine use in older adults: dangers, management, and alternative therapies. Mayo Clin Proc. 2016;91(11):1632–9.

McHugh RK, Votaw VR, Taghian NR, et al. Benzodiazepine misuse in adults with alcohol use disorder: Prevalence, motives, and patterns of use. J Subst Abuse Treat. 2020;117:108061.

McLaren J, Swift W, Dillon P, Allsop S. Cannabis potency and contamination: a review of the literature. Addiction. 2008;103(7):1100–9. https://doi.org/10.1111/j.1360-0443.2008.02230.x. Epub 2008 May 20. PMID: 18494838.

McQuade BM, Koronkowski M, Emery-Tiburcio E, et al.: SAFE—Home Opioid Management Education (SAFE-HOME) in older adults: a naloxone awareness program for home health workers. Drugs Context 10: 2021.

Mehmedic Z, Chandra S, Slade D, et al. Potency trends of Δ9-THC and other cannabinoids in confiscated cannabis preparations from 1993 to 2008. J Forensic Sci. 2010;55(5):1209–17.

Mojtabai R. National trends in long-term use of prescription opioids. Pharmacoepidemiol Drug Saf. 2018;27(5):526–34.

Mulkey MA, Olson DM. Delirium tremens in the older adult. J Neurosci Nurs. 2020;52(6):316–21.

National Institute of Drug Abuse (NIDA). Substance Use in older adults drug facts. National Institute on Drug Abuse website. 2020. https://www.drugabuse.gov/publications/substance-use-in-older-adults-drugfacts. Accessed 20 Mar 2022.

National Institute on Alcohol Abuse and Alcoholism (NIAAA) Alcohols effects on health. special populations co-occurring disorders in older adults. 2020. https://www.niaaa.nih.gov/alcohols-effects-health/special-populations-co-occurring-disorders/older-adults. Accessed 20 Mar 2022.

National Surveys on Drug Use and Health (NSDUH). Using 2010 U.S. Census for 2015–2018 based population estimates. Substance Abuse and Mental Health Services Administration Center for Behavioral Health Statistics and Quality Rockville, Maryland 20,857 August 26, 2019. 2019. https://www.samhsa.gov/data/data-we-collect/nsduh-national-survey-drug-use-and-health. Accessed 20 Mar 2022.

Ogbonna CI, Lembke A. Substance use among older adults: ethical issues. Focus (Am Psychiatr Publ). 2019;17(2):143–7.

Ogbonna CI, Lembke A. Tapering patients off of benzodiazepines. Am Fam Physician. 2017;96(9):606–10.

Perpétuo C, Plácido AI, Rodrigues D, et al. Prescription of potentially inappropriate medication in older inpatients of an internal medicine ward: concordance and overlap among the EU (7)-PIM List and Beers and STOPP Criteria. Front Pharmacol. 2021;12:676020.

Reeve E, Ong M, Wu A, et al. A systematic review of interventions to deprescribe benzodiazepines and other hypnotics among older people. Eur J Clin Pharmacol. 2017;73(8):927–35.

Rieb LM, Samaan Z, Furlan AD, Rabheru K, Feldman S, Hung L, Budd G, Coleman D. Canadian Guidelines on Opioid Use Disorder Among Older Adults. Can Geriatr J. 2020;23(1):123–34. https://doi.org/10.5770/cgj.23.420. PMID: 32226571; PMCID: PMC7067148.

Sachdeva A, Choudhary M, Chandra M. Alcohol withdrawal syndrome: benzodiazepines and beyond. J Clin Diagn Res. 2015;9(9):VE01-VE07.

Santo L, Rui P, Ashman JJ. Physician office visits at which benzodiazepines were prescribed: findings from 2014–2016 National Ambulatory Medical Care Survey. Natl Health Stat Report. 2020;137:1–16.

Saunders KW, Dunn KM, Merrill JO, et al. Relationship of opioid use and dosage levels to fractures in older chronic pain patients. J Gen Intern Med. 2010;25(4):310–5.

Scholl L, Seth P, Kariisa M, et al. Drug and opioid-involved overdose deaths—United States, 2013–2017. MMWR Morb Mortal Wkly Rep. 2019;67(5152):1419–27.

Smith PC, Schmidt SM, Allensworth-Davies D, Saitz R. Primary care validation of a single-question alcohol screening test. J Gen Intern Med. 2009;24(7):783–8.

Stitt D, Kumar N. Drugs of abuse, and the nervous system. Continuum (Minneap Minn). 2020;26(3):765–84.

SAMHSA. U.S. Department of Health and Human Services, Substance Abuse and Mental Health Services Administration. Substance Abuse and Mental Health Services Administration (SAMHSA): 2018 National Survey on Drug Use and Health Detailed Tables. Rockville, MD: Center for Behavioral Health Statistics and Quality, Substance Abuse and Mental Health Services Administration, 2019. https://www.samhsa.gov/data/report/2018-nsduh-detailed-tables. Accessed 30 Mar 2021.

SAMHSA. U.S. Department of Health and Human Services, Substance Abuse and Mental Health Services Administration. Substance Abuse and Mental Health Services Administration (SAMHSA): Substance abuse among older adults. Treatment Improvement Protocol (TIP) Series, no 26. HHS Publication No. (SMA) 12–3918. Rockville, MD, Substance Abuse and Mental Health Services Administration, 2012.

SAMHSA. U.S. Department of Health and Human Services, Substance Abuse and Mental Health Services Administration. Substance Abuse and Mental Health Services Administration (SAMHSA). Key substance use and mental health indicators in the United States: Results from the 2019 National Survey on Drug Use and Health (HHS Publication No. PEP20-07-01-001, NSDUH Series H-55). Rockville, MD: Center for Behavioral Health Statistics and Quality, Substance Abuse and Mental Health Services Administration. 2020. https://www.samhsa.gov/data/. Accessed 20 Mar 2022.

Substance Abuse and Mental Health Services Administration. (2019). TIP 63: Medications for Opioid Use Disorder. Retrieved from https://store.samhsa.gov/product/TIP-63-Medications-for-Opioid-Use-Disorder

Turner AR, Spurling BC, Agrawal S. Marijuana Toxicity. [Updated 2020 Jul 19]. In: StatPearls [Internet]. Treasure Island (FL): StatPearls Publishing; 2021 Jan-. Available from: https://www.ncbi.nlm.nih.gov/books/NBK430823/.

Weiss AJ, Heslin KC, Barrett ML, et al. Opioid-related inpatient stays and emergency department visits among patients aged 65 years and older, 2010 and 2015. HCUP Statistical Brief #244. Rockville, MD: Agency for Healthcare Research and Quality; 2018. www.hcup-us.ahrq.gov/reports/statbriefs/sb244-Opioid-InpatientStays-ED-Visits-Older-Adults.pdf. Accessed 20 Mar 2022

Wilkins JN, Danovitch I, & Gorelick DA: Management of stimulant, hallucinogen, marijuana, phencyclidine, and club drug intoxication and withdrawal. In R.K. Ries, D.A. Fiellin, S.C. Miller, & R. Saitz (Eds.), The ASAM Principles of Addiction Medicine (pp. 685-709). Philadelphia, PA: Wolters Kluver, 2014.

Wu LT, Blazer DG. Illicit and nonmedical drug use among older adults: a review. J Aging Health. 2011;23(3):481–504.

Yang KH, Kaufmann CN, Nafsu R, et al. Cannabis: an emerging treatment for common symptoms in older adults. J Am Geriatr Soc. 2021;69(1):91–7.

8 Sleep

Kate Marie Richards and Shannon Suo

Abstract
Disturbances of sleep are detrimental to the quality of life for the aging individual. Sleep disorder studies among adults above age 50 found that approximately 57% complained of significant sleep disruption; 45% reported periodic limb movements during sleep, 29% reported insomnia, 24% reported obstructive sleep apnea (OSA), 19% experienced early morning awakening, and 12% had restless legs syndrome (RLS) (Bloom et al. J Am Geriatr Soc 57(5): 761–789, 2009). Among over 9,000 participants aged 65 years and older, between 23% and 34% had symptoms of insomnia, and between 7% and 15% rarely or never felt rested after waking up in the morning (Foley et al. Sleep: 425–432, 1995). These sleep complaints were associated with an increasing number of respiratory symptoms, physical disabilities, nonprescription medications, depressive symptoms, and poorer self-perceived health (Foley et al. Sleep: 425–432, 1995). This chapter provides an overview of disorders of sleep and parasomnias and *age-adjusted* recommendations.

Because patients often wish for an immediate solution, and clinicians have limited time to assess sleep problems in depth, a medication prescription is frequently the first and only clinical intervention. The result can be increasingly complicated medication regimens, which include potentially inappropriate medications (PIM) with redundant pharmacological properties, and a greater risk of adverse drug–drug interactions (Wastesson et al. Expert Opin Drug Saf 17(12): 1185–1196, 2018). Recommended interventions include *first-line* behavioral approaches such as cognitive behavior therapy for insomnia, (CBT-I), followed by *second-line* age-adjusted psychopharmacological approaches.

K. M. Richards (✉)
Department of Psychiatry and Behavioral Sciences/
Department of Family and Community Medicine,
UC Davis Health, Sacramento, CA, USA
e-mail: kmrichards@ucdavis.edu

S. Suo
Call Psych, Sacramento, CA, USA

Case Example: Non-pharmacological Approach to Insomnia

A 68-year-old retired small business owner reported initial insomnia and intermittent awakenings for 4 years. She took 2 hours to fall asleep, woke up every 3 hours, and felt unrefreshed each morning. She lived alone for 6 years after her husband's death and did not know if she snored. Daytime drowsiness made it difficult to concentrate on her business, and sometimes she would fall asleep for an hour in the afternoon. She was treated by her primary care physician for hyper-

H. H. Fenn et al. (eds.), *Age-Adjusted Psychiatric Treatment for the Older Patient*,
https://doi.org/10.1007/978-3-031-53976-3_8

tension, osteoarthritis, type 2 diabetes mellitus, and hyperlipidemia. She had tried diphenhydramine 50 mg each night but felt groggy the next day. She added melatonin 5 mg each night for several months without benefit. She did not take energy drinks.

Medications and supplements included hydrochlorothiazide, lisinopril, acetaminophen, insulin, atorvastatin, and fish oil. She had one glass of wine daily with dinner, one cup of coffee each morning, and no substance misuse or illegal drug use. She woke up to urinate 2–3 times per night. BMI was 36 kg/m^2 with a gain of 20 pounds in the previous 3 years. At least five times a week, she watched TV for hours past her desired bedtime.

A sleep study and sleep medicine consultation ruled out obstructive sleep apnea (OSA), narcolepsy, other primary sleep disorders, and/or parasomnia disorders. No significant cognitive deficits or other psychiatric symptoms were found. Zolpidem 5 mg at bedtime as needed helped her to initiate sleep for few months, but one morning neighbors found her asleep in her car and the patient was unaware how she got there.

Zolpidem was discontinued, and her medication regimen was changed to take hydrochlorothiazide *in the morning* to decrease nighttime awakenings for urination. She reduced alcohol and caffeine use, began walking an hour each morning, avoided napping, and stopped computer work/TV after 6:00 PM. Six sessions of weekly Cognitive Behavioral Therapy for Insomnia (CBT-I) helped her consolidate sleep and initiate sleep readily. Daytime drowsiness resolved, and she became more productive and more rested.

Discussion: Improved sleep hygiene and non-pharmacological interventions were sufficient in this case because the patient was motivated and well-informed .

Structure of Sleep and Aging

The spectrum of normal sleep is broad and heterogeneous (Ohayon and Vecchierini 2005). Most older adults have normal alertness and are not symptomatic for sleep disorders (Lin and Suurna 2018). Total sleep time on average decreases from *6.5– 8.9 h a night for younger adults to 5.0– 7.4 h a night* for aged adults; age-dependent sleep changes plateau after age 60 in the absence of comorbidities. Impairments in sleep may occur, however, as older adults try behaviors that *further* disrupt sleep (see Table 8.1). For example, daytime napping may sabotage efforts to sleep by creating a sleep surplus, which reduces the drive to fall asleep later that night. If significant symptoms or a decline in functioning emerge, then underlying causes of sleep deprivation can be considered.

Two phases of sleep occur in 90-min cycles during the night:

- NREM (non-rapid eye movement) sleep—proportionally more initially. NREM is further divided between *light sleep* and *deep sleep.*
- REM (rapid eye movement) sleep—greater amount later in the night.

The duration of time since the person last slept is one driving factor for sleep. Circadian rhythm also drives sleep: the daily sleep-wake cycle is affected by the response of the suprachiasmatic nucleus in the hypothalamus to bright light, lead-

Table 8.1 Sleep parameters that change with age

Changes in sleep with aging	Increased	Decreased
Sleep onset or latency (time to fall asleep)	✓	
Duration of light sleep		✓
Duration of deep sleep (associated with restoration and repair)		✓
Duration of REM sleep (associated with memory consolidation and well-being)		✓
Sleep inefficiency (frequent awakenings and periods not asleep)	✓	
Natural shift to earlier circadian rhythm (feeling tired and waking earlier)	Shifts to earlier	
Average total sleep time plateaus (≥ 60 years and no comorbidities)	5.0–7.4 h per night	

Adapted from Gooneratne and Vitiello 2014; Ohayon et al. 2004; Bloom et al. 2009 ing to sleepiness as the sun sets and waking as the sun rises. LED/LCD screens (e.g., TVs, smartphones, tablets, and computers) emit blue light, simulating daytime and suppressing the release of the hormone melatonin, secreted by the pineal gland to initiate sleep.

Assessment

Even if the patient does not initially report sleep problems, disrupted sleep may be contributing to presenting complaints. An evaluation for a sleep disorder is indicated in the context of (see Table 8.2):

Table 8.2 Screening tools for sleep disorders

Description	Measurement	Interpretation	Application
Epworth sleepiness scale (ESS)			
ESS is a: • Licensed rating scale measuring average sleep propensity and likelihood of falling asleep during 8 daily activities • Does not indicate causality of insomnia • Able to detect types of sleep disorders resulting in "excessive" daytime sleepiness (e.g., sleep apnea, narcolepsy, periodic limb movements of sleep, and restless legs syndrome)	Daily activities include: • Sitting & reading • Watching TV • Sitting in a public place (inactive). • Riding as a passenger in a care for 1 h • Lying down to rest in the afternoon • Sitting and talking to someone • Sitting quietly after lunch • Sitting in a car stopped for a few minutes	Positive ESS findings are associated with: • Sleep-related breathing disorders (such as sleep apnea) • Circadian rhythm sleep-wake disorders • Sleep-related movement disorders • Hypersomnia (e.g., narcolepsy associated with excessive daytime sleepiness (EDS))	Consideration in geriatrics: • Validated by Spira et al. (2012) in a study of 3059 older men (mean age = 76.4 years) • Should not be used if patient has "serious cognitive impairment"
STOP-bang scale			
• Simple screening tool which estimates risk for obstructive sleep apnea (OSA)	Total of 8 factors the each factor with worth 1 point, including: • Snoring • Feeling tired • Observations of stopping breathing or choking/gasping in sleep • Medications for hypertension • Body mass index (BMI) > 35 kg/m^2 • Age > 50 • Neck size • Male gender	STOP-bang • Score > 2 for the general population indicates intermediate risk for obstructive sleep apnea and a sleep study can be considered • Score > 4 or score ≥ 2 with either male gender, BMI > 35 kg/m^2, or neck circumference > 17″ in males or > 16″ in females indicates high risk for obstructive sleep apnea and a referral is recommended for a sleep study (Rebelo-Marques et al. (2018))	Medicare will approve treatment with continuous positive airway pressure (CPAP) with: • Apnea-hypopnea index of ≥15 per hour (indicating moderate OSA) alone • Score 5–14 (mild OSA) with excessive daytime sleepiness, impaired neurocognitive function, mood disorder, history of stroke, insomnia, hypertension, or ischemic heart disease

(continued)

Table 8.2 (continued)

Description	Measurement	Interpretation	Application
Pittsburgh sleep quality index (PSQI)			
The PSQI is • Copyrighted self-administered questionnaire of bedtime, sleep latency, duration, and wake-up time • Does not differentiate etiology of the poor sleep	A 4-point scale: • Overall sleep quality • Frequency of over-the-counter or prescribed medication for sleep • Daytime sleepiness during activity • Enthusiasm for activities • Frequency of observed sleep disturbances (e.g., snoring, movement, or apnea)	The self-rated answers and ratings from bed partner (if available) produce a: • "Global PSQI score" • Score ≥ 5 is defined as consistent with "poor sleep" Buysse et al. (1989)	Valid in: • Older men and women (≥ 70 years) • Able to identify insomnia Beaudreau et al. (2012), Spira et al. (2012)

Table 8.3 Current sleep history from patient or observer

	Sleep hygiene	Sleep quality	Behavior during sleep	Environment	Intake
Factors	• Caffeine use • Napping during day • TV and digital device use before bed • Activities and exercise before bed • Activities in bed (except sleep and sex)	• Time to fall asleep • Tiredness before sleep • Waking frequency and cause (e.g., urination, pain or leg discomfort) • Number of hours of sleep • Restfulness upon waking	• Snoring • Interrupted breathing • Gasping for air • Leg and limb movements • Vocalizations	• Noise • Lighting • Temperature • Bed partners • Interruptions	• Medications and over-the-counter supplements (herbals, nutraceuticals), time of ingestion • Greasy and spicy foods before bed

Richards et al. 2018

- New symptoms, including systemic medical, surgical, psychiatric, medication, pain, and substance use history.
- Co-morbid systemic medical conditions, such as osteoarthritic pain, neurological or cardio-pulmonary disorders.
- Adverse effects and/or sleep disruption associated with prescribed and over-the-counter medications.
- Alcohol, caffeine, nicotine, and cannabis use can interfere with sleep.

A thorough evaluation for a sleep disorder includes vital signs, body mass index, physical examination of the mouth and nose, neck, thyroid, heart, and lungs, and labs such as CBC, vitamin levels (Vitamin B12, folate, Vitamin D), and thyroid levels (TSH with Free T4) (see Tables 8.3 and 8.4).

Table 8.4 Assessment tools and resources

Clinician screening tools	Patient resources
• STOP-banghttp://www.stopbang.ca/osa/screening.php • Pittsburgh sleep quality index https://www.sleep.pitt.edu/instruments/#psqi • Epworth sleepiness scalehttps://epworthsleepinessscale.com/about-the-ess/ • Patient health questionnaire 9 https://www.uspreventiveservicestaskforce.org/Home/GetFileByID/218 • Mood disorder questionnaire https://www.ncbi.nlm.nih.gov/pmc/articles/PMC314375/	• Sleep loghttps://www.sleepfoundation.org/sites/default/files/inline-files/SleepDiaryv6.pdf • Sleep hygiene handouthttps://www.cci.health.wa.gov.au/-/media/CCI/Mental-Health-Professionals/Sleep/Sleep%2D%2D-Information-Sheets/Sleep-Information-Sheet%2D%2D-04%2D%2D-Sleep-Hygiene.pdf • Sleep safety/fall precautions • Education about moving feet, sitting slowly, lingering at edge of bed before standing to prevent orthostatic hypotension • Adequate and accessible lighting • Smooth floor surfaces, without area rugs • Grab bars in bathrooms and by bed • Sleep apnea mask that can be easily removed • Bedside commode or handheld urinal • Doorway gate for pet to prevent tripping over pet

Contributors to Disrupted Sleep

Systemic Medical Conditions

Several factors and medical conditions should be explored for sleep complaints. A survey from the National Sleep Foundation found that *40%* of adults aged >65 years with medical comorbidities reported fair or poor sleep quality. Medical conditions included cardiovascular disease, musculoskeletal disease, diabetes mellitus, major depressive disorder, cancer, lung disease, memory problems, stroke, and benign prostatic hyperplasia. Approximately 10% *without* these comorbidities reported fair or poor quality of sleep (Foley et al. 2004).

Individuals with sleep disorders have been shown, even after adjusting for body mass index, to be at increased risk for major depressive disorder and vascular disease. Sleep deprivation can increase cortisol stress hormone, which increases risk of exacerbating diabetes mellitus, confusion, and accidents (Bloom et al. 2009).

Nocturia (awakening to urinate) can be due to drinking water close to bedtime, iatrogenic effects of diuretics, bladder weakness or numbness due to diabetic neuropathy, incomplete emptying of the bladder with benign prostatic hyperplasia or vaginal prolapse, incontinence, or urinary tract infection. *Pain or discomfort* in the legs (feeling the urge to move) while falling asleep may be related to electrolyte imbalances, anemia/iron deficiency, or restless legs syndrome (RLS). *Cardiovascular and pulmonary diseases* can impair breathing, especially while reclining, causing variable blood oxygen levels, and/or nighttime flares of symptoms. *Gastroesophageal reflux* can also be more symptomatic when reclining. Pain from musculoskeletal, endocrine, and autoimmune disorders is exacerbated in uncomfortable positions (see Table 8.5).

Medications

Timing and half-life of medications can affect the sleep-wake cycle. Prescriptions, therefore, should include times of administration (AM and PM) with clear directions. Beta-blockers (e.g., propranolol and metoprolol) and alpha-2-agonists (e.g., clonidine) can cause insomnia *or* sedation. Other medications can be stimulating, including bronchodilators. Corticosteroids can promote arousal and impair sleep and are thus best taken in the morning (see Table 8.6). Diuretics, when given in the *morning,* can decrease nocturia.

Decongestants or allergy medications with pseudoephedrine, pain or headache medications with caffeine, or nicotine products (cigarettes, vape, patches, gum, and lozenges) can impair sleep. Withdrawal from these medications can precipitate anxiety, cravings, and restlessness, prompting use and perpetuating a cycle of sleep

Table 8.5 Systemic medical conditions which contribute to insomnia

Diagnosis	Key sleep-disrupting symptoms
Congestive heart failure	Paroxysmal nocturnal dyspnea and orthopnea
Chronic lung disease (e.g., asthma, chronic obstructive pulmonary disease, pulmonary hypertension)	Coughing, oxygen desaturation, and shortness of breath
Coronary artery disease	Nocturnal angina pectoris
Gastroesophageal reflux disease	Heartburn worse while lying down or eating too close to bedtime; nocturnal cough
Anemia	Fatigue, poor sleep quality, restless legs
Major neurocognitive disorder (MNCD) (Alzheimer's and Parkinson's disease, vascular dementia)	Sleep disturbances with dementia-related sleep behaviors, cognitive decline, hypoxia, confusion and shifted sleep-wake cycle; increased association of REM sleep behavior disorder with Parkinson's disease
Delirium	Fluctuating attention/concentration/arousal in mental status; disrupted sleep-wake cycles
Post-stroke	Increased risk of obstructive sleep apnea and hypersomnia (increased daytime sleepiness)
Obstructive sleep apnea	Waking or arousals with apneic episodes and daytime fatigue despite adequate time asleep
Acute or chronic pain (e.g., arthritis, gout, neuropathy, fibromyalgia, musculoskeletal)	Delay in falling asleep, waking frequently, and difficulty finding a comfortable position
Benign prostatic hyperplasia	Nocturia and urinary retention
Renal disease	Excessive daytime sleepiness and restless legs
Endocrine (e.g., menopause, thyroid disease)	Hot flashes, night sweats, nocturnal awakenings, daytime fatigue
Diabetes	Polyuria, polydipsia and polyphagia; glucose levels (hyperglycemic and hypoglycemic episodes); neuropathic pain
Cancer	Waking due to pain, nausea, vomiting, chemotherapy side effects, mood changes, anxiety

Richards et al. 2018

Table 8.6 Medications which contribute to insomnia

Class	Medication examples
Acetylcholinesterase inhibitors	Donepezil, rivastigmine
Anti-epileptics	Lamotrigine, phenytoin
Antidepressants	Bupropion, SSRIs, SNRIs
Beta-blockers	Propranolol, metoprolol
Bronchodilators	Theophylline
Decongestants	Pseudoephedrine
Diuretics	Hydrochlorothiazide, furosemide, spironolactone
Corticosteroids	Dexamethasone, prednisone
Stimulants	Dextroamphetamine, methamphetamine, methylphenidate, modafinil

Richards et al. 2018

interruption. Istradefylline, a xanthine derivative which antagonizes adenosine A_{2A} receptors and is used in treatment of Parkinson's disease, also has insomnia as an adverse effect.

Substances

Alcohol within a few hours of bedtime can lead to sleep fragmentation from dehydration, sugar breakdown, nocturia, worsening Obstructive Sleep Apnea, decreased deep sleep, and early morning awakenings. Caffeinated beverages (coffee, soda, teas, and energy drinks) close to bedtime can retain a stimulant effect up to 8–14 h, as hepatic clearance of caffeine decreases with age (Wolkove et al. 2007).

Psychiatric Disorders and Disrupted Sleep

When sleep problems occur *only* in association with psychiatric symptoms, it is more likely that they are *secondary* to the psychiatric disorder.

Depressive disorders, bipolar disorder with mania or hypomania, post-traumatic stress disorder (PTSD), and generalized anxiety disorder (GAD) all include sleep disturbance as a DSM-5-TR diagnostic criterion. Panic attacks at night can also disrupt sleep. However, if symptoms persist *despite improvement or resolution* of the psychiatric illness, a *primary* sleep disorder may be considered, prompting further evaluation.

Depressive disorders may present with difficulty initiating or maintaining sleep, or complaints about the quality of sleep. Major depressive disorder (MDD) shows longer sleep latency, increased number and duration of awakenings, decreased sleep efficiency, and early morning awakenings. In addition, "atypical" major depressive disorder (MDD) presents with *hypersomnia* and psychomotor slowing. A 2-year cohort study of patients over 60 found that depressive disorder was almost 5 times more likely to recur in those with baseline insomnia, even after controlling for other depressive symptoms, antidepressant use, and level of education (Cho et al. 2008). Inadequate sleep and sleep deprivation can initiate or exacerbate psychiatric disorders and may contribute to suicidality. A 10-year study of people over 65 years with poor quality sleep at baseline reported that the risk of death by suicide was increased by 40% (Bernert et al. 2014).

Mania or hypomania are associated with decreased need for sleep, which can be misidentified as primary *insomnia.* Absence of fatigue or lack of tiredness despite lack of sleep is consistent with mania, distinct from *inability to sleep* when *sleep is desired.*

Disrupted sleep associated with *PTSD* is often accompanied by hyperarousal, nightmares, or reliving traumatic events at night. *Generalized anxiety disorder* (GAD) symptoms may include excessive worries and restlessness, with difficulty falling or staying asleep. *Panic disorder* and panic episodes may appear as spontaneous panic attacks disrupting sleep. *Bereavement and grief* may include sleep complaints which correlate with feelings of guilt, sadness, and loss. For further discussion, see Chaps. 10, 11, 12 and 13.

Neurocognitive Disorders

Sleep disruption may precede a clinical diagnosis of Alzheimer's disease (AD) or major neurocognitive disorders (MNCD) by years (Ferini-Strambi et al. 2020), and insomnia may be an independent risk factor for Alzheimer's disease. A 6-year study of aged patients *without MNCD* found that sleep fragmentation by actigraph at night showed a 1.5-fold increased risk of later developing Alzheimer's disease (Lim et al. 2013). Baseline complaints of insomnia led to a 49% increased risk of cognitive decline 3 years later among men 65 years and older compared to older men with no baseline cognitive problems (Cricco et al. 2001).

Disrupted sleep is a common symptom which accompanies MNCD and mild neurocognitive disorder (mNCD). Factors associated with sleep disruption and cognitive function include:

- When sleep apnea *and* neurocognitive disorders co-occur, effects on cognition can be compounded, and improved with treatment of sleep apnea.
- Disordered sleep prevents tau protein clearance in the brain and may hasten the progression from mild cognitive impairment to Alzheimer's disease (AD) (Romanella et al. 2020).
- Disruptions of sleep-wake cycle and circadian rhythms in Alzheimer's disease can result in loss of REM (restorative) sleep and increased daytime sleep, as well as sleep apnea, restless legs syndrome (RLS), and REM behavior disorder (RBD) (Gosney et al. 2012).
- *Sundowning,* or agitated behavior late in the day, is associated with MNCD. Light therapy, melatonin, daytime activity, and acetylcholinesterase inhibitors can have mild-to-moderate beneficial effects on circadian rhythm (Khachiyants et al. 2011). For further discussion, see Chap. 5.

Geriatric patients have reported cognitive problems due to insomnia, such as "trouble remembering things" (59%) and confused thinking or judgment (43%). However, several studies have shown *no differences in cognitive or executive function* testing between older people *with* insomnia as opposed to those reporting good sleep (Sivertsen et al. 2013) (see Table 8.7).

Table 8.7 Approaches for patients with cognitive impairment

Approach	Application
Cognitive restructuring	Addresses unhelpful thought patterns including: • Beliefs around quantity of sleep needed and impact on life (which affects anticipatory anxiety and expectations)
Sleep hygiene	• Improve sleep promoting activities. See Tables 8.4 and 8.8
Stimulus control	• Remove negative associations between bed and sleep • Go to bed only when tired, and avoid other activities in bed • If lying awake or anxious, get up, and do a soothing activity; return to bed when sleepy
Sleep restriction	• Use sleep log (see Table 8.4) to limit time in bed, increasing sleep efficiency (e.g., if spending 9 h in bed, and only sleeping 5 h, then limit time in bed to 5 h and gradually increase as progress is sustained.)
Relaxation (decrease stress and overthinking)	• Progressive muscle relaxation • Diaphragmatic breathing • Biofeedback • Listening to music • Meditation • Guided imagery
For chronic insomnia[a]	• Exercise (e.g., walking, yoga, tai chi) • Acupuncture • Massage therapy • Bright light therapy

[a]Interventions with potential positive benefits and low risk of harm. Evidence is limited by confounders inherent in the studies.

Specific Sleep Disorders

Insomnia Disorder

Prevalence of insomnia in the general population ranges from 10% to 20%. One study found that of 9,000 adults over age 65, 42% had difficulty initiating and maintaining sleep. Difficulty initiating and/or maintaining sleep, early awakenings, and/or poor quality of sleep are symptoms of insomnia. Those with many systemic medical conditions and those taking several medications have reported a higher prevalence of difficulty initiating and maintaining sleep (Bloom et al. 2009).

Primary insomnia is a term used when no underlying cause of the insomnia is found.

Chronic primary insomnia constitutes *persistent* difficulty with sleep at least three nights per week for over 3 months that impairs functioning despite an adequate opportunity for sleep and is not due to the other causes.

Secondary insomnia is due to systemic medical, psychiatric, and/or substance use disorders. Insomnia is more prevalent in men and people who live alone, but other factors such as reduced physical activity, acute life stressors, medication changes, and/or systemic medical conditions can increase the risk of developing insomnia (Gooneratne and Vitiello 2014). Compensatory behavioral changes, such as pre-sleep anxiety, watching TV before bed, or napping, may perpetuate chronic insomnia.

Narcolepsy

Daytime sleepiness, hallucinations while falling asleep, emotionally triggered loss of muscle tone without loss of consciousness, and sleep paralysis characterize narcolepsy. It is often diagnosed in a bi-modal distribution for onset from ages 10–15 and ages 35–40, but 15% of patients are diagnosed 16 years *after* symptom onset in men, and 28 years *after* symptom onset in women (Won et al. 2014). If narcolepsy is suspected, or if there are occupational risks from excessive fatigue, a *Multiple Sleep Latency Test* (MSLT) can measure the tendency to fall asleep, while the *Maintenance of Wakefulness Test* can measure the ability to stay awake.

Interventions for narcolepsy include scheduling one or two 20-min daytime naps per day, maintaining a regular nighttime sleep schedule, avoiding sedative medications and substances, and pharmacotherapy. The United States Food and Drug Administration (FDA)-approved medications for narcolepsy include modafinil, armodafinil, solriamfetol, pitolisant, sodium oxybate, and amphetamines (and their derivatives).

Sleep-disordered breathing (SDB) and Obstructive Sleep Apnea (OSA)

The prevalence of SDB and related conditions such as OSA increases with age. Loud snoring, episodes of not breathing or gasping for air, and frequent micro-awakenings are indicative of

SDB. A sleep study is important for evaluation, and sleep specialty consultation should be considered for patients with comorbidities, especially obesity-hypoventilation syndrome, central sleep apnea, and cardiovascular, neuromuscular, and pulmonary conditions.

Interventions for SDB and OSA. An international task force of 11 experts in geriatric sleep medicine reviewed available evidence and provided treatment recommendations (Netzer et al. 2016):

- The first-line treatment for OSA is Continuous Positive Airway Pressure (CPAP), shown in older adults to decrease daytime sleepiness, decrease apnea-hypopnea, improve oxygenation, increase cognitive function, and reduce morbidity (Gooneratne and Vitiello 2014).
- Positive airway pressure (PAP) should be used *routinely* for the treatment of SDB in older persons and in the frail elderly, particularly those with stroke but without major heart failure (heart failure defined as ejection fraction $\leq$45%). PAP leads to a significant improvement of oxygenation in patients with SDB and COPD (overlap syndrome), though adherence to PAP treatment is variable; one study showed only about 70% of older people used CPAP regularly (6+ nights/week) (Parish et al. 2000).
- Frail aged adults and patients with Alzheimer's or Parkinson's disease *can* tolerate PAP.
- *Positional treatment* (night-time positioning to improve breathing) is *not supported* as effective for OSA in the elderly.
- Pharmacotherapy is not recommended to treat SDB in geriatric patients.
- No specific pharmacologic treatments have yet been FDA approved for OSA.
- Alcohol, sedatives, or muscle relaxants, which can worsen obstruction and compromise breathing, should be minimized.

Medications such as donepezil, melatonergic drugs (e.g., ramelteon and agomelatine), mirtazapine, erythropoietin, and ACE inhibitors can help to alleviate clinical symptoms of comorbidities of SDB (e.g., MNCD, Parkinson's disease, stroke, heart failure, chronic obstructive pulmonary disease (COPD)). However, these drugs cannot be recommended for the treatment of SDB per se in the aging adult.

While CPAP offers the greatest benefit for SDB and OSA, behavioral and surgical recommendations can be considered. Observational studies show improvement in OSA for older patients with morbid obesity after bariatric surgery (Gooneratne and Vitiello 2014; Netzer et al. 2016). Despite the association between obesity and sleep apnea in the geriatric patient, sometimes excess weight in the frail elderly can be *beneficial* during acute illnesses. Oral appliances, such as mandibular advancement devices to move the lower jaw, can be helpful as second-line treatment (Netzer et al. 2016). These remedies can be costly, can increase temporary jaw pain, and cannot be used in edentulous patients. Noncompliance with CPAP and oral appliances in the aging patient is common despite potential benefit (Bloom et al. 2009).

Circadian Rhythm Disorders

- *Delayed sleep phase type*: sleep onset shifted *later* (going to bed later and awakening later).
- *Advanced sleep phase type*: sleep onset is shifted *earlier* (going to bed earlier and awakening earlier). Older people more often experience this phase type.

Optimized sleep hygiene and bright light (2500–10,000 lux) between 7:00 and 9:00 P.M. can help delay sleep onset, improving sleep efficiency and total sleep time. Blue light works the best in younger patients.

Bright light therapy (BLT) is a safe option for sleep disorders in Alzheimer's Disease. In ophthalmologic diseases, pre-existing bipolar I disorder, and migraines, light therapy can trigger adverse effects, even manic episodes. Pushing bedtime later every few days may be impractical due to limited follow-up, compliance, and length of treatment (Bloom et al. 2009). Use of melatonin in the *morning* to prolong sleep is not recommended. Behavioral interventions may benefit, with little risk, although the data is mixed.

Parasomnias

These conditions occur during entry into sleep, during sleep itself, or during arousals from sleep. The most common in the geriatric age-group are REM Sleep Behavior Disorder (RBD) and Restless Legs Syndrome (RLS). For further discussion, see Chap. 5.

Rapid Eye Movement (REM) Sleep Behavior Disorder (RBD)

RBD is present in 0.5% of the general population and may be secondary to neurodegenerative diseases, especially α-synucleinopathies such as Parkinson's disease (PD), major neurocognitive disorder with Lewy bodies, and multiple system atrophy (MSA) (Howell and Schenck 2015). Patients lack the atonia typical of normal REM and instead engage in physical movements during dreams.

Hallmarks include unpleasant dreams or nightmares with loss of expected atonia during REM, resulting in dream enactment, violent behavior, and vocalizations. During episodes, the individual may not respond to the environment, but when awakened, become fully alert and recall dream content. Increased electromyographic activity is found on polysomnography. The activity and/or vocalizations can be injurious to both bed partners and patients, e.g., swinging, thrashing, and falling out of bed (Zdanys and Steffens 2015).

RBD is associated with destruction of the REM-related sleep centers (locus coeruleus, amygdala, and limbic system) involving several neurotransmitter pathways, including the GABA, glutamate, and monoaminergic (dopamine) systems that control REM and wakefulness (Howell and Schenck 2015). Neuroimaging studies have documented dopaminergic, cholinergic, and cortical abnormalities in RBD like those in patients with α-synucleinopathies. Idiopathic RBD may reflect another, milder form of neurodegenerative disease. However, dopamine deficiency does not cause RBD. Melatonin (3–15 mg at bedtime) has been shown to improve REM sleep atonia and reduce RBD symptoms and is a gentle, safe alternative to clonazepam for the geriatric patient (Boeve et al. 2003; Jung and St Louis 2016).

Dementia with Lewy Bodies (DLB) is associated with both insomnia and RBD.

Approximately 81–90% of patients with RBD will eventually develop a neurodegenerative disorder and about 50% of patients with spontaneous onset of RBD will be identified with a Parkinsonian disorder within a decade. RBD, therefore, may be a prodromal syndrome of Parkinson's disease (or related disorder) and may predict a more severe, aggressive course; it can serve as a marker of heightened risk of PD and help families prepare for the patient's future needs. For further discussion, see Chap. 5.

Pseudo-RBD

This condition has been reported in other sleep disorders, such as obstructive sleep apnea (OSA), periodic limb movements of sleep (PLMS), restless legs syndrome (RLS), and insufficient sleep syndrome. Medications which alter cholinergic, serotoninergic, and monoamine neurotransmitters may also be associated with RBD-like symptoms. One study of patients on antidepressants who had dream enactment behavior also demonstrated symptoms associated with the α-synucleinopathies, including loss of sense of smell, constipation, and mild motor impairments. It is not known if antidepressants cause or unmask RBD in individuals predisposed to develop neurodegenerative disorders (Postuma et al. 2013). Older adults who later show problematic alterations in dreams or sleep behavior may need discontinuation of antidepressants.

Sleep Attacks

These events mimic narcolepsy, are more common in people >65 years old, and can result in falls while upright, or accidents while driving. Episodes may occur when the patient is already somnolent. They can be induced by dopamine agonists such as pramipexole, ropinirole, and apomorphine, dopamine promoters like tolcapone, amantadine, and MAOIs (safinamide, rasagiline, selegiline), or dopamine precursors (levodopa, carbidopa/levodopa). "Falling Asleep During Activities of Daily Living and Somnolence" provides more details on accessdata.fda.gov . Unfortunately, reduction of the offending medications may result in worsening of the movement disorder.

Restless Legs Syndrome (RLS)

Hallmarks include the sensation of a burning or painful urge to move one's legs, often worse in the evenings while trying to sleep, and which improves with activity. It is *not* caused by neuropathy or radiculopathy. History can be sufficient for diagnosis, bolstered by polysomnography (PSG) and/or information from a bed partner. Cognitively impaired individuals may demonstrate leg discomfort with groaning, fidgeting, kicking, or rubbing legs. Medications which can contribute to RLS include tricyclic antidepressants, SSRIs, lithium, and antipsychotics. Obesity, lack of activity, caffeine, and smoking can also increase risk of RLS.

First-line pharmacological treatment for RLS includes dopaminergic agents. FDA-approved ropinirole or pramipexole have less rebound and less symptom augmentation than carbidopa/levodopa (Bloom et al. 2009), although they increase the risk of orthostatic hypotension, nausea, headache, sedation, compulsive behaviors, and drug–drug interactions. *Second-line agents* include opioids, benzodiazepines, and anticonvulsants, with caution. Treating iron deficiency anemia can improve symptoms.

Treatment of Insomnia Disorder

A necessary amount of sleep is not fixed, and decreased sleep is not per se pathologic, especially if the person is asymptomatic and functional. Occasional nights of poor sleep or periods of insomnia often resolve spontaneously or are situation-specific. For the aging patient, determine first if there have been any recent, time-limited factors which may interfere with sleep, such as travel, medical/surgical procedures, acute pain, changes in living situation/bed partners, or stressful events. Patients without daytime symptoms or impairment of functioning can be reassured without offering medication.

Non-pharmacological Interventions

Many cases of insomnia are secondary to a combination of systemic medical and psychiatric disorders, medications, substances, or environmental factors. Correction of contributors to insomnia is a *first-line intervention*.

Sleep Hygiene and Cognitive Behavioral Therapy for Insomnia (CBT-I)

Cognitive behavioral therapy for insomnia (CBT-I). Randomized controlled trial (RCT) evidence supports the superiority of CBT-I over medications for short- and long-term management of insomnia in older adults, with reliable, durable benefits in 70–80% of patients. CBT-I consists of 6–10 manualized sessions with a psychotherapist, clinician, or self-guided resource to reduce counterproductive thoughts, optimize sleep hygiene, reassociate the bed with sleep, improve sleep efficiency, and promote relaxation. It can improve sleep latency, continuity, restfulness, and duration of sleep, with increased sleep efficiency and decreased time awake during the night (Roepke and Ancoli-Israel 2010; Trauer et al. 2015). Brief Behavioral Treatment for Insomnia (BBT-I) is a condensed version of CBT-I with one session and two or three quick follow-ups which emphasize sleep consolidation (Buysse et al. 2017) (see Tables 8.8 and 8.11).

Some studies have reported that CBT-I showed greater treatment effects and more lasting benefits than pharmacotherapy (Gosney et al. 2012). One RCT of CBT-I combined *with*

Table 8.8 Sleep hygiene recommendations

Category	Goals	Details
Schedule	• Consistent regular schedule for sleep and awakening	• Use an alarm to wake up regardless of sleep, vacations, and weekends • Set a consistent bedtime late enough to avoid early morning awakenings
Environment	• Cool, comfortable, quiet, dark	• Use earplugs, fan/air conditioning, white noise.
Pre-bedtime routine	• Calm, consistent	• Meditate or take a hot bath • Make a to-do list for the next day that can be set aside when sleepy
Diet/nutrition	• Minimize caffeine (e.g., coffee, tea, soda, energy drinks) • Avoid stimulating medications after morning • Improve diet	• Alcohol, nicotine, and cannabis can disrupt sleep architecture • Finish large meals and fluids several hours before bed • If hungry before bed, have a light non-sugary snack
Activity	• Increase exercise and activities in the morning and early afternoon	• Minimize heavy exercise within 2 h of bedtime
Reduce/avoid	• Naps • Looking at clock • Light from TV/screens/computers • Interruptions from pets, noisy/restless bed partners • Sleeping in locations other than bed/bedroom • Reading, watching TV, working in bed	• Keep naps <30 min. or before 2:00 P.M. if unavoidable • Bed is for sleep and sexual activity only

short-term pharmacological treatment in older adults noted that "combination therapy was effective for short-term management of insomnia in late life, but sleep improvements were better sustained over time with behavioral treatment" for over 2 years (Bloom et al. 2009). Another RCT found that patients who completed combination therapy with CBT-I and pharmacotherapy were able to taper off pharmacotherapy with improved remission rates, compared to those with pharmacotherapy alone (Gooneratne and Vitiello 2014). CBT-I has been reported as effective for patients with comorbid chronic pain, psychiatric disorders, and/or cancer (Gooneratne and Vitiello 2014). For patients with cognitive impairment, a combined approach can incorporate sleep hygiene, stimulus control, and sleep restriction.

Digital technology and CBT-I. In 2020, the FDA approved the first digital CBT-I treatment for insomnia, *Somryst*, which is a prescription-only phone or other mobile-based application that is used for 9 weeks and may be renewed in 9-week increments. *Somryst* is based on SHUTi, an app that was available to the public for purchase until it was approved by the FDA. It requires sleep restriction, so should not be used in patients with bipolar disorder or psychotic disorders which may be exacerbated by decreased sleep. It is contraindicated in those with untreated OSA, parasomnias, epilepsy, pregnancy, or patients at high risk of falls, as sleepiness may increase in early treatment. Treatment consists of six modules that are intended to be completed once every 7 days. A positive study of technology-based CBT-I in older adults with SHUTi was presented at the World Sleep Congress in 2022, showing reductions in Insomnia Severity Index from 15.9 ± 5.2 to 10.0 ± 5.2 during active treatment and at 6- (9.1 ± 5.0) and 12-month (8.9 ± 5.1) follow-up intervals (Ritterband et al. 2022). Safety data regarding this trial was not available at time of publication of this chapter, but *Somryst* has been approved for adults 22 years and older.

Pharmacologic Interventions for Insomnia

Guidance from RCTs and drug efficacy data is sparse for insomnia in the geriatric population, with short follow-up, small samples, and comparisons of the active drug to placebo or to no treatment, rather than to *standard* treatment. The physiological changes of aging contribute to potential adverse effects: pharmacokinetic changes can increase the half-life of medication due to decreased hepatic and renal clearance, increased adipose tissue, and smaller volume of distribution; medications remain active longer than expected and the peak serum level can be higher. As a result, drug–drug interactions due to polypharmacy are prevalent, as the duration of drug action can be prolonged (Wastesson et al. 2018). Adverse effects of a medication can outweigh the benefits. The American Academy of Sleep Medicine published clinical guidelines, based upon an expert task force's systematic review of RCTs, which showed *weak* clinical evidence for treatment of insomnia with many medications or supplements (see Table 8.9) compared to no treatment (Sateia et al. 2017). FDA-approved medications for insomnia have been associated with significant adverse events, such as falls, hip fractures, delirium, and dizziness in older patients.

Medications only should be used *concurrently* with evidence-based behavioral therapy when benefits outweigh risks; environmental changes and sleep hygiene can maximize treatment benefit. Drugs with a shorter half-life can decrease daytime drowsiness. In addition, the lowest dose (or half of the usual adult starting dose), and short-term use (up to 4 weeks), can minimize rebound insomnia and discontinuation symptoms. *As-needed* medication use may be appropriate for highly reliable, cognitively intact, or monitored patients (see Table 8.9).

Sedative-Hypnotics

A meta-analysis of 2,414 participants with a mean age of 60 across 24 studies compared sedative medications with placebo. The number needed to treat (NNT) was 13, versus the number

Table 8.9 Medications for insomnia

Medication	Recommendation	Selected risks	Considerations[a]
FDA-Approved			
Benzodiazepines			
• Estazolam • Flurazepam • Quazepam • Temazepam[b] • Triazolam[b]	• Frequent awakenings • Short-term use only	• Rebound insomnia, complex sleep-related behaviors, daytime withdrawal, long-term effects unknown • Dependence and tolerance • Not recommended for patients with respiratory disorders (risk of respiratory depression) or substance use disorders (potential tolerance or addiction)	• Cognitive impairment, delirium, falls, unsteady gait, syncope, accidents, fractures
Benzodiazepine receptor agonists			
• Zolpidem[b] • Zolpidem CR[b] • Zaleplon[b] • Eszopiclone[b]	• Increased sleep duration and rapid onset to decrease sleep latency • Not shown to decrease number of awakenings	• Rebound insomnia and adverse effects like benzodiazepines • Long-term effects unknown • Not recommended for patients with respiratory disorders (risk of respiratory depression) or substance use disorders (potential for tolerance or addiction) • Residual daytime sedation and next-day impairment	• Cognitive impairment • Delirium • Falls • Syncope • Motor vehicle accidents • Fractures • Minimal benefit

(continued)

Table 8.9 (continued)

Medication	Recommendation	Selected risks	Considerations[a]
Melatonin receptor agonist			
• Ramelteon[b]	• For sleep onset and maintenance • Less risk of tolerance, dependence, or falls compared with benzodiazepines • Study reported 8 mg/day for 7 days in older patients in acute care protected against delirium (Hatta et al. 2014)	• Do not take with melatonin	• Has not been tested in frail older adults
Tricyclic antidepressant			
• Doxepin[b]	• Sleep maintenance • Less risk of tolerance or addiction	• Dizziness and heart arrhythmia • Nausea/vomiting • Ringing in ears • Weight gain • Breast swelling • Decreased libido	• Confusion/ delirium • Cognitive impairment and sedation • Orthostatic hypotension • Urinary retention • SIADH • Constipation • Dry mouth
Orexin receptor antagonists			
• Suvorexant[b] • Lemborexant • Daridorexant	• Sleep maintenance	• Next-day impairment • Headache and dizziness • Abnormal dreams • Diarrhea	• Do not use in narcolepsy
Not FDA-Approved			
Antihistamines			
• Diphenhydramine[b] Hydroxyzine, Doxylamine	• Inexpensive; some over-the-counter	• Reduced clearance in the elderly • Limit in patients >60 or with closed-angle glaucoma, prostatic hyperplasia, severe asthma, COPD • Limited data regarding efficacy and safety • Residual daytime sedation and weight gain	• Confusion/delirium • Cognitive impairment and sedation • Orthostatic hypotension • Urinary retention • Constipation • Dry mouth
Antidepressants			
• Trazodone[b]	• Consider in patients with comorbid depressive disorder	• Residual daytime sedation • Headache • Dizziness • Orthostatic hypotension • Cardiac arrhythmias • Elderly psychomotor impairment • Some evidence of tolerance	• SIADH • Priapism in males
• Mirtazapine	• Consider in patients with comorbid depressive disorder	• Sedation is inversely dose dependent (higher doses are less effective for sleep) • Increased appetite and weight gain	• SIADH

Table 8.9 (continued)

Medication	Recommendation	Selected risks	Considerations[a]
Tricyclic antidepressants			
• Amitriptyline • Imipramine • Nortriptyline • Desipramine	• Consider in patients with comorbid depressive disorder	• High risk in the elderly due to anticholinergic, antihistamine, and cardiovascular adverse effects • May reduce seizure threshold	• Confusion/delirium • Cognitive impairment • Orthostatic hypotension • Sedation • Urinary retention • Constipation • SIADH
Antipsychotics			
• Quetiapine	• Consider in patients with comorbid psychotic or bipolar disorder	• Residual daytime sedation • Orthostatic hypotension and syncope • Unsteady gait and falls • Cognitive impairment • Constipation • Metabolic changes (dyslipidemia, glucose dysregulation, weight gain)	• Increased risk of stroke and death in patients with dementia • SIADH • Prolonged QTc • Neuroleptic Malignant Syndrome
Other			
• Melatonin[b] • Tryptophan[b] • Valerian[b]	• Physiologic analog • Inexpensive • Over-the-counter (OTC) • Inexpensive	• Delayed onset of action • Potential for serotonin syndrome with tryptophan and serotonergic antidepressants • Rare cases of hepatotoxicity with valerian	• Ongoing studies • Limited data • Limited regulation of OTC drugs

SIADH Syndrome of Inappropriate Antidiuretic Hormone Secretion, *COPD* Chronic Obstructive Pulmonary Disease
Adapted From Richards et al. (2018)
[a]American Geriatrics Society 2019 Updated AGS Beers Criteria® for Potentially Inappropriate Medication Use in Older Adults (2019)
[b]American Academy of Sleep Medicine clinical guidelines showed *weak* clinical evidence for treatment of insomnia compared to no treatment (Sateia et al. 2017)

needed to harm, which was 6; thus, a sedative drug was *twice as likely to be harmful* as beneficial (Gosney et al. 2012). In addition, people over 65 years are at increased risk of delirium and behavioral disinhibition with sedative-hypnotics (Paton 2002). Alcohol and other CNS depressants potentiate these effects and should be avoided in combination with sedative-hypnotics.

Suvorexant, lemborexant, eszopiclone, zaleplon, zolpidem. These sedative-hypnotics are prescribed with warnings about worsening of depressive disorders and completed suicides, as well as agitation/disinhibition, auditory and visual hallucinations, and anterograde amnesia which leads to so-called sleep-driving and other complex behaviors (accessdata.fda.gov). Abnormal sleep behaviors in geriatric patients during the night are problematic given the risk for falls and injury. *Zolpidem* has been implicated in more than one-fifth of all emergency department visits for psychotropic adverse drug events in older adults (Hampton et al. 2014).

Suvorexant and lemborexant are dual orexin receptor antagonists, a class of hypnotic that works by selectively blocking the binding of the wakefulness-promoting neuropeptides orexin A and B. Suvorexant has a half-life of 12 h and *lemborexant* has a half-life of 18 h, making them useful in patients with sleep-onset as well as sleep-maintenance insomnia. Suvorexant has been used in patients with mild to moderate chronic obstructive pulmonary disease without negative effect on oxygenation.

Benzodiazepines. The risks of benzodiazepines for the aging adult, especially the oldest-old, need to be weighed against the benefits. Yet time-limited use of benzodiazepines can be beneficial for insomnia after events such as bereavement, psychosocial disruptions, and medical/surgical stressors. Several benzodiazepines are FDA-approved for insomnia but should be used with caution because of their long half-life, e.g., flurazepam, quazepam, and estazolam (Gooneratne and Vitiello 2014). Benzodiazepine and non-benzodiazepine GABA-receptor agonists can contribute to delirium, falls, dependence, and rebound anxiety upon abrupt discontinuation.

Temazepam, clonazepam (used to treat some parasomnias), and other benzodiazepines or benzodiazepine receptor agonists act on the central nervous system, depressing mood, and impacting cognition, alertness, and respiratory drive. Prescribing information for benzodiazepines includes warnings about depressive disorders, withdrawal symptoms upon abrupt discontinuation, increase in suicide risk, agitation and disinhibition, auditory and visual hallucinations, and anterograde amnesia leading to "sleep-driving" and other complex behaviors.

Antihistamines

Diphenhydramine and other antihistamines should be avoided or used only in very low doses in the oldest-old and frail elderly, due to their anticholinergic effects on cognition. They can also induce nocturia and perpetuate insomnia due to associated dry mouth and thirst at night.

Antipsychotics (APs). Medication risks associated with cerebrovascular accidents and increased risk of death in patients with MNCD led to the *black box* warning by the FDA for all second-generation antipsychotics (SGA) (as well as the first-generation antipsychotics haloperidol and perphenazine) in 2005. Quetiapine, risperidone, and olanzapine are *not* FDA-approved for primary insomnia but are prescribed often for insomnia and sleep disorders secondary to psychosis and neuropsychiatric symptoms of MNCD. While these drugs are usually sedating, aging adults are also susceptible to orthostatic hypotension via alpha-1 blockade (Gugger 2011). Aged patients on APs should be monitored for cardiovascular symptoms such as prolonged QTc, light-headedness, metabolic derangements, and symptoms of cerebrovascular events.

Antidepressants. Some data supports short-term use of some tricyclic antidepressants, such as low-dose doxepin and trazodone; there is inconclusive evidence of efficacy for amitriptyline, although it is widely used (Everitt et al. 2018). Doxepin does have a FDA indication for maintaining sleep. Antidepressants such as bupropion, fluoxetine, or venlafaxine can cause insomnia as a side effect, and most antidepressants disrupt or restore sleep architecture. The selective serotonin reuptake inhibitors (SSRIs) have little evidence of benefit for *primary* insomnia or sleep disorders but can be helpful in the treatment of secondary insomnia resulting from depressive or anxiety disorders. For further discussion, see Chap. 11.

Table 8.10 displays the effect of depressive disorders and antidepressants on sleep architecture.

Trazodone: A systematic review of 45 clinical studies reported that there is adequate data supporting the efficacy and general safety of low-dose trazodone for the treatment of insomnia (Jaffer et al. 2017). However, trazodone has also been shown to increase the risk of orthostatic hypotension and falls in older adults, without evidence of *sustained* efficacy (Bloom et al. 2009).

Mirtazapine: Medications that elicit blocking of the histamine H1 receptor, such as mirtazapine (primarily at doses ≤15 mg), dampen cortical activity and cause sedation. But no conclusive evidence has emerged to date that mirtazapine provides benefits in sleep disorders in aging adults (Ferini-Strambi et al. 2020).

Acetylcholinesterase inhibitors: Cholinesterase inhibitors are the first-line treatment for major neurocognitive disorders such as AD but may cause vivid dreams or nightmares that disrupt sleep, possibly related to shortened REM latency, increased REM density, and increased time spent in REM sleep (Zdanys and Steffens 2015).

Table 8.10 Effects of depressive disorders and antidepressants on sleep architecture

Medication category or depressive disorder	Sleep quantity and continuity	Slow wave sleep	REM latency	REM sleep
Depressive disorders	Decreased	Shifted to second sleep cycle from first	Decreased	Increased
Sedating tricyclic antidepressants (e.g., amitriptyline, doxepin)	Increased	Increased	Increased	Decreased
Activating tricyclic antidepressants (e.g., imipramine, desipramine)	Decreased	Decreased	Increased	Decreased
SSRIs (selective serotonin reuptake inhibitors) (e.g., fluoxetine, citalopram, escitalopram, sertraline)	Decreased/neutral	Neutral/increased	Increased	Decreased
SNRIs (serotonin/norepinephrine reuptake inhibitors) (e.g., venlafaxine, duloxetine)	Decreased	Neutral/increased	Increased	Decreased
Bupropion	Neutral/decreased	Neutral/increased	Neutral/ decreased	Neutral/ increased
Sedating antidepressants (e.g., mirtazapine, trazodone)	Increased	Increased	Neutral	Neutral
Vortioxetine	Neutral/decreased	Unknown	Increased	Decreased

Adapted from Wichniak et al. 2017

Insomnia also occurs in up to 9% of patients taking donepezil or rivastigmine (accessdata.fda.gov).

Anti-epileptics: Lamotrigine, oxcarbazepine, topiramate, phenytoin, and valproic acid derivatives can cause insomnia as an adverse effect. Any of these medications *can*, however, ameliorate insomnia when it is secondary to manic, hypomanic, depressive, or mixed episodes.

Melatonin/Ramelteon: Ramelteon is a selective agonist of MT1 and MT2, which are melatonin receptors located in the suprachiasmatic nucleus in the hypothalamus. Activation of MT1 receptors decreases the alerting signal in the evening, and activation of MT2 receptors can shift the phase of the circadian system. A RCT of melatonin given 2 h before bedtime showed efficacy for older adults for up to 6 months, likely due to a shift of the circadian phase, although the effects may not have been directly from the medication (Gooneratne and Vitiello 2014). Ramelteon is well-tolerated and reduces the time to onset of sleep in healthy older adults with insomnia, but there is sparse evidence of its effect in frail older adults (Gosney et al. 2012). Ramelteon is associated with lower risk of falls, withdrawal, and tolerance, compared with benzodiazepine hypnotics, but may take several days to show any improvement in sleep initiation.

Cannabis: Medical marijuana and other forms are commonly used by patients to aid sleep, but evidence remains mixed. Long-term use may result in withdrawal phenomena and/or an effect on sleep architecture. In jurisdictions where medical use of cannabis requires a prescription, clinicians should consider the risks and benefits given lack of available data. Note that marijuana prescriptions vary from traditional prescriptions as they do not specify quantity, strength, or directions for use, but are an endorsement of the patient's use and ability to obtain cannabis from a dispensary.

Conclusions

Inadequate or disrupted sleep, insomnia, sleep deprivation, and daytime drowsiness are all common among aging adults. A first step is to rule out and/or address treatable systemic medical contributors and improve environmental factors which interrupt sleep. A thorough review and adjustment of medication regimens, along with deprescribing of potentially inappropriate medications (PIM), is important. These interventions, coupled with psychotherapeutic approaches such as CBT-I, and behaviors which promote restful sleep, constitute age-*adjusted* practice. Pharmacotherapy may add risks of misuse, excessive use, dependence, discontinuation symptoms upon sudden withdrawal, adverse effects, sedation, and even *exacerbation* of sleep problems. The goal is to balance psychotherapeutic and behavioral techniques with safety-focused pharmacological practice.

Age-Adjusted Recommendations

- Consider non-pharmacological as first approaches for insomnia, including Cognitive Behavioral Therapy for Insomnia (CBT-I) and improvement of sleep hygiene.
- Explore the contribution of chronic systemic medical conditions, such as pain of osteoarthritis and congestive heart failure, to sleep deprivation.
- Encourage reduction of alcohol and other substances.
- Refer to sleep medicine specialists to rule out and treat obstructive sleep apnea (OSA) for sleep-disordered breathing (SDB).
- Consider bright light therapy for circadian rhythm disorders.
- Treat psychiatric disorders which have associated symptoms of sleep disruption.
- Search for hypomanic or manic symptoms (often accompanied by *decreased need* for sleep or absence of sleepiness).
- Scrutinize medication regimens for impact on sleep, e.g., medications which alter cholinergic, serotonergic, and monoamine neurotransmitters and which may be associated with RBD-like symptoms.
- Specific medication recommendations:
  - Only use sedative-hypnotics short-term (under 4 weeks) to minimize rebound insomnia.
  - Avoid abrupt discontinuation of sedative-hypnotics which can cause rebound anxiety.
  - Determine the time of medication/supplement use to identify any contribution to sleep disruption.
  - Use medications with shorter half-lives for insomnia to minimize daytime drowsiness.

Resources

Screening Tools

- STOP-BANG http://www.stopbang.ca/osa/screening.php
- Pittsburgh Sleep Quality Index https://www.sleep.pitt.edu/instruments/#psqi
- Epworth Sleepiness Scale https://epworthsleepinessscale.com/about-the-ess/
- Patient Health Questionnaire-9 https://www.uspreventiveservicestaskforce.org/Home/GetFileByID/218
- Mood Disorder Questionnaire https://www.ncbi.nlm.nih.gov/pmc/articles/PMC314375/

Sleep Log

https://www.sleepfoundation.org/sites/default/files/inline-files/SleepDiaryv6.pdf

Sleep Hygiene Handout

https://www.cci.health.wa.gov.au/-/media/CCI/Mental-Health-Professionals/Sleep/Sleep%2D%2D-Information-Sheets/Sleep-Information-Sheet%2D%2D-04%2D%2D-Sleep-Hygiene.pdf

Sleep Safety/Fall precautions

- Education regarding moving feet/sitting slowly/lingering at edge of bed before standing to prevent orthostatic hypotension.
- Adequate and accessible lighting.
- Smooth floor surfaces, without area rugs.
- Grab bars in bathrooms and by bed.
- Sleep apnea mask that can be easily removed.
- Bedside commode or handheld urinal.
- Doorway gate for pet to prevent tripping over pet.

CBT-I Resources: (Table 8.11)

Table 8.11 CBT-I resources for patients

Type	Suggested
Book	• Jacobs, Gregg D. *Say good night to insomnia: The 6-week, drug-free program developed at Harvard Medical School.* Holt paperbacks revised 9/15/2009
Websites	• National Sleep Foundation "Cognitive Behavioral Therapy for Insomnia" https://sleepfoundation.org/sleep-news/cognitive-behavioral-therapy-insomnia • Stanford Health Care "CBT-I" https://stanfordhealthcare.org/medical-treatments/c/cognitive-behavioral-therapy-insomnia.html
Phone apps	• CBT for Insomnia—This website offers 5-sessions of online cognitive behavioral therapy (CBT) program for insomnia. Cost associated. http://www.cbtforinsomnia.com • CBT-I coach—This provides a structured program that teaches strategies to improve sleep and help alleviate symptoms of insomnia. http://t2health.dcoe.mil/apps/CBT-I • Sleepio—An evidence-based CBT-I online and mobile app program. Cost associated. https://www.sleepio.com/ • SlumberPRO—A4–8-week self-help program based out of Australia that requires about 30–60 min each day. Cost associated. http://www.sleeptherapy.com.au/index.php?page=6 • Go! To sleep—A 6-week CBT-I program available through Cleveland Clinic of Wellness. A mobile app is also available. Cost associated. http://www.clevelandclinicwellness.com/Programs/Pages/Sleep.aspx • SHUTi—6-week CBT-I program that has been evaluated in 2 randomized trials involving adults with insomnia & cancer survivors. Cost associated. http://www.myshuti.com/ • Restore CBT-I—A 6-week CBT-I program evaluated in a randomized trial. http://restore.cbtprogram.com/ • Sleep training system—A 6-week online CBT-I program with personalized feedback. Cost associated. http://www.sleeptrainingsystem.com/index.php • Meditation Oasis—Relax & Rest Guided Mediation apps. Cost associated. http://www.meditationoasis.com/apps/ • Pocket CBT—Self-guided app for multiple conditions, including chronic fatigue, with thought records. Cost associated. http://www.pocketcbt.com/

References

American Geriatrics Society Beers Criteria ® Update Expert Panel. American Geriatrics Society 2019 Updated AGS Beers criteria® for potentially inappropriate medication use in older adults. J Am Geriatr Soc. 2019;67(4):674–94.

Beaudreau SA, Spira AP, Stewart A, et al. Study of osteoporotic fractures validation of the Pittsburgh sleep quality index and the Epworth sleepiness scale in older black and white women. Sleep Med. 2012;13(1):36–42.

Bernert RA, Turvey CL, Conwell Y, Joiner TE. Association of poor subjective sleep quality with risk for death by suicide during a 10-year period: a longitudinal, population-based study of late life. JAMA Psychiatry. 2014;71(10):1129–37.

Bloom HG, Ahmed I, Alessi CA, et al. Evidence-based recommendations for the assessment and management of sleep disorders in older persons. J Am Geriatr Soc. 2009;57(5):761–89.

Boeve BF, Silber MH, Ferman TJ. Melatonin for treatment of REM sleep behavior disorder in neurologic disorders: results in 14 patients. Sleep Med. 2003;4(4):281–4.

Buysse DJ, Reynolds CF, Monk TH, et al. The Pittsburgh Sleep Quality Index: a new instrument for psychiatric practice and research. Psychiatry Res. 1989;28(2):193–213.

Buysse DJ, Rush AJ, Reynolds CF. Clinical management of insomnia disorder. JAMA. 2017;318(20):1973–4.

Cho HJ, Lavretsky H, Olmstead R, et al. Sleep disturbance and depression recurrence in community-dwelling older adults: a prospective study. Am J Psychiatry. 2008;165(12):1543–50.

Cricco M, Simonsick EM, Foley DJ. The impact of insomnia on cognitive functioning in older adults. J Am Geriatr Soc. 2001;49(9):1185–9.

Everitt H, Baldwin DS, Stuart B, et al. Antidepressants for insomnia in adults. Cochrane Database Syst Rev. 2018;5:CD010753.

Ferini-Strambi L, Galbiati A, Casoni F, Salsone M. Therapy for insomnia and circadian rhythm disorder in Alzheimer disease. Curr Treat Options Neurol. 2020;22:4.

Foley DJ, Monjan AA, Brown SL, et al. Sleep complaints among elderly persons: an epidemiologic study of three communities. Sleep. 1995;18(6):425–32.

Foley D, Ancoli-Israel S, Britz P, Walsh J. Sleep disturbances and chronic disease in older adults: results of the 2003 National Sleep Foundation Sleep in America Survey. J Psychosom Res. 2004;56(5):497–502.

Gooneratne NS, Vitiello MV. Sleep in older adults: normative changes, sleep disorders, and treatment options. Clin Geriatr Med. 2014;30(3):591–627.

Gosney M, Harper A, Conroy S, editors. Geriatric Medicine (Oxford Desk Reference). Oxford, UK: Oxford University Press; 2012. https://oxfordmedicine.com/view/10

Gugger JJ. Antipsychotic pharmacotherapy and orthostatic hypotension. CNS Drugs. 2011;25(8):659–71.

Hampton LM, Daubresse M, Chang HY, et al. Emergency department visits by adults for psychiatric medication adverse events. JAMA Psychiatry. 2014;71(9):1006–14.

Hatta K, Kishi Y, Wada K, et al. Preventive effects of ramelteon on delirium: a randomized placebo-controlled trial. JAMA Psychiatry. 2014;71(4):397–403.

Howell MJ, Schenck CH. Rapid eye movement sleep behavior disorder and neurodegenerative disease. JAMA neurol. 2015;72(6):707–12.

Jaffer KY, Chang T, Vanle B, et al. Trazodone for insomnia: a systematic review. Innov Clin Neurosci. 2017;14(7–8):24–34.

Jung Y, St Louis EK. Treatment of REM sleep behavior disorder. Curr Treat Options Neurol. 2016;18(11):1–12.

Khachiyants N, Trinkle D, Son SJ, Kim KY. Sundown syndrome in persons with dementia: an update. Psychiatry Investig. 2011;8(4):275–87.

Lim AS, Kowgier M, Yu L, et al. Sleep fragmentation and the risk of incident Alzheimer's disease and cognitive decline in older persons. Sleep. 2013;36(7):1027–32.

Lin J, Suurna M. Sleep Apnea and Sleep-Disordered Breathing. Otolaryngologic clinics of North America. 2018;51(4):827–33.

Netzer NC, Ancoli-Israel S, Bliwise DL, et al. Principles of practice parameters for the treatment of sleep disordered breathing in the elderly and frail elderly: the consensus of the International Geriatric Sleep Medicine Task Force. Eur Clin Respir. 2016;J48(4):992–1018.

Ohayon MM, Vecchierini MF. Normative sleep data, cognitive function, and daily living activities in older adults in the community. Sleep. 2005;28(8):981–9.

Ohayon MM, Carskadon MA, Guilleminault C, Vitiello MV. Meta-analysis of quantitative sleep parameters from childhood to old age in healthy individuals: developing normative sleep values across the human lifespan. Sleep. 2004;27(7):1255–73.

Parish JM, Lyng PJ, Wisbey J. Compliance with CPAP in elderly patients with OSA. Sleep Med. 2000;1(3):209–14.

Paton C. Benzodiazepines, and disinhibition: a review. Psychiatri Bull. 2002;26(12):460–2.

Postuma RB, Gagnon JF, Tuineaig M, et al. Antidepressants and REM sleep behavior disorder: isolated side effect or neurodegenerative signal. Sleep. 2013;36(11):1579–85.

Rebelo-Marques A, Vicente C, Valentim B, et al. STOP-Bang questionnaire: the validation of a Portuguese version as a screening tool for obstructive sleep apnea (OSA) in primary care. Sleep Breath. 2018;22(3):757–65.

Richards K, DeMartini J, Xiong G. Understanding sleep disorders in older adults. Psychiatr Times. 2018;35(2):17–20.

Ritterband L, Shaffer K, Thorndike F, et al. An RCT of an internet intervention for insomnia tailored for older adults (SHUTi-OASIS). Rome, Italy: Presented at World Sleep Congress; March 2022.

Roepke SK, Ancoli-Israel S. Sleep disorders in the elderly. IndianJ Med Res. 2010;131:302–10.

Romanella SM, Roe D, Paciorek R, et al. Sleep, noninvasive brain stimulation, and the aging brain: challenges and opportunities. Ageing Res Rev. 2020;61:101067.

Sateia MJ, Buysse DJ, Krystal AD, et al. Clinical practice guideline for the pharmacologic treatment of chronic insomnia in adults: an American Academy of Sleep Medicine clinical practice guideline. J Clin Sleep Med. 2017;13(2):307–49.

Sivertsen B, Hysing M, Wehling E, et al. Neuropsychological performance in older insomniacs. Neuropsychol Dev Cogn B Aging Neuropsychol Cogn. 2013;20(4):34–48.

Spira AP, Beaudreau SA, Stone KL, et al. Osteoporotic fractures in men study. Reliability and validity of the Pittsburgh Sleep Quality Index and the Epworth Sleepiness Scale in older men. J Gerontol A Biol Sci Med Sci. 2012;67(4):433–9.

Trauer JM, Qian MY, Doyle JS, et al. Cognitive behavioral therapy for chronic insomnia: a systematic review and meta-analysis. Ann Intern Med. 2015;163(3):191–204.

Wastesson JW, Morin L, Tan ECK, Johnell K. An update on the clinical consequences of polypharmacy in older adults: a narrative review. Expert Opin Drug Saf. 2018;17(12):1185–96.

Wichniak A, Wierzbicka A, Walęcka M, Jernajczyk W. Effects of antidepressants on sleep. Cur Psychiatry Rep. 2017;19(9):63.

Wolkove N, Elkholy O, Baltzan M, Palayew M. Sleep and aging: 2. Management of sleep disorders in older people. Can Med Assoc J. 2007;176(10):1449–54.

Won C, Mahmoudi M, Qin L, et al. The impact of gender on timeliness of narcolepsy diagnosis. J Clin Sleep Med. 2014;10:89–95.

Zdanys KF, Steffens DC. Sleep disturbances in the elderly. Psychiatr Clin North Am. 2015;38(4):723–41.

Psychotic Symptoms and Syndromes

9

William B. Smith, Peter J. Ureste, Christa DeFries, and Andreea L. Seritan

Abstract

Approximately 15% of older adults report psychotic symptoms, and primary psychotic disorders account for less than half. Onset of psychosis and other psychiatric symptoms after age 40, atypical presentations, or symptoms resistant to treatment may indicate a non-primary psychiatric etiology and should prompt a thorough medical work-up. Neurodegenerative diseases can be associated with psychiatric (commonly anxiety, mood, or psychotic) symptoms, along with cognitive deficits. For this reason, cognitive screening tests should be conducted with all patients presenting with late-onset psychotic symptoms. In this chapter, we will discuss a step-by-step approach to the evaluation and differential diagnosis of psychosis in older adults, review primary psychotic disorders and common neurodegenerative and other neurological diseases that can present with psychosis, and outline pharmacological and non-pharmacological management approaches.

W. B. Smith · P. J. Ureste · A. L. Seritan (✉)
Department of Psychiatry and Behavioral Sciences, University of California, San Francisco, San Francisco, CA, USA

UCSF Weill Institute for Neurosciences, San Francisco, CA, USA
e-mail: william2.smith@ucsf.edu; peter.ureste@ucsf.edu; andreea.seritan@ucsf.edu

C. DeFries
Talkiatry, New York City, NY, USA

Case Vignette

A 67-year-old woman with no history of psychosis began accusing her spouse of exchanging seductive glances with others. The spouse denied this, and his behavior was not consistent with these suspicions. The patient had a history of recurrent major depressive disorder (MDD) since her 30s, hyperlipidemia, hypertension, a left cerebellar stroke, and Parkinson's disease (PD), diagnosed 6 years prior. She became withdrawn and spent most of the day in her room, staring out the window. She had poor appetite, disrupted sleep, and poor concentration. She had no auditory or visual hallucinations but was convinced that her husband had an affair, despite evidence to the contrary. She planned to move out and sought a divorce attorney.

The patient's medications included aspirin 81 mg at bedtime, atorvastatin 10 mg daily, carbidopa-levodopa 25–100 mg, 2 capsules four times a day, metoprolol 100 mg daily, and sertraline 100 mg daily. No recent medication changes were identified. She did not drink alcohol or use any illicit substances. Her Montreal Cognitive Assessment (MoCA) score was 24/30 (missing two points for attention, one point for language, two points for recall, and one point for orientation). No localized neurological deficits could be demonstrated, and routine laboratory studies were negative. A non-contrast head computerized tomography (CT) scan showed mild generalized cerebral atrophy and an old lacunar lesion

H. H. Fenn et al. (eds.), *Age-Adjusted Psychiatric Treatment for the Older Patient*,
https://doi.org/10.1007/978-3-031-53976-3_9

in the left cerebellar hemisphere, with no acute changes.

This example illustrates the broad differential diagnosis of new-onset psychotic symptoms in older adults, including PD psychosis, levodopa-induced psychosis, MDD with psychotic features, very late-onset schizophrenia-like psychosis (VLOSLP), a new stroke (with cognitive, mood, and psychotic symptoms), delirium, or delusional disorder. The MoCA score can be impacted by inattention, poor effort (especially in patients with depression), psychosis, or preexisting cognitive deficits. After ruling out other etiologies and considering the type of delusion (infidelity), PD psychosis was the most likely diagnosis. Treatment strategies range from reducing levodopa dose (if motor symptoms allow it) to starting quetiapine 12.5–25 mg daily, titrated slowly to an effective dose.

Overview

Psychosis encompasses delusions, hallucinations, disorganized thinking or speech, grossly disorganized or catatonic behavior, and negative symptoms (APA 2022a). Approximately 15% of older adults report psychotic symptoms, with a higher lifetime prevalence in women (6.6%) compared to men (5%) (Belbeze and Gallarda 2020; McGrath et al. 2015). The overall lifetime prevalence of schizophrenia is approximately 1%, with an estimated rate of 0.1–0.5% among older adults (Howard et al. 2000). By 2025, more than 25% of persons with schizophrenia will be 55 years of age or older (Cohen et al. 2008).

Primary psychotic disorders that first occur in late life are infrequent and can manifest with distinctive clinical, genetic, and neuropsychological characteristics. The International Late-Onset Schizophrenia Group proposed the nomenclature designating late-onset schizophrenia (LOS) as schizophrenia with onset between 40 and 59 years of age, and VLOSLP for symptoms presenting in individuals 60 years old or older (Howard et al. 2000). Neither LOS nor VLOSLP are included in the Diagnostic and Statistical Manual of Mental Disorders, fifth edition, Text Revision (DSM-5-TR) (APA 2022a). Only 40% of older adults who experience psychosis have primary psychotic disorders (Reinhardt and Cohen 2015). Neurodegenerative diseases account for most of the remainder (Lyketsos et al. 2002; Ropacki and Jeste 2005; Tampi et al. 2019a) and should be kept in mind when evaluating patients with late-onset psychotic symptoms. Each category will be discussed in detail in this chapter.

Assessment

The American Psychiatric Association (APA) Practice Guideline for the Treatment of Patients with Schizophrenia (Keepers et al. 2021) provides direction, but there are few, if any, evidence-based guidelines for the evaluation of psychosis in older adults. A thorough history, physical examination, and medical work-up can aid in identifying possible reversible causes of psychosis, especially for symptoms with onset in late life (Freudenreich et al. 2009; Reinhardt and Cohen 2015; Tampi et al. 2019a). Onset of psychosis after age 40, atypical presentations, or symptoms resistant to treatment may indicate a non-primary psychiatric etiology and should prompt a thorough medical work-up. Age at symptom onset, past psychiatric history, and family history of neurodegenerative or psychiatric diseases can guide clinical reasoning (Gournellis et al. 2011). Collateral history can elucidate chronology, particularly in patients with cognitive impairment or disorganized thinking. Cognitive screening tests such as the MoCA (Nasreddine et al. 2005) or Mini-Mental State Examination (MMSE) (Folstein et al. 1975) should be performed for all patients with late-onset psychosis, followed by neuropsychological evaluation, if indicated.

Recommendations for laboratory testing for older adults with new-onset psychosis vary, with little consensus on standardized algorithms. Initial work-up includes complete blood count, basic metabolic panel (electrolytes, glucose, renal function), liver-associated enzymes, thyroid stimulating hormone, vitamin B_{12}, vitamin D, folate, and urine drug screen (Freudenreich et al. 2009; Keepers et al. 2021;

Reinhardt and Cohen 2015). Testing for human immunodeficiency virus (HIV) or rapid plasma reagin is indicated only for those at high risk for HIV or syphilis infection, respectively (also see Chap. 4).

Lumbar puncture or electroencephalogram may be indicated in certain clinical scenarios. Head CT or brain magnetic resonance imaging (MRI) have a limited diagnostic yield in first-episode psychosis but may be useful in adults older than 50 or patients with neurological exam findings (Goulet et al. 2009). Neuroimaging studies can uncover cerebrovascular disease, mass lesions (e.g., infectious, tumors), or white matter diseases associated with psychosis.

Late-Life Primary Psychotic Disorders

A broad variety of etiologies may result in psychotic symptoms, ranging from primary psychotic spectrum illnesses, major depressive or bipolar disorders, neurodegenerative or other systemic medical diseases, to delirium, toxins, and substances of abuse. Rarely, psychotic symptoms can be associated with obsessive-compulsive disorder or posttraumatic stress disorder.

Table 9.1 summarizes characteristics of late-life primary psychiatric disorders that can manifest with psychotic features.

Delusional Disorder

DSM-5-TR defines delusional disorder as the presence of one or more delusions for ≥1 month, without meeting diagnostic criteria for schizophrenia or schizoaffective disorder; additionally, symptoms cannot be explained by another illness (APA 2022a). Delusional disorder presents, on average, around 40–49 years old in men and 60–69 years old in women, with a female-to-male ratio of 1.6:1 (APA 2022a; de Portugal et al. 2010). Studies suggest a prevalence of 0.03% in older adults, similar to that in the general population (Meesters et al. 2012; Tampi et al. 2019a). Delusions are non-bizarre and not accompanied by hallucinations (APA 2022a). Patients' daily functioning is not significantly impaired, which makes it difficult to establish the true prevalence of this disorder. Late-onset (>65 years) delusional disorder (LODD) has recently been described (González-Rodríguez et al. 2022). Harris et al. (2014) characterized 19 community-dwelling aging adults (mean age, 83.5 years) with LODD. Delusions of partition (the belief that people, objects, or radiation can pass through barriers), persecution, theft, and being spied on were most frequent (Harris et al. 2014).

Delusional parasitosis is more common in older adults (particularly women) than younger individuals, and it can be associated with systemic medical conditions such as hyperthyroidism, hypoparathyroidism, or neurodegenerative diseases (Bailey et al. 2014; Ozten et al. 2013). This condition may pose treatment challenges, as patients are often reluctant to accept antipsychotic medications (Moriarty et al. 2019).

Early-Onset Schizophrenia (EOS) in Older Adults

Schizophrenia which first begins before the age of 40, typically in late adolescence (APA 2022a) is classified as early-onset schizophrenia (EOS). A Dutch Catchment Area study found the 1-year prevalence of EOS among adults older than 60 to be 0.35% (Meesters et al. 2012). The EOS and LOS symptom constellations overlap, but there are also differences. Aging adults with EOS are more likely to have a thought disorder and affective blunting compared to those with LOS or VLOSLP (Mason et al. 2013; Suen et al. 2019). Adults with EOS may also experience cognitive decline over time, with age-dependent deficits in verbal fluency, vocabulary, and executive function compared to healthy controls (Fett et al. 2020). Patients with LOS have less premorbid educational, occupational, and social functioning impairment and a lower prevalence of current or lifetime substance misuse, although they have higher rates of systemic medical comorbidities and unemployment compared to older adults with EOS (Chen et al. 2018; Tampi et al. 2019a).

Table 9.1 Late-life primary psychotic disorders

Psychiatric disorders	Onset age (years)	Sex ratio	Prevalence in older adults	Distinctive features	Risk factors
Early-onset schizophrenia (EOS)	Median 25 Men: Early-to-mid 20s Women: Late 1920s	M:F = 1.4:1	One-year prevalence in adults >60: 0.35%	AH > VH, although less frequent AH than in young adults with EOS Thought insertion/withdrawal and affective blunting more frequent than in LOS	Family history of schizophrenia Earlier onset age is associated with worse prognosis
Late-onset schizophrenia (LOS)	40–59	F > M[a]	One-year prevalence in adults >60: 0.14%	More severe positive symptoms than in EOS[b] Paranoid, partition delusions AH > VH	Family history of schizophrenia less common than in EOS Premorbid paranoid or schizoid personality traits
Very late-onset schizophrenia-like psychosis (VLOSLP)	≥ 60	F:M = 1.5:1[a]	One-year prevalence in adults >60: 0.05%	Significantly more severe positive symptoms, but less episodes than in EOS or LOS Paranoid, partition, grandiose, or referential delusions Rare hallucinations Rare/no negative symptoms Rare/no thought disorder Neuroimaging abnormalities	Family history of schizophrenia less common than in EOS Family history of avoidant, paranoid, or schizoid personality disorder Sensory deficits Social isolation Immigrant status
Delusional disorder	Men: 40–49 Women: 60–69 Late-onset: ≥ 60	F:M = 1.6:1	0.04%	Non-bizarre delusions: paranoid, partition, theft No hallucinations May have cognitive deficits and cerebrovascular disease, with poor treatment response	Family history of schizophrenia Family history of avoidant, paranoid, or schizoid personality disorder
Schizoaffective disorder	Late 20s	F = M	One-year prevalence in adults >60: 0.14%	Depressive symptom severity comparable with adults >50 years with bipolar disorder Thought disorder severity comparable to adults >50 years with schizophrenia	Earlier age at onset associated with higher severity of psychotic symptoms

Major depressive disorder with psychotic features	Peak 20; median 30[c]; 51 for psychotic depression	F > M[d]	9.8% MDD in adults >65; 15–34% may have psychotic symptoms	Psychotic symptoms more common in older than in younger adults with MDD, but no difference in rate of psychotic symptoms between early-onset (< 60 years) and late-onset (>60 years) MDD Delusions most common: Somatic; mood-congruent Hallucinations less common (typically AH)	Family history of psychosis and bipolar disorder Cerebrovascular disease Physical and/or sexual trauma, rural residence, acute medical problems, poorer social skills
Bipolar disorder with psychotic features	Peak 20; median 33[c,e]	F:M = 2.3:1	0.5–1% bipolar disorder in older adults; 64% may have psychotic symptoms	OABD: More depressive, less manic or psychotic symptoms (but more frequent paranoid delusions) than in younger adults with bipolar disorder Hallucinations less common (typically AH)	Family history of bipolar or major depressive disorder less common in late-onset (>50 years) than early-onset (<50 years) bipolar disorder Neurological disease

APA 2022a; Belbeze and Gallarda 2020; Chen et al. 2018; Cohen et al. 2014; de Portugal et al. 2010; Depp and Jeste 2004; Forlani et al. 2014; González-Rodríguez et al. 2022; Gournellis et al. 2011; Hanssen et al. 2015; Harris et al. 2014; Hirschfeld et al. 2003; Howard et al. 2000; Jääskeläinen et al. 2018; Kessler et al. 2010; Meesters et al. 2012; Reeves et al. 2002; Reinhardt and Cohen 2015; Rolin et al. 2017; Sajatovic et al. 2015; Solmi et al. 2022; Stafford et al. 2018; Suen et al. 2019; Tampi et al. 2019a; Vahia et al. 2010; Van Assche et al. 2019

AH auditory hallucinations, *EOS* early-onset schizophrenia, *F* female, *LOS* late-onset schizophrenia, *M* male, *MDD* major depressive disorder, *OABD* older-age bipolar disorder, *VH* visual hallucinations, *VLOSLP* very late-onset schizophrenia-like psychosis

[a]This sex ratio increases with age

[b]Vahia et al. (2010) found less positive symptoms in patients with LOS than with EOS

[c]Represents the mood disorder onset age in the general population

[d]This gender ratio narrows with age

[e]There is great heterogeneity across studies in defining age cutoff for late-onset bipolar disorder

Late-Onset Schizophrenia (LOS)

The proportion of individuals with LOS and VLOSLP among all people with schizophrenia has been estimated at 20–25%, with an incidence of new-onset schizophrenia of 0.3% per year in the 45–64 years old age-group (Köhler et al. 2007; Tampi et al. 2019a). Women make up 60% of the adults with onset of schizophrenia after age 40, and this sex ratio significantly increases with age (Chen et al. 2018; Hanssen et al. 2015; Howard et al. 2000).

Older adults with LOS and VLOSLP are significantly less likely than those with EOS to have a family history of schizophrenia, but significantly more likely to report positive symptoms (Chen et al. 2018; Hanssen et al. 2015; Stafford et al. 2018). Persecutory and partition delusions are predominant in both LOS and VLOSLP, while hallucinations are less common (Mason et al. 2013; Suen et al. 2019). Hallucinations can be visual, tactile, olfactory, or auditory hallucinations of third-person running commentary or multiple voices (Howard et al. 2000).

Very Late-Onset Schizophrenia-like Psychosis (VLOSLP)

VLOSLP has been shown to be distinct from the psychosis associated with neurodegenerative diseases, although the validity and stability of this diagnosis have been questioned (Belbeze and Gallarda 2020; Van Assche et al. 2019). The prevalence of VLOSLP ranges from 0.1 to 0.5% (Howard et al. 2000; Stafford et al. 2018). Onset of psychotic symptoms in a centenarian has been reported (Cervantes et al. 2006).

In a study comparing 338 patients with early, late, and very late-onset schizophrenia-spectrum disorders, those with very late-onset psychosis had significantly more severe positive symptoms (although less psychotic episodes) and significantly lower remission rates, were less likely to take medication, and needed significantly lower antipsychotic doses compared to the other two groups (Hanssen et al. 2015). In another study of 26 inpatients with VLOSLP, 69% endorsed paranoid thoughts and delusions, while only 15% of patients reported hallucinations (Reeves et al. 2002). Hallucinations can be auditory, visual, tactile, or olfactory (Reinhardt and Cohen 2015). The co-occurrence of paranoid and partition delusions is thought to be highly predictive of a VLOSLP diagnosis (Belbeze and Gallarda 2020; Van Assche et al. 2019).

Neurodegenerative Diseases Associated with Psychotic Symptoms

Common neurodegenerative diseases such as Alzheimer's disease (AD) (Bassiony and Lyketsos 2003; Jeste and Finkel 2000; Mizrahi et al. 2006; Ropacki and Jeste 2005), dementia with Lewy bodies (DLB) (McKeith et al. 2017; Nagahama et al. 2007; Perini et al. 2016), Huntington's disease (HD) (Orth et al. 2010; Paulsen et al. 2001), and PD (Kataoka and Sugie 2018; Kulick et al. 2018; Warren et al. 2018) can all be associated with psychotic symptoms. Delusions typically occur in mid-to-late stages of disease although they can also occur as part of neurodegenerative disease prodromes (Seritan 2023). Visual hallucinations (VH) are far more common than auditory hallucinations (AH). In PD, psychotic symptoms can also be caused or exacerbated by dopaminergic agents (Lee and Weintraub 2012). Although often encountered in patients with cognitive impairments, psychotic symptoms also be present in cognitively intact people with PD (Lee and Weintraub 2012).

Psychotic symptoms are a later manifestation in *AD* and *PD* but occur early in *DLB* (Jeste and Finkel 2000; Tampi et al. 2019b; Warren et al. 2018). Vivid, recurrent, and well-formed VH are a core clinical feature for probable DLB, along with fluctuating cognition and parkinsonism and REM sleep behavior disorder. Severe sensitivity to antipsychotics is a supportive clinical feature (McKeith et al. 2017).

Although initially believed to be uncommon in *frontotemporal dementia (FTD)*, psychotic symptoms are currently recognized as part of its clinical picture (Landqvist Waldö et al. 2015; Benussi et al. 2021). In a large series of patients with autopsy-confirmed FTD, almost a third had psychosis (Landqvist Waldö et al. 2015). The discovery of chromosome 9 open reading frame 72 (*C9orf72*) gene has led to a more sophisticated characterization of FTD phenotypes. *C9orf72* gene mutations are now known to be the most common genetic abnormality associated with behavioral variant (bv) FTD and familial amyotrophic lateral sclerosis (Shinagawa et al. 2015; Sha et al. 2012; Snowden et al. 2012). The bvFTD phenotype in *C9orf72* mutation carriers is consistent with slower progression of disease, but a higher incidence of delusions and hallucinations compared to non-carriers (Sha et al. 2012; Devenney et al. 2017). Psychosis was the presenting symptom in 38% of *C9orf72* mutation carriers with FTD-motor neuron disease (Snowden et al. 2012).

Patients with *HD* can have prominent psychiatric manifestations, including apathy (noted in approximately 70% of patients), depression (ranging from 33 to 69%), agitation or aggression (45%), anxiety (34%), obsessive-compulsive symptoms (27%), psychosis (6–12%), and mania (9%) (Orth et al. 2010; Paulsen et al. 2001). Twelve percent of patients with HD may have delusions (often paranoid or grandiose), and 2% endorse hallucinations (Paulsen et al. 2001).

Spinocerebellar ataxias (SCAs) are adult-onset, autosomal dominant neurodegenerative diseases of the cerebellum and connected areas. SCAs manifest primarily with neurological symptoms, although several (e.g., SCA type 2, 3—Machado-Joseph disease, 6, 7, 10, 14, and 17) can also be associated with cognitive deficits and/or psychiatric disturbances including anxiety, aggression, depression, and psychosis (Liszewski et al. 2004; Rottnek et al. 2008; Braga-Neto et al. 2016; Seritan 2023; Stevanin and Brice 2008). SCA17, also known as Huntington's disease-like 4, can manifest with psychosis, along with anxiety, depressive symptoms, chorea, dystonia, or parkinsonism (Stevanin and Brice 2008). Table 9.2 displays the prevalence and phenomenology of psychotic symptoms associated with the four most common neurodegenerative diseases.

Table 9.2 Psychotic symptoms in common neurodegenerative diseases

Psychotic symptoms	AD	DLB	FTD	PD
Delusions[a]				
Overall prevalence and phenomenology	31% (9–59%) Simple, non-bizarre. Typically occur in the middle stage and resolve (or are no longer expressed) in advanced disease stages	50% Systematized delusions are a supportive feature for the diagnosis of probable DLB; insight is gradually lost	2%–23% (57% in *C9orf72* carriers with bvFTD)	7–10% Typically occur later than hallucinations in the disease course. Delusions induced by dopaminergic agents have grandiose, exalted themes (e.g., "having superpowers") and may be associated with DDS, ICD, elevated mood, poor sleep, pressured speech, and disorganized thought process (flight of ideas, loosening of associations)
• Misidentification[b]	16–34%	33-52%	30%	11%
– Capgras	4–14%	6–17%	Case reports	Case reports
• Paranoid	14–46%	11–25%	20%	4–5%
• Spousal infidelity	1–26%	1–26%	Case reports	1–5%
• Theft	22%	14%	10%	1–2%

(continued)

Table 9.2 (continued)

Psychotic symptoms	AD	DLB	FTD	PD
Hallucinations[a]				
Overall prevalence	16% (6–41%)	75%	18% (36% in *C9orf72* carriers with bvFTD)	53–60%
• Auditory	8–12%	35%; often co-occur with VH	9–10%	0–22%; often co-occur with VH
• Visual	7–23% Simple	60–75% Detailed, recurrent, vivid, well-formed (people, children, small animals). Occur early in the disease course	7–9%	16–38% Well-formed (e.g., people, animals, patterns, lines). Often occur in dim light, when alone in the room. Typically late in the disease course and may predict cognitive impairment
• Other	9% passage[c] hallucinations; 5% extracampine[d] hallucinations	60% extracampine hallucinations Rare tactile hallucinations	Rare tactile, olfactory hallucinations	17% passage[c] hallucinations; 16–50% extracampine[d] hallucinations Rare tactile, olfactory, gustatory hallucinations

Bassiony and Lyketsos 2003; Belbeze and Gallarda 2020; Benussi et al. 2021; Cannas et al. 2017; Devenney et al. 2017; Harciarek and Kertesz 2008; Jeste and Finkel 2000; Josephs 2007; Kulick et al. 2018; Landqvist Waldö et al. 2015; Lee and Weintraub 2012; Mizrahi et al. 2006; Nagahama et al. 2007; Paulsen et al. 2001; Pereira and de Oliveira 2019; Perini et al. 2016; Ruiz et al. 2018; Seritan 2023; Shinagawa et al. 2015; Warren et al. 2018; Wood et al. 2015

AD Alzheimer's disease, *AH* auditory hallucinations, *bvFTD* behavioral variant frontotemporal dementia, *C9orf72* chromosome 9 open reading frame 72, *DDS* dopamine dysregulation syndrome, *DLB* dementia with Lewy bodies, *FTD* frontotemporal dementia, *ICD* impulse control disorders, *PD* Parkinson's disease, *VH* visual hallucinations

[a]Prevalence ranges represent data compiled from different studies

[b]Misidentification delusions include: Capgras syndrome (false belief that a familiar person, often a close family member or caregiver, has been replaced by an identical-looking impostor), Fregoli syndrome (false belief that different individuals are actually the same person, in disguise), and reduplicative paramnesia (false belief that a familiar person, place, object, or body part has been duplicated)

[c]Passage hallucinations = brief visions of a person or an animal passing in the periphery of the visual field

[d]Extracampine hallucinations (sense of presence) = feeling like another person is in proximity

Other Etiologies Associated with Psychosis

The differential diagnosis of late-life psychosis also includes Charles Bonnet syndrome, stroke, cerebral autosomal dominant arteriopathy with subcortical infarcts and leukoencephalopathy (CADASIL), delirium, epilepsy, metabolic and other systemic medical conditions, substances, toxins, and vascular major neurocognitive disorder (MNCD). See Reinhardt and Cohen (2015) and Seritan (2023) for a review of systemic medical etiologies and medication- and substance-induced psychotic disorders in older adults. Here we discuss common non-neurodegenerative neurological conditions that can present with psychosis in the geriatric population.

Charles Bonnet Syndrome (Visual Release Hallucinations)

This is one of the most common causes of VH in older adults, occurring in up to 30% of visually impaired individuals, although it may be underreported (Pang 2016; Scott et al. 2001). VH occur as a result of damage anywhere along the visual pathways, most often due to age-related macular degeneration, glaucoma, or cataracts (Pang 2016). Insight and cognition are typically intact, and there are no other psychotic symptoms (Pang 2016; Scott et al. 2001). VH due to chronic ocular disease may occur 1 year or later after the visual impairment, whereas VH secondary to acute cerebral or optic nerve injury (e.g., stroke, optic neuritis, and surgery) manifest within a few hours to days and can remit spontaneously in 25% of cases (Pelak 2021).

Poststroke Psychosis

Poststroke psychosis (also see Chap. 7) can occur after ischemic or hemorrhagic strokes or transient ischemic attacks, usually alongside neurological symptoms, although isolated psychotic features can occur (Almeida and Xiao 2007; Stangeland et al. 2018). Psychiatric symptoms occur within days to 6 months of the cerebrovascular accident (CVA), and symptoms are usually stable over time unless a subsequent stroke occurs (Almeida and Xiao 2007). Both cortical and subcortical CVAs can be associated with psychosis, with a recent systematic review implicating mainly right hemisphere lesions (McMurtray et al. 2014; Stangeland et al. 2018; Seritan 2023).

Psychosis of Epilepsy

Older adults have the highest incidence of new-onset epilepsy of all age groups, and the risk increases with age (Qin et al. 2005). The prevalence of psychosis among patients with epilepsy is 4–7% and is even higher (7–11%) in those with temporal lobe epilepsy (TLE) (Falip et al. 2009; Clancy et al. 2014; Irwin and Fortune 2014). The phenomenology of psychotic symptoms may help identify the location of the epileptogenic focus (Adachi et al. 2000). Olfactory or gustatory hallucinations are suggestive of TLE (APA 2022a).

Psychotic disorders in epilepsy are classified according to their temporal relationship to seizure activity:

- *Ictal psychosis* is concurrent with seizures, lasts for hours to days, and is associated with impaired consciousness (Irwin and Fortune 2014; Kim et al. 2008). Hallucinations and delusions are uncommon; patients may have stereotypical behaviors, such as picking at clothes, and are amnesic for the episode (Irwin and Fortune 2014).
- *Postictal psychosis (PIP)* occurs in about 6% of patients with epilepsy and can account for 25% of psychotic symptoms in this population (Falip et al. 2009; Pollak et al. 2014). PIP has an abrupt onset following seizures, after a "lucid interval" of 24–72 h during which patients have preserved consciousness and no behavioral changes. PIP lasts from one to 18 days (mean, 3–4 days), although it can persist for up to a month (Pollak et al. 2014). PIP may start with anxiety and insomnia and progress to delusions (paranoid, grandiose, or religious), hallucinations, catatonia, or depressive or manic episodes (Irwin and Fortune 2014; Pollak et al. 2014). PIP can recur several times a year (Kim et al. 2008).
- *Interictal psychosis (IIP)* occurs in about 5% of patients with epilepsy during seizure-free periods and does not appear to be directly related to seizure activity (Clancy et al. 2014; Kim et al. 2008). IIP episodes can last days to weeks and manifest with AH, paranoid delusions, and mystical experiences (Irwin and Fortune 2014). Approximately 14–20% of patients with IIP go on to develop *chronic* interictal psychosis, also termed schizophrenia-like psychosis of epilepsy (SLPE) (Kaufman et al. 2017; Pollak et al. 2014). SLPE is associated with paranoid and religious-themed delusions, AH of a menacing quality, and rare VH (Kandratavicius et al. 2014). Patients have relatively preserved affect and typically do not deteriorate over time.

Common non-neurodegenerative neurological conditions that can manifest with psychosis in older adults are summarized in Table 9.3.

Table 9.3 Non-neurodegenerative neurological conditions with psychotic symptoms

Condition	Onset age (years)	Prominent psychotic symptoms	Other features/associated symptoms	Risk factors
Charles Bonnet syndrome	>70	• Simple VH (lines, flashes of light, geometric shapes) • Complex VH (people, animals, scenes) • Seen more often when looking at white backgrounds • VH correspond to the underlying vision loss	Visual impairment No other psychotic symptoms No cognitive impairment	Female sex Worse visual acuity Bilateral or fluctuating unilateral visual impairment Social isolation Dim lighting, in the evening or at night
CADASIL	30–50	• Hallucinations: 44–71% (VH > AH) • Delusions: 57%	Migraine with aura, subcortical infarcts, seizures, focal neurological deficits, cognitive impairment	Autosomal dominant mutations in *NOTCH3* gene (on chromosome 19) that affect vascular smooth muscle cells
Psychosis of epilepsy	30 (10–20 years after epilepsy onset)	Ictal psychosis • Rare delusions or hallucinations Postictal psychosis • Delusions (paranoid, grandiose, religious, somatic) • AH Interictal psychosis • Delusions (paranoid) • AH Schizophrenia-like psychosis of epilepsy • Delusions (paranoid, religious) • AH • Rare VH • Social isolation	Cognitive disorders Depressive or bipolar disorders Suicide (4–5 times higher risk than in the general population) Violent behavior TLE interictal personality[a] (circumstantial, interpersonally "sticky," hyposexual, humorless, overly concerned with philosophical/religious questions, hypergraphia)	Age Family history of epilepsy, mood disorders, psychotic disorders TLE Neurodevelopmental disorders For postictal psychosis: • Cluster of seizures • Bilateral seizure foci For interictal psychosis: • Childhood onset of epilepsy • Structural abnormalities • Frequent seizures • Multiple seizure types • Seizures that require multiple AEDs • Postictal psychosis
Poststroke psychosis	Mean age 67	Overall incidence: 5–6.7% • Delusions (persecutory, jealousy, reduplicative paramnesia, somatic) • AH • VH	Cognitive disorders Depressive or bipolar disorders Personality changes	Predominantly right-sided cortical (frontal, temporal, parietal) and subcortical (midbrain, basal ganglia, cerebellar, thalamic) lesions

Table 9.3 (continued)

Condition	Onset age (years)	Prominent psychotic symptoms	Other features/associated symptoms	Risk factors
Vascular major neurocognitive disorder	> 65	• Delusions: 9–58% (paranoid, theft, misidentification) • Hallucinations: 4–67% – VH/visual illusions: 15% – AH/auditory illusions: 12%	Focal neurological deficits Apathy Depressive or manic symptoms Personality changes Stepwise cognitive decline	Age Male sex Hypertension Diabetes mellitus Hyperlipidemia Cardiac disease Cardiac surgery

Almeida and Xiao 2007; Drazyk et al. 2019; Irwin and Fortune 2014; Kandratavicius et al. 2014; Kaufman et al. 2017; Khanna et al. 2022; McMurtray et al. 2014; Pang 2016; Pelak 2021; Pollak et al. 2014; Qin et al. 2005; Reinhardt and Cohen 2015; Scott et al. 2001; Stangeland et al. 2018

AED antiepileptic drug, *AH* auditory hallucinations, *CADASIL* cerebral autosomal dominant arteriopathy with subcortical infarcts and leukoencephalopathy, *TLE* temporal lobe epilepsy, *VH* visual hallucinations

[a] This concept is controversial

Psychosocial Interventions for Late-Life Psychosis

The 2019 APA Practice Guideline for Treatment of Patients with Schizophrenia recommended psychosocial approaches such as psychoeducation and cognitive behavioral therapy for psychosis in addition to pharmacological management (Keepers et al. 2021).

- Cognitive behavioral social skills training (CBSST) is a manualized group therapy that combines cognitive behavioral therapy with social skills and problem-solving training and has been shown to improve daily functioning in older adults with schizophrenia. A randomized controlled trial (RCT) compared 24 weekly CBSST sessions to pharmacological treatment-as-usual in 76 outpatients aged 42 to 74 (mean age, 53.6 ± 7.5 years) with schizophrenia or schizoaffective disorder (Granholm et al. 2007). The CBSST group showed greater skill acquisition and reported improved community living skills compared to the control group; gains were maintained after 1 year.
- Functional Adaptation Skills Training (FAST) is a manualized intervention shown to significantly improve everyday living and social skills in older adults with schizophrenia and schizoaffective disorder (Patterson et al. 2006). A culturally adapted version of FAST improved everyday living skills in older Latino individuals with schizophrenia or schizoaffective disorder (Patterson et al. 2005).
- Psychosocial skills training combined with prophylactic health care intervention led to improved community living skills and increased use of preventive care among older adults with schizophrenia, even at 3-year follow-up (Bartels et al. 2014).

Pharmacological Treatment of Late-Life Psychosis

Pharmacological management is appropriate when psychotic symptoms do not respond to cognitive or behavioral strategies and patients are at risk of self-harm or harm to others (Reus et al. 2016). For older adults whose primary psychotic disorders began in young to middle age, continued pharmacological management must take into account age-related physiological changes such as slower hepatic metabolism, reduced glomerular filtration rate, complex medication regimens with higher risk of drug–drug interactions, and comorbidities such as diabetes mellitus, hypertension, and hyperlipidemia (also see Chap. 2).

The search for underlying causes of psychosis, such as medications (e.g., levodopa or corticosteroids) or systemic conditions is the first step of an age-adjusted approach. The second step is to reduce or discontinue the causative agent. For psychotic disorders due to systemic medical illness, the underlying conditions need to be identified and appropriately treated (e.g., thyroid replacement for hypothyroidism-related psychosis or tumor resection and/or immunotherapy for paraneoplastic limbic encephalitis). If these strategies do not alleviate psychotic symptoms, an antipsychotic should be considered. Standardized treatment guidelines have not been formulated.

Table 9.4 summarizes practical pharmacological management strategies.

Table 9.4 Strategies for pharmacological management of late-life psychosis

Dosing guidelines	
Starting dose	LOS/VLOSLP: 25–50% of younger adult starting dose
Target dose	Older adults with EOS/LOS: 25–50% of target dose in younger adults VLOSLP: 10% of target dose in younger adults AD psychosis: 15–25% of target dose for younger adults with schizophrenia DLB and PD psychosis: see Table 9.5 for specific dose recommendations
General principles for management of late-life psychosis • Use monotherapy as much as possible • In rare cases, two agents may need to be used concurrently; attempt to consolidate to monotherapy as soon as possible	
Principles for management of psychosis in major neurocognitive disorders • Use antipsychotics only if psychotic symptoms are severe, dangerous, or cause significant distress to the patient or their family • Titrate to lowest dose that controls symptoms • Discontinue if no improvement after 4 weeks • Attempt to taper off the medication within 4 months of initiation, if there was no symptom recurrence • Long-acting injectable agents should not be used first-line, unless there is a co-occurring chronic psychotic disorder • If injectable formulations were used acutely, convert to oral formulation as soon as possible	

Howard et al. 2000; Jeste and Finkel 2000; Reus et al. 2016

AD Alzheimer's disease, *DLB* dementia with Lewy bodies, *EOS* early-onset schizophrenia, *LOS* late-onset psychosis, *PD* Parkinson's disease, *VLOSLP* very late-onset schizophrenia-like psychosis

Antipsychotic Medications

A systematic Cochrane review found no trials upon which to base guidelines for the treatment of LOS and VLOSLP (Essali and Ali 2012). The Clinical Antipsychotic Trials of Intervention Effectiveness–Alzheimer's Disease (CATIE-AD) examined the benefits and safety of antipsychotic medications in patients with AD. This large double-blind, placebo-controlled trial was conducted between 2001 and 2004 at 42 sites: 421 outpatients with AD and psychosis, aggression, or agitation were randomly assigned to receive olanzapine (mean dose, 5.5 mg/day), quetiapine (mean dose, 56.5 mg/day), risperidone (mean dose, 1.0 mg/day), or placebo. Doses were adjusted as needed, and patients were followed for up to 36 weeks (Schneider et al. 2006). There were no significant differences among groups with regard to time to discontinuation due to either side effects or lack of benefit. There were no significant differences with regard to clinical improvement either: 32% of patients on olanzapine, 26% of patients taking quetiapine, and 29% of patients on risperidone showed improvement, compared to 21% of patients receiving placebo (Schneider et al. 2006). In a separate systematic review of RCTs or meta-analyses, olanzapine and risperidone showed modest, yet statistically significant effects on reducing aggression, hallucinations, and delusions associated with AD or vascular MNCD (Sink et al. 2005).

A double-blind RCT compared risperidone (median dose 2 mg/day) to olanzapine (median dose 10 mg/day) in 175 adults ≥60 years with schizophrenia or schizoaffective disorder (Jeste et al. 2003). Patients in both groups experienced significant reduction in Positive and Negative Syndrome Scale (PANSS) scores over the 8-week study period. In an open-label study, over half of 180 older adults with schizophrenia (mean age, 73 years) experienced a significant reduction in their PANSS scores with risperidone at a mean dose of 3.7 mg/day (Davidson et al. 2000). Both oral and long-acting injectable risperidone preparations have been well tolerated and effective in older adults with psychotic disorders (Davidson et al. 2000; Jeste et al. 2003; Lasser et al. 2004). Paliperidone (9-hydroxy-risperidone) is an active metabolite of risperidone available in an oral extended-release as well as long-acting injectable formulation. The oral formulation was relatively well tolerated at 3–12 mg/day, although not more effective than placebo, in a trial of 114 older adults (mean age, 70 years) with schizophrenia (Tzimos et al. 2008).

Olanzapine, at a median dose of 10 mg/day, also demonstrated improvement in Clinical Global Impressions (CGI)—Improvement and Brief Psychiatry Rating Scale (BPRS) scores in an open-label, 4-week trial of older adults (mean age, 74.2 years) with psychotic disorders (Hwang et al. 2003). Olanzapine and clozapine have anticholinergic properties and may worsen cognitive deficits; as such, they should be used cautiously in patients with MNCDs. Moretti and colleagues followed 68 outpatients (mean age, 71.2 ± 2.9 years) with AD, bvFTD, vascular MNCD, DLB, and PDD for up to 24 months and demonstrated benefits of olanzapine in doses ranging from 2 to 10 mg daily for psychosis and behavioral disturbances (e.g., verbal or physical aggression, anxiety, and weeping) (Moretti et al. 2003).

Quetiapine was well tolerated and effective in improving psychosis in older adults (mean age, 76.1 years) over a 52-week period, at a median dose of 137.5 mg/day, although only 28% of participants had primary psychotic disorders (Tariot et al. 2000). Significant reductions in BPRS and CGI-Severity of Illness scores were observed. A small open-label study of 12 older adults aged 63–85 years (mean age, 71.8 years) with schizophrenia, schizoaffective disorder, or bipolar disorder confirmed tolerability for quetiapine doses up to 250 mg three times daily (Jaskiw et al. 2004).

Clozapine is used to treat schizophrenia refractory to other antipsychotic agents. Clozapine has been shown to improve psychotic symptoms, reduce rehospitalization rates, and is also FDA-approved for reducing the risk of recurrent suicidal behavior in patients with schizophrenia or schizoaffective disorder (Clozaril (clozapine) [package insert] 2023). Doses up to 600 mg/day can be used in older adults with schizophrenia who have been on this medication for many years. However, mean doses used in studies were lower (264 mg/day) and experts recommend maximum 150–200 mg/day (Mukku et al. 2018; Pridan et al. 2015).

Aripiprazole showed mixed results in case reports including 10 adults with schizophrenia aged 62–86 years old (Madhusoodanan et al. 2004). A randomized, placebo-controlled, double-blind study of 256 nursing home residents with psychosis associated with AD used aripiprazole in doses of 0.7–15 mg/day (mean dose at endpoint, 8.6 mg/day) was negative for the primary outcome measure, the Neuropsychiatric Inventory-Nursing Home (NPI-NH) Psychosis subscale, although there was significant improvement in agitation and depression (Streim et al. 2008). In another large study of 487 nursing home residents, patients were randomized to fixed doses of aripiprazole of either 2, 5, or 10 mg/day. The 10 mg daily dose showed a significant difference in NPI-NH Psychosis subscale score compared to placebo after 10 weeks (Mintzer et al. 2007).

In a study of 38 older adults with first-episode schizophrenia (mean age, 68.5 years), half were randomized to ziprasidone 40–120 mg (mean dose, 92.4 mg) daily, and half to olanzapine 5–20 mg (mean dose, 9.5 mg) daily (Chen et al. 2017). There were no significant differences in PANSS scores between the two groups. Ziprasidone has also been used for the treatment of psychosis or acute agitation in PD and is generally well tolerated in doses of up to 80 mg/day oral and

10–20 mg intramuscularly, with mixed results regarding efficacy (Younce et al. 2019).

Lurasidone 40 mg/day was studied in a 6-week multicenter randomized, double-blind, placebo-controlled study of adults 18–74 years old (mean age, 39.3 ± 11.4 years) hospitalized for acute exacerbation of schizophrenia (Iyo et al. 2021). There were significant PANSS score reductions. An open-label, flexible-dose (40–120 mg/day) extension of this study also showed sustained PANSS improvements for up to 24 months (Correll et al. 2016). Results were not shown by age group in either study, so it is difficult to draw conclusions regarding target dose for the older patients. A secondary analysis from a trial of lurasidone monotherapy up to 120 mg/day also revealed efficacy for bipolar depression in adults ≥55 years old (Sajatovic et al. 2016).

Insufficient data exist regarding the efficacy, safety, and tolerability of asenapine and iloperidone in older adults with psychosis.

Pimavanserin, considered a third-generation antipsychotic, is a serotonin 5HT2A receptor inverse agonist and the only FDA-approved agent for treating delusions and hallucinations in PD currently. Due to its lack of dopaminergic receptor antagonism, pimavanserin does not worsen PD motor symptoms. In a 6-week randomized, double-blind, placebo-controlled trial of 199 adults (mean age, 72.4 years) with PD psychosis, there was significant score improvement in a PD-adapted version of the Scale for Assessment of Positive Symptoms in the active treatment arm compared to placebo (Cummings et al. 2014). It is recommended to continue the previous antipsychotic, if one was used, for at least 2 weeks after starting pimavanserin, because this drug takes 10 days to reach steady state. Its safety in older adults has not been fully established. A retrospective cohort study of adults 65 years or older with PD revealed a significantly higher risk of hospitalization at 1 month and a higher risk of death for up to 1 year after initiation of treatment with pimavanserin, compared to patients not taking this agent (Hwang et al. 2021).

Table 9.5 shows antipsychotic medication recommended doses and dose adjustments for older adults.

Adverse Effects of Antipsychotics

Older adults, especially the oldest old, are more susceptible to extrapyramidal side effects (EPS) and tardive syndromes, such as dystonia and dyskinesia (Jeste 2004; Musco et al. 2019; Tampi et al. 2019a). Tardive dyskinesia (TD) is characterized by choreoathetoid movements that occur after at least several months of exposure to offending agents and last longer than 8 weeks (APA 2022b). Older age, female sex, white or African American race, high-potency dopamine blocking agents (including antiemetics such as prochlorperazine or metoclopramide), medication dose and exposure interval, longer illness duration, intellectual disability, neurological disease, and concurrent mood disorders increase risk of TD (Solmi et al. 2018a). All antipsychotics can cause TD, with a prevalence of 23.4% in patients exposed to first-generation antipsychotics and 7.2% of patients treated with second-generation agents, except for clozapine, which appears to have a lower risk (Carbon et al. 2017). The 1-year cumulative TD incidence in younger adults is 5%, increasing by about 5% per year. However, the 1-year cumulative TD incidence in older adults can reach 29%, rising by 25% each year (Jeste 2004).

When TD occurs, slow taper of the antipsychotic agent is key (abrupt discontinuation may actually worsen symptoms). Patients may not desire treatment for mild TD manifestations; in about 13% of cases, symptoms spontaneously remit (Zutshi et al. 2014). If TD symptoms persist for several months and are bothersome, pharmacological treatment is recommended. The newer vesicular monoamine transporter 2 (VMAT2) inhibitors, valbenazine and deutetrabenazine, are both effective, with lower risk for increasing depression and suicidal ideation than tetrabenazine (Solmi et al. 2018b). Valbenazine clinical trials included individuals up to 85 years old. Pooled data from three 6-week, randomized, double-blind, placebo-controlled studies of valbenazine (40 mg/day or 80 mg/day) found a robust improvement in Abnormal Involuntary Movement Scale (AIMS) scores and no difference in response or side effect rates in older

Table 9.5 Antipsychotic medications used in older adults

Medication	Formulation	Initial dose (mg/day)	Target dose (mg/day)	Dose adjustment for special conditions	Other information/adverse effects[a]
Aripiprazole	Tablet, ODT, solution, IM, LAI	2	10–20	Not recommended in PD No dose adjustment for renal or hepatic impairment	Akathisia; may cause or worsen impulse control disorders
Brexpiprazole[b]	Tablet	0.5	2–3	Not recommended in PD Maximum dose 2 mg/day for patients with moderate-severe renal or hepatic impairment	Weight gain, orthostatic hypotension; may cause or worsen impulse control disorders
Cariprazine	Capsule	1.5	1.5–6	No dose adjustment for mild-to-moderate renal or hepatic impairment Not recommended in severe renal or hepatic impairment	Akathisia, weight gain Limited evidence in older adults
Clozapine[c]	Tablet, ODT, solution	12.5	250–600	For PD psychosis: Start 6.25 mg/day, maximum dose 125 mg/day (up to 225 mg/day reported) Use with caution in renal or hepatic impairment	Agranulocytosis, weight gain, sedation, diabetes mellitus, dyslipidemia, sialorrhea, orthostatic hypotension, constipation, intestinal obstruction, myocarditis, cardiomyopathy, tachycardia,[d] seizures
Haloperidol	Tablet, solution, IM[e], LAI	0.5	1–5	Contraindicated in PD No dose adjustment for renal or hepatic impairment	EPS, QTc interval prolongation (with IV use), neuroleptic malignant syndrome
Lurasidone	Tablet	20–40	40–120	In moderate-to-severe renal or hepatic impairment, start 20 mg/day; maximum dose 80 mg/day for renal impairment and moderate hepatic impairment and 40 mg/day for severe hepatic impairment	Akathisia, dizziness, nausea, somnolence Administer with food (>350 Cal)
Olanzapine	Tablet, ODT, IM[e]	2.5–5	7.5–20	Not recommended in PD Avoid in patients with diabetes mellitus	Weight gain, diabetes mellitus, dyslipidemia
Paliperidone	Tablet, LAI	3	3–12	In mild renal impairment, start 3 mg/day; maximum dose 6 mg/day. In moderate-to-severe renal impairment, start 1.5 mg/day, maximum dose 3 mg/day. No dose adjustment for mild-to-moderate hepatic impairment; not studied in severe hepatic impairment	EPS, weight gain, metabolic changes, hyperprolactinemia, tachycardia
Pimavanserin	Tablet, capsule	10–34	20–34	Indicated for PD psychosis No dose adjustment in mild-to-severe renal impairment or hepatic impairment. Use with caution in ESRD	QTc interval prolongation, hallucinations, peripheral edema

(continued)

Table 9.5 (continued)

Medication	Formulation	Initial dose (mg/day)	Target dose (mg/day)	Dose adjustment for special conditions	Other information/adverse effects[a]
Quetiapine	Tablet	12.5–25	100–300 (max 750)	Preferred in PD and DLB; maximum recommended dose in PD 200 mg/day Reduce dose in patients with hepatic impairment	Orthostatic hypotension, weight gain, diabetes mellitus, dyslipidemia QTc interval prolongation
Risperidone	Tablet, ODT, solution, LAI	0.5–1	1.5–4 (LAI: 25–50 mg every 14 days)	Not recommended in PD In severe renal or hepatic impairment, start 0.5 mg/day and titrate in at least 1-week intervals	EPS, weight gain, metabolic changes, hyperprolactinemia, orthostatic hypotension
Ziprasidone	Capsule, IM	20–40	80–160	No dose adjustment for renal impairment with oral use. Use with caution for hepatic impairment	EPS, QTc interval prolongation Administer with food (>500 Cal)

Clozaril (clozapine) [package insert] 2023; Davidson et al. 2000; Devanand et al. 2011; Eng and Welty 2010; FDA 2016; Geodon (ziprasidone) [package insert] 2022; Grossberg et al. 2020; Invega (paliperidone) [package insert] 2022; Iyo et al. 2021; Jeste et al. 2003; Latuda (lurasidone HCl) [package insert] 2022; Lee et al. 2023; Mintzer et al. 2007; Nuplazid (pimavanserin) [package insert] 2023; Preskorn 2012; Reinhardt and Cohen 2015; Reus et al. 2016; Rexulti (brexpiprazole) [package insert] 2023; Seritan 2023; Seritan and Seritan 2015; Tariot et al. 2000; Tzimos et al. 2008; Vraylar (cariprazine) [package insert] 2022; Younce et al. 2019

DLB dementia with Lewy bodies, *EPS* extrapyramidal side effects, *ERSD* end-stage renal disease, *IM* intramuscular, *IV* intravenous, *LAI* long-acting injectable, *ODT* orally disintegrating tablet, *PD* Parkinson's disease

[a]Older adults with major neurocognitive disorder-related psychosis treated with antipsychotic medications are at an increased risk of death

[b]FDA-approved for treatment of agitation associated with dementia due to Alzheimer's disease; not approved for psychosis without agitation in dementia

[c]Requires use of Clozapine Risk Evaluation and Mitigation Strategy (REMS) program

[d]Reported in adults >60 years old

[e]Also used for IV administration for acute agitation

(≥55 years) compared to younger (<55 years) adults (Sajatovic et al. 2020). In a 3-year, open-label study of deutetrabenazine (mean dose, 39.5 mg daily), 76% of adults aged <55 years and 62% of those 55 years or older achieved at least a 50% reduction in AIMS scores (Sajatovic et al. 2022).

Conclusions

Psychotic symptoms are due to primary psychiatric conditions in less than half of older adults; neurodegenerative and other neurological or systemic medical diseases account for up to 60% of cases. Prompt recognition and treatment of medical conditions which contribute to, or cause the psychotic symptoms is imperative. Psychosis may remit spontaneously (e.g., Charles Bonnet syndrome due to acute cerebral or optic nerve injury, postictal psychosis), although in general a chronic or recurring course is observed.

Older adults, particularly those with neurodegenerative diseases, are more sensitive to adverse effects of medications. Patients with LOS and VLOSLP may respond to lower doses of antipsychotics (10–25% of doses used in younger adults with schizophrenia). Although there is limited evidence for the efficacy and tolerability of APs in older adults, guidelines recommend lower initial and target doses, dose adjustments for specific conditions, and shorter duration of treatment.

Age-Adjusted Recommendations

- Psychosis with onset in late life is often a manifestation of an underlying neurodegenerative disease or another neurological or systemic medical condition. A cognitive screening exam is recommended, followed by additional work-up as necessary.
- Onset of psychosis and other psychiatric symptoms after age 40, atypical presentations, or difficult-to-treat symptoms may indicate a non-primary psychiatric etiology and should prompt a thorough medical work-up.
- Specific types of psychotic symptoms can point to certain underlying etiologies.
- Behavioral strategies and psychosocial interventions should be a part of every treatment plan.
- Pharmacological management may be limited by adverse effects, in particular for people with LOS, VLOSLP, and DLB.

References

Adachi N, Onuma T, Nishiwaki S, et al. Inter-ictal and post-ictal psychoses in frontal lobe epilepsy: a retrospective comparison with psychoses in temporal lobe epilepsy. Seizure. 2000;9:328–35.

Almeida OP, Xiao J. Mortality associated with incident mental health disorders after stroke. Aust N Z J Psychiatry. 2007;41:274–81.

American Psychiatric Association. Schizophrenia Spectrum and Other Psychotic Disorders. In Diagnostic and statistical manual for mental disorders. 5th ed, Text Revision: Washington, DC, American Psychiatric Association; 2022a. pp 101–35.

American Psychiatric Association. Tardive Dyskinesia. In Diagnostic and statistical manual for mental disorders. 5th ed, Text Revision: Washington, DC, American Psychiatric Association; 2022b. pp 814–6.

Bailey CH, Andersen LK, Lowe GC, et al. A population-based study of the incidence of delusional infestation in Olmsted County, Minnesota, 1976-2010. Br J Dermatol. 2014;170:1130–5.

Bartels SJ, Pratt SI, Mueser KT, et al. Long-term outcomes of a randomized trial of integrated skills training and preventive health care for older adults with serious mental illness. Am J Geriatr Psychiatry. 2014;22:1251–61.

Bassiony MM, Lyketsos CG. Delusions and hallucinations in Alzheimer's disease: a review of the decade of the brain. Psychosomatics. 2003;44:388–401.

Belbeze J, Gallarda T. Very late onset psychotic symptoms: psychosis or dementia? A phenomenological approach. A systematic review. Geriatr. Psychol Neuropsychiatr Vieil. 2020;18:77–87.

Benussi A, Premi E, Gazzina S, et al. Progression of behavioral disturbances and neuropsychiatric symptoms in patients with genetic frontotemporal dementia. JAMA Netw Open. 2021;4:e2030194.

Braga-Neto P, Pedroso JL, Gadelha A. Psychosis in Machado-Joseph disease:clinical correlates, pathophysiological discussion, and functional brain imaging. Expanding the cerebellar cognitive affective syndrome. Cerebellum. 2016;15: 483–90.

Cannas A, Meloni M, Mascia MM, et al. Capgras syndrome in Parkinson's disease: two new cases and literature review. Neurol Sci. 2017;38:225–31.

Carbon M, Hsieh CH, Kane JM, Correll CU. Tardive dyskinesia prevalence in the period of second-generation antipsychotic use: a meta-analysis. J Clin Psychiatry. 2017;78:e264–78.

Cervantes AN, Rabins PV, Slavney PR. Onset of schizophrenia at age 100. Psychosomatics. 2006;47:356–9.

Chen J, Pan X, Qian M, Yang S. Efficacy and metabolic influence on blood-glucose and serum lipid of ziprasidone in the treatment of elderly patients with first-episode schizophrenia. Shanghai Arch Psychiatry. 2017;29:104–10.

Chen L, Selvendra A, Stewart A, Castle D. Risk factors in early and late onset schizophrenia. Compr Psychiatry. 2018;80:155–62.

Clancy MJ, Clarke MC, Connor DJ, et al. The prevalence of psychosis in epilepsy; a systematic review and meta-analysis. BMC Psychiatry. 2014;14:75.

Clozaril (clozapine) [package insert]. Rosemont, PA: HLS Therapeutics; 2023. https://www.hlstherapeutics.com/wp-content/uploads/monograph_pdf/HLS-Clozaril-PM-US.pdf. Accessed 9 Oct 2023.

Cohen CI, Vahia I, Reyes P, et al. Focus on geriatric psychiatry: schizophrenia in later life: clinical symptoms and social Well-being. Psychiatr Serv. 2008;59:232–4.

Cohen CI, Izediuno I, Yadack AM, et al. Characteristics of auditory hallucinations and associated factors in older adults with schizophrenia. Am J Geriatr Psychiatry. 2014;22:442–9.

Correll CU, Cucchiaro J, Silva R, Hsu J, Pikalov A, Loebel A. Long-term safety and effectiveness of lurasidone in schizophrenia: a 22-month, open-label extension study. CNS Spectr. 2016;21:393–402.

Cummings J, Isaacson S, Mills R, et al. Pimavanserin for patients with Parkinson's disease psychosis: a randomised, placebo-controlled phase 3 trial. Lancet. 2014;383:533–40.

Davidson M, Harvey PD, Vervarcke J, et al. A long-term, multicenter, open-label study of risperidone in elderly patients with psychosis. In J Geriatr Psychiatry. 2000;15:506–14.

de Portugal E, González N, Miriam V, et al. Gender differences in delusional disorder: evidence from an outpatient sample. Psychiatry Res. 2010;177:235–9.

Depp CA, Jeste DV. Bipolar disorder in older adults: a critical review. Bipolar Disord. 2004;6:343–67.

Devanand DP, Pelton GH, Cunqueiro K, et al. A 6-month, randomized, double-blind, placebo-controlled pilot discontinuation trial following response to haloperidol treatment of psychosis and agitation in Alzheimer's disease. Int J Geriatr Psychiatry. 2011;26:937–43.

Devenney EM, Landin-Romero R, Irish M, et al. The neural correlates and clinical characteristics of psychosis in the frontotemporal dementia continuum and the C9orf72 expansion. Neuroimage Clin. 2017;13:439–45.

Drazyk AM, Tan RYY, Tay J, et al. Encephalopathy in a large cohort of British cerebral autosomal dominant arteriopathy with subcortical infarcts and leukoencephalopathy patients. Stroke. 2019;50:283–90.

Eng ML, Welty TE. Management of hallucinations and psychosis in Parkinson's disease. Am J Geriatr Pharmacother. 2010;8:316–30.

Essali A, Ali G. Antipsychotic drug treatment for elderly people with late-onset schizophrenia. Cochrane Database Syst Rev. 2012;2:CD004162.

Falip M, Carreño M, Donaire A, et al. Postictal psychosis: a retrospective study in patients with refractory temporal lobe epilepsy. Seizure. 2009;18:145–9.

Fett AJ, Velthorst E, Reichenberg A, et al. Long-term changes in cognitive functioning in individuals with psychotic disorders: findings from the Suffolk County mental health project. JAMA Psychiatry. 2020;77:387–96.

Folstein M, Folstein S, McHugh P. "Mini-mental state": a practical method for grading the cognitive state of patients for the clinician. J Psychiatr Res. 1975;12:189–98.

Food and Drug Administration: FDA Drug Safety Communication: FDA warns about new impulse-control problems associated with mental health drug aripiprazole (Abilify, Abilify Maintena, Aristada). 2016. https://www.fda.gov/Drugs/DrugSafety/ucm498662.htm. Accessed 9 Oct 2023.

Forlani C, Morri M, Ferrari B, et al. Prevalence and gender differences in late-life depression: a population-based study. Am J Geriatr Psychiatry. 2014;22:370–80.

Freudenreich O, Schulz SC, Goff DC. Initial medical work-up of first-episode psychosis: a conceptual review. Early Interv Psychiatry. 2009;3:10–8.

Geodon (ziprasidone) [package insert]. New York, NY: Pfizer; 2022. https://labeling.pfizer.com/ShowLabeling.aspx?id=584. Accessed 9 Oct 2023.

González-Rodríguez A, Seeman MV, Izquierdo E, et al. Delusional disorder in old age: a hypothesis-driven review of recent work focusing on epidemiology, clinical aspects, and outcomes. Int J Environ Res Public Health. 2022;19:7911.

Goulet K, Deschamps B, Evoy F, Trudel JF. Use of brain imaging (computed tomography and magnetic resonance imaging) in first-episode psychosis: review and retrospective study. Can J Psychiatr. 2009;54:493–501.

Gournellis R, Oulis P, Rizos E, et al. Clinical correlates of age of onset in psychotic depression. Arch Gerontol Geriatr. 2011;52:94–8.

Granholm E, McQuaid JR, McClure FS, et al. Randomized controlled trial of cognitive behavioral social skills training for older people with schizophrenia: 12-month follow-up. J Clin Psychiatry. 2007;68:730–7.

Grossberg GT, Kohegyi E, Mergel V, Josiassen MK, Meulien D, Hobart M, et al. Efficacy and Safety of Brexpiprazole for the Treatment of Agitation in Alzheimer's Dementia: Two 12-Week, Randomized, Double-Blind, Placebo-Controlled Trials. Am J Geriatr Psychiatry. 2020;28(4):383–400.

Hanssen M, van der Werf M, Verkaaik M, et al. Comparative study of clinical and neuropsychological characteristics between early-, late and very-late-onset schizophrenia-spectrum disorders. Am J Geriatr Psychiatry. 2015;23:852–62.

Harciarek M, Kertesz A. The prevalence of misidentification syndromes in neurodegenerative diseases. Alzheimer Dis Assoc Disord. 2008;22:163–9.

Harris BS, Kotsopoulos EJ, Yamin S. Phenotypic cognitive impairment in late-onset delusional disorder. Int Psychogeriatr. 2014;26:965–75.

Hirschfeld RM, Calabrese JR, Weissman MM, et al. Screening for bipolar disorder in the community. J Clin Psychiatry. 2003;64:53–9.

Howard R, Rabins PV, Seeman MV, Jeste DV. Late-onset schizophrenia and very-late-onset schizophrenia-like psychosis: an international consensus. The international late-onset schizophrenia group. Am J Psychiatry. 2000;157:172–8.

Hwang JP, Yang CH, Lee TW, Tsai SJ. The efficacy and safety of olanzapine for the treatment of geriatric psychosis. J Clin Psychopharmacol. 2003;23:113–8.

Hwang YJ, Alexander GC, An H, Moore TJ, Mehta HB. Risk of hospitalization and death associated with pimavanserin use in older adults with Parkinson disease. Neurology. 2021;97:e1266–75.

Invega (paliperidone) [package insert]. Titusville, NJ: Janssen Pharmaceuticals, Inc.; 2022. http://www.janssenlabels.com/package-insert/product-monograph/prescribing-information/INVEGA-pi.pdf. Accessed 9 Oct 2023.

Irwin LG, Fortune DG. Risk factors for psychosis secondary to temporal lobe epilepsy: a systematic review. J Neuropsychiatry Clin Neurosci. 2014;26:5–23.

Iyo M, Ishigooka J, Nakamura M, et al. Efficacy and safety of lurasidone in acutely psychotic patients with schizophrenia: a 6-week, randomized, double-blind, placebo-controlled study. Psychiatry Clin Neurosci. 2021;23(75):227–35.

Jääskeläinen E, Juola T, Korpela H, et al. Epidemiology of psychotic depression - systematic review and meta-analysis. Psychol Med. 2018;48:905–18.

Jaskiw GE, Thyrum PT, Fuller MA, et al. Pharmacokinetics of quetiapine in elderly patients with selected psychotic disorders. Clin Pharmacokinet. 2004;43:1025–35.

Jeste DV. Tardive dyskinesia rates with atypical antipsychotics in older adults. J Clin Psychiatry. 2004;65(Suppl 9):21–4.

Jeste DV, Finkel SI. Psychosis of Alzheimer's disease and related dementias. Diagnostic criteria for a distinct syndrome. Am J Geriatr Psychiatry. 2000;8:29–34.

Jeste DV, Barak Y, Madhusoodanan S, et al. International multisite double-blind trial of the atypical antipsychotics risperidone and olanzapine in 175 elderly patients with chronic schizophrenia. Am J Geriatr Psychiatr. 2003;11:638–47.

Josephs KA. Capgras syndrome and its relationship to neurodegenerative disease. Arch Neurol. 2007;64:1762–6.

Kandratavicius L, Hallak JE, Leite JP. What are the similarities and differences between schizophrenia and schizophrenia-like psychosis of epilepsy? A neuropathological approach to the understanding of schizophrenia spectrum and epilepsy. Epilepsy Behav. 2014;38:143–7.

Kataoka H, Sugie K. Delusional jealousy (Othello syndrome) in 67 patients with Parkinson's disease. Front Neurol. 2018;9:129.

Kaufman DM, Geyer HL, Milstein MJ, editors. Epilepsy, in Kaufman's clinical neurology for psychiatrists. 8th ed. Philadelphia: PA, Elsevier; 2017. p. 197–220.

Keepers GA, Fochtmann LJ, Anzia J, et al. The American Psychiatric Association practice guideline for the treatment of patients with schizophrenia. 3rd ed. VA, American Psychiatric Association: Arlington; 2021.

Kessler RC, Birnbaum H, Bromet E, et al. Age differences in major depression: results from the National Comorbidity Survey Replication (NCS-R). Psychol Med. 2010;40:225–37.

Khanna R, White L, Bessey FY, et al. Barriers to treatment of hallucinations and delusions in people with dementia residing in long-term care. J Clin Psychiatry. 2022;83(2):21m14050.

Kim HF, Yudofsky SC, Hales RE, Tucker GJ. Neuropsychiatric aspects of seizure disorders. In: Yudofsky SC, Hales RE, editors. The American Psychiatric Publishing textbook of neuropsychiatry and behavioral neurosciences. 5th ed. Arlington, VA, American Psychiatric Publishing, Inc.; 2008. p. 649–75.

Köhler S, van Os J, de Graaf R, et al. Psychosis risk as a function of age at onset: a comparison between early- and late-onset psychosis in a general population sample. Soc Psychiatry Psychiatr Epidemiol. 2007;42:288–94.

Kulick CV, Montgomery KM, Nirenberg MJ. Comprehensive identification of delusions and olfactory, tactile, gustatory, and minor hallucinations in Parkinson's disease psychosis. Parkinsonism Relat Disord. 2018;54:40–5.

Landqvist Waldö M, Gustafson L, Passant U, Englund E. Psychotic symptoms in frontotemporal dementia: a diagnostic dilemma? Int Psychogeriatr. 2015;27:531–9.

Lasser RA, Bossie CA, Zhu Y, et al. Efficacy and safety of long-acting risperidone in elderly patients with schizophrenia and schizoaffective disorder. Int J Geriatr Psychiatry. 2004;19:898–905.

Latuda (lurasidone hydrochloride) [package insert]. Marlborough, MA: Sunovion Pharmaceuticals Inc.; 2022. https://www.latuda.com/LatudaPrescribingInformation.pdf. Accessed 9 Oct 2023.

Lee AH, Weintraub D. Psychosis in Parkinson's disease without dementia: common and comorbid with other non-motor symptoms. Mov Disord. 2012;27:858–63.

Lee D, Slomkowski M, Hefting N, Chen D, Larsen KG, Kohegyi E, et al. Brexpiprazole for the Treatment of Agitation in Alzheimer Dementia: A Randomized Clinical Trial. JAMA Neurol. 2023;80(12):1307–16.

Liszewski CM, O'Hearn E, Leroi I, et al. Cognitive impairment and psychiatric symptoms in 133 patients with diseases associated with cerebellar degeneration. J Neuropsychiatry Clin Neurosci. 2004;16:109–12.

Lyketsos CG, Lopez O, Jones B, et al. Prevalence of neuropsychiatric symptoms in dementia and mild cognitive impairment: results from the cardiovascular health study. JAMA. 2002;288:1475–83.

Madhusoodanan S, Brenner R, Gupta S, et al. Clinical experience with aripiprazole treatment in ten elderly patients with schizophrenia or schizoaffective disorder: retrospective case studies. CNS Spectr. 2004;9:862–7.

Mason O, Stott J, Sweeting R. Dimensions of positive symptoms in late versus early onset psychosis. Int Psychogeriatr. 2013;25:320–7.

McGrath JJ, Saha S, Al-Hamzawi A, et al. Psychotic experiences in the general population: a cross-national analysis based on 31,261 respondents from 18 countries. JAMA Psychiatry. 2015;72:697–705.

McKeith IG, Boeve BF, Dickson DW, et al. Diagnosis and management of dementia with Lewy bodies: fourth consensus report of the DLB consortium. Neurology. 2017;89:88–100.

McMurtray A, Tseng B, Diaz N, et al. Acute psychosis associated with subcortical stroke: comparison between basal ganglia and mid-brain lesions. Case Rep Neurol Med. 2014;428-425:2014.

Meesters PD, de Haan L, Comijs HC, et al. Schizophrenia spectrum disorders in later life: prevalence and distribution of age at onset and sex in a Dutch catchment area. Am J Geriatr Psychiatry. 2012;20:18–28.

Mintzer JE, Tune LE, Breder CD, et al. Aripiprazole for the treatment of psychoses in institutionalized patients with Alzheimer dementia: a multicenter, randomized, double-blind, placebo-controlled assessment of three fixed doses. Am J Geriatr Psychiatry. 2007;15:918–31.

Mizrahi R, Starkstein SE, Jorge R, Robinson RG. Phenomenology and clinical correlates of delusions in Alzheimer's disease. Am J Geriatr Psychiatry. 2006;14:573–81.

Moretti R, Torre P, Antonello RM, et al. Olanzapine as a treatment of neuropsychiatric disorders of Alzheimer's disease and other dementias: a 24-month follow-up of 68 patients. Am J Alzheimers Dis Other Dement. 2003;8:205–14.

Moriarty N, Alam M, Kalus A, O'Connor K. Current understanding and approach to delusional infestation. Am J Med. 2019;132:1401–9.

Mukku SSR, Sivakumar PT, Varghese M. Clozapine use in geriatric patients—challenges. Asian J Psychiatr. 2018;33:63–7.

Musco S, Ruekert L, Myers J, et al. Characteristics of patients experiencing extrapyramidal symptoms or other movement disorders related to dopamine receptor blocking agent therapy. J Clin Psychopharmacol. 2019;39:336–43.

Nagahama Y, Okina T, Suzuki N, et al. Classification of psychotic symptoms in dementia with Lewy bodies. Am J Geriatr Psychiatry. 2007;15:961–7.

Nasreddine ZS, Phillips NA, Bédirian V, et al. The Montreal cognitive assessment, MoCA: a brief screening tool for mild cognitive impairment. J Am Geriatr Soc. 2005;53:695–9.

Nuplazid (pimavanserin) [package insert]. San Diego, CA: ACADIA Pharmaceuticals Inc.; 2023. https://www.nuplazidhcp.com/pdf/NUPLAZID_Prescribing_Information.pdf. Accessed 9 Oct 2023.

Orth M, Handley OJ, Schwenke C, et al. Observing Huntington's disease: the European Huntington's disease Network's REGISTRY. PLoS Curr. 2010;2:RRN1184.

Ozten E, Tufan AE, Cerit C, et al. Delusional parasitosis with hyperthyroidism in an elderly woman: a case report. J Med Case Rep. 2013;7:17.

Pang L. Hallucinations experienced by the visually impaired. Optom Vis Sci. 2016;93:1466–78.

Patterson TL, Bucardo J, McKibbin CL, et al. Development and pilot testing of a new psychosocial intervention for older Latinos with chronic psychosis. Schizophr Bull. 2005;31:922–30.

Patterson TL, Mausbach BT, McKibbin C, et al. Functional adaptation skills training (FAST): a randomized trial of a psychosocial intervention for middle-aged and older patients with chronic psychotic disorders. Schizophr Res. 2006;86:291–9.

Paulsen JS, Ready RE, Hamilton JM, et al. Neuropsychiatric aspects of Huntington's disease. J Neurol Neurosurg Psychiatry. 2001;71:310–4.

Pelak VS: Visual release hallucinations (Charles bonnet syndrome). 2021. https://www.uptodate.com/contents/visual-release-hallucinations-charles-bonnet-syndrome. Accessed 29 Sep 2023.

Pereira GCM, de Oliveira GC. Prevalence of Capgras syndrome in Alzheimer's patients: a systematic review and metaanalysis. Dement Neuropsychol. 2019;13:463–8.

Perini G, Carlini A, Pomati S, et al. Misidentification delusions: prevalence in different types of dementia and validation of a structured questionnaire. Alzheimer Dis Assoc Disord. 2016;30:331–7.

Pollak TA, Nicholson TR, Mellers JD, et al. Epilepsy-related psychosis: a role for autoimmunity? Epilepsy Behav. 2014;36:33–8.

Preskorn SH. Clinically important differences in the pharmacokinetics of the ten newer "atypical" antipsychotics: part 3. Effects of renal and hepatic impairment. J Psychiatr Pract. 2012;18:430–7.

Pridan S, Swartz M, Baruch Y, et al. Effectiveness and safety of clozapine in elderly patients with chronic resistant schizophrenia. Int Psychogeriatr. 2015;27:131–4.

Qin P, Xu H, Laursen TM, et al. Risk for schizophrenia and schizophrenia-like psychosis among patients with epilepsy: population based cohort study. BMJ. 2005;331:23.

Reeves S, Stewart R, Howard R. Service contact and psychopathology in very-late-onset schizophrenia-like psychosis: the effects of gender and ethnicity. Int J Geriatr Psychiatry. 2002;17:473–9.

Reinhardt MM, Cohen CI. Late-life psychosis: diagnosis and treatment. Curr Psychiatry Rep. 2015;17:1.

Reus V, Fochtmann L, Eyler AE, et al. The American Psychiatric Association practice guideline on the use of antipsychotics to treat agitation or psycho-

sis in patients with dementia. Am J Psychiatry. 2016;173:543–6.
Rexulti (brexpiprazole) [package insert] 2023. Otsuka U.S. Revised 5, 2023. https://www.otsuka-us.com/sites/g/files/qhldwo7866/files/media/static/Rexulti-PI.pdf. Accessed March 14, 2024.
Rolin SA, Aschbrenner KA, Whiteman KL, et al. Characteristics and service use of older adults with schizoaffective disorder versus older adults with schizophrenia and bipolar disorder. Am J Geriatr Psychiatry. 2017;25:941–50.
Ropacki SA, Jeste DV. Epidemiology of and risk factors for psychosis of Alzheimer's disease: a review of 55 studies published from 1990 to 2003. Am J Psychiatry. 2005;162:2022–30.
Rottnek M, Riggio S, Byne W, et al. Schizophrenia in a patient with spinocerebellar ataxia 2: coincidence of two disorders or a neurodegenerative disease presenting with psychosis? Am J Psychiatry. 2008;165:964–7.
Ruiz M, Arias A, Sánchez-Llanos E, et al. Minor hallucinations in Alzheimer's disease. J Alzheimers Dis. 2018;64:543–9.
Sajatovic M, Strejilevich SA, Gildengers AG, et al. A report on older-age bipolar disorder from the international society for bipolar disorders task force. Bipolar Disord. 2015;17:689–704.
Sajatovic M, Forester BP, Tsai J, et al. Efficacy of lurasidone in adults aged 55 years and older with bipolar depression: post hoc analysis of 2 double-blind, placebo-controlled studies. J Clin Psychiatry. 2016;77:e1324–31.
Sajatovic M, Alexopoulos GS, Burke J, Farahmand K, Siegert S. The effects of valbenazine on tardive dyskinesia in older and younger patients. Int J Geriatr Psychiatry. 2020;35:69–79.
Sajatovic M, Finkbeiner S, Wilhelm A, et al. Long-term safety and efficacy of deutetrabenazine in younger and older patients with tardive dyskinesia. Am J Geriatr Psychiatry. 2022;30:360–71.
Schneider LS, Tariot PN, Dagerman KS, et al. Effectiveness of atypical antipsychotic drugs in patients with Alzheimer's disease. N Engl J Med. 2006;355:1525–38.
Scott IU, Schein OD, Feuer WJ, Folstein MF. Visual hallucinations in patients with retinal disease. Am J Ophthalmol. 2001;131:590.
Seritan AL. Advances in the diagnosis and management of psychotic symptoms in neurodegenerative diseases: a narrative review. J Geriatr Psychiatry Neurol. 2023;36:435–60.
Seritan AL, Seritan S. Geriatric psychopharmacology in acute settings. Curr Psychopharmacol. 2015;4:112–8.
Sha SJ, Takada LT, Rankin KP, et al. Frontotemporal dementia due to C9ORF72 mutations: clinical and imaging features. Neurology. 2012;79:1002–11.
Shinagawa S, Naasan G, Karydas AM, et al. Clinicopathological study of patients with *C9ORF72*-associated frontotemporal dementia presenting with delusions. J Geriatr Psychiatry Neurol. 2015;28:99–107.
Sink KM, Holden KF, Yaffe K. Pharmacological treatment of neuropsychiatric symptoms of dementia: a review of the evidence. JAMA. 2005;293:596–608.
Snowden JS, Rollinson S, Thompson JC, et al. Distinct clinical and pathological characteristics of frontotemporal dementia associated with C9ORF72 mutations. Brain. 2012;135(Pt 3):693–708.
Solmi M, Pigato G, Kane JM, Correll CU. Clinical risk factors for the development of tardive dyskinesia. J Neurol Sci. 2018a;389:21–7.
Solmi M, Pigato G, Kane JM, Correll CU. Treatment of tardive dyskinesia with VMAT-2 inhibitors: a systematic review and meta-analysis of randomized controlled trials. Drug Des Devel Ther. 2018b;12:1215–38.
Solmi M, Radua J, Olivola M, et al. Age at onset of mental disorders worldwide: large-scale meta-analysis of 192 epidemiological studies. Mol Psychiatry. 2022;27:281–95.
Stafford J, Howard R, Kirkbride JB. The incidence of very-late-onset psychotic disorders: a systematic review and meta-analysis, 1960-2016. Psychol Med. 2018;48:1775–86.
Stangeland H, Orgeta V, Bell V. Poststroke psychosis: a systematic review. J Neurol Neurosurg Psychiatry. 2018;89:879–85.
Stevanin G, Brice A. Spinocerebellar ataxia 17 (SCA17) and Huntington's disease-like 4 (HDL4). Cerebellum. 2008;7:170–8.
Streim JE, Porsteinsson AP, Breder CD, et al. A randomized, double-blind, placebo-controlled study of aripiprazole for the treatment of psychosis in nursing home patients with Alzheimer disease. Am J Geriatr Psychiatry. 2008;16:537–50.
Suen YN, Wong SMY, Hui CLM, et al. Late-onset psychosis and very-late-onset-schizophrenia-like-psychosis: an updated systematic review. Int Rev Psychiatry. 2019;31:523–42.
Tampi RR, Young J, Hoq R, et al. Psychotic disorders in late life: a narrative review. Ther Adv Psychopharmacol. 2019a;9:1–13.
Tampi RR, Young JJ, Tampi D. Behavioral symptomatology and psychopharmacology of Lewy body dementia. Handb Clin Neurology. 2019b;165:59–70.
Tariot PN, Salzman C, Yeung PP, et al. Long-term use of quetiapine in elderly patients with psychotic disorders. Clin Ther. 2000;22:1068–84.
Tzimos A, Samokhvalov V, Kramer M, et al. Safety and tolerability of oral paliperidone extended-release tablets in elderly patients with schizophrenia: a double-blind, placebo-controlled study with 6-month open label extension. Am J Geriatr Psychiatry. 2008;16:31–43.
Vahia IV, Palmer BW, Depp C, et al. Is late-onset schizophrenia a subtype of schizophrenia? Acta Psychiatr Scand. 2010;122:414–26.
Van Assche L, Van Aubel E, Van de Ven L, et al. The neuropsychological profile and phenomenology of late onset psychosis: a cross-sectional study on the differential diagnosis of very-late-onset schizophrenia-like psychosis, dementia with Lewy bodies and

Alzheimer's type dementia with psychosis. Arch Clin Neuropsychol. 2019;34:183–99.

Vraylar (cariprazine) [package insert]. Dublin, IE: Forest Laboratories Ireland Limited; 2022. https://media.allergan.com/actavis/actavis/media/allergan-pdf-documents/product-prescribing/vraylar_pi.pdf. Accessed 9 Oct 2023.

Warren N, O'Gorman C, Hume Z, et al. Delusions in Parkinson's disease: a systematic review of published cases. Neuropsychol Rev. 2018;28:310–6.

Wood RA, Hopkins SA, Moodley KK, Chan D. Fifty percent prevalence of extracampine hallucinations in Parkinson's disease patients. Front Neurol. 2015;6:263.

Younce JR, Davis AA, Black KJ. A systematic review and case series of ziprasidone for psychosis in Parkinson's disease. J Parkinsons Dis. 2019;9:63–71.

Zutshi D, Cloud LJ, Factor SA: Tardive syndromes are rarely reversible after discontinuing dopamine receptor blocking agents: Experience from a university-based movement disorder clinic. Tremor Other Hyperkinet Mov (N Y) 4:266, 2014. eCollection 2014.

Anxiety Disorders

10

Uma Suryadevara, Meena Nuthi,
Amanda Mihalik-Wenger, Rita Hitching,
and Howard H. Fenn

Abstract

Clinically relevant symptoms of anxiety in aging adults have been estimated to range between 15% and 52% in a community sample, and between 15% and 56% in medical settings (Jayasinghe et al. Clin Gerontol 40:141–58, 2017). This chapter reviews common anxiety syndromes and age-appropriate treatment strategies.

In spite of its prevalence, the identification of anxiety in the aging patient is challenging. Distinguishing anxiety from *apprehension* of normal aging is difficult; aging by itself may bring worries and increased caution, such as concern over the realistic risk of falling, avoidance of activities such as walking outside, or preoccupation with somatic symptoms or disabled partners. Geriatric individuals may focus on somatic symptoms rather than their anxiety. They may underreport psychological symptoms or use vague terms to describe anxiety, such as "concerns". And experts differ about how anxiety typically presents in older versus younger adults.

Finally, symptoms or signs of systemic medical comorbidities, substance abuse, medication misuse, and medication adverse effects overlap with anxiety disorders. Systemic medical conditions which contribute to anxiety are covered elsewhere (see Chaps. 3, 7, and 13).

U. Suryadevara (✉)
University of Florida, College of Medicine, Gainesville, FL, USA

NFSG VAMC, Gainesville, FL, USA

M. Nuthi
NFSG VAMC, Gainesville, FL, USA

University of Florida, College of Medicine, Gainesville, FL, USA

A. Mihalik-Wenger
University of Washington, Department of Psychiatry, Seattle, WA, USA

University of Florida, College of Medicine, Gainesville, FL, USA

R. Hitching
University of Newcastle, Newcastle, Australia

H. H. Fenn
VA Health Care System, Palo Alto, CA, USA

Department of Psychiatry and Behavioral Sciences, Stanford University, Stanford, CA, USA
e-mail: hhfenn@aol.com, howard.fenn@va.gov

Case Example: Family Support Minimized Emergency Department Visits

A 70-year-old accountant with no cardiac history began experiencing episodes of chest pain and palpitations which convinced him that he was having a heart attack. The episodes occurred approximately once a week, accompanied by excessive perspiration, shortness of breath, tingling sensations in both arms, and lightheaded-

H. H. Fenn et al. (eds.), *Age-Adjusted Psychiatric Treatment for the Older Patient*,
https://doi.org/10.1007/978-3-031-53976-3_10

ness. He would then immediately call 911, and an ambulance would transport him to the emergency department (ED). One of his three daughters would always meet him there.

Evaluations in the ED included extensive cardiology workups which were consistently negative or nonspecific. Cardiac monitoring for 1 week revealed occasional but very short bursts of supraventricular tachycardia. An echocardiogram showed normal cardiac functioning and left ventricular ejection fraction of 55%. A stress EKG was negative for any pathology. A calcium study of the coronary arteries found non-hemodynamically significant 40% obstruction in the coronary arteries. Non-cardiac chest pain (NCCP) and panic disorder were the working diagnoses; the risk of a myocardial infarction or cardiac event was considered low.

The patient never felt reassured by these results and was convinced he had a life-threatening cardiac condition with a high risk of a massive MI. After each ED visit, he became more worried about his own health and apprehensive about his family's reactions. He said, "My family thinks I am doing this for attention."

During one ED visit, the psychiatric consultant explored the onset of cardiac symptoms, which began around the time the patient moved from his own apartment, located within walking distance of one of two daughters, to an assisted living unit more than 20 miles away. After the move, the patient did not see his daughters as frequently. The patient declined referral for cognitive behavioral therapy (CBT), explaining that this confirm "it was all in my head."

However, he agreed to brief weekly visits with a nurse practitioner (NP) at the cardiologist's office to monitor the cardiac condition. During these appointments, the NP performed an EKG, auscultated the chest, and listened to complaints and fears. This regular attention seemed to reassure the patient that the physical symptoms were *not* indicative of a heart attack. Weekly visits continued for 3 months. A trial of sertraline 100 mg was initiated after a psychiatric consultation was ordered. The patient then agreed to a course of weekly CBT for 2 months to address anxiety and coping skills.

His daughters were encouraged to call every night without any prompting, and the patient was asked to call each daughter, instead of calling 911, whenever he experienced chest pain or palpitations. The frequency of ED visits declined over the next 6 months. Although benign palpitations continued, within 1 year, anxiety symptoms diminished, and episodes of panic resolved.

Discussion: The cardiac presentation of panic disorder led to an assessment to rule out the need for further cardiology interventions. The outpatient cardiology follow-up convinced the patient that his symptoms were taken seriously. This was supplemented by psychiatric management of panic disorder, which included a course of SSRI and CBT. The cardiology staff, family involvement, and psychotherapeutic interventions facilitated a successful *age-adjusted* outcome.

Early Versus Late-Onset Anxiety

Two-thirds of the aged with anxiety have developed anxiety disorders early in life, and the other one-third have new onset anxiety later in life (Chou et al. 2011; Le Roux et al. 2005). Adults with *early-onset* anxiety that has persisted into late life can have more severe anxiety and pathological worry than those with *late-onset* anxiety (Le Roux et al. 2005). If the onset is in *later* life, exploration of recent stressors or events can help guide psychosocial interventions and age-appropriate psychopharmacological treatment.

Assessment

The following instruments for the assessment of anxiety in the geriatric population have demonstrated good psychometric properties (Balsamo et al. 2018) following instruments Fig. 10.1

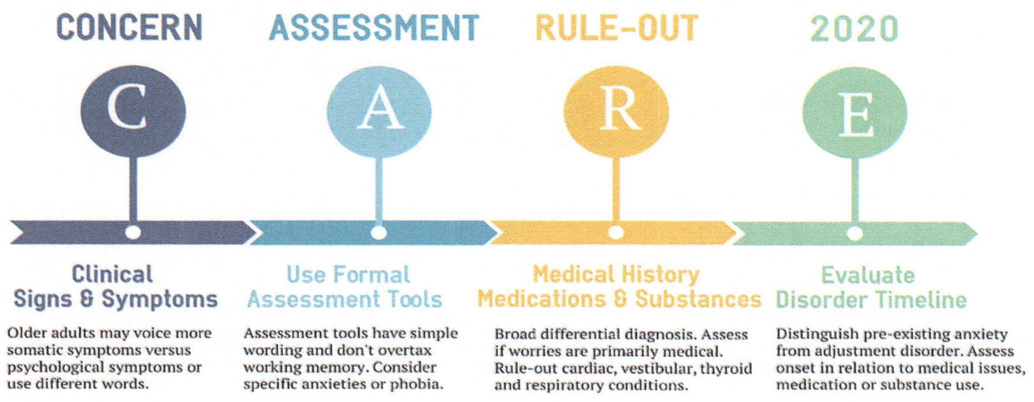

(Rita Hitching, MSc)

Fig. 10.1 Assessment of anxiety symptoms (Rita Hitching, MSc)

Geriatric Anxiety Inventory (GAI) and -Short-Form (GAI-SF)

The GAI-SF is a simple screening instrument for generalized anxiety disorder in aging. It is easy to administer, does not include somatic symptom items, and has only five items on a yes/no response scale. Psychometric properties of the Geriatric Anxiety Inventory (GAI) and its short-form (GAI-SF) have been validated in a clinical and non-clinical sample of older adults (Johnco et al. 2015). The GAI-SF consists of yes/no answers to:

- Worrying a lot of the time
- Being bothered by little things
- Thinking of oneself as a worrier
- Often feeling nervous
- Whether or not thoughts often make one nervous (Balsamo et al. 2018). A cutoff score of three correlates well with the DSM-IV diagnosis of generalized anxiety disorder (Byrne and Pachana 2011)

The Geriatric Anxiety Scale has been validated on community-dwelling older adults. It is a 30-item self-report questionnaire with 25 scoreable questions rated on a 4-point Likert scale; 5 items query specific content areas of worry and three subscales for somatic, cognitive, and affective symptoms. Respondents rate statements based on the prior week (Segal et al. 2010). A brief version, the GAS10, has good reliability and validity. Table 10.1

Table 10.1 Geriatric Anxiety Scale (GAS) items

Geriatric Anxiety Scale (GAS)			
	Somatic subscale	Cognitive subscale	Affective subscale
My heart raced or beat strongly	x		
My breath was short	x		
I had an upset stomach	x		
I felt like things were not real or like I was outside of myself		x	
I felt like I was losing control		x	
I was afraid of being judged by others			x
I was afraid of being humiliated or embarrassed			x
I had difficulty falling asleep	x		
I had difficulty staying asleep	x		
I was irritable			x
I had outbursts of anger			x
I had difficulty concentrating		x	
I was easily startled or upset			x
I was less interested in doing something I typically enjoy			x
I felt detached or isolated from others			x
I felt like I was in a daze		x	
I had a hard time sitting still	x		
I worried too much		x	
I could not control my worry		x	
I felt restless, keyed up, or on edge			x
I felt tired	x		
My muscles were tense	x		
I had back pain, neck pain, or muscle cramps	x		
I felt like I had no control over my life		x	
I felt like something terrible was going to happen to me		x	

Source: Segal et al. (2010)

Differential Diagnosis and Prevalence

All anxiety disorders have been found to decrease in prevalence with increasing age (Byers et al. 2010). Core symptoms such as muscle tension, irritability, autonomic response diminish with increasing age, while worry and concentrating abilities worsen with age. Sleep disturbances appear to stay stable (Wolitzky-Taylor et al. 2010). This apparent decline in prevalence has been explained by a decrease in *reporting* by older adults, or the possibility that one manages symptoms of anxiety better at an older age (Wolitzky-Taylor et al. 2010).

Generalized Anxiety Disorder (GAD)

GAD is the most prevalent anxiety disorder among aging individuals. It is a chronic disease, with waxing and waning symptomology and a prevalence of 1.2–4.6% in community-based samples (MacKenzie et al. 2014). In older adulthood, it is often correlated with life-threatening events, arrhythmia, heart failure, respiratory disorders, cognitive disorders, dysautonomia, and disease of hypothalamic-pituitary-adrenal axis (Chou et al. 2011). Late-onset GAD (after age 50) is associated with greater functional limitations which persist into older adulthood (Le Roux et al. 2005).

Social Anxiety Disorder and Specific Phobia

Social anxiety disorder has been reported to be present among approximately 2% of aging adults (Chou 2009); its profile and core symptoms are stable across the lifespan. Symptoms have been reported to decrease with age, making the diagnosis difficult to detect.

Specific phobia is characterized by an excessive and unreasonable fear of a specific situation or trigger. Estimates of prevalence vary from 4.5 to 11% in community-dwelling older adults and its prevalence with decreases in advanced age (Chou et al. 2009). Factors which can contribute include changes in sensory function, mental decline, decreased well-being of loved ones, isolation, separation from loved ones, inability to care for oneself, loss of control of bodily functions, and vulnerability to physical attack.

Panic Disorder

The 12-month prevalence of panic disorder in community-dwelling older adults has been reported as 1% (Byers et al. 2010). New onset panic disorder after the age of 40 is uncommon, and the prevalence of panic disorder decreases in aging adults. New onset panic attacks should prompt exploration for systemic medical or medication-related causes or other psychiatric disorders, such as anxiety disorders, alcohol use disorder, substance use disorder, substance withdrawal symptoms, and depressive disorders, all highly comorbid with panic disorder (Mohlman et al. 2004).

Panic disorder includes apprehension about further attacks, with avoidance of situations associated with past episodes. In addition, higher measures of sympathetic arousal, comorbid somatization, alcohol dependence, and agoraphobic avoidance are reported than those with GAD (Mohlman et al. 2004) as well as a significantly lower health-related quality of life.

The *fear of falling* out of proportion to a person's mobility limitations can contribute to avoidance of activities of which one is capable. Its reported prevalence varies by population surveyed and ranges from 3 to 85%. Risk factors include female gender, older age, and previous falls, although 50% of aging adults with it have not had a previous fall (Scheffer et al. 2008). Consequences of this fear include decreased physical functioning, imbalance and gait problems, avoidance of social activities, increased risk of falls, and decreased quality of life (Scheffer et al. 2008).

Obsessive-Compulsive Disorder (OCD)

Research into obsessive-compulsive disorder (OCD) in aging adults to date consists largely of case reports. Its prevalence has been noted to decrease with age, with estimates of 0.8% (Canuto et al. 2018). *Late-onset* OCD after age 60 is rare; case reports have associated it with medical causes, especially intracerebral pathology (Jazi and Asghar-Ali 2020). The obsessive-compulsive inventory-revised is a screening tool validated in older adults (Calamari et al. 2014). In contrast to OCD, rates of *hoarding disorder, characterized by inability to discard possessions,* increase with age, with a reported prevalence of more than 6% in adults over age 70 (Cath et al. 2017).

Subthreshold Anxiety

Individuals with subthreshold anxiety do not fulfill DSM-5 criteria for an anxiety disorder. Yet more chronic physical health problems occur in the aged *with subthreshold* patterns as well as *full anxiety disorder* symptoms than those *without* symptoms of anxiety. Those with subthreshold anxiety are prone to use various medications, including benzodiazepines (Grenier and Richer 2021). Subthreshold anxiety may also place the person at risk for developing a full anxiety disorder with morbidity and functional decline (Grenier and Richer 2021).

Anxiety Associated with Neurocognitive Disorders

The prevalence of anxiety in patients with neurocognitive disorders is estimated to range from 5% to 52% (van der Linde et al. 2016). Anticipatory anxiety and behavioral disturbance can also be markers of prodromal AD in those with mild neurocognitive disorder (mNCD). Comorbid anxiety in MNCD is associated with poorer functioning and increased likelihood of future nursing home placement (Seignourel et al. 2008).

Parsing out anxiety from other MNCD-related symptoms and from behavioral and psychological symptoms of dementia (BPSD) is challenging. The clinical determination of anxiety relies largely on self-report, but a patient with cognitive impairment may distort, enhance, or minimize the symptoms. A caregiver's report may not be accurate because information depends upon the relationship with the patient.

The anxiety subscale of the Neuropsychiatric Inventory (NPI) includes items like *shortness of breath, sighing, being unable to relax, feeling tense, or getting upset when separated.* The Rating Anxiety in Dementia scale is a 20-item questionnaire which includes symptoms both specific to anxiety disorder and symptoms attributed to MNCD (Seignourel et al. 2008).

Anxiety can also interfere with cognitive function and contribute to results which show up as cognitive deficits, especially during formal neurocognitive testing. A patient with anxiety may score low on *digit span backwards.* This test, which requires short-term attention, storage, and manipulation of information, might improve after several trials, suggesting that anxiety contributed to poor initial performance, low effort, and distractibility. A false positive finding of a major MNCD or mild neurocognitive disorder (mNCD) can result. For further discussion, see Chap. 5.

Anxiety and Depressive Disorders

About15%–37% of older adults with anxiety have been estimated to have a comorbid depressive disorder (King-Kallimanis et al. 2009). Patients with both major depressive disorder and GAD may have a more prolonged course as well as more severe functional impairment. Aging patients with depressive and anxiety disorders may also be at higher risk for suicide. In a study of 218 older adults diagnosed with a depressive disorder using ICD-10 criteria, higher anxiety scores on the Geriatric Anxiety Inventory were significantly correlated with scores on the Montgomery-Asberg Depression Rating Scale (MADRS) and with current suicidality (Bakkane et al. 2018).

Anxiety Symptoms Due to Another Medical Condition

A DSM-5 diagnosis of *anxiety disorder due to another medical condition* requires physical symptoms of anxiety which are a *direct physiologic consequence* of the medical condition. However, anxiety may be indistinguishable from apprehension *about* somatic symptoms (Hellwig and Domschke 2019). *Anxiety disorder due to another medical condition* is supported by:

- A clear temporal association between the onset, exacerbation, or remission of the medical condition and the anxiety symptoms.
- Features atypical of a primary anxiety disorder (e.g., atypical age at onset or course).
- Evidence from scientific literature that a known physiological mechanism (e.g., hyperthyroidism) causes anxiety.

Medical Conditions Associated with Anxiety Disorders

The systemic medical conditions most commonly comorbid with anxiety disorders include chronic obstructive pulmonary disease (prevalence 13–46%) (Willgoss and Yohannes 2013) and cardiovascular disease. GAD has been associated with a 62% higher rate of cardiovascular events such as cardiovascular mortality and coronary heart disease (Martens et al. 2010). Anxiety has been reported as a risk factor in the development of diabetes mellitus, cardiovascular disease, stroke, obesity, and physical and cognitive decline (Lever-van Milligen et al. 2019). Geriatric patients with physical disabilities also have a high prevalence of anxiety disorders. A study of disabled aged women conducted over a two-to-three-year period, found 41% had intermittent anxiety and 10% had chronic anxiety (Brenes 2006). If new onset of anxiety is associated with a recently diagnosed medical condition, an *adjustment disorder with anxious features* should be considered.

One study of adults aged >65 reported that having 2 systemic medical conditions was associated with a 1.79-fold increased incidence in anxiety, and three or more systemic medical conditions was associated with a 3.04-fold increased incidence of anxiety, measured by the Beck Anxiety Inventory (Gould et al. 2016). Aging adults with anxiety and chronic somatic symptoms may limit their activities, pursue unnecessary or extensive clinical workups, and avoid medications due to adverse effects (Lenze et al. 2005). Fear of pain and a tendency to catastrophize can lead to greater pain intensity, activity restriction, and further disability (Bierman and Lee 2018). Table 10.2.

Non-pharmacological Treatment

Randomized clinical trials (RCT) for treatment of anxiety in geriatric individuals have not to date provided widely accepted guidelines about which non-pharmacological interventions are most beneficial for specific anxiety disorders. Nevertheless,

Table 10.2 Medical conditions and symptoms which overlap with anxiety

System	Diagnosis	Somatic symptoms
Endocrine	Hyperthyroid Pheochromocytoma Hypoglycemia Hyperadrenocortisolism	Tachycardia, sleep disturbance Tachycardia, heat sensation Lightheadedness Trembling Difficulty concentrating
Cardiovascular	Congestive heart failure Pulmonary embolism Coronary artery disease Arrhythmia	Shortness of breath, tachycardia, sleep disturbance Air hunger, tachycardia, chest pain Chest pain, shortness of breath Tachycardia, palpitations
Respiratory	Chronic obstructive pulmonary disease Asthma Pneumonia Obstructive and central sleep apnea	Shortness of breath Chest pain Fatigue, difficulty concentrating, Palpitations, sleep disturbance, Drowsiness
Metabolic	Vitamin B12 deficiency Porphyria	Peripheral neuropathy, fatigue Palpitations, tingling, Shortness of breath
Neurologic	Stroke Parkinson's disease Neoplasms Vestibular dysfunction Delirium Seizure disorder Migraine	Paresthesias, loss of motor function, Loss of consciousness Pounding Vertigo, dizziness Confusion, disorientation, Clouded consciousness Muscle tension, altered vision, nausea
Autoimmune	Rheumatoid arthritis Lupus	Muscle tension, fatigue, Apprehension with joint movement, Muscle tension, fatigue
Infection	Influenza, COVID	Mental fogginess, disorientation
Musculoskeletal	Orthopedic injuries	Muscle tension, Excessive fear of re-injury

Source: Willgoss and Yohannes (2013)

non-pharmacological modalities can be beneficial (Subramanyam et al. 2018).

One meta-analysis reviewed 4 RCTs whose subjects (total $n = 255$, mean age range 67–71 years) had clinically significant anxiety and depressed mood (Wuthrich et al. 2021).

Psychological interventions *cognitive behavioral therapy* (CBT) and *mindfulness* showed improvement in both anxiety and depression over control conditions (active, waitlist). The pooled effect sizes indicated that psychological interventions may be efficacious for treating co-occurring anxiety and depression in older adults, with moderate benefit for *depression* in the presence of anxiety, and moderate benefit for *anxiety* in the presence of depression. Stronger conclusions could not be drawn due to the small number of studies, the low quality of some, small sample sizes, and heterogeneity across studies (Wuthrich et al. 2021).

Education & Lifestyle Modifications

Providing information to patients about their anxiety and its precipitants can minimize its adverse impact (Moreno-Peral et al. 2017). Changes in lifestyle factors that perpetuate anxiety, structured daily activities, modifications to diet, exercise, and sleep can all help ameliorate medical and non-medical triggers of anxiety. Paced activity, swimming, aquatic exercises, and stretching, including upper body only exercises for wheelchair-bound patients, can benefit (Subramanyam et al. 2018). Relaxation and yoga include modifications such as chair yoga and pranayama.

If the anxiety is focused on systemic medical illness, interventions to increase awareness, self-monitor, and relaxation (e.g., Jacobson's progressive muscle relaxation) can help. A 10-year systematic review and meta-analysis found relaxation training effective. A self-guided 4-week video-delivered relaxation intervention (BREATHE) in group and individual settings was found feasible for aging adults with anxiety disorders. The BREATHE intervention reduced anxiety, depressive, and somatic symptoms relative to waitlist control (Gould et al. 2019).

Behavioral, Cognitive Approaches, and Cognitive Behavior Therapy (CBT)

CBT integrates cognitive aspects, such as understanding and reformulating maladaptive beliefs about threats, with behavioral aspects of exposure and relaxation training. Evidence for CBT compared to other psychotherapeutic interventions for anxiety in geriatric individuals, however, is mixed. For *late-life* anxiety, unlike anxiety in younger populations, CBT has not shown superiority over other psychological treatments such as supportive counseling or group psychotherapy (Hendriks 2014). CBT shows efficacy in older adults, albeit with smaller effect sizes, but few studies include those >70 years of age (Gould et al. 2012). Evidence of efficacy of CBT in aging adults with GAD could be due to modifying cognitive schemata and promoting techniques, such as controlled breathing and muscle relaxation (Subramanyam et al. 2018). The hope is that CBT may establish coping strategies and skills that manage stressors after treatment ends.

Non-pharmacological Treatment of Anxiety in Patients with Cognitive Impairment

Results for CBT have been limited to cognitively intact, relatively healthy, educated, and independent older adults, and are difficult to generalize to the cognitively impaired or frail older patients. However, one systematic review of 14 RCTs (Kishita et al. 2020) of non-pharmacological interventions to improve anxiety, depression, and quality of life (QoL) in people with MNCD concluded that CBT was effective at reducing anxiety and depression (anxiety: MD = −4.57 depression: SMD = −0.22). Cognitive stimulation resulted in improved quality of life (QoL: standardized mean difference [SMD] = 0.38).

Augmentation of pharmacological treatment with modular cognitive-behavioral therapy (mCBT) has been shown to reduce anxiety symptoms and pathological worry. Moreover, SSRI and mCBT treatment has resulted in full remission, and sustained remission in some instances after all treatments ceased (Wetherell et al. 2011). CBT has also been reported, combined with medications, to be *more effective* than psychotherapy or pharmacotherapy alone, and associated with a decrease in the relapse of anxiety symptoms after the medication is discontinued (Wetherell et al. 2013). There is hope that psychotherapeutic modalities and CBT may improve online accessibility (Hobbs et al. 2017).

The ABC Model (Antecedents-Behavior-Consequences)

The ABC approach promotes the identification and modification of maladaptive behaviors or cognitions using cognitive restructuring (Subramanyam et al. 2018). However, long-established behaviors and thoughts are difficult to change.

Exposure Techniques (ET) and Adaptation of CBT

A review and meta-analysis of 54 studies concluded that in vivo and imaginal exposure were the mainstay approaches with associated reductions in severity of anxiety symptoms (Jayasinghe et al. 2017).

Acceptance and Commitment Therapy (ACT)

ACT uses principles based on CBT and assumes that distress is associated with psychological inflexibility. The goal is to assist older adults to accept life stressors or changes of aging rather than avoid them. One feasibility and acceptability study indicated its potential benefit (Gould et al. 2021).

Mindfulness-Based Therapies

This strategy focuses on the "now" to harmonize mind and body to target anxiety, depression, concurrent chronic pain, and insomnia. Mindfulness-based therapies support awareness of physical and mental sensations without a need to attend or change them and include *Mindfulness-Based Stress Reduction (MBSR)* and *Mindfulness-Based Cognitive Therapy (MBCT).* MBCT showed greater specificity in reducing anxiety and depression symptoms, with improvements to cognitive function (Hazlett-Stevens et al. 2019).

Art and Music Therapy

Unstructured art (e.g., painting, drawing, and sketching) and formal art therapy, in group or individually, can be beneficial for anxiety, regardless of levels of cognitive impairment or physical abilities. Listening to music, playing an instrument, singing and dancing, encourages movement in older adults, including wheelchair or bedridden older adults. These activities foster social interaction and improve mood, well-being, and quality of life, all of which reduce anxiety (Kishita et al. 2020). The benefits of music have also been demonstrated for mild to moderate Alzheimer's disease (AD) (Guetin et al. 2009). For further discussion, see Chaps. 15 and 16.

Psychopharmacological Treatment

The pharmacotherapy of anxiety for aging has not been studied extensively with RCTs; findings are often extrapolated from studies of middle-aged adults (Lenze and Wetherell 2011).

Antidepressants (AD)

Selective serotonin reuptake inhibitors (SSRIs) are first-line for generalized anxiety disorder (GAD) in geriatric patients. However, one study has reported a meager (7%) use of antidepressants in aging adults with anxiety, compared to 27% use of benzodiazepines (Schuurmans et al. 2005), which may be due to concern about anticholinergic effects. Yet escitalopram, which has few clinically significant drug–drug interactions, and citalopram have proven effective for treatment of generalized anxiety disorder, social anxiety, and panic disorder in the aging adult (Lenze et al. 2005). In pharmacokinetic studies, the half-life of escitalopram was increased by 50% in older compared to young adults, but the C_{max} was equivalent. The FDA recommends dosing escitalopram at 10 mg daily in older adults. Citalopram is the racemic mixture of the R and S-citalopram enantiomers, and due to the reported effect of prolonged QTc, doses greater than 20 mg daily are not recommended in adults older than age 60.

Paroxetine is FDA approved for generalized anxiety disorder and panic disorder. Its adverse effects such as weight gain and anticholinergic effects like dry mouth, constipation, urinary retention, blurry vision, and confusion are more prevalent than in other SSRIs. Its strong 2D6 inhibition of the cytochrome pathway can cause significant drug–drug interactions. Fluoxetine and fluvoxamine are also inhibitors of the cytochrome P450 pathways with the potential for drug–drug interactions.

Serotonin/norepinephrine reuptake inhibitors (SNRIs) are often second-line treatments for anxiety disorders. Venlafaxine and duloxetine are common SNRIs for anxiety disorders, especially when anxiety is accompanied by comorbid pain conditions (Katz et al. 2002). A retrospective pooled analysis of RCTs reported the efficacy of venlafaxine 37.5–225 mg daily for anxiety disorders in older adults. Duloxetine should be avoided in patients with hepatic insufficiency or end stage renal disease. Vortioxetine can increase serotonin, norepinephrine, and dopamine levels and has a favorable side effect profile in aging adults (Baldwin et al. 2018).

Tricyclic antidepressants (TCA) have demonstrated efficacy for generalized anxiety disorder, panic disorder, and social anxiety disorder. However, because of the unfavorable side effect profile (including their anticholinergic effects), TCAs have lost favor as primary treatment options. Monoamine oxidase inhibitors such as phenelzine and tranylcypromine have been used for panic disorder and social anxiety disorder with some benefit, but they are not recommended for aging adults due to significant risk for orthostatic hypotension, falls, and hypertensive crises. For further discussion, see Chaps. 2 and 11.

Benzodiazepines

Benzodiazepines can be beneficial for anxiety which is associated with acute and overwhelming stressors in short term (weeks to months). The best evidence for their benefit is treatment of insomnia (Gerlach et al. 2018). However, benzodiazepines treatment in aging adults requires close attention to the risk-benefit ratio. The US FDA in September of 2020 issued a warning about "abuse, addiction, physical dependence, and withdrawal reactions" with benzodiazepines (Hirschtritt et al. 2021). Benzodiazepines can cause slowed processing speed, poor concentration, and impaired memory, disinhibition, and aggressive behavior although no direct causal relationship with MNCD has been firmly established. Sedation is the most common adverse effect and is dose-dependent; patients should avoid complex tasks such as driving or operating dangerous implements (e.g., electric knives) when starting or increasing the dose of a benzodiazepine.

Current guidelines for prescribing to geriatric patients include "beginning with the end in mind:" setting proactive expectations for a brief duration of treatment (weeks rather than months) and frequently re-evaluating the need for continued use (Gerlach et al. 2018). In the geriatric population, long term benzodiazepine use without re-evaluation, can lead to tolerance, dependence and other negative outcomes. When discontinued abruptly, withdrawal symptoms can result in one study of adults 65 and older who had sustained a hip fracture, use of benzodiazepines in the month prior had an odds ratio of 3.73 for a fall with hip fracture (Machado-Duque et al. 2018). Long-acting but not short or intermediate-acting, benzodiazepines have been associated with a higher risk of falls (Berdot et al. 2009).

Aging adults taking benzodiazepines for years without reassessment should be informed about sedative properties, impact on cognition, impairment of psychomotor functioning, and the risks of abrupt discontinuation. A reduction in benzodiazepine use is best accomplished by a combination of supervised gradual withdrawal and adjunct pharmacotherapy and/or psychotherapy (Gould et al. 2014). For further discussion, see Chap. 7.

Buspirone

Buspirone is an anxiolytic that does not share the same side effect profile. A double-blind, placebo-controlled trial of buspirone (mean dose of 18 mg/day) in older adults with anxiety or neurotic depression demonstrated a statistically significant reduction in the Hamilton Rating Scale for Anxiety at 4 weeks. (Böhm et al. 1990).

Antipsychotics (APs)

Among the second-generation antipsychotics (SGAs), quetiapine has the most evidence as a monotherapy and adjunctive therapy for generalized anxiety disorder in adults ages 18–65 (Kreys and Phan 2015). Risperidone, olanzapine, and ziprasidone do not have consensus support for anxiety (Hershenberg et al. 2014). SGAs carry an FDA black box warning for increased risk of death in geriatric individuals with MNCD. Recent meta-analyses indicate that the increased risk of all-cause mortality in older adults treated with antipsychotics also includes *non-dementia* patients (Ralph and Espinet 2018). For further discussion, see Chaps. 2, 5, and 9.

Mood Stabilizers

Antiepileptics (AED)/mood stabilizers have not shown conclusive evidence of efficacy for anxiety, and they are not FDA approved for this indication. Lamotrigine has demonstrated some benefit for panic disorders with agoraphobia and for depressive disorders with anxiety (Zavodnick and Ali 2012). Valproate, gabapentin, and pregabalin have been used to treat anxiety disorders, especially when concurrent with certain pain syndromes or bipolar disorder (Crocco et al. 2017).

Antihypertensive Medications

Beta blockers like propranolol, or clonidine, an alpha-2 agonist, have been used to treat anxiety disorders, especially performance anxiety, yet have been associated in aging adults with onset of depressive disorder, fatigue, and increased sedation (Byrne 2021). Clonidine has precipitated hypotension, rebound hypertension, dizziness, drowsiness, dry mouth, bradycardia, heart block, and syncope, which limit its use for geriatric patients, especially the oldest-old and frail.

Hydroxyzine

Hydroxyzine, a mild antihistamine H1 antagonist with anticholinergic properties, has not been studied extensively in the geriatric population. It is prescribed off-label on an as-needed basis for anxiety because it has minimal sedative properties and no risk of physiological dependence. For further discussion, see Chap. 2.

Conclusions

Anxiety symptoms in the geriatric individual are common, under-studied, and challenging to assess. Somatic symptoms may appear to be anxious complaints which the aging patient may not identify or describe as *anxiety*. Conversely, an older patient's natural *apprehension and uncertainty* in the face of somatic symptoms, pain, and other stressors may be mis-identified as an anxiety disorder and unnecessarily treated with anti-anxiety medications. Apprehension may respond to reassurance and other non-pharmacological interventions. An *age-adjusted* practice emphasizes the early search for factors which contribute to anxiety. Treatment starts with psychotherapeutic techniques, followed, if necessary, by step-wise and cautious pharmacotherapy.

Age-Adjusted Recommendations

- Obtain a thorough history of anxiety symptoms, including prior treatments, response, and associated psychiatric disorders.
- Recognize those psychosocial and other factors which contribute to anxiety.
- Rule out and treat medical comorbidities which precipitate or exacerbate anxiety.
- Encourage the delivery of psychiatric/psychological interventions in settings outside of formal psychiatric practice.
- Enlist other health care providers to participate in the treatment plan.
- Use non-pharmacological interventions first-line while pursuing systemic medical work-up.
- Validate anxiety symptoms as distressing and needing attention.
- Prescribe medications in *age-adjusted* doses.
- Involve family members or other caregivers in treatment planning.

References

Baldwin D, Stein MB, Hermann R. Generalized anxiety disorder in adults: epidemiology, pathogenesis, clinical manifestations, course, assessment, and diagnosis. UpToDate; 2018.

Balsamo M, Cataldi F, Carlucci L, Fairfield B. Assessment of anxiety in older adults: a review of self-report measures. Clin Interv Aging. 2018;13:573–93.

Bakkane Bendixen A, Engedal K, Selbæk G, Hartberg CB. Anxiety Symptoms in Older Adults with Depression Are Associated with Suicidality. Dement Geriatr Cogn Disord. 2018;45(3-4):180–189. https://doi.org/10.1159/000488480. Epub 2018 Jun 1. PMID: 29860257

Berdot S, Bertrand M, Dartigues JF, Fourrier A, et al. Inappropriate medication use and risk of falls–a prospective study in a large community-dwelling elderly cohort. BMC Geriatr. 2009;9(1):1–10.

Bierman A, Lee Y. Chronic pain and psychological distress among older adults: a national longitudinal study. Res Aging. 2018;40(5):432–55.

Böhm C, Robinson DS, Gammans RE. Buspirone therapy for elderly patients with anxiety or depressive neurosis. J Clin Psychiatry. 1990;51(7):309.

Brenes GA. Age differences in the presentation of anxiety. Aging Ment Health. 2006;10(3):298–302.

Byers AL, Yaffe K, Covinsky KE, et al. High occurrence of mood and anxiety disorders among older adults: the National Comorbidity Survey Replication. Arch Gen Psychiatry. 2010;67(5):489–96.

Byrne GJ. Pharmacological treatment of anxiety in later life. In Anxiety in older people: clinical and research perspectives, pp 189; 2021.

Byrne GJ, Pachana NA. Development and validation of a short form of the geriatric anxiety inventory—the GAI-SF. Int Psychogeriatr. 2011;23:125–31.

Calamari JE, Woodard JL, Armstrong KM, et al. Assessing older adults' obsessive-compulsive disorder symptoms: psychometric characteristics of the obsessive-compulsive inventory-revised. J Obsessive Compuls Relat Disord. 2014;3(2):124–31.

Canuto A, Weber K, Baertschi M, et al. Anxiety disorders in old age: psychiatric comorbidities, quality of life, and prevalence according to age, gender, and country. Am J Geriatr Psychiatry. 2018;26(2):174–85.

Cath DC, Nizar K, Boomsma D, Mathews CA. Age-specific prevalence of hoarding and obsessive-compulsive disorder: a population-based study. Am J Geriatr Psychiatry. 2017;25(3):245–55.

Chou KL. Social anxiety disorder in older adults: evidence from the National Epidemiologic Survey on alcohol and related conditions. J Affect Disord. 2009;119(1–3):76–83.

Chou KL. Specific phobia in older adults: evidence from the national epidemiologic survey on alcohol and related conditions. Am J Geriatr Psychiatry. 2009;17(5):376–86. https://doi.org/10.1097/JGP.0b013e3181943214. PMID: 19390295.

Chou KL, Mackenzie CS, Liang K, Sareen J. Three-year incidence and predictors of first-onset of DSM-IV mood, anxiety, and substance use disorders in older adults: results from Wave 2 of the National Epidemiologic Survey on Alcohol and related Conditions; 2011.

Crocco EA, Jaramillo S, Cruz-Ortiz C, Camfield K. Pharmacological management of anxiety disorders in the elderly. Curr Treat Options Psychiatry. 2017;4(1):33–46.

Gerlach LB, Maust DT, Leong SH, et al. Factors associated with long-term benzodiazepine use among older adults. JAMA Intern Med. 2018;178(11):1560–2.

Gould RL, Coulson MC, Howard RJ. Efficacy of cognitive behavioral therapy for anxiety disorders in older people: a meta-analysis and meta-regression of randomized controlled trials. J Am Geriatr Soc. 2012;60(2):218–29.

Gould R, Coulson M, Patel N, et al. Interventions for reducing benzodiazepine use in older people: meta-analysis of randomised controlled trials. Br J Psychiatry. 2014;204(2):98–107.

Gould CE, O'Hara R, Goldstein MK, Beaudreau SA. Multimorbidity is associated with anxiety in older adults in the Health and Retirement Study. Int J Geriatr Psychiatry. 2016;31(10):1105–15.

Gould CE, Kok BC, Ma VK, et al. Video-delivered relaxation intervention reduces late-life anxiety: a pilot

randomized controlled trial. Am J Geriatr Psychiatry. 2019;27(5):514–25.
Gould RL, Wetherell JL, Serfaty MA, et al. Acceptance and commitment therapy for older people with treatment-resistant generalised anxiety disorder: the FACTOID feasibility study. Health Technol Assess. 2021;25(54):1–150.
Grenier S, Richer MJ. Subthreshold epidemiology and anxiety treatment in later strategies life. In: Anxiety in older people: clinical and research perspectives, pp 33; 2021.
Guetin S, Portet F, Picot MC, et al. Effect of music therapy on anxiety and depression in patients with Alzheimer's type dementia: randomised, controlled study. Dement Geriatric Cogn Disord. 2009;28(1):36–46.
Hazlett-Stevens H, Singer J, Chong A. Mindfulness-based stress reduction and mindfulness-based cognitive therapy with older adults: a qualitative review of randomized controlled outcome research. Clin Gerontol. 2019;42(4):347–58.
Hellwig S, Domschke K. Anxiety in late life: an update on pathomechanisms. Gerontology. 2019;65(5):465–73.
Hendriks GJ. Therapeutics in late-life anxiety disorders—an update. Curr Treat Options Psychiatry. 2014;1(1):27–36.
Hershenberg R, Gros DF, Brawman-Mintzer O. Role of atypical antipsychotics in the treatment of generalized anxiety disorder. CNS Drugs. 2014;28:519–33.
Hirschtritt ME, Olfson M, Kroenke K. Balancing the risks and benefits of benzodiazepines. JAMA. 2021;325(4):347–8.
Hobbs MJ, Mahoney AEJ, Andrews G. Integrating iCBT for generalized anxiety disorder into routine clinical care: treatment effects across the adult lifespan. J Anxiety Disord. 2017;51:47–54.
Jayasinghe N, Finkelstein-Fox L, Sar-Graycar L, et al. Systematic review of the clinical application of exposure techniques for late life anxiety. Clin Gerontol. 2017;40(3):141–58.
Jazi AN, Asghar-Ali AA. Obsessive-compulsive disorder in older adults: a comprehensive literature review. J Psychiatr Pract. 2020;26(3):175–84.
Johnco C, Knight A, Tadic D, Wuthrich VM. Psychometric properties of the Geriatric Anxiety Inventory (GAI) and its short-form (GAI-SF) in a clinical and nonclinical sample of older adults. Int Psychogeriatr. 2015;27:1089–97.
Katz IR, Reynolds CF, Alexopoulos GS, Hackett D. Venlafaxine ER as a treatment for generalized anxiety disorder in older adults: pooled analysis of five randomized placebo-controlled clinical trials. J Am Geriatr Soc. 2002;50:18–25.
King-Kallimanis B, Gum AM, Kohn R. Comorbidity of depressive and anxiety disorders for older Americans in the national comorbidity survey-replication. Am J Geriatr Psychiatry. 2009;17(9):782–92.
Kishita N, Backhouse T, Mioshi E. Nonpharmacological interventions to improve depression, anxiety, and quality of life (QoL) in people with dementia: an overview of systematic reviews. J Geriatr Psychiatry Neurol. 2020;33(1):28–41.
Kreys TJM, Phan SV. A literature review of quetiapine for generalized anxiety disorder. Pharmacotherapy. 2015;35(2):175–88.
Le Roux H, Gatz M, Wetherell JL. Age at onset of generalized anxiety disorder in older adults. Am J Geriatr Psychiatry. 2005;13(1):23–30.
Lenze EJ, Wetherell JL. Anxiety disorders: new developments in old age. Am J Geriatr Psychiatry. 2011;19(4):301–4.
Lenze EJ, Mulsant BH, Shear MK, et al. Efficacy and tolerability of citalopram in the treatment of late-life anxiety disorders: results from an 8-week randomized, placebo-controlled trial. Am J Psychiatry. 2005;162(1):146–50.
Lever-van Milligen BA, Verhoeven JE, Schmaal L, et al. The impact of depression and anxiety treatment on biological aging and metabolic stress: study protocol of the mood treatment with antidepressants or running (MOTAR) study. BMC Psychiatry. 2019;19(1):1–11.
van der Linde RM, Dening T, Stephan BC, et al. Longitudinal course of behavioural and psychological symptoms of dementia: systematic review. Br J Psychiatry. 2016;209(5):366–77.
Machado-Duque ME, Castaño-Montoya JP, Medina-Morales DA, et al. Association between the use of benzodiazepines and opioids with the risk of falls and hip fractures in older adults. Int Psychogeriatr. 2018;30(7):941–6.
Mackenzie CS, El-Gabalawy R, Chou KL, Sareen J. Prevalence and predictors of persistent versus remitting mood, anxiety, and substance disorders in a national sample of older adults. Am J Geriatr Psychiatry. 2014;22(9):854–65.
Martens EJ, de Jonge P, Na B, et al. Scared to death: generalized anxiety disorder and cardiovascular events in patients with stable coronary heart disease, the heart and soul study. Arch Gen Psychiatry. 2010;67(7):750–8.
Mohlman J, de Jesus M, Gorenstein EE, et al. Distinguishing generalized anxiety disorder, panic disorder, and mixed anxiety states in older treatment-seeking adults. J Anxiety Disord. 2004;18(3):275–90.
Moreno-Peral P, Conejo-Cerón S, Rubio-Valera M, et al. Effectiveness of psychological and/or educational interventions in the prevention of anxiety: a systematic review, meta-analysis, and meta-regression. JAMA Psychiatry. 2017;74(10):1021–9.
Ralph SJ, Espinet AJ. Increased all-cause mortality by antipsychotic drugs: updated review and meta-analysis in dementia and general mental health care. J Alzheimers Dis Rep. 2018;2(1):1–26.
Scheffer AC, Schuurmans MJ, van Dijk N, et al. Fear of falling: measurement strategy, prevalence, risk factors and consequences among older persons. Age Ageing. 2008;37(1):19–24.
Schuurmans J, Comijs HC, Beekman ATF, et al. The outcome of anxiety disorders in older people at 6-year follow-up: results from the Longitudinal

Aging Study Amsterdam. Acta Psychiatr Scand. 2005;111(6):420–8.
Segal DL, June A, Payne M, et al. Development and initial validation of a self-report assessment tool for anxiety among older adults: the Geriatric Anxiety Scale. J Anxiety Disord. 2010;24(7):709–14.
Seignourel PJ, Kunik ME, Snow L, et al. Anxiety in dementia: a critical review. Clin Psychol Rev. 2008;28(7):1071–82.
Subramanyam AA, Kedare J, Singh OP, Pinto C. Clinical practice guidelines for geriatric anxiety disorders. Indian J Psychiatry. 2018;60(Suppl 3):S371.
Wetherell JL, Stoddard JA, White KS, et al. Augmenting antidepressant medication with modular CBT for geriatric generalized anxiety disorder: a pilot study. Int J Geriatr Psychiatry. 2011;26(8):869–75.
Wetherell JL, Petkus AJ, White KS, et al. Antidepressant medication augmented with cognitive-behavioral therapy for generalized anxiety disorder in older adults. Am J Psychiatry. 2013;170(7):782–9.
Willgoss TG, Yohannes AM. Anxiety disorders in patients with COPD: a systematic review. Respir Care. 2013;58(5):858–66.
Wolitzky-Taylor KB, Castriotta N, Lenze EJ, et al. Anxiety disorders in older adults: a comprehensive review. Depress Anxiety. 2010;27(2):190–211.
Wuthrich VM, Meuldijk D, Jagiello T, et al. Efficacy and effectiveness of psychological interventions on co-occurring mood and anxiety disorders in older adults: a systematic review and meta-analysis. Int J Geriatr Psychiatry. 2021;36(6):858–72.
Zavodnick AD, Ali R. Lamotrigine in the treatment of unipolar depression with and without comorbidities: a literature review. Psychiatric Q. 2012;83(3):371–83.

Depressive Disorders

11

Amanda Mihalik-Wenger, Uma Suryadevara, Justin Wenger, Meena Nuthi, Rita Hitching, and Howard H. Fenn

Abstract

About one in three cases of depressive disorders in the geriatric population have their onset in *late* life; many more cases are recurrences of depressive disorders which began *earlier* in life. This chapter reviews the diagnosis and treatment of depressive disorders in late life to facilitate their differentiation from other conditions and recommend non-pharmacological treatment and age-adjusted pharmacological interventions.

Both *early-onset* and *late-onset* categories may be unreported or missed. *Late-life* depressive disorders have been under-recognized and inadequately treated in primary care, especially among Hispanic and African American men in the United States (Hasin et al. JAMA Psychiatry 75:336–46, 2018)).

Many factors may account for missed depressive disorders among aging individuals. The geriatric patient may present with more somatic complaints, greater social isolation, and reduced access to medical care (especially for underserved minority populations) and be hesitant to report depressive symptoms. The impact of psychosocial stressors on the patient may not be fully appreciated nor is clinical time often adequate to explore them. The number of systemic medical comorbidities increases with age and correlates with the increased prevalence of depressive disorders as patients age. Teasing out depressive symptoms among somatic complaints in the elderly patient is a challenge. Complex medication regimens, in the context of pharmacodynamic and pharmacokinetic effects of aging, can contribute to an increased risk of adverse effects, which can also contribute to depressive symptoms.

A. Mihalik-Wenger
University of Washington, Department of Psychiatry, Seattle, WA, USA

University of Florida, College of Medicine, Gainesville, FL, USA

J. Wenger
Seattle VA Medical center, Seattle, WA, USA

University of Florida, College of Medicine, Gainesville, FL, USA

M. Nuthi
Malcom Randall VA Medical Center, Gainesville, WA, USA

University of Florida, College of Medicine, Gainesville, FL, USA

U. Suryadevara (✉)
University of Florida, Gainesville, FL, USA

Malcom Randall VA Medical Center, Gainesville, FL, USA

R. Hitching
University of Newcastle, Newcastle, Australia

H. H. Fenn
VA Health Care System, Palo Alto, CA, USA

Department of Psychiatry and Behavioral Sciences, Stanford University, Stanford, CA, USA
e-mail: hhfenn@aol.com, howard.fenn@va.gov

H. H. Fenn et al. (eds.), *Age-Adjusted Psychiatric Treatment for the Older Patient*,
https://doi.org/10.1007/978-3-031-53976-3_11

Case Example: Depressive Symptoms Improved After Several Medication Trials

An 82-year-old retired health-care administrator, with a history of recurrent depressive episodes beginning in early life, was admitted to a skilled nursing facility (SNF) for rehabilitation of a fractured hip leading to total hip replacement. Over the course of the first 3 months, she began to develop morbid thoughts, irritable mood, and lost motivation to engage in treatment. She refused rehabilitation and did not eat full meals. The family explained that she was overwhelmed with challenges of the new environment. The patient complained of forgetfulness (e.g., missing appointments) and insomnia. A Montreal Cognitive Assessment (MoCA) scored 24 out of 30 with deficits in digit span and concentration items. The Geriatric Depression Scale (GDS) scored was 5/5.

Her first psychiatric hospitalization for depression was at age 30; she was treated successfully with nortriptyline. Upon full recovery, she went on to earn a BA at a prestigious university. She stopped nortriptyline after 1 year and had 2 subsequent depressive episodes, with improvement on fluoxetine, and full remission with 12 sessions of electroconvulsive therapy (ECT). The patient was maintained on a dose of fluoxetine 40 mg daily for 20 years before another depressive episode. When she stopped responding to fluoxetine 40 mg daily, the dosage was increased to 80 mg daily without benefit. Consequently, bupropion was added and increased to 300 mg daily. She improved and was stable without depressive symptoms until the relapse at the time admission to the SNF.

On admission to the SNF, the attending physician discontinued the fluoxetine and bupropion and initiated a regimen of citalopram 10 mg daily, which was increased to 20 mg daily after 4 weeks. A psychiatric consultant recommended discontinuation of citalopram and started venlafaxine XR, gradually increased from 75 mg daily to 300 mg daily.

After 6 weeks on venlafaxine, her oppositional behavior, isolation, angry mood, and insomnia continued, and she became more irritable. Aripiprazole 10 mg per day was added as an augmenting agent. The patient became restless, which was attributed to akathisia, and insomnia worsened. Aripiprazole was discontinued. Mirtazapine was started, and increased to 30 mg at bedtime which improved initiation of sleep and appetite, but without any improvement in mood. After another 4 weeks, the mood symptoms were not improved, and she became isolative, avoiding any groups.

Approximately 3 months from the initial contact, a treatment-resistant depression (TRD) was diagnosed due to a lack of meaningful improvement following treatment with ≥2 different antidepressant agents at adequate doses for sufficient duration.

The patient then received flexibly dosed esketamine nasal spray (up to 84 mg), twice weekly for 4 weeks. After 2 weeks she reported some improvement in mood, but this was not sustained and esketamine was discontinued. The full complement of depressive symptoms returned.

Augmentation with olanzapine 5 mg at bedtime was well tolerated. The patient reported more restful sleep and over 4 weeks appeared less irritable, more willing to engage with others. She had been an avid reader and now joined a book club which she attended by ZOOM. Her GDS now rated as 2/5.

Discussion: Treatment-resistant depression (TRD) is present in at least 2% of the general population and represents at least one-third of all depressed patients (Gaynes et al. 2020). The patient's improved socialization was facilitated by stabilization of mood through a medication regimen which included an SNRI (serotonin-norepinephrine reuptake inhibitor) (venlafaxine), a second antidepressant (mirtazapine), and a second-generation antipsychotic (olanzapine).

Epidemiology

The prevalence of depressive disorders in geriatric population varies by setting, definition of late-*life*, severity of symptoms, method of assessment, and subject sample. In community samples, the aged have generally shown lower prevalence of depressive disorder than the general adult population. One study estimated major depressive disorders in aging individuals as approximately 2% of

12-month prevalence compared to an estimate of 4.6% among the general *non-geriatric* population (Thornicroft et al. 2017). A nationally representative survey of *non-geriatric* adults in the United States found that the a 12-month prevalence of unipolar major depression was 10% and the lifetime prevalence was 21% (Hasin et al. 2018).

Among the highest rates of depression are those reported for geriatric patients in settings wherein medical comorbidity is also high. In long-term nursing home (LTNH) residents, 54.4% had a depressive episode diagnosed over the course of the first year, 32.8% at admission, and a further 21.6% later during the first year (Hoover et al. 2010).

Phenomenology

Depressive symptoms in late life may be more difficult to recognize than earlier in life. Late-life depressive disorder symptoms may be obscured by systemic medical comorbidities and other factors (Haigh et al. 2018) In addition, irritable mood, anxiety, and somatic symptoms often dominate the presentation more than depressed mood and tearfulness. Apathy, lethargy, fatigue, social withdrawal due to chronic pain, sleep deprivation, and cognitive deficits can be misidentified as part of, or overlap with, depressive disorder symptoms. There is also evidence that depression predisposes to the onset of major neurocognitive disorder (MNCD)/dementia, suggesting that depressive symptoms in their early stages may be *prodromes* of later MNCD/dementia (Alexopoulos 2021).

Many factors of aging can precipitate or obscure depressive symptoms. Medication regimens are often extensive in the geriatric patient, adding to the risk of adverse effects such as sedation, lethargy, or reduced energy which can mimic depressive symptoms. The losses and psychosocial stressors in the aged can precipitate adjustment disorders or symptoms of bereavement that resemble major depressive episodes but have a different course and respond to different approaches. Depressive episodes of *shorter* duration may be less responsive to antidepressants than a depressive episode of longer duration (greater than 10 years) (Nelson et al. 2013).

Differential Diagnosis and Assessment

The diagnostic criteria for major depressive disorder in the DSM-5-TR require either sadness or anhedonia, with a total of five or more depressive symptoms over a two-week period. Yet only two questions from the Patient Health Questionnaire-2 (PHQ-2) are sufficient to screen for a depressive disorder:

- During the past month, have you been bothered by feeling down, depressed, or hopeless?
- During the past month, have you been bothered by little interest or pleasure in doing things?

The PHQ-2 had a sensitivity of 100% and specificity of 77% in this population; specificity increased with age, male gender, and varied with racial and ethnic groups has been found valid in a sample of over 8000 noninstitutionalized adults aged 65 years and older (Grossberg et al. 2017).

The Geriatric Depression Scale (GDS)—short form—requires of two out of five positive answers to be considered a depressive disorder. Other rating scales which track depressive symptoms are the following:

- Hamilton Rating Scale for Depression (HAM-D)
- Beck Depression Inventory-II (BDI-II)
- Montgomery–Asberg Depression Rating Scale (MADRS)

A *comprehensive assessment* should be considered for any aging adult who presents with symptoms suggestive of a depressive disorder. Specifiers of major depressive disorder are reviewed below (Table 11.1).

Vascular Depressive Disorder (VaD)

Late-onset depressive disorder (LODD) has been associated with cardiovascular disease (CVD), cognitive deficits, psychomotor retardation, apathy, lack of insight, disability, and greater sever-

Table 11.1 Comprehensive assessment of depressive disorders in late life

Comprehensive assessment of depression in late life	
Assessment and diagnostic	• Severity, onset, duration of presenting symptoms, and prior depressive symptoms/episodes • Pre-morbid level of functioning & social support
Screening and rating scales	• Geriatric Depression Scale (GDS) *Are you basically satisfied with your life?* *Do you often get bored?* *Do you often feel helpless?* *Do you prefer to stay at home rather than going out and doing new things?* *Do you feel pretty worthless the way you are now?* Two out of five depressive responses ("no" to question 1 or "yes" to questions 2 through 5) suggests depressive disorder. • Hamilton Rating Scale for Depression (HAM-D) • Beck Depression Inventory-II (BDI-II) • Montgomery–Asberg Depression Rating Scale (MADRS)
Suicidal intent	• Geriatric depression scale suicide subscale (GDS-SI) • Patient Health Questionnaire-9 (PHQ-9) (for use in primary care settings) • Suicide risk assessment including access to firearms • Self-destructive, reckless behaviors, and suicide attempts
Psychiatric history	• Hospitalizations and emergency department visits. • Medication doses, duration, adverse effects, and response. • Manic, hypomanic, or mixed episodes.
Substance use history	• Use of alcohol, substances, non-prescribed, OTC (OTC)/medications, and treatments for abuse • Short Michigan Alcoholism Screening Test–Geriatric Version (SMAST-G) • Alcohol Use Disorders Identification Test (AUDIT) • CAGE-AID
Screening for delirium and neurocognitive disorder	• MoCA, MMSE, Mini-Cog, and SLUMS • Confusion assessment method (CAM) for delirium
Medication review	• Use of or withdrawal from psychotropics, antidepressants, antipsychotics, opioids, barbiturates, benzodiazepines, over-the-counter (OTC) substances, steroids, and stimulants • Medications which contribute to depressive symptoms
Laboratory and relevant studies	Systemic medical/laboratory work-up, for example: • Thyroid function tests • B12 and folate levels • Complete blood count and differential • Metabolic panel, including serum creatinine and eGFR = estimated glomerular filtration rate • Liver-associated enzymes • Lipid panel • Urine drug screen and urinalysis • EKG • CT/MRI to rule out stroke, trauma, or neurodegenerative disease Serum levels of lithium, valproic acid, and carbamazepine

ity of depressive symptoms (Aizenstein et al. 2016). Some authors have recommended screening all cardiovascular disease patients for depressive disorder (Zhang et al. 2018). Patients with severe depressive symptoms who responded well to psychiatric treatment have been shown to have *fewer* white matter lesions (Paranthaman et al. 2012), which suggests that CVD may be less likely benefit from treatment. Indeed, LODD has been shown to respond less robustly to antidepressants than earlier-onset depressive disorders.

A combination of systemic medical factors (hypertension, diabetes mellitus, obesity, vascular and hormonal changes, amyloid deposition, and inflammatory markers) has been hypothesized to contribute to an executive dysfunction which starts in mid-life and progresses (Alexopoulos 2021). This *depression-executive dysfunction syndrome (DED)* has been characterized by anhedonia, psychomotor retardation, pronounced disability, lack of insight, and suspiciousness. Although these symptoms appear more prominent in DED, patients often show less evidence of depressed mood, per se. DED has been reported to respond less completely and more slowly to conventional antidepressant pharmacotherapy (Alexopoulos 2019), higher rates of relapse, difficulty achieving remission, and worse treatment outcomes (Sözeri-Varma 2012). Poststroke depression (PSD) is a depressive condition associated with CVD. For further discussion, see Chap. 3.

Early-Onset Depressive Disorder (EODD)

A depressive disorder during old age is *three times more likely* to be a *recurrent* episode of a depressive disorder that began earlier in life than later in life. As mentioned above, an *early-onset* depressive disorder may respond better to antidepressant treatment than late-onset depressive disorder; history therefore is important (Luijendijk et al. 2008).

Late-Life Treatment-Resistant Depression (LLTRD)

Almost one-third of aging patients with depressive disorders are considered resistant to available treatments (McIntyre et al. 2014; Souery et al. 2006). Consensus criteria used to define treatment-resistant depression (TRD) among patients diagnosed with MDD (Gaynes et al. 2020; Gronemann et al. 2021) include inadequate response to at least *two* consecutive treatments with antidepressants at adequate doses with full compliance for an adequate length of time.

Adjustment Disorder with Depressed Mood

This disorder is diagnosed if symptoms of depressive disorder do not meet diagnostic criteria for MDD and appear within 3 months of the onset of severe psychosocial stressor(s) such as a significant loss, a serious or worsening medical condition, a clinically disabling illness, a change in financial or living situation, or any other impactful event. Adjustment disorders have been associated with physical decline, disability, and death. Non-pharmacological approaches are first-line and include supportive psychotherapy, family therapy, CBT, or psychosocial interventions.

Many conditions in the aging individual can give rise to symptoms which mimic depression, such as lethargy, sleep disruption, apathy, social withdrawal, and failure to thrive. Sadness and grief are normal responses to life events such as bereavement, adjustment to changes in social status with retirement and loss of income, transition from independent living to assisted or residential care, and loss of physical, social, or cognitive function from illness.

Socialization and other supportive therapies can mitigate the vicious cycle of greater isolation and decline, hopefully avoiding antidepressants, especially if loneliness can be addressed and resilience fortified (Perissinotto et al. 2012). For further discussion, see Chap. 13.

Persistent Depressive Disorder (Dysthymia)

DSM-5-TR criteria for *persistent depressive disorder* in old age require depressive symptoms that occur on most days for at least 2 years but fewer symptoms than for MDD. The *late-onset* variant of persistent depressive disorder has been associated with higher prevalence of cardiovascular disease (Devanand et al. 2004). Both pharmacological and non-pharmacological interventions are the same as for MDD. See *Stepwise Pharmacological Treatment* below.

Bipolar I or Bipolar II Disorder: Prior Manic or Hypomanic Episodes

If a pre-existing manic or hypomanic episode can be confirmed, a diagnosis of bipolar disorder I or II, with a mixed or manic episode, is appropriate. Pharmacotherapy is usually indicted, with the addition of mood stabilizers and/or second-generation antipsychotics (SGAs). For further discussion, see Chap. 12.

Substance/Medication-Induced Depressive Disorder

DSM-5-TR *criteria for substance/medication-induced depressive disorder* include a mood disturbance dominated by depressed mood or markedly diminished interest or pleasure in almost all activities. There must also be evidence of (1) symptoms which developed during or soon after the substance intoxication or withdrawal or after exposure to the medication and (2) the substance or medication that can produce the mood disturbance symptoms. A history of alcohol or illegal substance abuse, misuse of prescribed medications, or inappropriate use of over-the-counter OTC substances should be sought.

Changes in medication regimens, prescribers, abrupt discontinuation, or adequacy about the medication delivery system can provide indirect evidence of misuse of medications or substance use disorders.

An overlap of depressive symptomatology with substance-induced depressive symptoms is challenging to parse. Details and accurate history of medication or substance use or its onset may be difficult to obtain because of the following reasons:

- The cognitively impaired patient may be unaware, may deny, or may have forgotten details of substance or alcohol abuse.
- The patient may be unaware of any misuse of prescribed medications.
- A geriatric patient living alone may not have observers to provide information.

The substance/medication-induced depressive disorder diagnosis is not offered if the depressive symptoms arose *before* the onset of the substance use or if they continue approximately 1 month after cessation of substance use or if they are better explained by history of a depressive disorder *independent* of substance/medication use.

A full list of medications from all of the patient's prescribers can be crucial to treatment of *substance/medication-induced depressive disorder*. The risk of not pursuing this information can challenge concerns about privacy and confidentiality of health records. Families, caregivers, or other practitioners can be enlisted to provide evidence of medication misuse or substance abuse. A brief inpatient hospitalization may also be necessary to ensure safe withdrawal from substances, especially if the patient is cognitively impaired or unreliable.

If the use or misuse of common medications can be recognized and addressed through medication adjustment or better delivery process, depressive symptoms can be alleviated and unnecessary pharmacotherapy can be avoided. See below for a list of common medications which can cause symptoms of depressive disorder (Grossberg et al. 2017). For further discussion, see Chap. 7 (Table 11.2).

Table 11.2 Common medications that can contribute to depressive symptoms

Hydralazine
Estrogens
Progesterone
Tamoxifen
Vinblastine
Vincristine
Opioids
Benzodiazepines
Interferon-alpha
Corticosteroids
Anti-parkinsonian medications
Beta-blockers
Cimetidine
Clonidine
Corticosteroids
Tamoxifen

Depressive Disorder Due to Another Medical Condition

The contribution of comorbid medical conditions to the onset of depressive symptoms can be established with a comprehensive medical work-up. Appropriate laboratory studies, physical examination, history, and prior medical records, such as TSH, T3, and T4, can rule out hypothyroidism or vitamin B12 and folate levels to rule out lethargy/cognitive impairment. Stroke, loss of hearing, loss of vision, cardiac disease, and chronic lung disease all substantially increase the risk of depressive disorders in old age (Huang et al. 2010). For further discussion, see Chaps. 3 and 4.

Neurocognitive Disorders and Neurodegenerative Disorders

Any patient over the age of 65 carries an increased risk of a neurocognitive disorder, major or mild. It has been estimated that 30% of depressed older adults show abnormal performance on tests of verbal fluency, response inhibition, novel problem-solving, cognitive flexibility, working memory, and/or ideomotor planning, findings of a prodromal MNCD (Tables 11.3 and 11.4). Therefore, identification of a MNCD or a neurodegenerative disorder, previously diagnosed as TRD, can avoid unnecessary medications and inappropriate interventions. If MNCD is diagnosed, behavioral and psychological symptoms

Table 11.3 Early-onset major depressive disorder (EODD) versus late-onset depressive disorder (LODD)

Features	Early-onset depressive disorder (EODD)	Late-onset depressive disorder (LODD) (first episode occurs in late life)
Prognosis	Good	Greater number of relapses Prognosis poor in presence of comorbid anxiety, fatigue, chronic pain, and loneliness
Severity of symptoms	Mild, moderate, or severe	• *Moderate-severe* (46.5%) • *Severe-melancholic* (38.4%): decreased appetite, weight loss, decreased sleep, and more psychomotor changes • *Atypical-severe* in 15.0%: weight gain and increased appetite (Veltman et al. 2017; Lamers et al. 2013)
Comorbid disorders	High prevalence: • Comorbid psychiatric illnesses • Substance abuse	High prevalence: • Chronic pain • Systemic medical conditions • Anxiety disorders • Neurocognitive disorders • Cerebrovascular disease
Risk factors	Family history of depressive disorders	Loneliness/isolation Loss of significant other
Somatic symptoms	Not predominant over depressive symptoms	Predominant among other complaints
Guilt	Common	Not common
Psychosis	Not common	Common, especially somatic delusions
Agitation	Not common	Common
Cognitive impairment and changes	Deficits in social cognition	Deficits in executive function (EF), verbal learning, memory, motor speed (Thomas and Elliott 2009), and + white matter lesions
Non-pharmacological strategies or other interventions	CBT and other psychotherapies neuromodulation interventions Bright light therapy Exercise ECT	CBT and other psychotherapy modalities Rule out and address contributing factors: systemic medical conditions, sleep deprivation, and pain Bright light therapy Exercise ECT
Psychopharmacological	Likely to respond to medications	Less likely to respond to medications than EODD

References: Hegeman et al. (2012), Hasin et al. (2018), Kessler et al. (2005), Weinberger et al. (2018), Jeuring et al. (2018), Maarsingh et al. (2018), Thomas and Elliott (2009), Nelson et al. (2013)

Table 11.4 Disorders in late life with depressive features

Disorder	Mean age of onset	Prevalence in aging adults	Distinctive features	Risk factors
Early-onset depressive disorder (EODD)	26	Three times more common than late-onset MDD	High prevalence of comorbid psychiatric illnesses, alcohol, or drug use Limited social support and higher residual symptoms	Family history of depressive disorders and earlier age of onset
Late-onset depressive disorder (LODD)	60	0.9–14% depending on setting. Prevalence is higher in in LTC	Impairment in executive function, increased mortality and suicide, more white matter changes, more apathy, and higher relapse rate	Neuroticism/anxiety disorders, cognitive impairment, loss of spouse, loneliness, and comorbid systemic medical illness
Adjustment disorder with depressed mood	Adolescence	2.3%	Older adults with adjustment disorders rarely seek help. Distress is out of proportion to severity of stressor	Medical illness, loss, disabilities, relocation, financial problems, illness in a relative, and family conflicts
Persistent complex bereavement disorder	60	>70% of bereaved experienced symptoms over a span of 2.5 years from loss	Increased morbidity; increased mortality especially in men; and increased use of health care Severe and persistent grief and mourning beyond culturally accepted norms Grief includes moods of emptiness, loneliness, and preoccupation with loss, Self-esteem preserved Older adults prone to complicated grief	Death of a loved one or impending loss of a loved one
Depressive disorder due to another medical condition	0–2 years from diagnosis of the medical condition	5–42% depending on setting	Untreated depressive disorder increases mortality rates in these systemic medical conditions	Cardiovascular diseases, endocrine disturbances, Parkinson's disease, stroke, and cancer common medical conditions wherein depressive disorder is comorbid
Major depressive disorder (MDD) with psychotic features	32	9.8% of aging adults with MDD have psychotic symptoms	Somatic delusions common	Family history of bipolar disorder and psychosis

Aziz and Steffens (2013), Volkert et al. (2013), Hegeman et al. (2012), Djernes (2006), Sözeri-Varma (2012), Kok and Reynolds (2017)

of dementia (BPSD), including depressive symptoms, can also be suspected. For further discussion, see Chaps. 3, 5, 9, and 13.

Non-pharmacological Treatment and Somatic Modulation Modalities

Exercise

Adding exercise to SSRI (selective serotonin reuptake inhibitor) treatment can improve symptoms of depressive disorder. A study compared 121 subjects (mean age 75.6), on sertraline alone versus subjects on sertraline (S) + progressive aerobic exercise (S + PAE) versus subjects on a nonprogressive exercise regimen. The S + NPE arm additionally attended three supervised group non-progressive exercise sessions (NP) per week (60-min duration). Patients in the S + PAE group exercised on bikes with a preplanned increase of the workload over the course of the 24-week study. All patients received sertraline at a starting dosage of 50 mg, with later increases according to the clinical course. Participants in the S + NPE arm additionally attended three supervised group nonprogressive exercise sessions (NP) per week. Patients in the S + PAE group attended exercise sessions with a similar schedule to that of NP but exercised on bikes with a preplanned increase of the workload over the course of the study.

The primary outcome was remission from depression, defined as a total score of ten or less on the HAM-D at study end. The two groups receiving sertraline plus exercise displayed similar rates of remission from depression (S + PAE, 81%, S + NPE, 73%). These results were combined into a sertraline plus exercise group (S + EX, $n = 79$, remission rate: 77%), which was contrasted with the sertraline-only group (S, $n = 42$, remission rate: 45%). In sum, the S + EX groups displayed significantly greater improvements of depressive symptom dimension (total effect size = 0.79), with largest changes in the first 4 weeks and the last 12 weeks. Improvements were noted primarily in symptoms of depressed mood and psychomotor retardation (Murri et al. 2018). Similar results were found when exercise (endurance, muscle strengthening, and stretching twice per week for 10 weeks) was compared to antidepressants alone (Mather et al. 2002).

Bright Light Therapy (BLT)

BLT is delivered through a light box that is equipped with fluorescent tubes and a reflector or diffusing screen. The modality poses little risk and has shown potential to benefit both mood and sleep in geriatric patients *without* seasonal affective disorder. In a RCT (randomized controlled trial) of 89 outpatients (60 years or older) with MDD, bright light treatments (pale blue approximately 7500 lux) improved mood, enhanced sleep efficiency, and increased the upslope melatonin level both after 3 weeks of treatment. The active intervention was a pale blue or dim red light treatment therapy at home using two light boxes (Lieverse et al. 2011). Concealed within the light boxes, a single-layer filter was wrapped around the fluorescent tubes, a mist-blue filter (Model 061; Lee Filters, Andover, England) with high-throughput pale blue (7500 lux) for the active condition; a blood-red filter (Model 789; Lee Filters) with low-throughput red (50 lux) was chosen for placebo condition. Dim red light is biologically inactive. Subjects were exposed for 60 min in the early morning at about 7500 lux (Lieverse et al. 2011). Other factors like changes in intervention intensity, light type, duration of intervention, and measuring scales did not have any statistically significant moderating effects on depression (Zhao et al. 2018).

Psychotherapies

Cognitive-behavioral therapy CBT, problem-solving therapy (PST), interpersonal therapy (IPT), and engage therapy (ET) (Alexopoulos et al. 2016) have been found effective for symptoms of depressive disorders, although more high-quality RCTs for geriatric patients are needed (Gould et al. 2012). For further discussion, see Chap. 15.

Repetitive Transcranial Magnetic Stimulation (rTMS)

rTMS is a safe intervention for geriatric depression, with fewer cognitive side effects than ECT. However, remission rates are lower when compared to remission rates for ECT (McDonald 2016). For further discussion, see Chap. 14.

Deep Brain Stimulation (DBS)

DBS for treatment-resistant depression (TRD) in aging adults has to date not been studied thoroughly enough to draw conclusions. Its putative mechanism is not understood. There is evidence that DBS can be relatively safe and well tolerated (Dandekar et al. 2018). One study has shown effectiveness in relief of depressive symptoms and reducing the incidence of major depressive disorder (van't Veer-Tazelaar et al. 2009).

Electroconvulsive Therapy (ECT)

ECT is a safe, effective, well-established treatment for aging patients who are resistant to psychotherapy and medications or who cannot tolerate medications due to medical comorbidities (Riva-Posse et al. 2013). Efficacy rate has been demonstrated at over 60% (Meyer et al. 2020), and greater rates of improvement have also been reported. The cognitive side effects are mostly transient even in patients with pre-existing cognitive deficits (Hausner et al. 2011). ECT is usually safe and well tolerated in patients with systemic medical comorbidities. For further discussion, see Chap. 14.

Pharmacological Treatment of Depressive Disorders in Late Life

Many studies support antidepressant monotherapy for depressive disorders in late life (Beyer and Johnson 2018). One review concluded that outcomes of antidepressant treatment for major depressive disorder in aging adults are comparable to that for younger populations and that geriatric patients with a lifetime history of depressive disorder should be maintained on medication for at least 2 years following remission from a MDD episode (Kok and Reynolds 2017).

Other authors have noted that one-third of aged patients with depressive disorder are *resistant* to available treatments (Knöchel et al. 2015) and that the response of depressed aging patients to antidepressants is *less robust* than the response in younger patients (Tedeschini et al. 2011). Aging adults may have more adverse outcomes due to inability to tolerate medications, resulting in medication discontinuation prior to completion of a full course, and therefore a higher relapse rate of depressive symptoms. In addition, antidepressants can lose effectiveness over time (Targum 2014). This can occur within the continuation treatment phase and into the maintenance phase (Nierenberg et al. 2003).

Loss of effectiveness of an antidepressant and a recurrence of the original depressive symptoms can be indistinguishable from depressive and anxiety withdrawal symptoms which occur as part of an SSRI *discontinuation* syndrome. To help distinguish these syndromes, an SSRI *discontinuation* syndrome is marked by depressive symptoms and physiological symptoms of anxiety often within 2 weeks of stopping the antidepressant (Kinrys et al. 2019). After that timeline, depressive symptoms diminish.

Stepwise Pharmacological Treatment of Late-Life Depressive Disorder (LLDD)

Prior to initiating medications consider the following:

- Previous responses to, or tolerance of, medications
- Potential drug-drug interactions
- The medication adverse effect profile (Cleare et al. 2015), including risk of hyperlipidemia, cerebrovascular events, or sudden death

(Beyer and Johnson 2018; Espinoza et al. 2021; Mulsant et al. 2014; Pruckner and Holthoff-Detto 2017)

Step 1: If patient has been taking an antidepressant medication at an adequate dose for an adequate duration (over 8 weeks), without any significant benefit, consider discontinuing it. This can clarify the diagnosis, identify any medication adverse effects, and guide the choice of a new medication to target current symptoms. This process is consistent with *deprescribing* which can minimize polypharmacy and wean potential inappropriate medications (PIM) *(*Pravodelov 2020).

Step 2: Confirm adherence to prescribed medications; assess patient's motivation and the reliability of the medication delivery system. If the patient has been receiving the recommended prescription medications, and after 8 weeks, a 50% reduction in symptoms has not been achieved, proceed to Step 3.

Step 3: Augmentation strategies outperform switching strategies. Studies demonstrate that an absence of a 20% decrease in the baseline depression score by the end of week 2 of an antidepressant trial means less than a 10% chance of reaching remission by week 12 (Hicks et al. 2019). Augmentation has the benefit of avoiding risk of serotonin syndrome which can result from the combination of two antidepressants with serotonin-enhancing properties. There is a paucity of rigorous data to support the use of *T4 and T3 thyroid hormone* augmentation in aging individuals.

Step 3A. *Augment with a second-generation antipsychotic (SGA).*

Aripiprazole (Mulsant et al. 2014), quetiapine, ziprasidone, or olanzapine can benefit depressive symptoms even if the depressive disorder is *without* psychotic features (MacQueen et al. 2016; DeBattista and Hawkins 2009). Quetiapine XR has shown benefit for treatment of psychosis and insomnia as well as for treatment of depressive disorder in aging individuals (Katila et al. 2013).

—or—.

Step 3B. *Augment with lithium:* Geriatric patients may respond more favorably to lithium augmentation than non-geriatric patients (Buspavanich et al. 2019), although lithium increases the risk of hypothyroidism and hyperparathyroidism and has a narrow therapeutic window. Monitor lithium levels regularly, as well as renal function for insufficient renal clearance (serum creatinine 0.67–1.17 mg/dL BUN 8.0–23 mg/dL). Therapeutic serum lithium ranges from 0.5 mEq/L to 1.2 mEq/L.

For further discussion, see Chap. 2.

—or—

Step 3C. *Augment with a stimulant*: If the patient has been medically cleared of cardiovascular or other risk factors, consider methylphenidate or dextroamphetamine. Start methylphenidate at 2.5 mg every morning and increase slowly as tolerated to a typical dose of 5 mg twice daily. Do not administer late in the day to avoid interference with sleep. In a RCT of 143 older adults (69.7 (SD = 7.3) years), citalopram and methylphenidate *combined* demonstrated an enhanced clinical response profile in mood and well-being, as well as a higher rate of remission, compared with either medication alone (Lavretsky et al. 2015). To date, the addition of modafinil has not been studied in the geriatric population but has demonstrated effectiveness in younger populations (Fava et al. 2007). If augmentation does not result in remission, go to Step 4.

Step 4*: Switch to a different category of antidepressant—see Switching Strategies below.* Start an SNRI (e.g., duloxetine, venlafaxine, desvenlafaxine), at a dose adjusted for age, tolerance, and medical status. Increase dose gradually for a duration of up to 8 weeks to reach a maximum response. Depressive symptoms which are reduced by 50% from baseline can be considered an adequate response. A meta-analysis in 2015 demonstrated that SNRIs like duloxetine, venlafaxine, and desvenlafaxine were well tolerated and efficacy was comparable to SSRIs (Thorlund et al. 2015).

—or—

Start a non-SSRI/non-SNRI antidepressant such as bupropion, vortioxetine, or mirtazapine. The STAR*D (sequenced treatment alternatives to relieve depression) trial reported that the outcome for patients with depressive disorder who were *switched* to medications like bupropion or venlafaxine was not significantly different than for those where bupropion and venlafaxine were added as augmenting agents (Rush et al. 2008).

—or—

Start an SNRI (duloxetine, venlafaxine, desvenlafaxine) instead of the SSRI, or start an ***SSRI*** if the first medication is an ***SNRI.*** The doses should start low and increase slowly. For example, duloxetine is started at 20 mg per day and increased up to 60 mg per day over 4 weeks, and venlafaxine XR would be started at 37.5 mg per day and dose increased up to 225 mg per day over 4 weeks. Monitor closely for development of *serotonin syndrome.* If the regimen is not effective, taper and discontinue the second medication over a period of few weeks to avoid *discontinuation syndrome.*

—or—

If the aforementioned steps achieve 50% reduction in symptoms, go to **Step 5**.

If the aforementioned steps *do not* achieve 50% reduction in depressive symptoms after 8 weeks, see TRD protocol below.

Step 5: *Maintenance:* If depressive symptoms have responded adequately to medication, do the following:

- Continue antidepressant regimen in combination with psychotherapy to prevent relapse (Segal et al. 2003).
- Following a *first* episode of major depressive episode, continue treatment for 12 months after remission (Kato et al. 2021). If there is an increased risk of relapse based upon history, continue treatment for 2 years. Risk of relapse is higher in geriatric patients who have comorbid medical conditions.
- For patients at *highest risk* of relapse, including multiple previous episodes, continue treatment indefinitely (Geddes et al. 2003). If there is a substantial risk of suicide, consider continuation of treatment indefinitely (Gibbons et al. 2012).

Antidepressant Switching Strategies

1. **Direct substitution without a period of washout:** The abrupt withdrawal of an SSRI or SNRI *without tapering* and therefore the possibility of *discontinuation syndrome* due to absence of the medication binding to a specific receptor. SNRIs like duloxetine and venlafaxine have demonstrated withdrawal symptoms when discontinued abruptly (Fava et al. 2018).
2. **Cross-tapering.** Taper the current antidepressant, along with a gradual introduction of a second, *replacement antidepressant* at low doses. Consider this for aging individuals at high risk for relapse of depressive symptoms and/or at risk of a *discontinuation* syndrome. The original antidepressant can be decreased by 25% per week while adding the second medication in small increments. *Cross-tapering* adds the risk drug-drug interactions while the two medications are both active; frequent monitoring (at least weekly) can help discern *discontinuation* symptoms from *adverse effects* of the second, new antidepressant.

The pharmacokinetic properties of the drug, as well as pharmacodynamics and medical status of the patient, can guide the *cross-tapering* process. For example, if the current antidepressant is a potent CYP2D6 inhibitor and the aged patient is being switched to an antidepressant primarily metabolized by 2D6, the levels of the replacement antidepressant will be elevated, unless the *first* medication is washed out adequately (Espinoza et al. 2021; Kok and Reynolds 2017; Mulsant et al. 2014). Starting the *second* antidepressant at a low dose can mitigate the risk of adverse effects.

3. **Washout without overlap.** This is a gradual taper and discontinuation of the original antidepressant, followed by a washout period (1–2 weeks) *before* starting the second antidepressant. It may be safest to taper the first medication for at least 4 weeks, by 25% every week, before discontinuing it, and start the *replacement* medication after the first antidepressant has washed out completely. The dose increments of taper may be guided by patient tolerability. If an MAOI is the first medication, it is better to taper the MAOI for a minimum period of 2 weeks, before starting the replacement (serotonergic) antidepressant,

due to risk of serotonin syndrome. If switching from fluoxetine to an MAOI, wait at least *5 weeks after discontinuation* before starting an MAOI (Soreide et al. 2017).

Although criteria for treatment resistant depression (TRD) have not been standardized, a practical definition, mentioned above, refers to major depressive episodes that do not respond sufficiently after two trials of antidepressant monotherapy with adequate dose, for adequate duration. A partial or inadequate response is considered one in which appropriate treatment has not achieved 50% reduction of depressive symptoms after 8 weeks of treatment (Gadzhanova et al. 2018). A treatment algorithm for TRD follows below (Table 11.5).

Table 11.5 Medications for late-life depressive disorder

Medication selective serotonin reuptake inhibitors (SSRIs)	Formulation	Initial dose (mg/day)[a]	Target dose (mg/day)	Dose adjustment and monitoring	Adverse effects/other characteristics
Citalopram or escitalopram	Tablets and oral solution	5	10–20	Cautious use with poor CYP2C19 metabolizers or CYP2C19 inhibitors. Cautious use in patients with severe renal impairment	20 mg daily can prolong QTc interval. SIADH Serotonin syndrome
Fluoxetine	Capsules, tablets, oral solution, and weekly capsule	10	20–40	Dose decrease in renal and hepatic impairment	SIADH Serotonin syndrome Drug–drug interactions (DDI) Not associated with discontinuation syndrome
Paroxetine	Immediate release tablets, oral suspension, and controlled release	10	20–40	<40 mg in renal impairment Cautious use in patients with cognitive decline	Anticholinergic syndrome SIADH drug–drug interactions Serotonin syndrome
Sertraline	Tablet and oral concentrate	12.5–25	50–200	Dose decrease in mild hepatic impairment and caution in severe hepatic impairment	SIADH Serotonin syndrome
Fluvoxamine	Tablets	25	50–300	Decrease dose in hepatic impairment	SIADH Serotonin syndrome Drug-drug interactions
Serotonin-norepinephrine reuptake inhibitors (SNRIs)					
Desvenlafaxine	XR tablets	50	50	Dose adjustment in patients with renal impairment	Increased risk of orthostatic hypotension; renal clearance is decreased in older adults.
Duloxetine	Capsules	20	60	Avoid use in patients with hepatic insufficiency or severe renal impairment	Discontinuation syndrome Orthostatic hypotension, hepatotoxicity Serotonin syndrome increased risk of bleeding

(continued)

Table 11.5 (continued)

Medication selective serotonin reuptake inhibitors (SSRIs)	Formulation	Initial dose (mg/day)[a]	Target dose (mg/day)	Dose adjustment and monitoring	Adverse effects/other characteristics
Levomilnacipran	Capsules	20	40–120	Dose adjustment in patients with renal impairment	Discontinuation syndrome, elevated BP and HR, orthostatic hypotension, serotonin syndrome, increased risk of bleeding, and angle closure glaucoma
Venlafaxine	IR tablets XR capsules	50 37.5	75–225	Dose adjustment in patients with hepatic and renal impairment	Discontinuation syndrome, elevations in blood pressure, serotonin syndrome, increased risk of bleeding, and angle closure glaucoma
Others					
Bupropion	Tablets SR XL ER	150 (SR or XL) 174 (ER)	150–400 (SR) 150–450 (XL) 522	Renal and hepatic clearance is decreased in older adults; moderate inhibitor of CYP2D6: Dose adjustment if patient is on fluoxetine or paroxetine	Risk of seizures elevated in poststroke patients
Mirtazapine	Tablets Wafers (disintegrating tablets)	7.5 15	5–60 15–60	Oral clearance of mirtazapine is decreased in older adults especially in males. Use of mirtazapine with MAO inhibitors is contraindicated.	Risks in frail nursing home patients: Delirium Weight gain, somnolence, hyponatremia, and rare neutropenia or agranulocytosis
Vortioxetine	Tablets	5	5–20	Do not exceed 10 mg/day in poor CYP2D6 metabolizers. Increase or decrease dose if patient is on other CYP2D6 inducers or inhibitors.	Serotonin syndrome, increasled risk of bleeding, angle closure glaucoma, and hyponatremia
Trazodone	Tablets ER tablets	25–150	50–150	Dose adjustments in patients with renal or hepatic impairment	Used as a sedative. Dry mouth, orthostatic hypotension, priapism, and QT prolongation
Vilazodone	Tablets	20	20–40	Dose adjustments with strong CYP3A4 inhibitors	Discontinuation syndrome, seizures, serotonin syndrome, increased risk of bleeding, and angle closure glaucoma
Tricyclic antidepressants and others					
Desipramine	Tablets	10	10–150	Extreme caution in patients with cardiovascular disease, and impaired renal function. Obtain EKG	Delirium, cardiac side effects, and serotonin syndrome, Urinary retention, glaucoma, seizure disorders, and thyroid disorders

Table 11.5 (continued)

Medication selective serotonin reuptake inhibitors (SSRIs)	Formulation	Initial dose (mg/ day)[a]	Target dose (mg/ day)	Dose adjustment and monitoring	Adverse effects/other characteristics
Nortriptyline	Capsules Oral solution	10	25–75	Extreme caution in patients with cardiovascular disease, impaired renal function, urinary retention, glaucoma, seizure disorders, and thyroid disorders Obtain EKG, orthostatic blood pressures, pulse, electrolytes, serum creatinine, blood levels, and liver function tests every 6 months	Serotonin syndrome, delirium, cardiac side effects, urinary retention, glaucoma, seizure disorders, and thyroid disorders
Amitriptyline	Tablets	10	25–50	Extreme caution in patients with cardiovascular disease, impaired renal function, urinary retention, glaucoma, seizure disorders, and thyroid disorders Obtain EKG, orthostatic blood pressures, pulse, electrolytes, serum creatinine, and liver function tests every 6 months.	Serotonin syndrome, delirium, cardiac side effects, urinary retention, glaucoma, seizure disorders, and thyroid disorders
Doxepin	Capsules Oral solutions	3	150	Extreme caution in patients with cardiovascular disease, Urinary retention, glaucoma, seizure disorders, and thyroid disorders	Delirium, cardiac adverse effects, urinary retention, glaucoma, serotonin syndrome, seizure disorders, and thyroid disorders
Augmenting medications					
Aripiprazole	Tablet, ODT, solution, IM, and LAI	2	10–15	No dose adjustment for renal or hepatic impairment	Akathisia may worsen impulse control
Quetiapine	Tablet	12.5	300	Reduce dose in patients with hepatic impairment	Orthostatic hypotension, weight gain, diabetes mellitus, and hyperlipidemia
Brexpiprazole	Tablet	0.5	3	Reduce dose in patients with hepatic or renal impairment	Akathisia and weight gain

Olanzapine and fluoxetine—tablet—3/25 mg/d—12/50 mg/d

[a]Consider lower initial doses for the frail elderly or oldest-old; consultation with a compounding pharmacy may be needed

Suicidality

Unipolar depressive disorder is the most common psychiatric disorder in aging adults who complete suicide (Conwell 2014; Koo et al. 2017). Of concern is that a greater proportion of suicide attempts in the aged population are lethal, than among younger age groups (Kiosses et al. 2014). Several reasons have been offered: a high prevalence of comorbid medical conditions provides less resilience to any serious self-injury, isolation from others means less chance to rescue, and the aging individual may exert greater determination and planning prior to any suicide attempt (Van Orden et al. 2016).

Clinical vigilance, along with other observers, needs to be commensurate to this degree of risk. Primary prevention is best accomplished by obtaining current accurate information of risk factors, which include past attempts, reckless behavior, current suicidal ideation, use of alcohol and substances, and availability of lethal means. If a patient has credible, active suicidal ideation, immediate treatment through hospitalization is recommended along with preventing access to lethal means. Secondary prevention can often be started on the inpatient unit (Bachmann 2018) by collaboration between family, caregivers, and others. A treatment plan can be tailored appropriate to level of risk.

If there are no imminent safety concerns, ongoing outpatient monitoring with structured suicide risk rating scales and clinical interviews should continue, along with an effective and tolerable antidepressant regimen. If a patient has passive suicidal ideation, further evaluation is needed. A safety plan which addresses suicidality can be updated based on changing psychosocial circumstances (Grant and Lusk 2015; Raue et al. 2014).

Conclusions

A growing body of evidence supports the inclusion of *late-life* major depressive disorder into the next DSM iteration (Husain-Krautter and Ellison 2021). Hopefully, this will promote awareness of depressive disorders in the geriatric population and encourage clinicians to ferret out treatable contributors. This diagnosis may also stimulate research of non-pharmacological, somatic modalities, and pharmacological interventions with fewer adverse effects. Targeting medical comorbidities, reviewing medication regimens, adjusting doses, and de-prescribing can hopefully help avoid unnecessary interventions and develop more individualized treatment plans.

Somatic modalities such as DBS and rTMS hold promise, especially when the patient is among the oldest-old and frail and has multiple medical problems and complex medication regimens. Psychotherapeutic interventions can also build on innate coping mechanisms to mobilize an individual's resilience. Although some studies suggest that the elderly are less responsive to antidepressants, evidence shows that aging individuals with depression, under clinical scrutiny, can benefit substantially from a correct choice of medication, age-adjusted dosing, and adequate duration. In general, medication categories, such as lithium, SGAs, and stimulants, need not be categorically excluded but rather adjusted to aging physiology.

Age-Adjusted Recommendations

- Review and adjust medication regimens which adversely affect mood and behavior (e.g., corticosteroids, hypnotics, beta-blockers, benzodiazepines, opioids, anticholinergics).
- Consider non-pharmacological interventions as first-line.
- Employ a stepwise protocol for pharmacotherapy, with doses, administration, and combinations adapted to aging pharmacokinetics and pharmacodynamics.
- Perform a screening cognitive examination.
- Rule out and treat potential contributors to depressive symptoms, such as systemic medical conditions, stroke, hypothyroidism, diabetes mellitus, or cardiovascular disease.
- Search past history for age of onset, duration, and response to prior treatment.

- Conduct a neurological work-up to rule out neurological, neurodegenerative, or cerebrovascular disease.
- Reconsider any diagnosis of treatment-resistant depression (TRD) for validity.
- Screen for depression in patients with cardiovascular disease.

References

van't Veer-Tazelaar PJ, van Marwijk HW, van Oppen P, et al. Stepped-care prevention of anxiety and depression in late life: a randomized controlled trial. Arch Gen Psychiatry. 2009;66(3):297–304.

Aizenstein HJ, Baskys A, Boldrini M, et al. Vascular depression consensus report—a critical update. BMC Med. 2016;14(1):1–61.

Alexopoulos GS. Mechanisms and treatment of late-life depression. Transl Psychiatry. 2019;9:188.

Alexopoulos GS. Mechanisms and treatment of late-life depression. Focus. 2021;19(3):340–54.

Alexopoulos GS, Raue PJ, Gunning F, et al. "Engage" therapy: behavioral activation and improvement of late-life major depression. Am J Geriatr Psychiatry. 2016;24:320–6.

Aziz R, Steffens DC. What are the causes of late-life depression? Psychiatr Clin. 2013;36(4):497–516.

Bachmann S. Epidemiology of suicide and the psychiatric perspective. Int J Environ Res Public Health. 2018;15(7):1425.

Beyer JL, Johnson KG. Advances in pharmacotherapy of late-life depression. Curr Psychiatry Rep. 2018;20(5):1–11.

Buspavanich P, Behr J, Stamm T, et al. Treatment response of lithium augmentation in geriatric compared to non-geriatric patients with treatment-resistant depression. J Affect Disord. 2019;15(251):136–40.

Cleare A, Pariante CM, Young AH, et al. Evidence-based guidelines for treating depressive disorders with antidepressants: a revision of the 2008 British Association for Psychopharmacology guidelines. J Psychopharmacol. 2015;29(5):459–525.

Conwell Y. Suicide later in life: challenges and priorities for prevention. Am J Prev Med. 2014;47(3 Suppl 2):S244–50.

Dandekar MP, Fenoy AJ, Carvalho AF, et al. Deep brain stimulation for treatment-resistant depression: an integrative review of preclinical and clinical findings and translational implications. Mol Psychiatry. 2018;23(5):1094–112.

DeBattista C, Hawkins J. Utility of atypical antipsychotics in the treatment of resistant unipolar depression. CNS Drugs. 2009;23(5):369–77.

Devanand DP, Adorno E, Cheng J, et al. Late onset dysthymic disorder and major depression differ from early onset dysthymic disorder and major depression in elderly outpatients. J Affect Disord. 2004;78(3):259–67.

Djernes JK. Prevalence and predictors of depression in populations of elderly: a review. Acta Psychiatr Scand. 2006;113(5):372–87.

Espinoza RT, Unützer J, Schmader KE. Diagnosis and management of late-life unipolar depression. Waltham, MA: UptoDate; 2021.

Fava M, Thase ME, DeBattista C, et al. Modafinil augmentation of selective serotonin reuptake inhibitor therapy in MDD partial responders with persistent fatigue and sleepiness. Ann Clin Psychiatry. 2007;19(3):153–9.

Fava GA, Benasi G, Lucente M, et al. Withdrawal symptoms after serotonin-noradrenaline reuptake inhibitor discontinuation: systematic review. Psychother Psychosom. 2018;87(4):195–203.

Gadzhanova S, Roughead EE, Pont LG. Antidepressant switching patterns in the elderly. Int Psychogeriatr. 2018;30(9):1365–74.

Gaynes BN, Lux L, Gartlehner G, et al. Defining treatment-resistant depression. Depress Anxiety. 2020;37(2):134–45.

Geddes JR, Carney SM, Davies C, et al. Relapse prevention with antidepressant drug treatment in depressive disorders: a systematic review. Lancet. 2003;361(9358):653–61.

Gibbons RD, Brown CH, Hur K, et al. Suicidal thoughts and behavior with antidepressant treatment: reanalysis of the randomized placebo-controlled studies of fluoxetine and venlafaxine. Arch Gen Psychiatry. 2012;69(6):580–7.

Gould RL, Coulson MC, Howard RJ. Cognitive behavioral therapy for depression in older people: a meta-analysis and meta-regression of randomized controlled trials. J Am Geriatr Soc. 2012;60(10):1817–30.

Grant CL, Lusk JL. A multidisciplinary approach to therapeutic risk management of the suicidal patient. J Multidiscip Healthc. 2015;8:291–8.

Gronemann FH, Petersen J, Alulis S, et al. Treatment patterns in patients with treatment-resistant depression in Danish patients with major depressive disorder. J Affective Disord. 2021;287:204–13.

Grossberg GT, Beck D, Zaidi SYZ. Rapid depression assessment in geriatric patients. Clin Geriatr Med. 2017;33:383–91.

Haigh EAP, Bogucki OE, Sandra MA, et al. Depression among older adults: a 20-year update on five common myths and misconceptions. Am J Geriatr Psychiatry. 2018;26(1):107–22.

Hasin DS, Sarvet AL, Meyers JL, et al. Epidemiology of adult DSM-5 major depressive disorder and its specifiers in the United States. JAMA Psychiatry. 2018;75(4):336–46.

Hausner L, Damian M, Sartorius A, Frölich L. Efficacy and cognitive side effects of electroconvulsive therapy (ECT) in depressed elderly inpatients with coexisting mild cognitive impairment or dementia. J Clin Psychiatry. 2011;72(1):91–7.

Hegeman JM, Kok RM, van der Mast RC, Giltay EJ. Phenomenology of depression in older compared with younger adults: meta-analysis. Br J Psychiatry. 2012;200(4):275–81.

Hicks P, Sevilimedu V, Johnson GR, et al. Predictability of nonremitting depression after first 2 weeks of antidepressant treatment: AVAST-D trial. Report Psych Res Clin Pract. 2019;1:58–67.

Hoover DR, Siegel M, Lucas J, et al. Depression in the first year of stay for elderly long-term nursing home residents in the U.S.A. Int Psychogeriatr. 2010;22(7):1161–71.

Huang CQ, Dong BR, Lu ZC, et al. Chronic diseases and risk for depression in old age: a meta-analysis of published literature. Ageing Res Rev. 2010;9(2):131–41.

Husain-Krautter S, Ellison JM. Late life depression: the essentials and the essential distinctions. Focus. 2021;19(3):282–93.

Jeuring HW, Stek ML, Huisman M, et al. A six-year prospective study of the prognosis and predictors in patients with late-life depression. Am J Geriatr Psychiatry. 2018;26(9):985–97.

Katila H, Mezhebovsky I, Mulroy A, et al. Randomized, double-blind study of the efficacy and tolerability of extended-release quetiapine fumarate (quetiapine XR) monotherapy in elderly patients with major depressive disorder. Am J Geriatr Psychiatry. 2013;21(8):769–84.

Kato M, Hori H, Inoue T, et al. Discontinuation of antidepressants after remission with antidepressant medication in major depressive disorder: a systematic review and meta-analysis. Mol Psychiatry. 2021;26(1):118–33.

Kessler RC, Berglund P, Demler O, et al. Lifetime prevalence and age-of-onset distributions of DSM-IV disorders in the National Comorbidity Survey Replication. Arch Gen Psychiatry. 2005;62(6):593–602.

Kiosses DN, Szanto K, Alexopoulos GS. Suicide in older adults: the role of emotions and cognition. Curr Psychiatry Rep. 2014;16(11):495. https://doi.org/10.1007/s11920-014-0495-3. PMID: 25226883; PMCID: PMC4225125.

Kinrys G, Gold AK, Pisano VD, et al. Tachyphylaxis in major depressive disorder: a review of the current state of research. J Affect Disord. 2019;15(245):488–97.

Knöchel C, Alves G, Friedrichs B, et al. Treatment-resistant late-life depression: challenges and perspectives. Curr Neuropharmacol. 2015;13(5):577–91. https://doi.org/10.2174/1570159x1305151013200032.

Kok RM, Reynolds CF. Management of depression in older adults: a review. JAMA. 2017;317(20):2114–22.

Koo YW, Kõlves K, De Leo D. Suicide in older adults: a comparison with middle-aged adults using the Queensland Suicide Register. Int Psychogeriatr. 2017;29(3):419–30.

Lamers F, Vogelzangs N, Merikangas KR, et al. Evidence for a differential role of HPA-axis function, inflammation and metabolic syndrome in melancholic versus atypical depression. Mol Psychiatry. 2013;18(6):692–9.

Lavretsky H, Reinlieb M, St Cyr N, et al. Citalopram, methylphenidate or their combination in geriatric depression: a randomized, double-blind, placebo-controlled trial. Am J Psychiatry. 2015;172(6):561–9.

Lieverse R, Van Someren EJ, Nielen MM, et al. Bright light treatment in elderly patients with nonseasonal major depressive disorder: a randomized placebo-controlled trial. Arch Gen Psychiatry. 2011;68(1):61–70.

Luijendijk HJ, van den Berg JF, Dekker MJ, et al. Incidence and recurrence of late-life depression. Arch Gen Psychiatry. 2008;65(12):1394–401.

Maarsingh OR, Heymans MW, Verhaak PF, et al. Development and external validation of a prediction rule for an unfavorable course of late-life depression: a multicenter cohort study. J Affect Disord. 2018;235:105–13.

MacQueen GM, Frewy BN, Ismail Z, et al. Canadian Network for Mood and Anxiety Treatments (CANMAT) 2016 clinical guidelines for the management of adults with major depressive disorder: section 6. Special populations: youth, women, and the elderly. Can J Psychiatr. 2016;61:588–603.

Mather AS, Rodriguez C, Guthrie MF, et al. Effects of exercise on depressive symptoms in older adults with poorly responsive depressive disorder. Randomised controlled trial. Br J Psychiatry. 2002;180:411–5.

McDonald WM. Neuromodulation treatments for geriatric mood and cognitive disorders. Am J Geriatr Psychiatry. 2016;24(12):1130–41.

McIntyre RS, Filteau MJ, Martin L, et al. Treatment-resistant depression: definitions, review of the evidence, and algorithmic approach. J Affect Disord. 2014;156:1–7.

Meyer JP, Swetter SK, Kellner CH. Electroconvulsive therapy in geriatric psychiatry: a selective review. Clin Geriatr Med. 2020;36(2):265–79.

Mulsant BH, Blumberger DM, Ismail Z, et al. A systematic approach to pharmacotherapy for geriatric major depression. Clin Geriatr Med. 2014;30(3):517–34.

Murri MB, Ekkekakis P, Menchetti M, et al. Physical exercise for late-life depression: effects on symptom dimensions and time course. J Affective Disorders. 2018;230:65–70.

Nelson JC, Delucchi KL, Schneider LS. Moderators of outcome in late-life depression: a patient-level meta-analysis. Am J Psychiatry. 2013;170:651–9.

Nierenberg AA, Petersen TJ, Alpert JE. Prevention of relapse and recurrence in depression: the role of long-term pharmacotherapy and psychotherapy. J Clin Psychiatry. 2003;64(Suppl 15):13–7.

Paranthaman R, Greenstein A, Burns AS, et al. Relationship of endothelial function and atherosclerosis to treatment response in late-life depression. Int J Geriatr Psychiatry. 2012;27(9):967–73.

Perissinotto CM, Stijacic Cenzer I, Covinsky KE. Loneliness in older persons: a predictor of functional decline and death. Arch Intern Med. 2012;172:1078–83.

Pravodelov V. Thoughtful prescribing and deprescribing. Med Clin North Am. 2020;104:751–65.

Pruckner N, Holthoff-Detto V. Antidepressant pharmacotherapy in old-age depression—a review and clinical approach. Eur J Clin Pharmacol. 2017;73:661–7.
Raue PJ, Ghesquiere AR, Bruce ML. Suicide risk in primary care: identification and management in older adults. Curr Psychiatry Rep. 2014;16(9):466.
Riva-Posse P, Hermida AP, McDonald WM. The role of electroconvulsive and neuromodulation therapies in the treatment of geriatric depression. Psychiatr Clin North Am. 2013;36:607–30.
Rush A, Wisniewski S, Warden D, et al. Selecting among second-step antidepressant medication monotherapies: are clinical, demographic, or first-step treatment results informative? Arch Gen Psychiatry. 2008;65:870–80.
Segal ZV, Pearson JL, Thase ME. Challenges in preventing relapse in major depression. Report of a National Institute of Mental Health Workshop on state of the science of relapse prevention in major depression. J Affect Disord. 2003;77(2):97–108.
Soreide KK, Ward KM, Bostwick JR. Strategies and solutions for switching antidepressant medications. Psychiatr Times. 2017;34(12)
Souery D, Papakostas GI, Trivedi MH. Treatment-resistant depression. J Clin Psychiatry. 2006;67(Suppl 6):16–22.
Sözeri-Varma G. Depression in the elderly: clinical features and risk factors. Aging Dis. 2012;3(6):465–71.
Targum SD. Identification and treatment of antidepressant tachyphylaxis. Innov Clin Neurosci. 2014;3-4:24–8.
Tedeschini E, Levkovitz Y, Iovieno N, et al. Efficacy of antidepressants for late-life depression: a meta-analysis and meta-regression of placebo-controlled randomized trials. J Clin Psychiatry. 2011;72(12):1660–8.
Thomas EJ, Elliott R. Brain imaging correlates of cognitive impairment in depression. Front Hum Neurosci. 2009;3:30.
Thorlund K, Druyts E, Wu P, et al. Comparative efficacy and safety of selective serotonin reuptake inhibitors and serotonin-norepinephrine reuptake inhibitors in older adults: a network meta-analysis. J Am Geriatr Soc. 2015;63(5):1002–9.
Thornicroft G, Chatterji S, Evans-Lacko S, et al. Undertreatment of people with major depressive disorder in 21 countries. Br J Psychiatry. 2017;210(2):119–24.
Van Orden, et al. Issues in research on aging and suicide. Aging Ment Health. 2016;20(2):240–51.
Veltman EM, Lamers F, Comijs HC, et al. Depressive subtypes in an elderly cohort identified using latent class analysis. J Affect Disord. 2017;218:123–30.
Volkert J, Schulz H, Härter M, et al. The prevalence of mental disorders in older people in Western countries–a meta-analysis. Ageing Res Rev. 2013;12(1):339–53.
Weinberger AH, Gbedemah M, Martinez AM, et al. Trends in depression prevalence in the USA from 2005 to 2015: widening disparities in vulnerable groups. Psychol Med. 2018;48(8):1308–15.
Zhang Y, Chen Y, Ma L. Depression and cardiovascular disease in elderly: current understanding. J Clin Neurosci. 2018;47:1–5.
Zhao X, Ma J, Wu S, et al. Light therapy for older patients with non-seasonal depression: a systematic review and meta-analysis. J Affect Disord. 2018;232:291–9.

12 Bipolar and Related Disorders

Amanda Mihalik-Wenger, Uma Suryadevara, Justin Wenger, Meena Nuthi, Rita Hitching, and Howard H. Fenn

Abstract

Manic and hypomanic symptoms in late life are, more likely than not, recurrent episodes of bipolar disorder which began *early* in life. A manic or hypomanic episode which occurs for the *first time* in late life is often associated with, or due to, systemic medical comorbidity and can be considered *secondary* mania/hypomania. By similar reasoning, a patient with a pre-existing unipolar depressive disorder which first occurred *earlier* in life, and who subsequently develops a first manic episode in *late* life, may be re-diagnosed as bipolar I disorder. One study of a cohort with recurrent unipolar depressive disorders found that at least 1% per year converted to bipolar disorder with a manic episode over the course of their lifetimes, even beyond age 70 (Angst et al., J Affect Disord 84:149–57, 2005). A detailed history of mood episodes for the geriatric patient and a thorough medical evaluation is therefore essential.

This chapter provides an overview of the diagnosis and treatment of bipolar disorder and related disorders in late life. In the aging patient, mania or hypomania can emerge in the context of cognitive deficits, communication difficulties, systemic medical comorbidities, and medication effects, all of which can confound assessment and accurate diagnosis. Conditions which can present with mania or hypomania include behavioral and psychological symptoms of dementia (BPSD) and delirium with symptoms such as apathy, distractibility, labile mood, anxiety, and irritability (Cassel and Fulmer, JAMA 327:919–920, 2022). The search for causes of secondary manic or hypomanic symptoms which appear in late life can help minimize unnecessary or inappropriate treatment.

A. Mihalik-Wenger · J. Wenger · M. Nuthi
University of Florida, Gainesville, FL, USA
e-mail: amihalik@ufl.edu; jwenger1@ufl.edu; godiva86@ufl.edu

U. Suryadevara (✉)
University of Florida, Gainesville, FL, USA

Malcom Randall VA Medical Center, Gainesville, FL, USA

R. Hitching
University of Newcastle, Newcastle, NSW, Australia
e-mail: rita@hitching.net

H. H. Fenn
VA Health Care System, Palo Alto, CA, USA

Department of Psychiatry and Behavioral Sciences, Stanford University, Stanford, CA, USA
e-mail: hhfenn@aol.com, howard.fenn@va.gov

H. H. Fenn et al. (eds.), *Age-Adjusted Psychiatric Treatment for the Older Patient*,
https://doi.org/10.1007/978-3-031-53976-3_12

Case Example: Management of Bipolar Disorder I in a Geriatric Patient

A 71-year-old corporate CEO with a history of early-onset bipolar disorder (EOBD) presented to the emergency department (ED) following a fall, during which he briefly lost consciousness. He had no history of seizures, cardiovascular disease, or neurological disease. CBC (complete blood count) and lipid panel were WNL (within normal limit), but serum creatinine was elevated at 1.7 mEq/L, sodium was 139 mEq/L, eGFR (estimated glomerular filtration rate) was 45 mL/min/1.73m^2, BUN (blood urea nitrogen) was 25 mg/dL, and serum lithium was above therapeutic range at 2.1 mEq/L. CT (computed tomography) and MRI (magnetic resonance imaging) of brain were negative. Neurological examination revealed an unsteady gait and an intention tremor of both hands. The patient was distractible and disoriented, with a MoCA score of 24/30. He was admitted to internal medicine for one day of observation, where he remained irritable, dysphoric, and agitated. Confusion Assessment Method (CAM) was negative, and delirium was ruled out. After one day, he was transferred to inpatient psychiatry.

For the prior 2 years, the patient had been euthymic on lithium 900 mg BID with serum levels every 6 months, ranging 0.9–1.2 mEq/L, fluoxetine 60 mg per day, mirtazapine 15 mg at bedtime, pravastatin 40 mg daily, and lisinopril 20 mg per day. There were no episodes of orthostatic hypotension or syncope. A dose of 10 mg of amlodipine was added 6 months prior to the current admission to control hypertension.

His first manic episode occurred at age 23 when he was hospitalized for 2 weeks and stabilized on lithium 900 mg BID. Fluoxetine 60 mg daily was added when he developed depressive symptoms. He tolerated this regimen and depressive symptoms resolved.

The patient went on to earn an MBA, followed by a successful career, which was not interrupted by either depressive or manic symptoms for 30 years. The lithium 900 mg BID provided stable serum levels which ranged between 1.2 and 1.5 mEq/L. At age 50, his primary care physician noted the onset of hypertension and started lisinopril 20 mg.

At age 53, he developed a major depressive episode; a 21-item Hamilton Rating Scale for Depression (HRSD) scored at 29. He had morbid thoughts, self-blame for financial decisions, lethargy, and suicidal ideation. Marital discord followed an affair he had had with a co-worker. He was hospitalized for 3 weeks, during which fluoxetine was considered ineffective and was discontinued. Over the next 6 weeks, his depressive episode improved on a dose of lamotrigine 150 mg daily and lithium 900 mg BID. He was symptom-free and without adverse effects except for slight intention tremor. He returned to full-time work.

At age 65, he developed dysphoria, morbid thoughts, irritability, and social isolation over the course of 6 months. He had trouble initiating sleep but also said he did not need much sleep. He had excessive energy and inflexible thinking, and his judgment became dominated by unrealistic optimism at work. He became less interested in monthly fly-fishing trips or golf, and he refused to see friends or participate in family events. He was quarrelsome in board meetings, and he argued vociferously for an acquisition which was based upon unsubstantiated assumptions. He was asked to take time off for 6 months, after which he was terminated.

After termination, he said he was "worthless" and felt dead. He stopped taking all medications, followed by a suicide attempt by hanging. He was hospitalized with a diagnosis of bipolar I disorder, mixed episode, marked by irritable mood, grandiosity, impaired judgment, morbid thoughts, self-blame, and suicidality.

His lithium 900 mg BID and lamotrigine 150 mg daily were restarted, and aripiprazole 5 mg daily was added for depression but was withdrawn after he developed a parkinsonian gait and a resting tremor. After 2 weeks, he denied suicidality; he was discharged on lithium 900 mg BID and lamotrigine 150 mg daily. Over the next 3 months, his mood stabilized, but his gait was unsteady, and he fell three times. The third fall prompted the most recent ED visit. In the ED, his impairment in renal function was attributed to aging and the adverse effect of lithium. The symptoms of lithium toxicity and high serum lithium of 2.1 mEq/L were attributed in part to retention of lithium due to lisinopril. He was admitted to a psychiatric inpatient unit where lithium was discontinued and lisinopril decreased to 10 mg daily. Blood pressure was monitored daily and did not exceed 135/85 mmHg. He was observed without any mood stabilizer for one week to assess any cognitive effects due to his head injury. His MoCA returned to 27/30.

After five days on the inpatient unit, he became hyperactive, irritable, and distractible and had increased energy. Valproate-delayed release 500 mg at bedtime was started, which reached a serum level of 45 mcg/mL within 5 days. Racing thoughts and distractibility diminished, but he continued to have insomnia and irritability. Mirtazapine was discontinued and quetiapine 300 mg at bedtime was added. Within one more week, he was sleeping better, and the remaining manic symptoms improved. He no longer endorsed suicidal impulses.

At discharge, his medication regimen was lamotrigine at 150 mg/day, valproate delayed release 500 mg at bedtime daily, quetiapine 300 mg at bedtime, amlodipine 20 mg, lisinopril 10 mg daily, and pravastatin 40 mg daily. Over the next 10 years, his serum valproate levels ranged between 45 and 55 mcg/mL. Serum creatinine ranged between 1.3 and 1.5 mEq/L and eGFR stabilized at 55 mL/min/1.73m^2. Tremor and gait improved, and he remained free of any mood episode.

Discussion: This patient with early-onset bipolar disorder had an episode of recurrent mixed episode in late life. His renal function had declined due to aging and adverse effects of lithium, both of which, in combination with lisinopril, contributed to retention of lithium, toxicity, imbalance, and falls. A modest dose of valproate (VPA delayed release) in place of lithium reached therapeutic range and manic symptoms resolved. The adjunctive quetiapine improved sleep. Irritability diminished because of restful sleep. Lamotrigine prevented recurrent depressive symptoms. VPA stabilized his mood without further decline in renal function (Young et al. 2017).

Epidemiology

In the general population, BPD (borderline personality disorder) prevalence has been found as high 1% (Merikangas et al. 2011; Vieta et al. 2018). A systematic literature review of 1519 psychiatric inpatients ages 60–96 found the prevalence of early-onset bipolar disorder (EOBD) to be 6.0% and late-onset bipolar disorder (LOBD) to be 1.8% (Dols et al. 2014). Another survey of a nationally representative sample in the USA, ages 65 and older, reported a one-year prevalence of bipolar I disorder at approximately 0.4% and the lifetime rate is 0.8% (Blanco et al. 2017). The same survey found the prevalence of bipolar I disorder in *non-aging* adults as lower among Blacks, Hispanics, and Asians/Pacific Islanders than Whites but higher among Native Americans (Blanco et al. 2017).

Phenomenology

The definition of *late onset* differs, as ages 50, 55, 60, and 65 have all be used as cutoffs. Nevertheless, symptoms of bipolar disorder in late life, whether early-onset bipolar disorder (EOBD) or late-onset bipolar disorder (LOBD), have both been observed as *milder* in severity compared to symptoms in the younger population. An analysis of baseline, cross-sectional data from 19 international studies of bipolar patients ($N = 1377$), of which 72% had bipolar I disorder, with a mean sample age of 60.8 years (standard deviation [SD] 12.2 years), reported both manic and depressive symptom severities lower among older individuals ($p < 0.0001$). Greater depressive symptom severity was strongly associated with worse functioning (Sajatovic et al. 2022).

Phenomenology of Early-Onset Bipolar Disorder (EOBD)

Early history should be explored for episodes of mania, hypomania, anxious distress, mixed features, rapid cycling, or psychotic features.

Phenomenology of Late-Onset Bipolar Disorder (LOBD)

LOBD patients have shown a higher incidence of co-occurring cognitive deficits, more often with mixed features, less hypersexuality, and no relevant family history of bipolar disorder, compared to patients with an *early-onset* pattern (Chen et al. 2017). Systemic medical comorbidity is also more prevalent in the aged, with a median of seven systemic medical illness per elderly bipolar disorder patient (Brown 2001).

Manic symptoms of bipolar disorder in late life are similar to mood-related symptoms seen in MNCD (major neurocognitive disorder) of Alzheimer's disease (BPSD) which are more likely accompanied by the following:

- Rapid decline in cognitive functioning, mood fluctuation, changes in energy, and sleep
- Focal neurological findings, such as aphasia apraxia or impaired visuospatial functioning
- Night-time agitation and confusion
- A negative family history of BPD

Studies that directly compare older and younger adults with BPD show that the clinical presentation and the density of affective episodes are remarkably similar between the EOBD and LOBD, across the lifespan (Depp and Jeste 2004). Bipolar I disorder and bipolar II disorder may be less distinct from each other in the older patient (Leboyer et al. 2005). The intervals between mood episodes also become shorter and episodes may occur more frequently in older patients. Whether or not these differences are related to inter-interval pharmacologic treatment is unclear, but in later life, the episodes may meld into one another, presenting with mixed features.

Assessment and Differential Diagnosis

For a DSM-5-TR diagnosis, bipolar I disorder at least one manic episode is required. Other criteria include the following:

(a) A distinct period of abnormally and persistently elevated, expansive, or irritable mood, for at least one week.
(b) Three or four among seven symptoms of mania.
(c) Marked impairment of social or occupational functioning.
(d) The manic episode is not attributable to physiological effect of a substance or another medical condition. If the episode can be determined to be the direct pathophysiological consequence of another medical condition, it is diagnosed as *bipolar and related disorder due to another medical condition. Major depressive episode* of bipolar disorder is addressed in Chap. 11.

Manic or hypomanic symptoms which first manifest in late life are often *secondary* to other conditions such as delirium, medication effects, substance abuse or excessive alcohol use, multiple sclerosis, neurodegenerative disorders, temporal lobe epilepsy, HIV infection, major neurocognitive disorders, and traumatic brain injury (Wijeratne and Malhi 2007). Comorbid systemic medical conditions in the aging individual can also exacerbate symptoms of an early-onset BPD, for example, migraine headache, asthma, cancer, diabetes mellitus, hypertension, thyroid disease, cerebrovascular disease, or cardiac disease (Forty et al. 2014). Therefore, symptoms suggestive of manic, hypomanic, depressive, or mixed episodes in life deserve a complete medical, neurological, laboratory evaluation for causative factors.

The Comprehensive Evaluation for Bipolar Disorder in Table 12.1 lists the work-up to rule out conditions which may contribute to, exacerbate, or mimic bipolar disorder symptoms; substance abuse, medication effects, neurocognitive disorders, delirium, and other systemic medical illnesses (e.g., hypothyroidism) may exacerbate or precipitate a mood episode (Dols et al. 2014; Prabhakar and Balon 2010).

If manic or hypomanic episodes are found to be direct physiologic effects of a general medical condition, the diagnosis in DSM-5-TR is *bipolar and related disorder due to another*

Table 12.1 Early-onset (EOBD) vs. late-onset bipolar disorder (LOBD)

Features	Early-onset bipolar disorder (EOBD)	Late-onset bipolar disorder (LOBD)
Age of onset in years	Ages approximately 20–30	Different definitions of late-onset include over age 50, 55, 60, or 65
Prevalence	1–2% of general population	10% of aged bipolar patients are late onset, but this varies by definition of late onset
Family history of bipolar or a depressive disorder	History of BPD in first-degree relatives	No relevant family history
Common comorbid conditions	Substance use and anxiety disorders	Neurological conditions, including cerebrovascular disease
Presentation of symptoms	Duration of manic episodes may be longer than in LOBD	Hypersexuality and euphoria less common Mixture of manic, dysphoric, cognitive symptoms
Psychosis	Paranoid delusions	Not prevalent
Prognosis	Excellent response to appropriate treatment	Variable response to treatment; Burden of residual subsyndromal or hypomanic symptoms is higher than in EOBD
Cognitive deficits	Deficits in social cognition	Deficits in executive functioning, verbal memory, and processing speed, seen in around 30% of patients
Course of illness	Long intervals between acute episodes	Higher burden of residual symptoms More frequent mood episodes
Neuroimaging findings	Not contributory	Subcortical white matter hyperintensities

Sources. Besga et al. (2015); Chen et al. (2017); Depp and Jeste (2004); Dols et al. (2014); Goldstein et al. (2006); (Sajatovic et al. 2015)

medical condition. The World Health Organization's International Classification of Diseases—10th Revision (ICD-10)—for mood episodes secondary to general medical conditions uses the term *organic bipolar affective disorder*. Specifiers of a bipolar disorder diagnosis follow (Table 12.2).

Substance/Medication-Induced Bipolar and Related Disorders

Lifetime prevalence rates of comorbid substance misuse have been reported at 36.5% of patients with BPD substances, and medications can contribute to a recurrent episode of EOBD or LOBD. EOBD in late life can be associated with increased frequency of suicide attempts, depressive and mixed episodes, rapid cycling, and poor treatment compliance, and greater number of hospitalizations in old age can result (Carrà et al. 2014). For further discussion, see Chap. 7.

Neurocognitive Disorders and Neurodegenerative Disorders

Secondary mania should be suspected in aging patients who present with manic symptoms and neurological or cognitive deficits. Conditions to be ruled out include encephalitis, meningitis, HIV encephalopathy (HAND), tertiary syphilis, major or mild neurocognitive disorder, neurodegenerative disorders, brain tumors, traumatic brain injury, thyrotoxicosis, Cushing's disease, vitamin B12 deficiency, and niacin deficiency (Chen et al. 2017).

Behavioral and psychological symptoms of dementia (BPSD) can present with intense mood symptoms which are difficult to distinguish from bipolar manic or hypomanic episodes. This is especially true for dementias such as behavioral variant frontotemporal dementia (bvFTD) and Alzheimer's disease (Besga et al. 2015). Frontotemporal dementias, Huntington's disease, and basal ganglia calcification are often associated with change in social behavior, personality

Table 12.2 Comprehensive assessment of bipolar disorder in late life

Comprehensive assessment of bipolar disorder in late life	
Assessment and diagnostic	• Severity, onset, duration of presenting symptoms, prior manic, hypomanic, depressive, or mixed symptoms/episodes • Premorbid level of functioning and social support
Screening and rating scales	• Mania rating scale: Manic syndrome subscale score—Total of five items—Elevated mood, less need for sleep, excessive energy, and excessive activity, and grandiosity; possible scores: 0–25. The behavior and ideation subscale score—Five items –instability, motor hyperactivity, accelerated speech, racing thoughts, and poor judgment • Young Mania Rating Scale: 11-item clinician-administered instrument assesses the severity of mania. Items: elevated mood, increased motor activity/energy, sexual interest, sleep, irritability, speech, language/thought disorder, content, disruptive/aggressive behavior, appearance, and insight
Suicidal intent	• Geriatric Depression Scale Suicide Subscale (GDS-SI) • Patient Health Questionnaire-9 (PHQ-9) (for use in primary care settings) • Suicide risk assessment including access to firearms • Self-destructive, reckless behaviors, and suicide attempts
Psychiatric history	• Hospitalizations and emergency department visits • Medication doses, duration, adverse effects, and response • Manic, hypomanic, depressive, or mixed episodes
Substance use history	• Alcohol, illegal substances, and nonprescribed (OTC)/prescribed medications • Short Michigan Alcoholism Screening Test—Geriatric Version (SMAST-G) • Alcohol Use Disorders Identification Test (AUDIT) • CAGE-AID
Screening for delirium and neurocognitive disorder	• MoCA, MMSE, Mini-Cog, and SLUMS • Confusion assessment method (CAM) for delirium
Medication review	• Use of, or withdrawal from, psychotropics, antidepressants, antipsychotics, opioids, barbiturates, benzodiazepines, OTC substances, and stimulants • Medications which contribute to manic/hypomanic symptoms
Laboratory and relevant studies	Systemic medical/laboratory work-up, for example, • Thyroid function tests • B12 and folate levels • Complete blood count and differential • Metabolic panel, including serum creatinine and eGFR* • Liver-associated enzymes • Lipid panel • Urine drug screen and urinalysis • EKG • CT/MRI to rule out stroke, trauma, or neurodegenerative disease • Serum levels of lithium, valproic acid, and carbamazepine

traits, or aphasia. Patients with Huntington's disease, an inherited and untreatable progressive neurodegenerative disorder, display choreiform movements, psychiatric/behavioral symptoms, and dementia. One encouraging study of 38 patients using EEG and MRI in combination *was* able to delineate between LOBD and bvFTD with 87% accuracy (Metin et al. 2018). Although mania has been associated with strokes in the right orbital frontal lobe, temporal lobe, basal ganglia, or thalamus (Santos et al. 2011), a systematic review found that only 49 cases of manic or hypomanic episodes secondary to stroke were identified in the literature through 2010 (Saraiva et al. 2021). For further discussion, see Chap. 5.

Focal Brain Lesions, Tumors, Infection, Concussion, and Traumatic Brain Injury

Brain lesions and other insults can give rise to intense mood symptoms which can be considered episodes of secondary mania or hypomania.

Headache, seizures, nausea, focal neurologic symptoms, and manic or hypomanic episodes may indicate cerebral pathology such as brain tumor (Satzer and Bond 2016). An elderly patient with a traumatic brain injury after an unwitnessed fall may present with confusion, amnesia, and manic or hypomanic symptoms, even without full loss of consciousness.

Imaging, neurocognitive testing, neurological examination, and laboratory studies may be necessary to diagnose the underlying brain pathology. If neuroimaging is unremarkable, history and other investigations are essential to uncover the etiologies. Infections, including human immunodeficiency virus (HIV), and COVID-19 have been linked to manic symptoms. Delirious mania has been reported, and although these case reports are from the younger population, this risk also applies to aging individuals (Uvais and Moideen 2022). For further discussion, refer to Chap. 4.

Vascular mania. A causative relationship between cerebrovascular disease, mania, and depressive episodes has been proposed, based upon evidence of symptoms with late-age onset, associated vascular risk factors, and typical neuroimaging changes. To date, research has not confirmed biological markers for vascular mania, although neuroimaging holds promise Table 12.3.

Treatment

Non-pharmacological

Non-pharmacological and behavioral interventions for MDD of late-life bipolar disorder do not differ significantly from those for late-life depressive disorder. Refer to Chaps. 11 and 15.

Pharmacological

Antiepileptics, mood stabilizers, lithium, and/or second-generation antipsychotics (SGA), adjusted for age and frailty, can be as effective for mania and hypomania in geriatric patients as in younger patients. Given the paucity of RCTs of treatment for mania and hypomanic in late life, there is a need to rely on studies of younger subjects, with doses and combinations adjusted to aging pharmacokinetics, pharmacodynamics, individual frailty, and tolerance.

First-line medications. Lithium, valproate, carbamazepine, and lamotrigine and second-generation antipsychotics (SGAs) quetiapine and olanzapine are *first-line* treatments for bipolar disorder in both younger and older adults (Brooks et al. 2010). Lithium, valproate, carbamazepine, olanzapine, and quetiapine have demonstrated

Table 12.3 Categories of bipolar disorder in late life

Disorders	Onset (years)	Prevalence in older adults	Distinctive features	Risk factors
Early-onset bipolar disorder (EOBD)	20–29	1%	Reoccurring symptoms seen more commonly; duration of mania is typically longer	Family history, comorbid substance abuse and anxiety, and increased rates of suicide
Late-onset bipolar disorder (LOBD)	50–65	5% of aged bipolar patients have onset after age 60	Greater heterogeneity in presentation and course in older adults; cognitive impairment is common	Neurological illness and other medical comorbidities
LOBD manic episode	>55	4.6–18.5% of all geriatric admissions	Evaluation should start with an attempt to rule out secondary causes for manic episodes	Comorbid neurological disorder
EOBD with psychotic features	18–20	64% of patients with bipolar disorder have psychotic symptoms	Paranoid delusions are seen more commonly in older age than younger adults with bipolar disorders. Hallucinations less common, typically AH	Family history of bipolar disorder is less common in late-onset (>50) than early-onset (<50) bipolar disorders

efficacy for mania (Brooks et al. 2010; Young et al. 2017). Some authors recommend starting with a mood stabilizer and augmenting with SGAs if manic or hypomanic symptoms are not fully controlled. One population-based study of adults aged 66 and older with BPD reported 75.3% of patients were prescribed SGAs and 38.5% were prescribed antidepressants, 35.4% valproate, and 23.4% lithium (Rej et al. 2017).

Stepwise Pharmacological Treatment

Step 1: Stabilization of acute mania, hypomania, and mixed mood states. Approximately 50–80% of older adults with mania will respond to a first-line medication treatment (Young et al. 2004). The choice of a specific drug for acute mania or hypomania can be guided by past response to medications, current renal function and clearance, psychotic symptoms (e.g., grandiose delusions), side effect profiles, comorbid general medical conditions, potential for drug-drug interactions, and patient preference. Certain SGAs would not be first choice for a diabetic patient due to risk of hyperglycemia (Rej et al. 2017). Some authors recommend SGAs as *second line* if manic or hypomanic symptoms are not fully controlled or if mood-congruent or non-mood-congruent psychotic symptoms are present. FGAs, risperidone, and ziprasidone are contraindicated if there are parkinsonian symptoms. Other mood stabilizers are discussed below. Dosing principles are the following:

- Intervals between dose changes are guided by balancing the time needed to achieve steady state against the risk of adverse effects. The duration of intervals depends upon the pharmacokinetics of the agent in the particular patient.
- Dose adjustments and medication additions or discontinuations are best done one at a time, with at least 24–48 h between changes and primary effects (Fountoulakis and Vieta 2008). Assay serum levels and adjust doses to target the therapeutic serum level.

Step 1A. If psychotic features are present: If patients with mood-congruent or mood-incongruent psychotic features do not improve after Step 1 consider the addition of an SGA.

Step 2. If stabilization of acute symptoms is *not* achieved or if there is an inadequate response, switch from lithium to valproate (VPA) or from VPA to lithium

-or-

Step 3. If response is inadequate, add a second mood stabilizer (lithium, VPA, or carbamazepine) or add a SGA such as the following:

- Olanzapine starting 2.5 mg once daily at bedtime up to 15 mg as tolerated
- Quetiapine or quetiapine XR at starting dose of 12.5 mg once daily at bedtime, up to 250 mg as tolerated
- Risperidone starting at 0.5–1 mg once daily or in two divided doses, up to 4 mg daily once daily or in two divided doses
- Ziprasidone at starting dose of 20 mg once daily or 40 mg per day in two divided doses with a target dose 80–120 mg per day, in two divided doses
- Aripiprazole starting at 2.5–5 mg once daily with a target dose 5–15 mg once daily
- Asenapine starting dose 5 mg once or twice daily with target dose 10 mg twice daily (Sajatovic et al. 2020)

SGA adverse effects include orthostatic hypotension, sedation, weight gain, hyperglycemia, diabetes mellitus, hyperlipidemia, agranulocytosis, seizures, elevated prolactin, and sudden cardiac death (Schatzberg and Roose 2006; Kok and Reynolds 2017; Beyer and Johnson 2018).

Step 4A: Refractory mania or hypomania: *If stabilization not achieved* and assaultive/agitated/harmful behavior cannot be otherwise controlled, consider haloperidol, a first-generation antipsychotic (FGA), in age-adjusted doses, for example, 0.5–1 mg every 4 h as needed (PRN). Increase doses until improvement in symptoms, balanced against adverse effects, such as extrapyramidal symptoms.

Step 4B. If mania, hypomania, or mixed features are refractory to the above interventions, consider ECT. For further discussion, see Chap. 14.

-or-

Step 4C. Refractory mania or hypomania: refer to section on clozapine below.

Step 5. Maintenance treatment. After an acute mood episode has resolved, lithium, valproate, olanzapine, and quetiapine can be used for maintenance treatment. Regular monthly monitoring of antiepileptic serum levels is recommended, especially in frail and oldest-old patients.

Step 6. Treatment for specifiers of bipolar disorder. There are few treatment studies of bipolar disorder specifiers in late life. We rely upon RCTs of younger patients with mania with psychotic features, anxious distress, rapid cycling, or mixed features (which requires at least three of six symptoms which are consistent with depressive episode but must not be attributable to physiological effects of a substance, medication, or drug of abuse).

Specific Medications

Lithium. Lithium is a *first-line* treatment for acute mania and long-term maintenance in a geriatric patient if there is normal renal function (De Fazio et al. 2017). Aging adults with BPD have been found to have fewer depressive symptoms and greater improvement on lithium, with less frequent use of benzodiazepines, than patients *not* taking lithium (Morlet et al. 2019). Specific considerations are the following:

- Lithium is a first choice if there is adequate renal clearance and lithium serum level is monitored regularly. Start at 75 mg once or twice daily or 150 mg once daily to target a steady-state serum level 0.4–0.0.8 mEq/L. It is not recommended for a frail patient with renal insufficiency.
- Lower doses of lithium should be prescribed to geriatric patients, rarely more than 900 mg/day for adults ages 65–75 and seldom more than 450 mg/day in patients aged >80 years (Sproule et al. 2000). An expert consensus panel has recommended optimal lithium serum concentrations of 0.4–0.8 mmol/L for ages 60–79 years and 0.4–0.7 for ages >80 years, based on tolerability (De Fazio et al. 2017; Volkmann et al. 2020).
- The half-life of lithium increases from about 28–36 h as people age, so the dose of lithium needed to reach steady state is lower. Lithium can be started at 150 mg once or twice daily, monitored by a 12-h serum trough-level concentration taken 5–7 days after each dose and adjusted or increased every 1–5 days as tolerated, with serum levels targeted as follows (Shulman et al. 2019):
  - Patients 60–79 years—0.4–0.8 mEq/L (0.4–0.8 mmol/L)
  - Patients 80 years and older—0.4–0.7 mEq/L (0.4–0.7 mmol/L)

For patients with impaired renal clearance, frequent serum lithium-level monitoring is recommended, sometimes as often as weekly. Lithium, even at apparently therapeutic doses, can increase the risk of delirium, ataxia, tremor, renal insufficiency, hyperparathyroidism, and hypothyroidism. If the estimated glomerular filtration rate (eGFR) is below 30 mL/min/1.73m^2, lithium is not recommended (Fotso Soh et al. 2019; Lieber et al. 2020).

Monitoring of lithium treatment includes metabolic panel and thyroid function every 6 months, an annual complete blood count (CBC), and an annual cognitive exam (Shulman et al. 2019), as well as avoiding drugs that increase lithium levels such as NSAIDs, diuretics, and ACE inhibitors. Lithium may need to be held for at least 48–72 h before scheduled surgeries or ECT.

Valproate. Valproate/valproic acid/divalproex (VPA) appears to prevent and/or ameliorate mood *elevation* more than improvement of depressive symptoms. One randomized double-blind controlled trial of VPA compared the efficacy of lithium carbonate and divalproex in subjects over 60. Results indicated similar efficacy and tolerability of lithium and valproate, with greater reduction of symptoms of mania at 9 weeks using lithium (Young et al. 2017).

VPA Caveats

- Valproic acid ER formulation, a first-line medication, starting at 125–250 mg/day with a steady-state target serum level of 65–90 mcg/mL. Valproate should be avoided if there is hepatic or pancreatic disease.

VPA can cause delirium, hyperammonemia, liver toxicity, thrombocytopenia, and pancreatitis. It interacts with other medications:

- Aspirin can displace VPA from protein binding sites resulting in an increase in free VPA concentrations.
- VPA increases the unbound fraction of warfarin.
- VPA decreases clearance of amitriptyline and nortriptyline.
- VPA and lamotrigine (LTG) combined can double plasma LTG concentration due to inhibition of enzymes which metabolize LTG and is not recommended.

VPA Dosing Recommendations

- Assess complete blood count (CBC) pretreatment and during dose escalation or when VPA is used in combination with medications that influence platelet production.
- Assess baseline platelet count prior to treatment and thereafter as clinically indicated or every 6 months to identify thrombocytopenia.
- Encourage food prior to each dose.
- Prescribe enteric-coated formulations, which smooths absorption and minimizes gastric discomfort.
- Monitor unbound VPA concentrations if there are unexplained adverse effects, if clinical response is not adequate for the dose, or if the patient has reduced blood levels of albumin.
- Assess baseline cognitive function testing; repeat testing if cognitive changes emerge.
- Examine for rigidity, cogwheeling, tremor, and gait disturbance prior to and during VPA therapy. Begin VPA at 125 mg to 500 mg/day in divided doses; increase in increments 125–250 mg per day. In the frailest, old-old, consider a starting dose of 50 mg liquid elixir, within the range 10–20 mg/kg/24 h.
- Target serum levels (divalproex: 50–100 mcg/mL in patients with acute mania)
- Monitor ammonia (NH_3) levels especially if there is altered level of consciousness or symptoms of delirium.
- Monitor for adverse effects weekly or for increased levels of concomitant medications, especially warfarin, aspirin, phenobarbital, or phenytoin (Fenn et al. 2006).

Carbamazepine (CBZ). CBZ received FDA approval in 2004 for the treatment of acute manic and mixed episodes of BPD. CBZ may benefit aged patients with BPD who also have chronic pain and syndromes such as lumbar stenosis, trigeminal neuralgia, or any other neuropathic or radicular pain syndrome (Brooks et al. 2010). Carbamazepine can be started at 100 mg twice daily with a steady-state target serum level of 4–8 mcg/mL. CBZ is not often prescribed to older patients with BPD because of the following:

- CBZ side effects include severe headaches, mouth sores, fainting, irregular heartbeat, joint pain, rash, vision changes or nystagmus, liver and kidney problems, confusion, aplastic anemia, and hyponatremia due to SIADH.
- CBZ induces CYP 3A3/4 and conjugation, along with CYP isoforms not yet characterized.
- CBZ *decreases* serum concentrations of CBZ itself (autoinduction) and other medications (hetero-induction). It can undermine the effectiveness of several classes of medications.
- Anticonvulsants phenytoin, phenobarbital, primidone, and felbamate *decrease* serum CBZ concentrations.
- Medications that inhibit CYP 3A3/4 like erythromycin, diltiazem, ketoconazole, ritonavir, verapamil, grapefruit juice, itraconazole, and clarithromycin can cause *increased* serum CBZ concentrations, resulting in CBZ toxicity.

- Therapeutic range of serum levels is narrow (4–12 mcg/mL).

Lamotrigine (LTG). LTG was FDA-approved for the maintenance treatment of BPD in 2003 and stabilizes mood by ameliorating or preventing depressive symptoms (Fenn et al. 2006). In contrast to VPA and CBZ, LTG prevents recurrent depressive episodes more than it moderates or prevents recurrent mania in BPD. It is not associated with many drug-drug interactions that are common in geriatric patients taking multiple medications (Faught et al. 2018). Caution: pooled data from 13 clinical trials of LTG monotherapy (77% of the doses were between 50 and 100 mg/day) in epilepsy patients aged >65 years found an incidence of 49% drug-related adverse events over median exposure of 24 weeks (Giorgi et al. 2001).

Second-generation antipsychotic medications (SGAs). The effectiveness of SGAs in aging adults with bipolar disorder has not been studied extensively, and little evidence exists for their use in older adults in the depressed phase of bipolar disorder (Sajatovic et al. 2022). FDA-approved SGAs for treatment of mania include olanzapine, risperidone, quetiapine, quetiapine XR, ziprasidone, aripiprazole, and asenapine. Medications and combinations approved for acute bipolar depression (major depressive episodes in bipolar disorder) include quetiapine, quetiapine XR, olanzapine-fluoxetine combination, and lurasidone. For the maintenance phase, approved medications include olanzapine, quetiapine, quetiapine XR, aripiprazole, ziprasidone, and risperidone. (For further discussion see Chaps. 2, 3, and 10.)

Clozapine. Administration of clozapine is a reasonable choice for refractory mania, with slow titration upward, starting with 12.5 mg daily. The geriatric patient is particularly vulnerable to clozapine adverse effects:

- Severe neutropenia: Prior to initiating treatment, a baseline ANC must be at least 1500/mm^3 along with regular ANC monitoring. Severe neutropenia or infection can be identified by fever, weakness, lethargy, and sore throat. In the USA, a Risk Evaluation Mitigation Strategy (REMS) called the Clozapine REMS Program in the USA is required for prescribing.
- Orthostatic hypotension, bradycardia, syncope, myocarditis, cardiomyopathy, and cardiac arrest: During titration and dose escalation, these risks are highest even with the first dose of 12.5 mg/day; titration upward should be slow.
- Seizures: A dose-related risk is high if there is a history of seizures or risk factors for seizures and any episodes of loss of consciousness.
- Anticholinergic effects: Delirium, decreased peristalsis, fecal impaction, and urinary retention.
- Sedation: Reduced energy, impaired level of arousal, and delirium

Treatment of Major Depressive Episode of Bipolar Disorder

Steps for the treatment unipolar MDD in Chap. 11 apply also to MDD of bipolar disorder, with the following additions:

- The combination of olanzapine with fluoxetine was approved by the US FDA for treatment of bipolar depression. In comparison with lamotrigine, olanzapine-fluoxetine combination demonstrated statistically significantly greater improvement in depressive and manic symptoms but with a higher incidence of treatment-emergent adverse events, such as weight gain and elevation in metabolic factors (Citrome 2011), which require caution in aging patients.
- Escitalopram can be started at 10 mg per day, increased up to 20 mg per day. Venlafaxine can be started at 37.5 mg and gradually increased to 225 mg per day. The dose and side effects of olanzapine are discussed in Chap. 2.
- Lamotrigine has demonstrated effectiveness for maintenance treatment of bipolar disorder,

with a greater benefit in preventing recurrence of major depressive disorder (MDD) episodes than manic or hypomanic episodes. Caution is warranted in the aged patient because exposure to the drug is increased by 55% and renal clearance reduced by 37%. In addition, its serum level is affected in the presence of valproate or carbamazepine. For further discussion, see Chap. 3.

- ECT is an effective treatment modality for major depressive episodes of bipolar disorder. Efficacy rate has been demonstrated at the lower end over 60% (Meyer et al. 2020), and higher improvement rates have been reported. Cognitive side effects are transient even in patients with pre-existing cognitive deficits (Meyer et al. 2020). ECT is usually safe and well tolerated in patients with systemic medical comorbidities. For further discussion, see Chap. 14.

Conclusions

Pharmacotherapy using age-adjusted mood stabilizers and/or SGAs, combined with treatment of comorbid medical conditions and management of contributing factors, can successfully treat the geriatric patient with mania or hypomania. Ruling out causes of *secondary* mania can minimize the risk of unnecessary interventions. Psychotherapeutic strategies encourage insight and judgment which foster adherence to acute and maintenance treatment of bipolar disorder but cannot alone resolve an acute manic or hypomanic episode.

Evidence has been growing to support the inclusion of *late-life bipolar disorder* in a future iteration of DSM (Goldstein and Levitt 2006). Studies also show an association between mania and vascular disease in life late and may support another specifier for bipolar disorder. These diagnostic additions will hopefully spark more research into symptomatology of mania, hypomania, and bipolar disorders in the elderly (Wijeratne and Malhi 2007).

Age-Adjusted Recommendations

- When manic, hypomanic, or mixed episodes appear in the aging patient, search for and if possible rule out:
  - Evidence of pre-existing bipolar disorder earlier in life.
  - Causative factors of *secondary mania*, including systemic medical comorbidities, medication effects, substance use, delirium, neurocognitive disorder, or neurodegenerative disorder.
- Rule out abuse or misuse of medications, substances, or over-the-counter formulations.
- Explore age of onset, duration, prior treatments, and outcomes of manic/hypomanic/major depressive episodes.
- Review medication regimens and adjust or deprescribe medications which adversely affect psychiatric symptoms (e.g., corticosteroids, stimulants, hypnotics, beta-blockers, benzodiazepines, opioids, anticholinergics).
- Consider a neurological work-up for manic or hypomanic symptoms in late life, especially if accompanied by new neurological signs or symptoms.
- Prescribe pharmacotherapy as a *first-line* intervention for geriatric patients with acute mania, hypomania, or mixed features.

References

Angst J, Sellaro R, Stassen HH, Gamma A. Diagnostic conversion from depression to bipolar disorders: results of a long-term prospective study of hospital admissions. J Affect Disord. 2005;84(2–3):149–57.

Besga A, Gonzalez I, Echeburua E, et al. Discrimination between Alzheimer's disease and late onset bipolar disorder using multivariate analysis. Front Aging Neurosci. 2015;7:231.

Beyer JL, Johnson KG. Advances in pharmacotherapy of late-life depression. Curr Psychiatry Rep. 2018;20:34.

Blanco C, Compton WM, Saha TD, et al. Epidemiology of DSM-5 bipolar I disorder: results from the National Epidemiologic Survey on alcohol and related conditions—III. J Psychiatr Res. 2017;84:310.

Brooks JO, Sommer BR, Ketter TA. Management of bipolar disorders in older adults. In: Ketter TA, editor. Handbook of diagnosis and treatment of bipolar disorders. 2010. pp. 453–497.

Brown SL. Variations in utilization and cost of inpatient psychiatric services among adults in Maryland. Psychiatr Serv. 2001;52(6):841–3.

Carrà G, Bartoli F, Crocamo C, et al. Attempted suicide in people with co-occurring bipolar and substance use disorders: systematic review and meta-analysis. J Affect Disord. 2014;167:125–35.

Cassel C, Fulmer T. Achieving diagnostic excellence for older patients. JAMA. 2022;327(10):919–20.

Chen P, Dols A, Rej S, Sajatovic M. Update on the epidemiology, diagnosis, and treatment of mania in older-age bipolar disorder. Curr Psychiatry Rep. 2017;19(8):46.

Citrome L. Olanzapine–fluoxetine combination for the treatment of bipolar depression. Expert Opin Pharmacother. 2011;12(17):2751–8.

De Fazio P, Gaetano R, Caroleo M, et al. Lithium in late-life mania: a systematic review. Neuropsychiatr Dis Treat. 2017;13:755–66.

Depp CA, Jeste DV. Bipolar disorder in older adults: a critical review. Bipolar Disord. 2004;6(5):343–67.

Dols A, Kupka RW, van Lammeren A, et al. The prevalence of late-life mania: a review. Bipolar Disord. 2014;16(2):113–8.

Faught E, Szaflarski JP, Richman J, et al. Risk of pharmacokinetic interactions between antiepileptic and other drugs in older persons and factors associated with risk. Epilepsia. 2018;59(3):715–23.

Fenn HH, Sommer BR, Ketter TA, Alldredge B. Safety and tolerability of mood-stabilising anticonvulsants in the elderly. Expert Opin Drug Saf. 2006;5(3):401–16.

Forty L, Ulanova A, Jones L, et al. Comorbid medical illness in bipolar disorder. Br J Psychiatry. 2014;205(6):465–72.

Fotso Soh J, Klil-Drori S, Rej S. Using lithium in older age bipolar disorder: special considerations. Drugs Aging. 2019;36(2):147–54.

Fountoulakis KN, Vieta E. Treatment of bipolar disorder: a systematic review of available data and clinical perspectives. Int J Neuropsychopharmacol. 2008;11(7):999–1029.

Giorgi L, Gomez G, O'Neill F, et al. The tolerability of lamotrigine in elderly patients with epilepsy. Drugs Aging. 2001;18(8):621–30.

Goldstein BI, Levitt AJ. Further evidence for a developmental subtype of bipolar disorder defined by age at onset: results from the national epidemiologic survey on alcohol and related conditions. Am J Psychiatry. 2006;163(9):1633–6.

Goldstein BI, Herrmann N, Shulman KI. Comorbidity in bipolar disorder among the elderly: results from an epidemiological community sample. Am J Psychiatry. 2006;163(2):319–21.

Kok RM, Reynolds CF. Management of depression in older adults: a review. JAMA. 2017;317(20):2114–22.

Leboyer M, Henry C, Paillere-Martinot ML, Bellivier F. Age at onset in bipolar affective disorders: a review. Bipolar Disord. 2005;7(2):111–8.

Lieber I, Ott M, Öhlund L, et al. Lithium-associated hypothyroidism and potential for reversibility after lithium discontinuation: findings from the LiSIE retrospective cohort study. J Psychopharmacol. 2020;34(3):293–303.

Merikangas KR, Jin R, He JP, et al. Prevalence and correlates of bipolar spectrum disorder in the world mental health survey initiative. Arch Gen Psychiatry. 2011;68(3):241–51.

Metin SZ, Erguzel TT, Ertan G, et al. The use of quantitative EEG for differentiating frontotemporal dementia from late-onset bipolar disorder. Clin EEG Neurosci. 2018;49(3):171–6.

Meyer JP, Swetter SK, Kellner CH. Electroconvulsive therapy in geriatric psychiatry: a selective review. Clin Geriatr Med. 2020;36(2):265–79.

Morlet E, Costemale-Lacoste JF, Poulet E, et al.; CSA Study Group. Psychiatric and physical outcomes of long-term use of lithium in older adults with bipolar disorder and major depressive disorder: a cross-sectional multicenter study. J Affect Disord. 2019;259:210–217.

Prabhakar D, Balon R. Late-onset bipolar disorder: a case for careful appraisal. Psychiatry (Edgmont). 2010;7(1):34.

Rej S, Herrmann N, Shulman K, et al. Current psychotropic medication prescribing patterns in late-life bipolar disorder. Int J Geriatr Psychiatry. 2017;32(12):1459–65.

Sajatovic M, Chen P, Schmader KE. Geriatric bipolar disorder: general principles of treatment. UpToDate. 2020.

Sajatovic M, Dols A, Rej S, et al. Bipolar symptoms, somatic burden, and functioning in older-age bipolar disorder: analyses from the Global Aging and Geriatric Experiments in Bipolar Disorder Database project. Bipolar Disord. 2022;24(2):195–206.

Sajatovic M, Strejilevich SA, Gildengers AG, Dols A, Al Jurdi RK, Forester BP, Kessing LV, Beyer J, Manes F, Rej S, Rosa AR, Schouws SN, Tsai SY, Young RC, Shulman KI. A report on older-age bipolar disorder from the International Society for Bipolar Disorders Task Force. Bipolar Disord. 2015;17(7):689–704. https://doi.org/10.1111/bdi.12331. Epub 2015 Sep 19. PMID: 26384588; PMCID: PMC4623878.

Santos CO, Caeiro L, Ferro JM, Figueira ML. Mania and stroke: a systematic review. Cerebrovasc Dis. 2011;32:11–21.

Saraiva R, Proença F, Gonçalves M, et al. Poststroke bipolar disorder. J Nerv Ment Dis. 2021;209(11):851–4.

Satzer D, Bond DJ. Mania secondary to focal brain lesions: implications for understanding the functional neuroanatomy of bipolar disorder. Bipolar Disord. 2016;18(3):205–20.

Schatzberg A, Roose S. A double-blind, placebo-controlled study of venlafaxine and fluoxetine in geriatric outpatients with major depression. Am J Geriatr Psychiatry. 2006;14(4):361–70. https://doi.org/10.1097/01.JGP.0000194645.70869.3b.

Shulman KI, Almeida OP, Herrmann N, et al. Delphi survey of maintenance lithium treatment in older adults with bipolar disorder: SBD task force report. Bipolar Disord. 2019;21(2):117–23.

Sproule BA, Hardy BG, Shulman KI. Differential pharmacokinetics of lithium in elderly patients. Drugs Aging. 2000;16(3):165–77. https://doi.org/10.2165/00002512-200016030-00002.

Uvais NA, Moideen S. COVID-19 presenting with delirious mania: a case report. Bipolar Disord. 2022;24(3):332–3.

Volkmann C, Bschor T, Köhler S. Lithium treatment over the lifespan in bipolar disorders. Front Psychiatry. 2020;11:377.

Wijeratne C, Malhi GS. Vascular mania: an old concept in danger of sclerosing? A clinical overview. Acta Psychiatr Scand Suppl. 2007;(434):35–40.

Young RC, Gyulai L, Mulsant BH, et al. Pharmacotherapy of bipolar disorder in old age: review and recommendations. Am J Geriatr Psychiatry. 2004;12(4):342–57.

Young RC, Mulsant BH, Sajatovic M, et al.; GERI-BD Study Group. GERI-BD: a randomized double-blind controlled trial of lithium and divalproex in the treatment of mania in older patients with bipolar disorder. Am J Psychiatry. 2017;174(11):1086–1093.

13 Trauma- and Stressor-Related Disorders

Uma Suryadevara, Dawn Bruijnzeel, Justin Wenger, Rita Hitching, and Howard H. Fenn

Abstract

Aging adults experience many stressful events, and psychiatric symptoms associated with these events can exert a significant impact (Murayama et al., Geriatr Gerontol Int 20:297–303, 2020). Loss of loved ones, changes in living situation, impaired mobility, surgery, loss of employment, financial demands, acute medical conditions, and various physical disabilities are common. Psychological and social reserves in the geriatric patient may afford resilience and facilitate successful adaptation (Whitson et al., J Gerontol A Biol Sci Med Sci 71:489–495, 2016).

A thorough history from both the patient and reliable observers who know the patient's baseline can also aid in the early identification of stressors and maladaptive responses. The syndrome of post-traumatic stress disorder (PTSD) although often categorized under anxiety disorders is included here because it is the result of significant stressors which may have occurred earlier in life and may be overlooked in the aging adult (see Fig. 13.1).

Symptoms of adjustment disorder, acute stress disorder, posttraumatic stress disorder (PTSD), persistent complex bereavement, and/or bereavement may be overlooked by the busy clinician who must focus on the current medical symptomatology. This chapter provides an overview of stress-related syndromes in the geriatric patient to encourage early recognition and prompt *age-adjusted* interventions (see Table 13.1).

U. Suryadevara (✉) · D. Bruijnzeel
University of Florida College of Medicine, Gainesville, FL, USA

North Florida South Georgia VA Medical Center, Gainesville, FL, USA

J. Wenger
Seattle VA Medical center, Seattle, WA, USA

University of Florida College of Medicine, Gainesville, FL, USA

R. Hitching
University of Newcastle, Newcastle, NSW, Australia

H. H. Fenn
VA Health Care System, Palo Alto, CA, USA

Department of Psychiatry and Behavioral Sciences, Stanford University, Stanford, CA, USA
e-mail: hhfenn@aol.com, howard.fenn@va.gov

H. H. Fenn et al. (eds.), *Age-Adjusted Psychiatric Treatment for the Older Patient*,
https://doi.org/10.1007/978-3-031-53976-3_13

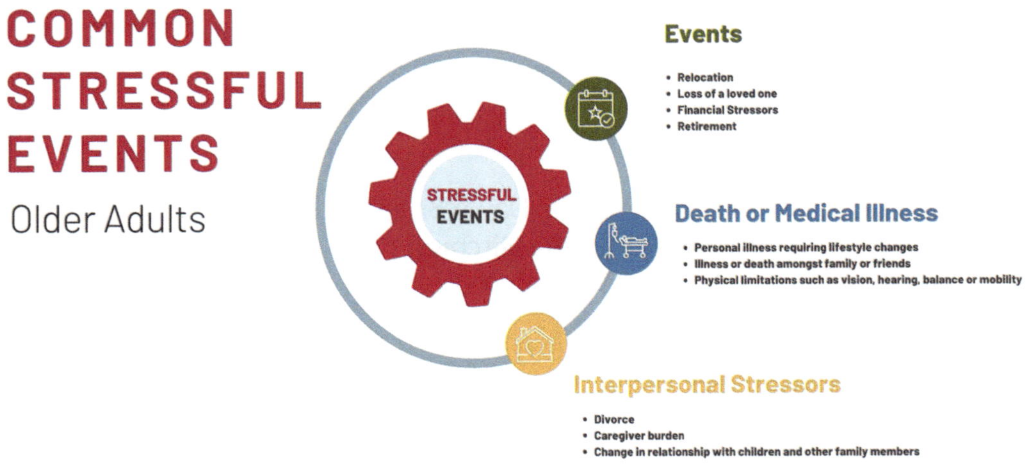

(Rita Hitching, MSc)

Fig. 13.1 Common stressful events in older adults (Rita Hitching, MSc)

Table 13.1 DSM-5 Diagnosis of trauma and stressor-related disorders

	Persistent complex bereavement disorder[a]	Adjustment disorder	Acute stress disorder	Posttraumatic stress disorder

Event or Stressor	Loss of a loved one	• Identifiable stressor(s) or consequences of stressor(s)
		• Major life event
		• Loss(es) which do not fulfill criteria for bereavement
			• Acute stress disorder: Symptom onset typically immediately after traumatic event
			• PSTD: Onset of some symptoms may be delayed 6 months after traumatic event
			• Criterion A event:
			  • Exposure to threatened death, serious injury, or sexual violation event(s) can have occurred at any time in past:
			    – Threat to life
			    – Combat trauma
			    – Sexual violence or rape
			    – Physical assault	

Table 13.1 (continued)

	Persistent complex bereavement disorder[a]	Adjustment disorder	Acute stress disorder	Posttraumatic stress disorder
DSM-5 criteria	• Severe or persistent grief and mourning • Rumination on deceased • Reluctance to accept loss • Worry about deceased • Shocked or numb • Anger • Reduced trust of others • Vivid recall of deceased • Avoidance of memory triggers	• Disproportionate stress response • Does not meet criteria for another disorder • Does not exacerbate pre-existing disorder • Symptoms do not represent normal bereavement • Onset of symptoms within 3 months of onset of stressor (s)	Acute stress disorder: Exposure to traumatic event • Witnessing or learning about threat of life/danger to others • Repeated exposure to traumatic events • Intrusions, negative mood, dissociation, avoidance, and arousal • Precursor to PTSD	PTSD: Exposure to traumatic event • Exposure to actual or threatened death, serious injury, and sexual violence • Shocked or numb • Presence of intrusion symptoms • Persistent avoidance of stimuli • Negative alterations in cognition and mood • Marked alterations in arousal and reactivity associated with traumatic event • Specify: With or without dissociative symptoms
Onset/ duration	Onset <3 months after stressor and continuing >12 months after	• Onset of symptoms within 3 months after stressor and resolving <6 months • Once stressor(s) or its consequences have terminated, symptoms do not persist for >6 months	Symptoms last >3 days but <1 month after the traumatic event	Symptoms last >1 month after the traumatic event
Severity	Any severity or level		Any severity or type of Criterion A	
Degree of impairment	Mild to severe		Severe and debilitating	

[a] DSM-5 diagnosis of major depressive disorder is possible in the context of bereavement even if the major depressive episode emerged as a result of, or concurrent with, the loss. These two diagnoses are not mutually exclusive

[b] In the absence of another primary diagnosis, other medical conditions or substance induced

Case Example: Maladaptive Adjustment to Proposed Open-Heart Surgery

A 74-year-old software engineer with a history of generalized anxiety disorder was not in any psychiatric treatment. He was followed with annual echocardiograms after a mechanical aortic valve replacement 5 years earlier. The patient was asymptomatic for congestive heart failure or other cardiac pathology, but 2+ mitral regurgitation (MR) was discovered on physical examination and echocardiography. The cardiologist recommended open-heart surgery for a mitral valve (MV) repair. The patient became overwhelmed with anxiety, ruminated about a *redo* sternotomy, and could not sleep throughout the night. He refused to consider surgery and insisted that he was asymptomatic, although he had progressive shortness of breath on minimal exercise. He would not discuss the issue with family or physicians.

Over the course of 6 months, the mitral regurgitation (MR) progressed to 4+ (severe), with a reduced left ventricular ejection fraction (LVEF) and significant increase in right ventricle systolic pressure (RVSP) (from 25.1 to 38.9 mmHg). Repeat echocardiogram demonstrated the left atrium was "severely dilated." Laboratory studies showed an increase in ntBNP to 628 pg/mL (normal range for age 0–229). The decline in cardiac function did not respond to treatment with olmesartan and carvedilol. He began to experience shortness of breath while walking and had frequent runs of extrasystolic contractions. These new symptoms precipitated even greater anxiety and he continued to refuse surgery.

His cardiologist requested a psychiatric consultation, which his wife, son daughter, and family members attended. An adjustment disorder with anxiety, in addition to GAD, was diagnosed. At the suggestion of the psychiatrist, the patient's wife and two adult children studied the literature of MR repair and open-heart surgery. The patient himself was too anxious to read about it. The psychiatrist offered suggestions to the family for discussing the risk-benefit ratio, while encouraging the patient to ventilate about worst case scenarios. Lorazepam 0.5 mg every 8 h as needed for anxiety was prescribed. Over the course of four weekly sessions of supportive psychotherapy and family discussions, the apprehension, rumination, and anxiety diminished, insomnia improved. The patient discussed the risks and benefits, and accepted a second open-heart surgery, which was successful. Lorazepam was discontinued over the course of 4 weeks postop.

Discussion: psychotherapeutic interventions ameliorated disabling anxiety symptoms of an adjustment disorder with anxiety (Table 13.1 and Fig. 13.1).

Adjustment Disorders

Prevalence

The prevalence of adjustment disorders in aging adults differs by setting. One study found a 1–2% prevalence in the general population (Zelviene and Kazlauskas 2018). Among a sample of aged individuals (65–96 years) assessed by standardized interviews or self-report questionnaires, a 2.3% prevalence of adjustment disorder was found (Maercker et al. 2008). Among aging adults who present to the emergency department for a psychiatric condition, the odds ratio of having an adjustment disorder was reported as 3.42 (Walsh et al. 2015).

Assessment

The diagnostic construct of an adjustment disorder prompts the clinician to search for and identify maladaptive responses to stressors (Strain 2020). DSM-5-TR criteria require that symptoms of an adjustment disorder begin *within 3 months of the stressor* and persist for no longer than an additional 6 months *after the termination of the stressor(s) or its consequences*. The symptoms must be either markedly out of proportion to the severity of the stressor and/or cause significant dysfunction in social, occupational, or other important areas of function. The *Adjustment Disorder New Module (ADNM)*, a self-report

Table 13.2 Symptoms of trauma and stressor-related disorders

Depression differential	Persistent complex bereavement disorder[a]	Adjustment disorder[a]	Acute stress disorder[a]	Posttraumatic stress disorder[a]
Overlapping features	• Extreme sadness • Anhedonia • Disrupted sleep and insomnia • Disengagement from world • Weight loss and poor appetite	• Low mood • Social withdrawal • Anxiety and worry • Agitation • Feel trapped • Cognitive impairment • Hopelessness • Sleep and appetite change • Lack of energy	• Anhedonia • Hopelessness • Low self-esteem • Anger • Emotional detachment • Agitation and anxiety • Changes to sleep and appetite • Social withdrawal and isolation • Blame self or others	• Anhedonia • Hopelessness • Low self-esteem • Anger • Cognitive impairment • Emotional detachment • Agitation and anxiety • Changes to sleep and appetite • Social withdrawal and isolation • Blame self or others
Distinguishing features	• Death-focused guilt • Yearning for loved one • Positive emotion associated with deceased • Emptiness • Waves and periods of grief • Self-esteem intact • No worthlessness or self-loathing • Maintain social connections • Sadness due to loss • Hopeful about future happiness • Absence of prior psychiatric history • Absence of weight gain or overeating • Humor • No excessive sleep	• Inability and preoccupation with change • Early suicidal ideation • Avoidance of routines • Impulsive or rebellious behavior • Palpitations • Prior psychiatric history uncommon	• Hypervigilance • Dissociation • Situational or stressor avoidance • Intrusive and negative thoughts • Avoidance behaviors • Fear of safety • Palpitations and panic attacks	• Hypervigilance • Dissociation • Situational or stressor avoidance • Intrusive and negative thoughts • Avoidance behaviors • Fear of safety • Palpitations and panic attacks

[a] All disorders can precipitate, trigger, co-occur, or exacerbate major depressive disorder

scale, which has not been validated for geriatric patients (Ben-Ezra et al. 2018), includes a list of stressors and the adjustment disorder symptom item list (see Table 13.2).

Non-pharmacological Treatment

An adjustment disorder diagnosis is not intended to "pathologize" normal human emotions or natural responses to adverse life events. The condition may be self-resolving and might not always warrant treatment. Some studies have supported the view that aging individuals may be *more resilient* to loss than younger patients and may adapt relatively well to stressors (Newson et al. 2011). However, it is also possible that adjustment disorders can last longer and remain unrecognized in the aging population because the functional and psychological *consequences* of stressors are prolonged. For example, reduced mobility, loss of a companion, isolation, and sensory and cognitive deficits may continue long after the initial stressful event resolves. Limited access to psychosocial support can also interfere with adaptive coping mechanisms.

Psychotherapy is a first-line intervention when symptoms of adjustment disorder are prolonged, severe, disruptive of social or occupational functioning, or dangerous to self/others (O'Connor 2012). Cognitive-behavioral therapy (CBT), psychodynamic psychotherapy, patient-centered psychotherapy, supportive psychotherapy, relaxation techniques like meditation, and progressive muscle relaxation can help. For further discussion, see Chap. 15.

Pharmacological Treatment

Although the term *adjustment disorder with depressed mood* may suggest less severe dysfunction than *major depressive disorder*, an adjustment disorder can be disabling, and its duration can continue beyond 6 months. If psychotherapeutic modalities have not mitigated the symptomatology, suicidality, or harmful behavior, then pharmacotherapy is indicated.

There are few randomized controlled trials (RCTs) of medications to for adjustment disorder in aging adults. Serotonin reuptake inhibitors (SSIs) and serotonin-norepinephrine reuptake inhibitors (SNRIs) are commonly prescribed for anxiety and/or depressive symptoms. Benzodiazepines or buspirone may be used for a time-limited duration of months but require assessment of the risks versus the benefits, especially for frail and oldest-old populations. (For further discussion, see Chap. 2)

Bereavement

Prevalence

The loss of spouse or partner and subsequent bereavement increase in prevalence with age. In the USA, for ages 85 and above, 73% of women and 34% of men are widowed. Between ages 75 and 84, 43% of women and 16% of men are widowed. From ages 65–74, 2% of women and 7% of men are widowed (Federal Interagency Forum on Aging-Related Statistics (NIFARS) 2016).

DSM-5-TR lists *persistent complex bereavement* as a specifier under "Other Specified Trauma and Stressor-Related Disorder," described as severe and persistent grief and mourning reactions. Such a course of bereavement can impair functioning beyond a culturally accepted norm of severity or duration and is marked by bereavement and psychiatric symptoms of intense yearning, painful memories, and inability to move on. Unique *culturally accepted* norms can be ascertained by consulting members who are familiar with the patient's particular culture. See discussion below.

A new DSM diagnosis, *Persistent Complex Bereavement Disorder*, has been proposed (Cozza et al. 2020). The ICD-11 has a construct, *Prolonged Grief Disorder* (Doering and Eisma 2016), which could serve as an example. The ICD-11 diagnosis requires only *6 months* of symptoms post-bereavement, and the DSM-5 provisional criteria require *one-year* symptom duration post-bereavement.

Bereavement after death of a loved one is easy to identify in the aged, but bereavement symptoms may be missed if the death of a loved one is anticipated but *has not yet happened*. A spouse, for example, may know that a partner's medical condition is terminal or that declining cognitive function diminishes any connection. Feelings of devastating loss may follow estrangement from children, terminal medical conditions, decline in capabilities, loss of attractiveness due to aging, and/or physical limitations.

Bereavement is associated with an increased risk of depressive symptoms, increased substance use, disturbed sleep, suicide attempts, and increased mortality (Prigerson and Jacobs 2001). The clinician who recognizes a patient with these maladaptive responses to loss can facilitate early referral of the patient and family to psychosocial supports and psychotherapeutic resources.

Assessment, Prevalence, and Treatment of Persistent Complex Bereavement

Inventory of complicated grief (ICG) is a validated, self-administered 19-point scale, developed to guide the clinical assessment. One study used the ICG to report a 4.8% prevalence of *complicated* grief in the general aging adult population; the 75- to 85-year-old age cohort experienced significantly more complicated grief than surrounding age groups (Newson et al. 2011). Variables associated with complicated bereavement include age and gender of the survivor, mode of death, presence of significant depressive symptoms after death, ability to accept loss, social support network, and previous close relationships. However, new complicated grief symptoms, like maladaptive self-appraisal and a patient's difficulty in positive reminiscing, are not assessed in the ICG.

Cultural Issues

Understanding culturally unique manifestations of bereavement can promote tailored interventions. Most cultures have rituals and beliefs that influence the way people grieve. These can vary depending on specific subgroup, geographic, ethnic, or religious backgrounds as well as individual past experiences. Normative bereavement behavior should be distinguished from behavior and reactions which are considered *outside* the range what is accepted within a specific cultural group (Clements et al. 2003). One study looked at cross-cultural similarities and differences between bereaved parents of Chinese and Swiss origins: the Chinese sample felt more like life was empty or meaningless, whereas Swiss parents went through more severe grief-related preoccupation (Xiu et al. 2016).

Treatment

Complicated grief therapy is the most studied psychotherapy for grief, followed by other therapeutic modalities like interpersonal psychotherapy (Wittouck et al. 2011). This modality helps the individual accept and cope with the loss while moving forward with life without the deceased. Its core themes include understanding and accepting loss, learning to manage painful emotions, working on a meaningful future with strong ongoing relationships, and living with the memories (Iglewicz et al. 2020). Receptiveness to psychotherapy may increase with age, since loss, such as the death of a loved or retirement, can lead to greater introspection and ability to review trauma (Ditlevsen and Elklit 2010). The goal for complicated grief therapy is to help the patient understand barriers to adaptation and integration of loss. Recognizing maladaptive ruminations like disbelief, self-blame, and protest while restoring the capacity to thrive is important in the treatment of prolonged grief disorder. Education of family members is also an important component. Antidepressants have shown to be beneficial and augment response to complicated grief therapy.

Acute Stress Disorder and Posttraumatic Stress Disorder (PTSD)

Prevalence

A *lifetime* prevalence of PTSD of 4.5% has been reported in older adults (Pietrzak et al. 2012). Between 2.8 and 4.5% aging adults meet full criteria for PTSD and up to 10% meet criteria for *subthreshold* PTSD, with comorbid depressive and anxiety disorders (Glaesmer et al. 2012). Up to 90% of adults aged 65 years and older have reported a traumatic or life-threatening event; men were significantly overrepresented (Kuwert et al. 2013). Unexpected death, serious illness, injury of a loved one, and sexual assault or intimate partner violence within the geriatric population are examples of traumatic events that are seen in full or partial PTSD syndromes (Pietrzak et al. 2012). A meta-analysis reported that older adults were 2.11 times more likely to experience PTSD symptoms and 1.73 times more likely to develop adjustment disorders when exposed to natural disasters, compared to younger adults (Siskind et al. 2016).

Compared to younger adults, the prevalence of PTSD in individuals 60 years and older has been reported to be significantly *lower*. However, large-scale studies have not included enough older adults to examine the effects of age on presentation, evaluations, and treatment (Reynolds et al. 2016; Cook and Simiola 2017). A previous year prevalence study from 2016 found PTSD significantly lower in older 65+ adults (2.6%), compared to young age 20–34 (4.3%) and middle age 35–64 (5.2%) (Reynolds et al. 2016). In aged male veteran populations, the lifetime incidence of PTSD was 8% with a *current* diagnosis prevalence 4.8% (Magruder et al. 2015). Regarding comorbid psychiatric conditions, aging adults with PTSD are more likely to meet criteria for generalized anxiety disorder and other anxiety disorders (Pietrzak et al. 2012).

Assessment of PTSD in the Aging Adult

The geriatric patient with PTSD may present with more sleep difficulties, more somatic complaints, or greater cognitive deficits than younger patients (Thorp et al. 2012). Geriatric individuals may not report experiences as "trauma" and are more likely to report somatic symptoms like gastrointestinal issues, sleep disturbance, or pain, rather than emotional problems. Of note, aging adults exposed to a serious illness or a traumatic event are three times more likely to endorse suicidal ideation (Beristianos et al. 2016). Symptoms of PTSD might persist for a lifetime or recur periodically, even though the traumatic event occurred when they were much younger (Chopra et al. 2014). Adverse events during childhood have been correlated in older adults with a higher chance of experiencing PTSD (Raposo et al. 2014).

In sum, acute stress disorder or PTSD in aging adults may be missed because of the following:

- Psychological distress and symptoms may be reported as *somatic* complaints.
- PTSD is associated with increased mortality and fewer aging adults with PTSD survive to late life.
- Many aging adults with trauma-related symptoms do not develop the full PTSD syndrome.
- The traumatic event(s) may have occurred many years earlier, its details not readily acknowledged, and the syndrome not adequately considered at its onset.
- Symptoms of anxiety, depressed mood, apprehension, isolation, and/or avoidance, which may accompany medical or other psychiatric conditions, can overlap with, or obscure, symptoms of acute stress disorder or PTSD (Owens et al. 2005).

The Clinician-Administered PTSD Scale (CAPS-5) is a 30-item questionnaire which corresponds to the DSM-5-TR diagnostic criteria (Weathers et al. 2018). *The PTSD Checklist (PCL)* is a self-report measure for PTSD which has been updated to reflect changes in DSM-5 (Bovin et al. 2016). The PCL has been noted to have high internal consistency, test-retest reliability, temporal validity, and convergent validity (Wilkins et al. 2011); lower cut-off scores for the PCL for older adults have been suggested (Cook et al. 2005).

Women

One study found that 7% of women aged 57–85 years reported a history of rape, a mean of 36 years since the trauma occurred (Sachs-Ericsson et al. 2014). Among female Vietnam-era veterans, 13.5% met current criteria, and 16.9% met lifetime criteria for PTSD (Cook et al. 2013). It has been reported that for women aged 65 years and over, 14% reported a lifetime history of sexual and physical assault. Women with a history of interpersonal violence were more likely to meet criteria for PTSD, depression, and anxiety in the past year and lifetime (Miles-McLean et al. 2021).

Systemic Medical Comorbidity and PTSD

Systemic medical comorbidities are prevalent in older adults with PTSD, including cardiovascular diseases, gastrointestinal ulcer disease, and diabetes mellitus type 2 (Pietrzak et al. 2011). Aging adults with a history of trauma have higher rates of cardiovascular disease, diabetes mellitus, and osteoarthritis (Glaesmer et al. 2012). Medical illness can also interfere with how a patient copes, such as cognitive deficits (Schuitevoerder et al. 2013) and physical limitations (Byers et al. 2014; Yaffe et al. 2010) which impair self-care. Stress from a traumatic event can also worsen the *perception* of pain and vice-versa in older adults (Alamdari and Laganà 2015).

Non-pharmacological Treatment of PTSD

Prolonged exposure (PE) therapy is recommended as one of the first-line treatments by clinical practice guidelines for PTSD (DOD guidelines is the Card 2018). Its core components include *imagined exposure*, designed to revisit the traumatic memory, and to talk about it. It can also include in vivo exposure, wherein the patient deals with triggers or situations that cause distress. With adaptation, PE has been noted as effective for aging adults with PTSD (Thorp et al. 2012).

Cognitive processing therapy (CPT) and eye movement desensitization reprocessing (EMDR). These evidence-based treatments for PTSD (Forbes et al. 2010) have been accompanied by a lower dropout rate in older adults compared to a younger population (Kehle-Forbes et al. 2016). Treatment modifications and adaptations to address comorbid conditions such as pain, chronic illness, and cognitive impairment may be needed (e.g., repetition of sessions for cognitively impaired patients or support from caregivers) (Kaiser et al. 2019).

Life-review and cognitive-behavioral therapy have been noted to benefit older cognitively intact individuals with PTSD (Böttche et al. 2012; Chan et al. 2011). Stress inoculation training (SIT), present-centered therapy (PCT) and interpersonal psychotherapy (IPT) have also been used for the treatment of PTSD in older adults. Acceptance and commitment therapy (ACT) or dialectical behavioral therapy (DBT) are not yet supported by sufficient evidence.

Digital technology and mobile health applications (apps) are usually based on cognitive behavioral therapy (CBT) principles and include psychoeducation, tracking depressive and anxiety symptoms, and cognitive restructuring, as well as relaxation exercises (Sander et al. 2020). For further discussion, see Chap. 16.

Pharmacological Treatment of PTSD

SSRIs such as sertraline, paroxetine, fluoxetine, or the SNRI venlafaxine are recommended first-line agents for adult patients (Ostacher and Cifu 2019), but there is limited RCT evidence for their use for PTSD in geriatric patients. The Veterans Administration and Department of Defense (DOD) VA/DoD Clinical Practice Guidelines for PTSD emphasize the avoidance of benzodiazepines for the treatment of PTSD (Raskind et al. 2018; Ostacher and Cifu 2019). For further discussion, see Chap. 2 (Table 13.3).

Table 13.3 Assessment/treatment of trauma and stressor-related disorders

	Persistent/complex bereavement disorder[a]	Adjustment disorder[a]	Acute stress disorder[a]	Posttraumatic stress disorder[a]
Prevalence	2–4%[b]	2–8%[c]	5–50%	1.5–4%[d]
Situations and locations	10–20% romantic partner or child[b]	• 7% of psychiatric units • 20% of acute medical care	• 13–21% of car accidents • 19% assault	• 2–17% military • 20–50% rape
Risk factors	• First-degree relationship • Loss of a child • Women >60 years • Unhappy marriage • Sudden loss • Inability say goodbye • Hospital death • Not prepared for death • Substance abuse • Prior depression	• Negative view of stress • Bereavement <6 months • Prolonged stressors • Recent unemployment • Unanticipated changes enforced transitioning • Financial strain • History of depression • Prior trauma or abuse	• Repeated stress exposure • Prior trauma or abuse • Acute medical disorder • Terminal illness	• Female • Prior trauma or abuse • Childhood adversity • Early or late-life trauma • Prior depression • History of substance abuse
Suicidality	Wish to join deceased	Less frequent	High prevalence	
Assessment**	• BGQ • ICG • AAG • GSIS	• DIAD • ADNM • PSQ-20 • GSIS	• GAD-7 • PHQ-9 • GSIS • P4	• CAPS • PCL • GSIS • P4
Treatments***	• First-line psychotherapy • CGT • Second-line SSRIs • Combination treatment	• First-line psychotherapy • BADI • CBT • SOLAR • IPT • PST • BGDT • Pharma limited evidence	• First-line psychotherapy • CISD • Narrative Therapy • Anxiolytic medication in extreme cases • Combination treatment	• First-line psychotherapy • PE • MBSR • EMDR • SIT • Second-line SSRIs • Combination treatment

Mini-mental state examination (MMSE)

• Brief Grief Questionnaire (BGQ) • Inventory of Complicated Grief (ICG) • Adult Attitude to Grief (AAG) • Clinician-Administered PTSD Scale (CAPS) • PTSD Checklist (PCL)	• Mini-Mental State Examination (MMSE) • Perceived Stress Questionnaire (PSQ) • Patient Health Questionnaire (PHQ-9) • Critical Incident Stress Debriefing (CISD) • P4 Suicide Risk Screener	• Generalized Anxiety Disorder (GAD7) • Diagnostic Interview for Adjustment Disorder (DIAD) • Adjustment Disorder New Module (ADNM) • Geriatric Suicide Ideation Scale (GSIS)

(continued)

Table 13.3 (continued)

	Persistent/complex bereavement disorder[a]	Adjustment disorder[a]	Acute stress disorder[a]	Posttraumatic stress disorder[a]
Treatment (adapt if cognitively impaired)***				
• Cognitive behavioral therapy (CBT) • Interpersonal therapy (IPT) • Problem-solving therapy (PST) • Brief goal-directed therapy (BGDT)	• Brief Adjustment Disorder Intervention (BADI) • Skills for Life Adjustment and Resilience (SOLAR) • Prolonged Exposure Therapy (PE) • Complicated Grief Treatment (CGQ)		• Mindfulness-Based Stress Reduction (MSR) • Eye Movement Desensitization Reprocessing (EMDR) • Stress Inoculation Training (SIT)	

[a] All disorders can precipitate, trigger, co-occur, or exacerbate major depressive disorder
[b] Federal Interagency Forum on Aging-Related Statistics (NIFARS) (2016)
[c] Sachs-Ericsson et al. (2014), Zelviene and Kazlauskas (2018), Maercker et al. (2008)
[d] Reynolds et al. (2016), Magruder et al. (2015), Pietrzak et al. (2012), Glaesmer et al. (2012)

Conclusions

Stress-associated psychiatric disorders among geriatric patients can be overlooked when symptoms are attributed primarily to aging. Systemic medical conditions, somatic complaints, cognitive deficits, reluctance to admit vulnerability, and communication barriers in the aging adult can also make it difficult to identify the impact of significant stressful factors. Exploration of the patient's history can help the clinician recognize stressors that are not fully acknowledged by the patient. This can facilitate *age-adjusted* effective interventions which can attenuate maladaptive coping or stress-related symptomatology.

Age-Adjusted Recommendations

- Determine a baseline level of functioning(s) to establish realistic goals of treatment.
- Probe for traumatic or stressful events, losses, or changes that impact quality of life.
- Do not underestimate the impact of stressful events even though patient may be reluctant to discuss them.
- After a loss, monitor for symptoms of bereavement or persistent complex bereavement.
- Recognize that symptoms of bereavement can begin *before* the death of a loved one.
- Determine cultural and ethnic attitudes and accepted behaviors in response to loss, bereavement, and other stressful events.
- Consider psychotherapeutic approaches tailored to the unique culture, beliefs, limitations, insight, and level of cooperation.
- Use age-adjusted psychopharmacology to avoid adverse effects.
- Elicit observations about the patient's coping style and behavior from family members, caregivers, and trusted others.

References

Alamdari G, Laganà L. The relationship of older adults' physical pain to depression and post-traumatic stress disorder (PTSD): a review. J Geriatr Med Gerontol. 2015;1(2):7.

Ben-Ezra M, Mahat-Shamir M, Lorenz L, et al. Screening of adjustment disorder: scale based on the ICD-11 and the adjustment disorder new module. J Psychiatr Res. 2018;103:91–6.

Beristianos MH, Maguen S, Neylan TC, Byers A. Trauma exposure and risk of suicidal ideation among older adults. Am J Geriatr Psychiatry. 2016;24(8):639–43.

Böttche M, Kuwert P, Knaevelsrud C. Posttraumatic stress disorder in older adults: an overview of characteristics and treatment approaches. Int J Geriatr Psychiatry. 2012;27(3):230–9.

Bovin MJ, Marx BP, Weathers FW, et al. Psychometric properties of the PTSD checklist for diagnostic and statistical manual of mental disorders-fifth edition (PCL-5) in veterans. Psychol Assess. 2016;28(11):1379–91.

Byers AL, Covinsky KE, Neylan TC, Yaffe K. Chronicity of posttraumatic stress disorder and risk of disability in older persons. JAMA Psychiatry. 2014;71(5):540–6.

Chan D, Fan MY, Unützer J. Long-term effectiveness of collaborative depression care in older primary care patients with and without PTSD symptoms. Int J Geriatr Psychiatry. 2011;26(7):758–64.

Chopra MP, Zhang H, Kaiser AP, et al. PTSD is a chronic, fluctuating disorder affecting the mental quality of life in older adults. Am J Geriatr Psychiatry. 2014;22(1):86–97.

Clements PT, Vigil GJ, Manno MS, et al. Cultural perspectives of death, grief, and bereavement. J Psychosoc Nurs Ment Health Serv. 2003;41(7):18–26.

Cook JM, Simiola V. Trauma and PTSD in older adults: prevalence, course, concomitants, and clinical considerations. Curr Opin Psychol. 2017;14:1–4.

Cook JM, Elhai JD, Areán PA. Psychometric properties of the PTSD checklist with older primary care patients. J Trauma Stress. 2005;18(4):371–6.

Cook JM, Pilver C, Dinnen S, et al. Prevalence of physical and sexual assault and mental health disorders in older women: findings from a nationally representative sample. Am J Geriatr Psychiatry. 2013;21(9):877–86.

Cozza SJ, Shear MK, Reynolds CF, et al. Optimizing the clinical utility of four proposed criteria for a persistent and impairing grief disorder by emphasizing core, rather than associated symptoms. Psychol Med. 2020;50(3):438–45.

Ditlevsen DN, Elklit A. The combined effect of gender and age on post-traumatic stress disorder: do men and women show differences in the lifespan distribution of the disorder? Ann Gen Psychiatry. 2010;9(1):1–12.

Doering BK, Eisma MC. Treatment for complicated grief: state of the science and ways forward. Curr Opin Psychiatry. 2016;29(5):286–91.

Federal Interagency Forum on Aging-Related Statistics (NIFARS). Older Americans 2016: key indicators of well-being. Federal Interagency Forum on aging-related statistics. Washington: U.S. Government Printing Office. 2016.

Forbes D, Creamer M, Bisson JI, et al. A guide to guidelines for the treatment of PTSD and related conditions. J Trauma Stress. 2010;23(5):537–52.

Glaesmer H, Kaiser M, Bräehler E, et al. Posttraumatic stress disorder and its comorbidity with depression and somatisation in the elderly—a German community-based study. Aging Ment Health. 2012;16(4):403–12.

Iglewicz A, Shear MK, Reynolds CF 3rd, et al. Complicated grief therapy for clinicians: an evidence-based protocol for mental health practice. Depress Anxiety. 2020;37(1):90–8.

Kaiser AP, Cook JM, Glick DM, Moye J. Posttraumatic stress disorder in older adults: a conceptual review. Clin Gerontol. 2019;42(4):359–76.

Kehle-Forbes SM, Meis LA, Spoont MR, Polusny MA. Treatment initiation and dropout from prolonged exposure and cognitive processing therapy in a VA outpatient clinic. Psychol Trauma. 2016;8(1):107.

Kuwert P, Pietrzak RH, Glaesmer H. Trauma and posttraumatic stress disorder in older adults. Can Med Assoc J. 2013;185(8):685.

Maercker A, Forstmeier S, Enzler A, et al. Adjustment disorders, posttraumatic stress disorder, and depressive disorders in old age: findings from a community survey. Compr Psychiatry. 2008;49:113–20.

Magruder K, Yeager D, Goldberg J, et al. Diagnostic performance of the PTSD checklist and the Vietnam Era Twin Registry PTSD scale. Epidemiol Psychiatr Sci. 2015;24(5):415–22.

Miles-McLean HA, LaMotte AD, Williams MR. Trauma exposure and PTSD among women receiving treatment for intimate partner violence perpetration. J Interpers Violence. 2021;36(13–14):6803–26.

Newson RS, Boelen PA, Hek K, et al. The prevalence and characteristics of complicated grief in older adults. J Affect Disord. 2011;132(1–2):231–8.

O'Connor H. Cartwright: adjustment disorder. In: Sturmey P, Hersen M, editors. Handbook of evidence-based practice in clinical psychology. Hoboken: Wiley; 2012. p. 493–506.

Ostacher MJ, Cifu AS. Management of posttraumatic stress disorder. JAMA. 2019;321(2):200–1.

Owens GP, Baker DG, Kasckow J, et al. Review of assessment and treatment of PTSD among elderly American armed forces veterans. Int J Geriatr Psychiatry. 2005;20(12):1118–30.

Pietrzak RH, Goldstein RB, Southwick SM, Grant BF. Medical comorbidity of full and partial posttraumatic stress disorder in United States adults: results from wave 2 of the National Epidemiologic Survey on alcohol and related conditions. Psychosom Med. 2011;73(8):697.

Pietrzak RH, Goldstein RB, Southwick SM, Grant BF. Psychiatric comorbidity of full and partial posttraumatic stress disorder among older adults in the United States: results from wave 2 of the National Epidemiologic Survey on alcohol and related conditions. Am J Geriatr Psychiatry. 2012;20(5):380–90.

Prigerson HG, Jacobs SC. Caring for bereaved patients: all the doctors just suddenly go. JAMA. 2001;286(11):1369–76.

Raposo SM, Mackenzie CS, Henriksen CA, Afifi TO. Time does not heal all wounds: older adults who experienced childhood adversities have higher odds of mood, anxiety, and personality disorders. Am J Geriatr Psychiatry. 2014;22(11):1241–50.

Raskind MA, Peskind ER, Chow B, et al. Trial of prazosin for post-traumatic stress disorder in military veterans. N Engl J Med. 2018;378(6):507–17.

Reynolds K, Pietrzak RH, Mackenzie CS, et al. Posttraumatic stress disorder across the adult lifespan: findings from a nationally representative survey. Am J Geriatr Psychiatry. 2016;24(1):81–93.

Sachs-Ericsson N, Kendall-Tackett KA, Sheffler J, et al. The influence of prior rape on the psychological and physical health functioning of older adults. Aging Ment Health. 2014;18(6):717–30.

Sander LB, Schorndanner J, Terhorst Y, et al. 'Help for trauma from the app stores?' a systematic review and standardised rating of apps for post-traumatic stress disorder (PTSD). Eur J Psychotraumatol. 2020;11(1):1701788.

Schuitevoerder S, Rosen JW, Twamley EW, et al. A meta-analysis of cognitive functioning in older adults with PTSD. J Anxiety Disord. 2013;27(6):550–8.

Siskind DJ, Sawyer E, Lee I, et al. The mental health of older persons after human-induced disasters: a systematic review and meta-analysis of epidemiological data. Am J Geriatr Psychiatry. 2016;24(5):379–88.

Strain JJ. The adjustment disorder diagnosis, its importance to liaison psychiatry, and its psychobiology. Int J Environ Res Public Health. 2020;16(23):4645.

Thorp SR, Stein MB, Jeste DV, et al. Prolonged exposure therapy for older veterans with posttraumatic stress disorder: a pilot study. Am J Geriatr Psychiatry. 2012;20(3):276–80.

VA/DOD Clinical Practice Guideline for the Management of Posttraumatic Stress Disorder and Acute Stress Disorder: Clinician Summary. Focus (Am Psychiatr Publ). 2018;16(4):430–448. https://doi.org/10.1176/appi.focus.16408. Epub 2018 Oct 18. PMID: 32021581; PMCID: PMC6996084.

Walsh PG, Currier GW, Shah MN, Friedman B. Older adults with mental disorders: what factors distinguish those who present to emergency departments for mental health reasons from those who do not? Am J Geriatr Psychiatry. 2015;23(11):1162–71.

Weathers FW, Bovin MJ, Lee DJ, et al. The clinician-administered PTSD scale for DSM-5 (CAPS-5): development and initial psychometric evaluation in military veterans. Psychol Assess. 2018;30(3):383–95.

Wilkins KC, Lang AJ, Norman SB. Synthesis of the psychometric properties of the PTSD checklist (PCL) military, civilian, and specific versions. Depress Anxiety. 2011;28(7):596–606.

Wittouck C, Van Autreve S, De Jaegere E, et al. The prevention and treatment of complicated grief: a meta-analysis. Clin Psychol Rev. 2011;31(1):69–78.

Xiu D, Maercker A, Woynar S, et al. Features of prolonged grief symptoms in Chinese and Swiss bereaved parents. J Nerv Ment Dis. 2016;204(9):693–701.

Yaffe K, Vittinghoff E, Lindquist K, et al. Posttraumatic stress disorder and risk of dementia among US veterans. Arch Gen Psychiatry. 2010;67(6):608–13.

Zelviene P, Kazlauskas E. Adjustment disorder: current perspectives. Neuropsychiatr Dis Treat. 2018;14:375–81.

Part IV

Therapeutics and Interventions

14 Neuromodulation Therapies

Amer M. Burhan, Daphne Goveas, Sama Thiab, and Mervin Blair

Abstract

Noninvasive brain stimulation (NiBS) techniques or therapeutic brain stimulation and modulation modalities (TBSM) have the potential to become first-line treatment options for depressive disorders and other common psychiatric conditions in geriatric patients. This chapter discusses their advantages and how these are consistent with an *age-adjusted* approach. NiBS and TBSM can minimize polypharmacy in treatment-resistant geriatric patients, provide an alternative for patients who cannot tolerate medications, or offer treatment to those who do not engage in psychotherapies. The non-pharmacological therapies discussed here include transcranial magnetic stimulation (rTMS), electroconvulsive therapy (ECT), magnetic seizure therapy (MST), and transcranial direct current stimulation (tDCS). The psychotomimetics ketamine and esketamine therapies are also reviewed.

The original version of the chapter has been revised. A correction to this chapter can be found at https://doi.org/10.1007/978-3-031-53976-3_19

A. M. Burhan (✉)
Psychiatry at University of Toronto, Ontario Shores Centre for Mental Health Sciences, Whitby, ON, Canada
e-mail: burhana@ontarioshores.ca

D. Goveas · S. Thiab
Lawson Health Research Institute/Parkwood Institute, London, ON, Canada

M. Blair
Ontario Shores Centre for Mental Health Sciences, Whitby, ON, Canada

Lawson Health Research Institute/Parkwood Institute, London, ON, Canada

Case Example: ECT for Bipolar Depressive Disorders

A 71-year-old kindergarten teacher was referred by geriatric medicine for diagnostic clarification for major neurocognitive disorder commingled with bipolar disorder type I. His score on the MoCA test was 18 out of 30. Geriatric psychiatry consultation established that the patient was severely depressed despite having been maintained on lithium carbonate 450 mg/day achieving a level of 0.6 mEq/L and bupropion long-acting 300 mg/day for over 10 years.

After discussion of treatment options, the patient requested ECT for more assured and quick response despite potential short-term memory side effects. A course of 12 right unilateral ultra-brief ECT sessions titrated to sixfold the individual seizure threshold was administered. After six sessions, he showed significant improvement in depression and anxiety symptoms (e.g., his HAMD-17 score went down from 24 to 8). His score on repeat MoCA test 3 months after

H. H. Fenn et al. (eds.), *Age-Adjusted Psychiatric Treatment for the Older Patient*, https://doi.org/10.1007/978-3-031-53976-3_14

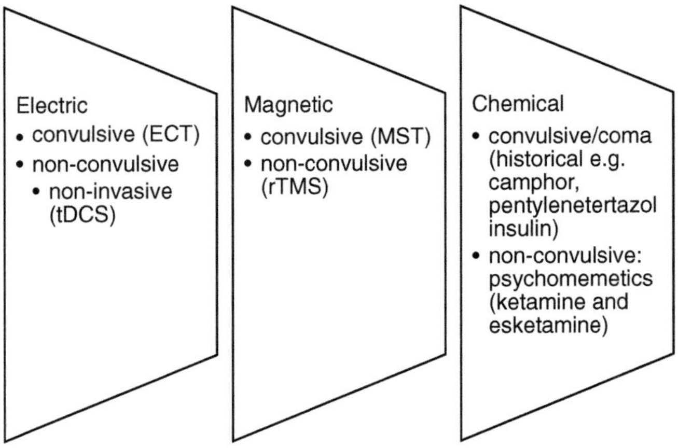

Fig. 14.1 Overview of brain stimulation/modulation modalities

initial testing rose to 25/30. He was moved to a schedule of weekly maintenance sessions of right unilateral ultra-brief ECT for four sessions and then was followed on maintenance doses of lithium 450 mg/day achieving a level of 0.7 mEq/L and bupropion 300 mg/day with occasional ECT sessions based on his mood scores.

Discussion

A course of ECT was administered successfully for recurrent major depressive disorder which presented with symptoms of cognitive impairment.

Overview of Neuromodalities (Fig. 14.1)

Electroconvulsive Therapy (ECT)

For patients over age 65 years, ECT has a high rate of success with low risk; remission rates for depressive disorders range between 73 and 90% (Spaans et al. 2015). ECT avoids common antidepressant-related adverse effects (e.g., cardiovascular, anticholinergic, serotonergic) (Stek et al. 2003; Tripathi 2013) and treats patients with symptoms such as weight loss, dehydration, frailty, and agitation (see Table 14.1 and Fig. 14.2). ECT has been recognized as the gold standard for severe major depressive disorder (most commonly medication-resistant) (Engel and Kayser 2016; Sabesan et al. 2015; van Dierman et al. 2018) and is faster in symptom relief than antidepressants (Gálvez et al. 2015; Geduldig and Kellner 2016). Its use is highest among aging adults, specifically the oldest-old population (80 years and older) (Gálvez et al. 2015; Geduldig and Kellner 2016; Kumar et al. 2016).

Indications for ECT in Geriatric Patients

Severe depression with suicidality and treatment-resistant depression (TRD) are the most common indications for ECT (Milev et al. 2016). TRD is often diagnosed after an inadequate response to treatment, defined as a lack of a reduction in depressive symptoms of at least 50%, as per scores on objective clinical scales (Rybak et al. 2021). Although a wide consensus for an operational definition of TRD has not yet been established, it is generally considered a heterogeneous condition marked by the following:

1. The absence of an adequate response after at least two evidence-based trials of antidepressant medication at full dose.
2. Adequate compliance with treatment.
3. For an adequate treatment duration.
4. Following one treatment course of evidence-based psychotherapy.

The following illnesses can benefit from ECT: less severely ill episodes of major depressive disorder, delirious mania, bipolar disorder (manic and depressive episodes), obsessive

Table 14.1 Three therapeutic brain stimulation and modulation modalities (TBSM)

	ECT	rTMS	Ketamine/esketamine
Anesthesia needed	Yes	No	No
General indication	Severe, life-threatening depressive disorder, for example, with psychotic features	Patients with MDD who have failed at least one antidepressant	Treatment-resistant depressive disorder
Effectiveness for specific indications	• Severe agitated, psychotic depressive disorder, and suicidal behavior with quick onset of action • Psychotic disorder, catatonia, treatment-resistant schizophrenia, manic episode, and other severe or treatment-resistant presentations	• Nonpsychotic TRD but require long course of treatment • Emerging efficacy in PTSD, OCD, among others	• Nonpsychotic TRD, with a rapid onset of action for suicidal ideation and behavior • Emerging role in illnesses like PTSD
Safety			
	• General anesthesia use (2–4 deaths per 100,000 treatment) • Avoid in the context of isolated neurocognitive disorders • Increased intracranial pressure • Recent stroke/cerebral hemorrhage • Amyloid angiopathies and aneurysms • Cardiovascular disease/ complications • Pheochromocytoma	• Seizure is most serious risk • Malfunctioning of metal implants following rTMS	• Potential interaction with other medications, such as amphetamines, antianxiety medications, MAOIs, and seizure medications • Embryo-fetal toxicity • Potential for abuse
Physiological side effects			
	Acute: • Elevated heart rate • Elevated blood pressure • Asystole (transient) • Postictal headaches • Nausea • Muscle aches • Vomiting • Prolonged seizures Long-term: • Arrythmias • Myocardial ischemia • Myocardial infarction • Severe heart block • Embolism	Generally, well tolerated but associated with few side effects Acute: • Light-headedness • Mild headaches • Tingling in the face, jaw, or scalp • Temporary hearing problems Long-term: • Seizures	Acute: • Psychomimetic adverse effects • Dizziness • Nausea • Lethargy • Increased blood pressure • Pounding in ears Long term (rare): • Cystitis and lower urinary tract symptoms • Bile duct injury

(continued)

Table 14.1 (continued)

	ECT	rTMS	Ketamine/esketamine
Cognitive adverse side effects			
	Acute: • Confusion • Delirium • Disorientation • Arousal disturbances • Slower processing speed Long-term: • Retrograde amnesia • Anterograde amnesia • Worsened verbal learning and executive functions Long-term prognosis: • Acute effects are typically transient • Recovery of memory functions observed 1–4 weeks post-ECT • No permanent structural or functional brain damage • May be prolonged by age, MNCD/dementia, other brain disease, bilateral placement, and excess stimulus intensity	No absolute cognitive side effects but possible deterioration in divided attention, problem-solving, planning, and verbal learning and memory	• Dissociation syndromes • Sense of detachment from self or body • Trouble speaking • Behavioral changes • May impair attention, judgement, thinking, reaction speed and motor skills • Not associated with long-term cognitive impairment to date
Focality	Non-focal (widespread electrical stimulation of the brain using electrodes applied to the scalp)	Focal (with direct precise measurements, stimulation is limited to an area of ~3 cm^2)	Non-focal (IV, nasal spray, subcutaneous or intramuscular administration; widespread network effect on brain cells involved in mood)
[a]Levels of evidence in general population for MDD			
	Level I evidence		
	• Acute efficacy, maintenance efficacy and safety, and tolerability as a second-line treatment • Acute efficacy, maintenance efficacy and safety, and tolerability as a first-line treatment in some clinical situations	Acute efficacy and safety and tolerability as a first-line treatment for patients who have failed at least one antidepressant	[b]As an adjunctive medication for nonresponse or partial response to an antidepressant
	Level II evidence		
		Maintenance efficacy as a first-line treatment for patients who have failed at least one antidepressant	
	Level III evidence		
Typical range of efficacy for seniors	Remission rates: 50–75% Relapse rates: 70% (nonresistant) and about 60% in treatment resistant	Response rates: 20–30% Remission rates: 40–50%	Response rates: 65–80% Remission rates: 50–60%

(continued)

Table 14.1 (continued)

	ECT	rTMS	Ketamine/esketamine
Putative mechanism of action	Depolarization of cerebral neurons by an electric current alters neuronal depression pathways: • GABAergic (enhancement) • Serotonergic • Dopaminergic • Adrenergic Dysregulation of hypothalamic–pituitary–adrenal axis	Speculation that it: • Alters synaptic plasticity, mainly the long-term potentiation/depression of excitatory synaptic transmission • Modulates functional networks, particularly the meso-cortico-limbic reward circuit • Increases glutamate, dopamine, and GABAa and GABAb synapse excitability	Not well known, but thought to: • Preferentially target and inhibit *N*-methyl-D-aspartate (NMDA) receptor on GABAergic neurons
Treatment course	2–3 times weekly	20–30 daily treatment sessions, each lasting 30–40 min	Once a week under strict medical supervision
Time/number of treatments to therapeutic effect	Case-by-case basis (usually 6–12 treatments)	4–6 weeks	Few hours–days
Feasibility	• Access to a specialized service with full level of staffing • Due to general anesthesia requirement, patients need to be accompanied and supervised by a responsible adult after treatment given the patient cannot drive or participate in any major instrumental activities for several hours after the procedure	No restrictions on patient activities and do not need to be supervised by a responsible adult after the procedure, but access in some areas might be an issue given the limited public funding for the procedure in some jurisdictions	
Work-up preparation	Full medical and anesthesia work-up, medical screening, and monitoring	Generally only requires some medical screening via questionnaires and clinical monitoring for seizures, side effects, and vital signs	

MDD major depressive disorder, *TRD* treatment-resistant depression
[a]Data referenced from Milev et al. (2016) where level I evidence indicates "meta-analysis with narrow confidence intervals and/or two or more RCTs with adequate sample size, preferably placebo controlled"; level II evidence indicates "meta-analysis with wide confidence intervals and/or one or more RCTs with adequate sample size"; level III evidence indicates "small sample RCTs or non-randomized controlled prospective studies or case series or high quality retrospective studies"; and level IV evidence indicates an expert opinion/consensus
[b]Referenced from Kennedy et al. (2016)

compulsive disorder, poststroke depressive disorder (PSD), major neurocognitive disorder (MNCD) with depressive symptoms, catatonia (including malignant/excited episodes), neuroleptic malignant syndrome (MNS), and psychotic disorders (Meyer et al. 2020).

ECT is also used as a first-line treatment to relieve high mortality rates linked to delirious mania, malignant catatonia, and neuroleptic malignant syndrome (NMS). ECT is preferentially used to treat severe major depressive disorder with suicidal ideation, with rapid alleviation of suicide risk (Fink et al. 2014; Park et al. 2021).

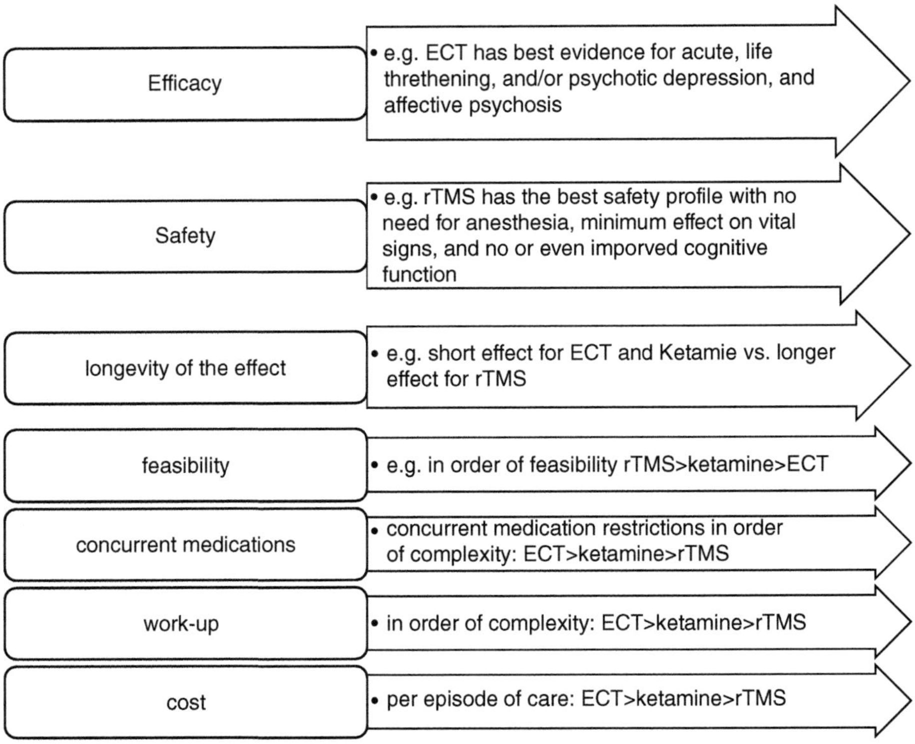

Fig. 14.2 Factors to consider in selection of TBSM

- ECT is considered a second-line treatment in schizophrenia-spectrum disorders and bipolar disorders (Meyer et al. 2020).
- ECT has been found particularly effective in resolution and reduction in relapse of major depressive disorder *with psychotic features*. In a prospective naturalistic follow-up study 110 patients with LLD, those with psychotic depression had a lower risk of relapse after successful ECT than patients without a psychotic illness. Of a total of 22 patients, 32.8% experienced a relapse, and subjects with psychotic depression were less likely to relapse (odds ratio = 0.32, $p = 0.047$) (Wagenmakers et al. 2020). In a meta-analysis of 34 studies, the presence of psychotic features was found to be a predictor of ECT remission [odds ratio (OR) = 1.47, $P = 0.001$]. ECT remission and response rates were positively associated with age (standardized mean difference of 0.26 and 0.35, respectively), and ECT was noted to be particularly effective in aged patients with depression (van Dierman et al. 2018).

For the geriatric population, ECT has unique advantages and for this reason is administered more frequently to older than to younger patients (Flint and Gagnon 2002; Meyer et al. 2018; van Schaik et al. 2012). This is in part due to the increased presence of systemic medical comorbidities and related vulnerabilities, such as cardiovascular disease, multi-drug regimens, and low tolerance of and high sensitivity to medication (Rosen et al. 2016; van Schaik et al. 2012). ECT has also proven more efficacious than tricyclic antidepressants (TCAs), monoamine oxidase inhibitors (MAOIs), or selective serotonin reuptake inhibitors (SSRIs), with faster remission rates than pharmacotherapy after 5 weeks of treatment in a randomized clinical trial (RCT) (63.8% and 23.5%, respectively) (Spaans et al. 2015). An ultra-brief pulse right unilateral (RUL) ECT combined with venlafaxine, administered in the Prolonging Remission in Depressed Elderly (PRIDE) study, revealed a 70% response rate and 62% remission rate in 240 patients aged 60 years and older (Kellner et al. 2016a).

ECT Parameters

Aging increases the seizure threshold (ST) during ECT. *Decreased excitability* of the brain and/or increased skull thickness with increased age may be underlying reasons (Gálvez et al. 2015; Meyer et al. 2018). A larger stimulus intensity is required for seizure initiation in aged patients, who may have shorter and weaker seizures, with a shorter duration of the slow wave phase (Meyer et al. 2018). Seizure threshold (ST) is most precisely determined through stimulus dosing, with the delivery of electrical stimulus subconvulsively until induction of a generalized seizure (of at least 20 s) occurs as documented by EEG (Flint and Gagnon 2002). Seizure duration beyond the minimum requirement of 20 s has been noted to have no effect on ECT efficacy (Flint and Gagnon 2002).

Electrode Placement

Choosing among three common electrode placements, *right unilateral* (RUL), *bilateral*, and *bifrontal* is dependent on factors, such as symptom severity, presence of systemic medical comorbidities, cognitive status, and trajectory of response (Meyer et al. 2018) (see Table 14.2). The risk of cognitive adverse effects, which is minimized by RUL placement, often needs to be balanced against the greater efficacy and speed of improvement seen with bilateral placement. Severity of symptoms and the urgent need for a response may suggest an initial trial of low-dose bilateral ECT. Less common placements include left anterior, right temporal, and left unilateral (for left-handed patients with right hemisphere language dominance) (Meyer et al. 2018). While the number of treatments needed for response may vary, 6–12 ECT treatments are often required to achieve maximal efficacy, and this must be determined by the individual case and clinical judgment. If there is little or no initial response, many experts recommend at least 10–12 bilateral treatments before the depressive episode is labelled nonresponsive. Treatment is usually discontinued if there is no improvement or remission after two consecutive courses of 12 treatments (Flint and Gagnon 2002).

Other ECT Parameters

- Current, pulse width, and frequency of the stimulus can influence both efficacy and adverse effects (Meyer et al. 2018). Depressive symptom amelioration can be similarly achieved using brief pulse stimulation or sine wave stimulation (Eser et al. 2007; Kho et al. 2003).
- Sine wave ECT results in increased cognitive impairment, rendering brief pulse stimulation the standard method of stimulus application (Eser et al. 2007; Kho et al. 2003; Meyer et al. 2018).
- Brief pulse stimulation has been noted to cause more cognitive effects than *ultra-brief pulse stimulation*, which may have a slower time to benefit than brief pulse (Milev et al. 2016).

Medications During ECT

Anticonvulsant medication must be monitored in patients undergoing a course of ECT. Benzodiazepines are to be avoided in geriatric patients, if possible, during ECT sessions (Gálvez et al. 2015), though a small dose (e.g., 2 mg total per 24 h) of lorazepam can be used cautiously for extreme anxiety but will need to be held for 12–15 h before planned ECT. General anesthesia is most often induced with methohexital (dose: 0.75–1.0 mg/kg) and succinylcholine (0.75–1.5 mg/kg), a depolarizing neuromuscular blocking agent used to prevent the motor manifestations of a seizure (Tripathi 2013). It is recommended to avoid lithium immediately pre-ECT due to delirium risk.

Table 14.2 Most common electrode placements in ECT

Electrode placement	Right unilateral (RUL)	Bilateral	Bifrontal
Order of treatment in geriatric patients	First-line[a]	Second-line[a]	First-line[a]
Seizure threshold (ST) maximal efficacy for antidepression achieved at stimulus X times seizure threshold (ST)	5–6 times[a,b]	1.5–2 times[a]	1.5–2 times[a]
Cognitive adverse effects	Low[b] (increasing dose risks cognitive impairment)[b] – No effect on the dominant (left) hemisphere language centers[b,d]	Modest[a,d,f] (typically transient)	Low[f] (comparable to RUL in elderly)
Remission rates for depression in geriatric patients	51.4% (RCT, 73 depressed elderly patients)[g] 88.2% (RCT, 39 depressed elderly patients)[h]	68.2% (RCT, 39 depressed elderly patients)[g] Limited data comparing bilateral and RUL in elderly[b] Determined on case-by-case basis, based on symptom severity, comorbidities and response	Comparable to RUL[f,g] 38.9% (RCT, 73 depressed elderly patients)[g]
Specific indications	PD and MNCD with depressive disorder[a,c]	Psychotic spectrum illnesses[e] Severe MDD requiring urgent response[b]	Requires better characterization for use in geriatric patients with MD[g]
Recommended number of treatments for optimum efficacy (more than three treatments may increase risk for adverse cognitive effects)[a]	Three times weekly[i,j]	2–3 times weekly (could be reduced to limit cognitive impairment)[i]	2–3 times weekly (could be reduced to limit cognitive impairment)[i]

[a]Milev et al. (2016)
[b]Meyer et al. (2018)
[c]Kumar et al. (2016)
[d]Flint and Gagnon (2002)
[e]Liu et al. (2014)
[f]Dybedal et al. (2016)
[g]Bjølseth et al. (2015b)
[h]Stoppe et al. (2006)
[i]Grover and Somaiya (2017)
[j]Flint and Gagnon (2002)

Maintenance ECT and Pharmacotherapy

Maintenance ECT (mECT) can decrease hospitalization periods in geriatric patients with medication-resistant depressive disorder and is found to be as efficacious as continuation pharmacotherapy in preventing relapse (van Schaik et al. 2012). Although relapse of depression after even a successful ECT course can occur, relapse has been reported in only 50% of patients prescribed continuation pharmacotherapy, as opposed to 85% of patients who were not on continuation pharmacotherapy within the first 6 months of a successful ECT trial (van Schaik et al. 2012). Antidepressants *during* a course of ECT (Milev et al. 2016) as well as continuation pharmacotherapy have been beneficial.

One review of nine studies of mECT for exclusively aging patients reported that mECT is generally as effective and well tolerated as continuation medication in severely depressed elderly patients after a successful course of ECT (van Schaik et al. 2012). mECT has also been found to decrease intervals between hospitalization in geriatric patients (van Schaik et al. 2012). One RCT found the period until relapse was longer in depressed patients over 60 years of age who received nortriptyline *with* maintenance ECT versus continuation pharmacotherapy alone (23 months vs. 16 months, respectively) (Navarro et al. 2008). Another RCT reported a greater relapse rate in the continuation pharmacotherapy group (nortriptyline only) versus the group of geriatric patients receiving mECT (54% vs. 17%, respectively) (Serra et al. 2006). The CORE study RCT also investigated relapse, using HDRS-24, in 184 unipolar depressed patients (mean age: 57.1) assigned to either mECT alone or lithium carbonate and nortriptyline. No significant difference was found in relapse rates between the two groups (37% vs. 32%, respectively) after 6 months (Kellner et al. 2006).

The recommended frequency of mECT is not well established, but most studies have suggested that after the acute course and when response is achieved, sustained benefit is achieved with weekly ECT for four times (1 month), followed by ECT every 2 weeks for a month, and then monthly afterward. Clinical factors may affect this; for example, some patients may show early relapse and need more frequent mECT while others can be treated every 3 months and remain stable (Luccarelli et al. 2020).

Adverse Effects and Cautions

Serious complications are a low risk with ECT, except for those risks accompanying general anesthesia, such as prolonged seizures and death (Eser et al. 2007; Tripathi 2013); mortality rate is about 2 deaths per 100,000 treatments (Fink and Taylor 2007). Cardiac dysfunction, cerebral abnormalities, and respiratory disease have a high incidence rate in older adults and increase this mortality rate (Geduldig and Kellner 2016; Meyer et al. 2018).

Cardiac

Autonomic response to ECT varies. Sympathetic tone increases during seizure initiation, and then parasympathetic (vagal) tone increases once the seizure terminates and during stimulus delivery (Meyer et al. 2018; Tripathi 2013). This shift may create a strain on the cardiovascular system, especially in geriatric patients, and it is considered the primary aspect of ECT-related somatic complications (Flint and Gagnon 2002; Meyer et al. 2018).

Downstream effects of the parasympathetic response may lead to bradycardia, hypotension, and atrial arrythmia (Flint and Gagnon 2002; Tripathi 2013). In addition, downstream effects of the *sympathetic* response may lead to hypertension and tachycardia (Tripathi 2013; Meyer et al. 2018). Transient asystole is also commonly observed upon parasympathetic activation through seizure induction in elderly depressed patients (Meyer et al. 2018; van der Wurff et al. 2003). Heart rate and blood pressure both increase at the beginning of seizure due to effects mediated by the sympathetic response (catecholamine release from the adrenal medulla) (Tripathi 2013). These effects may increase the risk for patients with ischemic heart disease by leading to arrythmias and raising oxygen demand, the latter of which can be mitigated by sufficient ventilation. Specifically, prolonged arrythmias, myocardial ischemia, myocardial infarction, and severe heart block may ensue in patients with pre-existing cardiac conditions (Meyer et al. 2018). High risk of embolism formation is also present in patients with atrial fibrillation. Prevention of adverse sympathetic and parasympathetic effects is achieved by using beta-blockers (e.g., esmolol) and anticholinergics (e.g., atropine), respectively (Meyer et al. 2018; Tripathi 2013).

Susceptibility to bradycardia, tachycardia, arrythmia, and other cardiovascular events must be assessed prior to administration. Despite the increased incidence of cardiac effects in geriatric patients, those complications are usually transient (Flint and Gagnon 2002). See Table 14.3 for medication utility and contra-indication in ECT versus other modalities and Fig. 14.3 for clinical considerations.

Table 14.3 Medication use and contraindications across TBSM

Modality	Potentially unsafe agents → consequence	Medications that affect cortical excitability/seizure threshold (CE-ST) → consequence (↑/↓ CE-ST)	Medications that impact efficacy → consequence (↑/↓ efficacy)	Medications to manage side effects → consequences
ECT[a]	MAOI → hypertensive crisis Lithium → delirium Insulin → hypoglycemia Choline esterase inhibitors → prolong paralysis from succinylcholine Agents that lower seizure threshold resulting in status epilepticus (see next column)	Benzodiazepines and other GABAergic agents → ↑ Xanthines (theophylline, caffeine, aminophylline) → ↓ Antidepressants (especially bupropion), antipsychotics (especially clozapine) and psychostimulants → ↓	Benzodiazepines and other GABAergic agents → ↓ Antidepressants → ↑ Antipsychotics → ↑	Antihypertensives → control hypertensive response Glycopyrrolate → ↓ secretions and bradycardia Antiemetics → ↓ nausea and vomiting Analgesics → ↓ muscle pain and headaches Antiacids → ↓ risk of aspiration pneumonitis Anti-angina Anti-arrhythmia → ↓ risk of angina and tachyarrhythmia Bronchodilators → control broncospasm
rTMS[b]	Agents that lower seizure threshold (see next column) Medical devices that can malfunction or can be displaced/heated (pacemaker, coils, etc.)		Psychostimulants → ↑ Benzodiazepines and other GABAergic agents → ↓	Analgesics → ↓ scalp pain and headaches
Ketamine[c]	MAOI → hypertension		Antidepressants →? ↑ Benzodiazepines→?↓ (hold for 12 h) Glutamate modulators (e.g., lamotrigine) →?↓	Benzodiazepines → treat anxiety and muscle spasm (short as needed use) Alpha-2 agonists → treat anxiety and hypertension Antipsychotics → treat psychotic dissociation Antiemetics → ↓ nausea and vomiting Antihistamine → help allergy like reaction

This table is meant to be a practical guide regarding concurrent use of medications and devices with therapeutic brain stimulation and modulation modalities and not a comprehensive list

MAOI monoamine oxidase inhibitor

[a]Burhan, Amer & Jarmain, Sarah & Sharma, Verinder. (2014). Burhan AM, Jarmain S and Sharma V. An evidence-informed model for the modern practice of electroconvulsive therapy. In electroconvulsive therapy: Clinical uses, efficacy and long-term health effects. Kathleen Braddock (Ed.). NOVA Science Publisher, August 2014

[b]*Hunter AM, Minzenberg MJ, cook IA, Krantz DE, Levitt JG, Rotstein NM, Chawla SA, Leuchter AF. Concomitant medication use and clinical outcome of repetitive transcranial magnetic stimulation (rTMS) treatment of major depressive disorder. Brain and behavior. 2019 may;9(5):e01275*

[c]Several case report of safe use of MAOI and ketamine for example: Katz RB, Toprak M, Wilkinson ST, Sanacora G, Ostroff R. Concurrent use of ketamine and monoamine oxidase inhibitors in the treatment of depression: a letter to the editor. General hospital psychiatry. 2018 Sep;54:62. And Dunner DL, Fugate RM, Demopulos CM. Safety and efficacy of esketamine nasal spray in a depressed patient who was being treated with tranylcypromine: A case report. Neurology, psychiatry and brain research. 2020 Jun 1;36:30–1

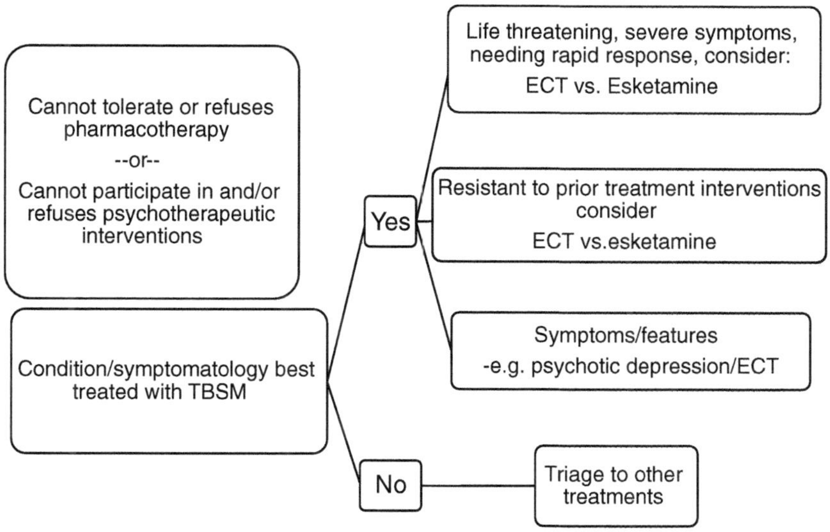

Fig. 14.3 Decision tree for TBSM

Somatic Adverse Effects After ECT

Headaches, nausea, muscle aches, and vomiting can occur after treatment (Meyer et al. 2018). Postictal headache symptoms can be alleviated using analgesics, such as acetylsalicylic acid and paracetamol, while regular migraine attacks can be treated with an oral or nasal administration of drugs such as sumatriptan (Eser et al. 2007). Nausea is a rare symptom of anesthesia and can be treated with metoclopramide (Eser et al. 2007). Generally prolonged seizures (up to 180 s) can also occur, especially in patients treated with theophylline. Benzodiazepines are then usually delivered IV to terminate the seizure with ictal and postictal EEG monitoring (Eser et al. 2007). Tongue injuries, bladder rupture, and joint dislocation are other possible complications of ECT (Tripathi 2013).

Comorbidities such as stroke, aneurysm, pheochromocytoma, myocardial infarction, and amyloid angiopathies increase the risk of neurological side effects (Tripathi 2013; Meyer et al. 2018; Milev et al. 2016). Brain tumors and other comorbidities causing a heightened intercranial pressure (ICP) also increase risk of ECT administration; however, if the tumors are stable, without increased ICP, ECT poses minimal risk (Meyer et al. 2018). In the event of a stroke, clinicians implement a 1–2-month delay before ECT to allow the strengthening of friable vessels (Meyer et al. 2018). However, ECT has been administered as early as 4 days following a stroke in extremely urgent cases.

Cognition and ECT

The aged individual is susceptible to cognitive adverse effects after ECT (van Schaik et al. 2012). The most common are retrograde amnesia, anterograde amnesia, and acute confusion. A state of confusion usually occurs immediately after a treatment (Eser et al. 2007; Tripathi 2013). The retrograde and anterograde amnesia tend to resolve in the hours following the ECT session but may worsen in the context of other brain disease, bilateral electrode placement, high stimulus intensity, and advanced age (Meyer et al. 2018). Disorientation and delirium risk can also be increased in association with age, stimulus dose, adverse effects of psychoactive drugs, and type of anesthetic (Eser et al. 2007). A study of 43 depressed elderly patients found that bilateral ECT caused retrograde memory impairment; however, this effect resolved completely 7 months following the ECT course, and cognitive improvement was observed in the follow-up period (Rosenberg et al. 2009).

Another study investigated cognitive adverse effects induced by ECT in 54 depressed non-demented geriatric patients (age range: 65–80) both with and without cognitive impairment. Both groups demonstrated cognitive adverse effects—without any permanent effect on neurocognitive function. Retrograde and anterograde memory impairments were not significantly different between the cognitively impaired and non-cognitively impaired patients (Dybedal et al. 2015). In contrast, neuropsychological functioning was examined in 65 depressed elderly patients (age range: 60–85) without major neurocognitive disorder/dementia, 27 of whom had a mild cognitive impairment. Following a twice-weekly administration of ECT (RUL or bifrontal placement), 55.6% of the cognitively impaired patients showed improvement in cognitive status. A word reading task had the only negative correlation with ECT remission rates out of all the assessments (e.g., processing speed, verbal learning, memory, executive function). No overall association was found between ECT remission rates and cognitive impairment in geriatric patients (Bjølseth et al. 2015a). The cognition of 62 depressed elderly patients (without dementia) before and after an ECT course was compared to 17 healthy controls (Dybedal et al. 2014). Letter fluency was the only cognitive function that was significantly worsened compared to the control group, whereas other measures showed stable or increased functioning. However, 11% of the patients treated with ECT displayed retrograde amnesia and 40% showed a deterioration in neuropsychological functioning—specifically anterograde impairment. These findings indicate a possibility of developing mild cognitive deficits throughout an ECT course.

Recovery from the cognitive effects of ECT is usually seen at 1–4 weeks following treatment (Eser et al. 2007; Tielkes et al. 2008). A meta-analysis showed resolution of cognitive adverse effects (e.g., arousal disturbances, orientation, ictal processing speed) as early as 3 days following an ECT treatment (Kumar et al. 2016). The presence of permanent adverse cognitive effects in depressed geriatric patients following an acute ECT course was not confirmed. Eser et al. (2007) also found no conclusive evidence on any long-lasting functional or structural damage to the brain because of ECT.

Some studies have reported an improved cognitive performance in depressed patients with major neurocognitive disorder (MNCD)/dementia following an ECT course (Liu et al. 2014; Tielkes et al. 2008). Verbal memory was the only MMSE component that worsened following ECT (Tielkes et al. 2008). In certain trials, cognitive impairment has been found to occur at a lower frequency in elderly patients than in younger adults (Kumar et al. 2016). This finding may reflect an overall improved global cognition in aging patients through the alleviation of depressive disorders.

Overall, MMSE scores of depressed patients exhibit an *improvement* in global cognition following an ECT course, a finding commonly seen when successfully treating late-life depressive disorders (Kumar et al. 2016). Some have speculated that this may be due to tension between the improvement of depressive symptoms and the adverse effect of ECT on cognition (Flint and Gagnon 2002; Kumar et al. 2016).

Maintenance ECT (mECT) may increase the deleterious impact of ECT on cognition in geriatric patients. One review examined the impact of mECT on cognitive functioning of depressed patients (mean age ≥55 years) in seven studies before and after treatment. No significant difference was found in MMSE scores prior to and after treatment; further, no significant difference was observed in mean MMSE scores between depressed patients prescribed with continuation pharmacotherapy and maintenance ECT (van Schaik et al. 2012).

No significant difference in global cognitive functioning has been reported between geriatric patients treated *with ECT* and those *never exposed to it*; however, a deterioration of verbal learning and executive functioning has also been noted (Rami-González et al. 2003). In the Consortium for Research in ECT (CORE) study, lower retrograde memory scores were observed with maintenance ECT as opposed to continuation pharmacotherapy in 85 patients after 12 weeks of their last ECT session (Smith et al. 2010).

However, those retrograde memory effects resolved 24 weeks after ECT completion.

In sum, the benefits of ECT to TRD, major depressive disorder (MDD), suicidality, and MDD with psychotic features usually outweigh any risks of cognitive impairment.

Remission

ECT may offer faster response and remission from major depressive disorder (MDD) for geriatric patients. One study of patients who completed ECT reported that the greatest mean age of patients was found in the rapid remission group (65.3 years) in comparison with the moderate response (57.6 years) and non-remitting (51.5 years) groups. The highest percentage of remitted patients (80%) and most favorable course trajectory was also observed in the rapid remission group (Rhebergen et al. 2015). The PRIDE study observed higher remission rates (69.7%) in patients aged 70 years and older than in patients aged 60–69 (55%) with a greater likelihood (1.89) of response in the former group (Kellner et al. 2016a). In 24 studies, the average age for ECT remitters was 59.7 years versus 55.4 years for patients who did not remit (van Dierman et al. 2018). Previous treatment resistance has a strong predictive effect on response to ECT, in that it may decrease response (Milev et al. 2016; Tripathi 2013).

The successful responses of geriatric patients to ECT have been attributed to many factors, including their increased risk of developing depressive disorders with psychotic features, increased medication intolerance, decreased prevalence of comorbid personality disorders, and, often, an *earlier referral* to ECT (Greenberg and Kellner 2005; Rhebergen et al. 2015). However, a confounding effect may be produced by this early referral, such that older adults may not be at severe levels of depressive symptoms at the time ECT is prescribed (Rhebergen et al. 2015). Aging by *itself* may not impact this strong influence on remission and response rates but rather clinical concomitants *associated* with aging.

Previous depressive episodes and comorbidities in aging adults increase susceptibility to relapse following ECT. This can prompt clinicians to prescribe mECT for aging adult patients (van Schaik et al. 2012). To prevent relapse, mECT is usually administered (along with pharmacotherapy) at reduced frequency over the 6-month period following an acute ECT course (Greenberg and Kellner 2005; van Schaik et al. 2012). After a 6-month period, elderly patients can receive maintenance ECT at a minimum level of frequency, guided by illness severity, resistance to medication, psychotic symptoms (or lack thereof), and severity of depressive disorder. Fewer rehospitalizations, shorter hospitalization periods, and reduced relapse rates have been observed in geriatric patients prescribed mECT, especially in those with a psychotic spectrum illness such as schizophrenia, or major depressive disorder with psychotic features (Meyer et al. 2018).

The PRIDE study prospectively examined 240 patients (age >60 years) receiving ultra-brief pulse RUL ECT along with venlafaxine, 62% of whom remitted and 70% who responded (mean ECT treatment number: 7.3) (Kellner et al. 2016a). In the second phase of that study, an RCT was conducted on 120 elderly depressed patients (age >60 years) administered with an acute ultra-brief RUL ECT course. Following remission, patients were prescribed either mECT (four treatments) with venlafaxine and lithium or continuation pharmacotherapy using only the same medication. The combined mECT + pharmacotherapy approach showed fewer depressive symptoms on the Hamilton Depression Rating Scale and a greater rating of "not ill at all" on the Clinical Global Impressions severity scale compared to pharmacotherapy alone (Kellner et al. 2016b).

Repetitive Transcranial Magnetic Stimulation (rTMS)

This noninvasive neuromodulatory treatment was initially introduced as an alternative to transcranial electrical stimulation, which was considered painful and uncomfortable (Fitzgerald and Daskalakis 2013). rTMS discharges brief (200–300 ms) and powerful (0.2–0.4 T) magnetic pulses repetitively and tangentially to the skull and create an electric current that abruptly changes the excitability of the underlying neuronal firing (Eldaief et al. 2013). Adverse cognitive effects are minimal with rTMS (Iriarte and George 2018); it has been shown safe for older patients with neurological disorders who also present with comorbid depressive symptoms, including cognitive impairment and Parkinsonism (Sabesan et al. 2015).

Current indications for rTMS are the following:

1. *Medication-resistant depressive disorder* is the only current FDA-approved indication for rTMS, supported by evidence from open trials, sham-controlled studies, and comparison studies. Yet only a few RCTs of rTMS in geriatric patients have been completed or are definitive. Study designs have often used different stimulation parameters (e.g., intensity, stimulation site, number of stimuli, frequency) which confounds comparisons across studies (Jorge and Robinson 2011; Lisanby et al. 2009; Conelea et al. 2017). High frequency to the left dorsolateral prefrontal cortex (DLPFC) and low-frequency stimulation to the right DLPFC have both shown similar antidepressant effect, but low-frequency rTMS stimulation of right DLPFC is better tolerated with lower risk of seizure (Gershon et al. 2003).
2. *Cognitive impairment:* rTMS shows promise for geriatric patients with cognitive impairment (Drumond Marra et al. 2015; Wu et al. 2015; Rabey et al. 2013). Evidence suggests a significant cognitive improvement in patients treated with rTMS (see Cognition and rTMS) (Guse et al. 2010).
3. *Chronic pain:* Aged patients are particularly susceptible to adverse effects of first-line pain medications (Iriarte and George 2018). High-frequency rTMS (HF-rTMS) may be an alternative for pain management in geriatric patients (Lefaucheur et al. 2014). One study of HF-rTMS over the affected region combined with pharmacological treatment reported significant reductions in pain 3 months posttreatment in patients with postherpetic neuralgia (Ma et al. 2015).
4. *Smoking cessation:* rTMS could potentially benefit older adults with smoking cessation (Iriarte and George 2018). It is suggested that rTMS manipulates regions of the brain involved in addiction, and HF-rTMS of the DLPFC can reduce nicotine consumption and craving in working-age adults (Amiaz et al. 2009; Li et al. 2013) with prolonged effects 6-month posttreatment (Dinur-Klein et al. 2014).

Positive predictors of beneficial response to rTMS among geriatric patients includes patients who are younger, nonpsychotic, with shorter duration of depressive episode, low level of treatment resistance, and a history of previous response to ECT and/or rTMS (Tatti et al. 2016).

rTMS for Depression

Current response rates of depressive disorders to rTMS range from 30 to 45% (Sabesan et al. 2015; Trevizol et al. 2019) with remission rates of 40% and 0% to bilateral and unilateral high-frequency rTMS (HF-rTMS), respectively (Trevizol et al. 2019). rTMS has been found effective for older patients with TRD (Sabesan et al. 2015) and for patients who cannot tolerate high doses of medications (Pallanti et al. 2012). Many older adults exhibit atrophy in the prefrontal cortex (Baena et al. 2010), minimizing the odds that the magnetic field of rTMS will reach the brain and produce its full desired effect. Age appears inversely correlated with low-frequency right-sided rTMS treatment response (Aguirre et al. 2011), suggesting that response to stimulation therapies may vary in subpopulations of treatment-resistant patients (Pallanti et al. 2012). Antidepressant response, cognition, and sleep benefit patients aged 65 years or older from an increased number of rTMS pulses compared with those younger than 65 years (Jorge and Robinson 2011). It is well known that there is a better response to higher frequency and intensity rTMS, and longer treatment protocols may also be more effective (Gálvez et al. 2015).

Treatment for Cognitive Impairment

In trials with a single target, primarily the dorsolateral prefrontal cortex (DLPFC), there was improvement in cognition after active rTMS (Drumond Marra et al. 2015; Wu et al. 2015). The effect is not significant among trials with multiple targets (Brem et al. 2013). Additionally, no significant rTMS effect was reported in trials with *concurrent* cognitive training (mental activities that improving cognitive abilities such as working memory and executive functioning); trials *without* cognitive training showed improvement in cognition after active rTMS (Brem et al. 2013; Wu et al. 2015).

There is good evidence that rTMS produces significant cognitive improvement in cognitively impaired geriatric patients (Iriarte and George 2018; Guse et al. 2010). Although results are still preliminary and more studies with larger sample sizes are needed, high-frequency rTMS shows considerable promise in reducing mild cognitive impairment in nondepressed older adults, with positive effects sustained at least 1-month posttreatment (Nardone et al. 2014; Drumond Marra et al. 2015).

A synergistic effect on cognition has been shown with a combination of rTMS and cognitive training in patients with Alzheimer's disease (Bentwich et al. 2011). Rabey et al. (2013) have shown improvements in Alzheimer Disease Assessment Scale-Cognitive and Clinical Global Impression of Change scores 6 weeks and 4.5 months posttreatment in patients with mild to moderate Alzheimer's disease who received rTMS plus cognitive training.

rTMS has been used as an alternative intervention to improve cognition and memory in older patients with cognitive impairment (Cheng et al. 2018; Liao et al. 2015) by targeting the cortical area of interest (Liao et al. 2015). rTMS has been shown to be effective in geriatric patients with mild cognitive impairment (Cheng et al. 2018). rTMS has shown beneficial effects on cognition following application over the DLPFC in patients with MNCD/dementia (Ahmed et al. 2012; Cotelli et al. 2006). High-frequency rTMS improved naming performance in older patients with mild to moderate Alzheimer's disease (Cotelli et al. 2008) and had a better effect than low-frequency rTMS (Ash et al. 2014), but optimal parameters of rTMS for this effect are not known (Cheng et al. 2018). rTMS treatment has improved memory and attention, with a sustained improvement in memory after 1 month (Kim et al. 2019).

rTMS is a powerful tool to demonstrate the involvement of the left or right DLPFC in high- and low-performing older individuals during encoding and retrieval. In one study, researchers divided two subgroups of older adults according to their performance in a word pairs memory task and compared rTMS of the left and right DLPFCs during encoding and retrieval (Manenti et al. 2011). The authors showed that high-performing older adults, whose scores were similar to younger adults, employed bilateral DLPFC regions equally, whereas low-performing older adults engaged *the left DLPFC* more frequently than the right during encoding. However, both groups employed the DLPFC symmetrically during retrieval, which differs from what is observed in younger adults. Therefore, at least during encoding, the reorganization of brain functions in high-performing older adults may protect against selective cognitive impairment, while low-performing older adults, like young adults, may recruit specific brain regions but use it inefficiently (Manenti et al. 2012).

rTMS has been applied to improve memory deficits in older adults in patients with amnesic mild cognitive impairment (Cotelli et al. 2011; Solé Pedullés et al. 2006). Using a combination of rTMS and functional magnetic resonance imaging (fMRI), Solé Pedullés et al. (2006) demonstrated an improvement in associative memory in older patients with memory impairment following high-frequency rTMS applied over the left and right DLPFC. Specifically, the participants exhibited a behavioral improvement in a face-name association memory task following a single session of rTMS. A significant improvement in memory was found using a face-name associations test in an individual with amnestic mild cognitive impairment following daily high-frequency rTMS to the left parietal area for 2 weeks (Cotelli et al. 2011). The duration of the improvement persisted at least for 30 days after the last rTMS session, indicating associative memory enhancement by rTMS (Manenti et al. 2012).

Overall, improvements in associative memory, attention, and naming performance have been observed in the application of high-frequency rTMS over the left and right DLPFC; high-performing aging adults have been shown to employ both equally during encoding. In Alzheimer's disease patients, improved language performance has been demonstrated with rTMS (Cotelli et al. 2011; Rabey et al. 2013).

Parameters and Technique of rTMS

The delivery of rTMS therapy must be customized for each patient. This is needed to elicit desired brain effects (either excitatory or inhibitory) which have been shown to be effective for various psychiatric illnesses (Manenti et al. 2012). Technical parameters include number, strength, and duration of the stimuli, the length of the interval between stimuli, coil orientation, site of the reference electrode, the targeted area of the brain, and the possible interactions among these factors and the physiological and cognitive state of the patient (Peterchev et al. 2012).

Most studies and treatments use a figure-of-eight coil and involve the DLPFC region, either unilaterally or bilaterally, as the target site (Zibman et al. 2019). The DLPFC is found using a non-imaging-based technique, known as the "5-cm anterior method" in which, in a parasagittal line, the rTMS coil is placed 5 cm anterior to the motor cortical site for hand muscle movement (Johnson et al. 2013). Herbsman et al. (2009) showed that more lateral and anterior coil placement was associated with better clinical response. Stimulus intensity is based on individually determined resting motor threshold (RMT—the minimum intensity to elicit muscle twitches at relaxed upper or lower extremities). The most common intensity in all trials to date is 110% RMT (Kedzior et al. 2014), but most recent large trials have used a 120% RMT. Stimulation above this level is deemed unsafe (Rossi et al. 2009).

MRI guided targeting of the DLPFC has shown a trend toward greater clinical improvement when compared with the standard method (Rusjan et al. 2010). As in ECT, treatments can be delivered unilaterally or bilaterally. Unilateral rTMS involves high-frequency stimulation (i.e., 5 Hz or more) applied over the left DLPFC or low-frequency stimulation (i.e., 1 Hz) applied over right DLPFC. The rationale for stimulating with high frequency over the left, and low frequency over the right, prefrontal cortex originates from the observation that patients who suffer a stroke in the left hemisphere become depressed and those who sustain a stroke in their right hemisphere become manic more commonly than the general population (Blumberger et al. 2016). Imaging studies have demonstrated that MDD is associated with deficient activity in the left DLPFC and increased activity in the right DLPFC (Shiozawa et al. 2015). With rTMS treatment, imaging studies demonstrate normalized DLPFC function in patients with MDD (Sabesan et al. 2015). High-frequency stimulation has an activating effect on stimulated brain tissue (Fitzgerald et al. 2006; Luo et al. 2017) and also potentiates inhibitory neurotransmission in the cortex (Barr et al. 2009). The standard figure-of-eight coils stimulate the cortex in a more focal manner, activating an area of about 3 cm^2 as opposed to the more intense, but diffuse, activation pattern produced by a circular coil (Lee et al. 2012).

Compared to ECT

The efficacy of ECT short term for geriatric depression has been reported superior to rTMS in older adults. ECT appears to provide an earlier response to treatment when compared to rTMS (Xie et al. 2013). rTMS was significantly inferior to ECT with less than 4 weeks of treatment. The medium- and long-term efficacies of comparing the two treatments remain inconclusive (Sabesan et al. 2015).

Older age does not appear to be a negative predictor of response to rTMS for depression; aging patients show comparable benefit as younger patients (Lisanby et al. 2009). No differences in response and remission rates were found in patients above and below the age of 60 (Conelea et al. 2017). However, more rTMS sessions may be needed to elicit a favorable antidepressant benefit in older versus younger patients (Janicak et al. 2017), and geriatric patients require a higher intensity stimulation (120%) to overcome age-related prefrontal atrophy (Nahas et al. 2004).

A typical course of rTMS is delivered daily (normally 5 days per week) for up to 30 sessions. Some patients show response earlier but, in general, most patients need 15 sessions or more, which typically translates to a 3–6-week course. A cost-utility analysis indicated that rTMS is cost-effective compared to ECT in treatment-resistant depressive disorder (Fitzgibbon et al. 2020). There is emerging evidence for "accelerated" rTMS courses, whereby several sessions are provided per day and, as such, deliver the full course of rTMS in 5 days (Cole et al. 2020).

A few small studies have addressed the question of maintenance rTMS. Benadhira et al. (2017) demonstrated significantly less relapse in those maintained on weekly rTMS after responding to acute treatment. More studies are needed to confirm these findings and to address the issue of cost-effectiveness especially since rTMS is not currently funded by all insurers or available in all jurisdictions (Rachid 2018).

Adverse Effects in rTMS

Transient headache, transient hearing loss, seizure induction, cervical and scalp pain, burning scalp, and nonspecific minor scalp discomfort have been reported (Biagioni et al. 2018). The risk of seizure, although rare, is higher among individuals with a history of seizures, higher frequency of stimulation, greater number of pulses, and rTMS as opposed to single- or paired-pulse stimulation (Rossi et al. 2009; Iriarte and George 2018). Another serious side effect, treatment-emergent manic episode, has been seen in patients treated with rTMS (Iriarte and George 2018), but there was no significant difference in the rates of treatment-emergent manic episode in the active versus the sham rTMS groups in one study (Xia et al. 2008). Transient hearing loss appears connected to transient trigeminal nerve stimulation in approximately 35–50% of patients receiving therapeutic doses but abates with repeated stimulation or acetaminophen administered prophylactically (Lee et al. 2012).

To determine changes in cognitive performance, effects of rTMS on task performance were studied by using the two frontal task tests—Trail Making Test Part B (TMT-B) and the verbal fluency test of animal naming. In TMT-B, there was an initial impairment in the active rTMS group, followed by a great improvement after 1 month. In the verbal fluency test, the sham group had a gain and then impairment at the last evaluation (Drumond Marra et al. 2015). A temporary deterioration in executive function and planning following high-frequency rTMS to bilateral PFC of patients with depression has also been found. Two years later, the same group showed a deterioration in the retention of verbal material (Loo et al. 2003).

Aftereffects of repeated rTMS sessions may persist for days to weeks, and rTMS is not indicated for treatment of depressive disorder in patients with a history of seizures or for individuals with a cardiac pacemaker, intra-cardiac lines, or the presence of a brain lesion, vascular, traumatic, neoplastic, infectious, or metabolic (the latter is a chemical imbalance in the blood leading to impaired cerebral metabolism) (Rossi et al. 2009). Furthermore, patients who have sustained ischemic damage in the frontal cortex should not receive rTMS in order to avoid stimulation of a potential epileptogenic site (Jorge and Robinson 2011).

Ketamine and Esketamine

The psychotomimetic agents ketamine and esketamine, *N*-methyl-D-aspartate (NMDA) antagonists, are included in this chapter because both are administered as single procedures under medical/psychiatric supervision, as rapid acting antidepressant interventions for treatment-resistant depression in aging adults (Subramanian and Lenze 2021).

Ketamine is a racemic mixture of its enantiomers, *S*-(+)-ketamine and *R*-(−)-ketamine. *S*-(+)-ketamine, or esketamine, has 3–4 times the receptor affinity than the *R*-(−)-ketamine enantiomer (Muller et al. 2016). Ketamine is given as a single infusion, as multiple infusions, or as adjunctive therapy to other antidepressants (George et al. 2017). One single infusion of 0.5 mg/kg over 40 min produced an antidepressant response within 2–4 h that lasted up to 7 days (Murrough et al. 2013). Intravenous (IV) ketamine infusion of 0.5 mg/kg over 40 min is commonly administered (Andrade 2017; da Frota et al. 2017). Ketamine infusions are not FDA-approved and thus remain an off-label treatment for TRD (Bahji et al. 2021).

Infusion of intravenous racemic ketamine is recommended at a dose of 0.5 mg/kg over a duration of 40 min per session (McIntyre et al. 2021), although not FDA-approved. While the ideal frequency of ketamine infusion has not been established in adults with TRD (McIntyre et al. 2021), a reduction in suicidal ideation is shown to persist up to 6 weeks in patients who have been treated with repeated infusions (0.5 mg/kg, 2–3 times a week) over a span of 2 weeks (Phillips et al. 2020; McIntyre et al. 2021). Currently, there is no established upper dosing limit for intravenous racemic ketamine, but higher doses (0.5–1.0 mg/kg) have been shown to be more effective at reducing depressive symptoms than lower doses (0.1–0.2 mg/kg) 1 day after administration (Fava et al. 2020; McIntyre et al. 2021). In patients with low medication tolerability, doses may be lowered, but treatment efficacy may then be compromised (Molero et al. 2018; McIntyre et al. 2021). However, a 0.5 mg/kg dose shows comparable efficacy to a 1.0 mg/kg dose, indicating that patients may equally benefit from a lower-dose treatment course (Fava et al. 2020; McIntyre et al. 2021). Although most patients respond to treatment after two ketamine infusions, some may only respond after 4–6 treatment sessions. A follow-up assessment is conducted following completion of the treatment course to determine overall efficacy and response (McIntyre et al. 2021).

Intranasal esketamine is typically started at a dose of 56 mg on Day 1 and is increased to a maximum dose of 84 mg, administered twice weekly for 4 weeks. After this first set of 4 weeks, intranasal esketamine can then be administered once weekly for another set of 4 weeks, followed by once every 1–2 weeks thereafter (Molero et al. 2018; McIntyre et al. 2021). Intravenous esketamine at doses of 0.20 mg/kg or 0.40 mg/kg administered over 40 min show comparable response rates (60–65%) to racemic intravenous ketamine, with better tolerability at 0.20 mg/kg (Singh et al. 2016; Molero et al. 2018).

Patients should be monitored for at least 2 h after treatment with intravenous ketamine or esketamine, to ensure they are hemodynamically stable, with a clear sensorium, and show few dissociative or psychotomimetic effects. Additionally, a psychiatric assessment must be conducted to determine tolerability and response (McIntyre et al. 2021).

Efficacy

The evidence for long-term efficacy of ketamine and esketamine in the geriatric patient, especially for TRD, remains inconclusive. One review of six studies of ketamine treatment, without focusing on geriatric patients, found that ketamine was not an equally effective treatment alternative to ECT in patients with TRD. There was some evidence for a more favorable short-term cognitive side effect profile after ketamine treatment (Veraart et al. 2021).

Another RCT examined the antidepressant effect of intranasal esketamine (56 mg and 84 mg) twice weekly, with clinically significant antidepressant effects at day 28. Adverse effects generally appeared shortly after dosing but resolved within 1.5 h (Popova et al. 2019). Intranasal esketamine, as of March 2019, is the only FDA-approved intervention for TRD (Bahji et al. 2021). Esketamine may also be associated with transient cognitive decline (e.g., slower performance time or greater error rates), but this effect returned to placebo levels after 2 h (Morrison et al. 2018).

A RCT of treatment for TRD with esketamine combined with an antidepressant versus placebo combined with an antidepressant in older patients (65 and over) showed no statistically significant difference in depressive symptoms 4 weeks posttreatment (Ochs-Ross et al. 2020). Treatments included flexibly dosed intranasal esketamine (+ antidepressant) and placebo nasal spray (+ antidepressant). However, secondary analysis showed greater differences in antidepressant effects of esketamine in patients between 65 and 74 years old or patients with earlier onset of depressive disorder (<55 years old). Response and remission rates at 8 weeks posttreatment resembled those in younger adults at 4 weeks. Improvements were also observed in patients 75 years of age and older (Ochs-Ross et al. 2020).

It has been proposed (McIntyre 2021) that TRD criteria should not require trials of SGAs prior to a use of esketamine. Limited data and comparative head-to-head studies have not demonstrated efficacy, safety, and tolerability of selected atypical antipsychotics nor neurostimulation modalities. Only olanzapine–fluoxetine combination (OFC) is currently approved by the US FDA for adults with treatment-resistant depression, and aripiprazole, brexpiprazole, and quetiapine each have US FDA approvals only as add-on strategies in adults with major depressive disorder. Intolerability remains a major limitation of atypical antipsychotics in adults with major depressive disorder. FDA-approved second- and third-generation antipsychotics for major depressive disorder are associated with clinically significant weight gain, metabolic dysregulation, acute extrapyramidal symptoms, and tardive dyskinesia. It is also notable that the evidence base for second-generation antipsychotics in major depressive disorder is comprised largely of acute studies with a paucity of long-term data characterizing tolerability and safety.

Maintenance data for esketamine has documented the long-term efficacy, safety, and tolerability of esketamine in adults with treatment-resistant depression up to 1 year, which would justify a trial of esketamine even if SGAs have not been tried (McIntyre 2021).

Adverse Effects, Including Cognition

Acute psychiatric and psychotomimetic effects, blurred vision, dizziness, anxiety, irritability, and headaches can appear but are transient (Corriger and Pickering 2019). Dissociative symptoms have also been shown to be greater with higher doses of ketamine, peaking immediately following drug administration, although they were transient and subsided within minutes up to 2 h following the treatment (Zarate et al. 2006).

Low-dose ketamine was associated with selective memory impairments immediately posttreatment (e.g., delayed recall); however, immediate recall and verbal fluency remained intact. A lower response rate was also associated with acute reductions in cognitive performance following ketamine treatment (Murrough et al. 2013).

Neuromodulation Interventions Under Study

Several neuromodulation modalities currently in the research realm are not covered thoroughly but mentioned here to underline their potential.

Transcranial direct current stimulation (tDCS) is a neuromodulation technique whereby a weak electrical current, used for brain stimulation techniques in the past, has been modified with higher-intensity stimuli (Loo et al. 2012). This modality is relatively safe, and the Canadian Network for Mood and Anxiety Treatments (CANMAT) guidelines recommended tDCS as a third-line treatment for MDD patients (Milev et al. 2016).

Magnetic seizure therapy (MST) is a technique whereby a high-frequency magnetic stimulus in

MST induces a generalized seizure, like that of ECT, but creates an electrical field restricted to the *superficial cortex* (Engel and Kayser 2016; Tang et al. 2020). In contrast to widespread brain stimulation in ECT, the magnetic stimulus of MST is unaffected by skull impedance; thus, the procedure offers more focal control over targeted brain regions (Cretaz et al. 2015; Engel and Kayser 2016).

Studies of MST efficacy for psychiatric disorders in geriatric patients are sparse, but because of the favorable cognitive profile, there are reports that MST may be beneficial to vulnerable populations with neuropsychiatric diseases and neurocognitive impairment (Luber et al. 2013). One RCT reported similar antidepressant effects and cognitive safety in TRD patients treated with MST compared to those treated with brief pulse RUL ECT (Kayser et al. 2011). The MST group had an earlier recovery and reorientation time and a lack of somatic side effects, such as headache, nausea, and muscle ache.

Although MST has been observed to be less effective for TRD than ECT (Cretaz et al. 2015), fewer cognitive side effects are generally observed with MST than ECT (Engel and Kayser 2016). Recovery and reorientation times are also shorter (by 15 min) following MST (Engel and Kayser 2016; Luber et al. 2013). MST has shown stable global cognition, decreased depressive symptoms, and no retrograde and anterograde memory effect (Luber et al. 2013).

Conclusions

Neuromodulation interventions, also called noninvasive brain stimulation (NiBS) techniques, may offer excellent *age-adjusted* treatment if they establish their efficacy and can overcome limitations such as access, feasibility, cost, and cognitive adverse effects (Tatti et al. 2016). Modalities such as tDCS, MST, and rTMS may prove to be alternatives to ECT for the aging adult, if long-term improvement can be demonstrated and their safety confirmed.

Age-Adjusted Recommendations

- Review past psychiatric history, prior treatments, and outcomes.
- Review health insurance coverage for the specific modality proposed.
- Liaison with sites which provide neuromodulation (NiBIS) techniques.
- Review inclusion and exclusion criteria for the specific neuromodulation technique.
- Identify the specific information and referral questions required at each site.
- Inform patients and family members of risk-benefit ratio and that evidence of *long-term* benefit from neuromodulation and esketamine for geriatric individuals is inconclusive.
- Maintain contact with patient's family (with patient consent as needed) and others throughout the process of referral, treatment, and posttreatment.
- Ensure follow-up and maintenance treatment after completion of initial treatment course.

References

Aguirre I, Carretero B, Ibarra O, et al. Age predicts low-frequency transcranial magnetic stimulation efficacy in major depression. J Affect Disord. 2011;130(3):466–9.

Ahmed MA, Darwish ES, Khedr EM, et al. Effects of low versus high frequencies of repetitive transcranial magnetic stimulation on cognitive function and cortical excitability in Alzheimer's dementia. J Neurol. 2012;259:83–92.

Amiaz R, Levy D, Vainiger D, et al. Repeated high-frequency transcranial magnetic stimulation over the dorsolateral prefrontal cortex reduces cigarette craving and consumption. Addiction. 2009;104(4):653–60.

Andrade C. Ketamine for Depression, 1: Clinical Summary of Issues Related to Efficacy, Adverse Effects, and Mechanism of Action. J Clin Psychiatry. 2017;78(4):e415–9.

Ash E, Bregman N, Moore O, et al. Transcranial magnetic stimulation of deep brain regions in Alzheimer's disease. Alzheimers Dement. 2014;10:P450.

Baena E, Allen PA, Kaut KP, Hall RJ. On age differences in prefrontal function: the importance of emotional/cognitive integration. Neuropsychologia. 2010;48(1):319–33.

Bahji A, Vazquez GH, Zarate CA Jr. Comparative efficacy of racemic ketamine and esketamine for depression: a systematic review and meta-analysis. J Affect Disord. 2021;278:542–55.

Barr MS, Farzan F, Rusjan PM, et al. Potentiation of gamma oscillatory activity through repetitive transcranial magnetic stimulation of the dorsolateral prefrontal cortex. Neuropsychopharmacology. 2009;34(11):2359–67.

Benadhira R, Thomas F, Bouaziz N, et al. A randomized, sham-controlled study of maintenance rTMS for treatment-resistant depression (TRD). Psychiatry Res. 2017;258:226–33.

Bentwich J, Dobronevsky E, Aichenbaum S, et al. Beneficial effect of repetitive transcranial magnetic stimulation combined with cognitive training for the treatment of Alzheimer's disease: a proof-of-concept study. J Neural Transm (Vienna). 2011;118(3):463–71.

Biagioni MC, Sharma K, Migdadi HA, Cucca A. Non-invasive neuromodulation therapies for Parkinson's disease. In: Yenisetti SC, editor. Parkinson's disease understanding pathophysiology and developing therapeutic strategies. InTech; 2018.

Bjølseth TM, Engedal K, Benth JŠ, et al. Baseline cognitive function does not predict the treatment outcome of electroconvulsive therapy (ECT) in late-life depression. J Affect Disord. 2015a;185:67–75.

Bjølseth TM, Engedal K, Benth JŠ, et al. Clinical efficacy of formula-based bifrontal versus right unilateral electroconvulsive therapy (ECT) in the treatment of major depression among elderly patients: a pragmatic, randomized, assessor-blinded, controlled trial. J Affect Disord. 2015b;175:8–17.

Blumberger DM, Maller JJ, Thomson L, et al. Unilateral and bilateral MRI-targeted repetitive transcranial magnetic stimulation for treatment-resistant depression: a randomized controlled study. J Psychiatry Neurosci. 2016;41(4):E58–66.

Brem AK, Schilberg L, Freitas C, et al. Effects of cognitive training and rTMS in Alzheimer's disease. Alzheimers Dement. 2013;9:P664.

Cheng CPW, Wong CSM, Lee KK, et al. Effects of repetitive transcranial magnetic stimulation on improvement of cognition in elderly patients with cognitive impairment: a systematic review and meta-analysis. Int J Geriatr Psychiatry. 2018;33(1):e1–e13.

Cole EJ, Stimpson KH, Bentzley BS, et al. Stanford accelerated intelligent neuromodulation therapy for treatment-resistant depression. Am J Psychiatry. 2020;177(8):716–26.

Conelea CA, Philip NS, Yip AG, et al. Transcranial magnetic stimulation for treatment-resistant depression: naturalistic treatment outcomes for younger versus older patients. J Affect Disord. 2017;217:42–7.

Corriger A, Pickering G. Ketamine and depression: a narrative review. Drug Des Dev Ther. 2019;13: 3051–67.

Cotelli M, Manenti R, Cappa SF, et al. Effect of transcranial magnetic stimulation on action naming in patients with Alzheimer disease. Arch Neurol. 2006;63:1602–4.

Cotelli M, Manenti R, Cappa SF, et al. Transcranial magnetic stimulation improves naming in Alzheimer disease patients at different stages of cognitive decline. Eur J Neurol. 2008;15:1286–92.

Cotelli M, Calabria M, Manenti R, et al. Improved language performance in Alzheimer's disease following brain stimulation. J Neurol Neurosurg Psychiatry. 2011;82:794–7.

Cretaz E, Brunoni AR, Lafer B. Magnetic seizure therapy for unipolar and bipolar depression: a systematic review. Neural Plast. 2015;2015:521398.

da Frota M, Ribeiro C, Riva-Posse P. Use of ketamine in elderly patients with treatment-resistant depression. Curr Psychiatry Rep. 2017;19(12):1–5.

Dinur-Klein L, Dannon P, Hadar A, et al. Smoking cessation induced by deep repetitive transcranial magnetic stimulation of the prefrontal and insular cortices: a prospective, randomized controlled trial. Biol Psychiatry. 2014;76(9):742–9.

Drumond Marra HL, Myczkowski ML, Maia Memória C, et al. Transcranial magnetic stimulation to address mild cognitive impairment in the elderly: a randomized controlled study. Behav Neurol. 2015;2015:287843.

Dybedal GS, Tanum L, Sundet K, et al. Cognitive side-effects of electroconvulsive therapy in elderly depressed patients. Clin Neuropsychol. 2014;28:1071–90.

Dybedal GS, Tanum L, Sundet K, Bjølseth TM. The role of baseline cognitive function in the neurocognitive effects of electroconvulsive therapy in depressed elderly patients. Clin Neuropsychol. 2015;29(4):487–508.

Dybedal GS, Bjølseth TM, Benth JS, Tanum L. Cognitive effects of bifrontal versus right unilateral electroconvulsive therapy in the treatment of major depression in elderly patients: a randomized, controlled trial. J ECT. 2016;32(3):151–8.

Eldaief MC, Press DZ, Pascual-Leone A. Transcranial magnetic stimulation in neurology: a review of established and prospective applications. Neurol Clin Pract. 2013;3(6):519–26.

Engel A, Kayser S. An overview on clinical aspects in magnetic seizure therapy. J Neural Transm. 2016;123:1139–46.

Eser D, Schüle C, Rupprecht R, Baghai TC. Electroconvulsive therapy: update and new research. In: Marcolin MA, Padberg F, editors. Transcranial brain stimulation for treatment of psychiatric disorders. Karger; 2007. p. 1–17.

Fava M, Freeman MP, Flynn M, et al. Double-blind, placebo-controlled, dose-ranging trial of intravenous ketamine as adjunctive therapy in treatment-resistant depression (TRD). Mol Psychiatry. 2020;25(7):1592–603.

Fink M, Taylor MA. Electroconvulsive therapy: evidence and challenges. JAMA. 2007;298(3):330–2.

Fink M, Kellner CH, McCall WV. The role of ECT in suicide prevention. J ECT. 2014;30(1):5–9.

Fitzgerald PB, Daskalakis ZJ. In: Fitzgerald PB, Daskalakis ZJ, editors. The history of TMS and rTMS treatment of depression in repetitive transcranial magnetic stimulation treatment for depressive disorders. Berlin: Springer; 2013. p. 7–12.

Fitzgerald PB, Fountain S, Daskalakis ZJ. A comprehensive review of the effects of rTMS on motor cortical excitability and inhibition. Clin Neurophysiol. 2006;117(12):2584–96.

Fitzgibbon KP, Plett D, Chan BC, et al. Cost-utility analysis of electroconvulsive therapy and repetitive transcranial magnetic stimulation for treatment-resistant depression in Ontario. Can J Psychiatry. 2020;65(3):164–73.

Flint AJ, Gagnon N. Effective use of electroconvulsive therapy in late-life depression. Can J Psychiatry. 2002;47:734–41.

Gálvez V, Ho K, Alonzo A, et al. Neuromodulation therapies for geriatric depression. Curr Psychiatry Rep. 2015;17(7):59.

Geduldig ET, Kellner CH. Electroconvulsive therapy in the elderly: new findings in geriatric depression. Curr Psychiatry Rep. 2016;18:40.

George D, Gálvez V, Martin D, et al. Pilot randomized controlled trial of titrated subcutaneous ketamine in older patients with treatment-resistant depression. Am J Geriatr. 2017;25(11):1199–209.

Gershon AA, Dannon PN, Grunhaus L. Transcranial magnetic stimulation in the treatment of depression. Am J Psychiatry. 2003;160:835–45.

Greenberg RM, Kellner CH. Electroconvulsive therapy: a selected review. Am J Geriatr Psychiatry. 2005;13(4):268–81.

Grover S, Somaiya M. Electroconvulsive therapy in the elderly. J. Geriatr. Ment. Health. 2017;4(2):74–82.

Guse B, Falkai P, Wobrock T. Cognitive effects of high-frequency repetitive transcranial magnetic stimulation: a systematic review. J Neural Transm (Vienna). 2010;117(1):105–22.

Herbsman T, Avery D, Ramsey D, et al. More lateral and anterior prefrontal coil location is associated with better repetitive transcranial magnetic stimulation antidepressant response. Biol Psychiatry. 2009;66(5):509–15.

Iriarte IG, George MS. Transcranial magnetic stimulation (TMS) in the elderly. Curr Psychiatry Rep. 2018;20(1):6.

Janicak PG, Dowd SM, Marcolin MA, Rosa MA. Transcranial magnetic stimulation versus electroconvulsive therapy for the treatment of more severe major depression. In: Marcolin M, Padberg F, editors. Transcranial brain stimulation for treatment of psychiatric disorders. Karger Publishers; 2017. p. 97–109.

Johnson KA, Baig M, Ramsey D, et al. Prefrontal rTMS for treating depression: location and intensity results from the OPT-TMS multi-site clinical trial. Brain Stimul. 2013;6(2):108–17.

Jorge RE, Robinson RG. Treatment of late-life depression: a role of non-invasive brain stimulation techniques. Int Rev Psychiatry. 2011;23(5):437–44.

Kayser S, Bewernick BH, Grubert C, et al. Antidepressant effects, of magnetic seizure therapy and electroconvulsive therapy, in treatment-resistant depression. J Psychiatry Res. 2011;45:569–76.

Kedzior KK, Azorina V, Reitz SK. More female patients and fewer stimuli per session are associated with the short-term antidepressant properties of repetitive transcranial magnetic stimulation (rTMS): a meta-analysis of 54 sham-controlled studies published between 1997–2013. Neuropsychiatr Dis Treat. 2014;10:727–56.

Kellner CH, Knapp RG, Petrides G, et al. Continuation ECT versus pharmacotherapy for relapse prevention in major depression: a multi-site study from the consortium for research in electroconvulsive therapy (CORE). Arch Gen Psychiatry. 2006;63:1337–44.

Kellner CH, Husain MM, Knapp RG, et al. Right unilateral ultrabrief pulse ECT in geriatric depression: phase 1 of the PRIDE study. Am J Psychiatry. 2016a;173(11):1101–9.

Kellner CH, Husain MM, Knapp RG, et al. A novel strategy for continuation ECT in geriatric depression: phase 2 of the PRIDE study. Am J Psychiatry. 2016b;173(11):1110–8.

Kennedy SH, Lam RW, McIntyre RS, et al. CANMAT Depression Work Group. Canadian Network for Mood and Anxiety Treatments (CANMAT) 2016 Clinical Guidelines for the Management of Adults with Major Depressive Disorder: Section 3. Pharmacological Treatments. Can J Psychiatry. 2016;62(5):356

Kho KH, van Vreeswijk MF, Simpson S, Zwinderman AH. A meta-analysis of electroconvulsive therapy efficacy in depression. J ECT. 2003;19: 139–47.

Kim TD, Hong G, Kim J, et al. Cognitive enhancement in neurological and psychiatric disorders using transcranial magnetic stimulation (TMS): a review of modalities, potential mechanisms and future implications. Exp Neurobiol. 2019;28(1):1–16.

Kumar S, Mulsant BH, Liu AY, et al. Systematic review of cognitive effects of electroconvulsive therapy in late-life depression. Am J Geriatr Psychiatry. 2016;24:547–65.

Lee JC, Blumberger DM, Fitzgerald PB, et al. The role of transcranial magnetic stimulation in treatment-resistant depression: a review. Curr Pharm Des. 2012;18(36):5846–52.

Lefaucheur JP, André-Obadia N, Antal A, et al. Evidence-based guidelines on the therapeutic use of repetitive transcranial magnetic stimulation (rTMS). Clin Neurophysiol. 2014;125(11):2150–206.

Li X, Hartwell KJ, Owens M, et al. Repetitive transcranial magnetic stimulation of the dorsolateral prefrontal cortex reduces nicotine cue craving. Biol Psychiatry. 2013;73(8):714–20.

Liao X, Li G, Wang A, et al. Repetitive transcranial magnetic stimulation as an alternative therapy for cognitive impairment in Alzheimer's disease: a meta-analysis. J Alzheimers Dis. 2015;48:463–72.

Lisanby SH, Husain MM, Rosenquist PB, et al. Daily left prefrontal repetitive transcranial magnetic stimulation in the acute treatment of major depression: clinical predictors of outcome in a multisite, randomized controlled clinical trial. Neuropsychopharmacology. 2009;34(2):522–34.

Liu AY, Rajji TK, Blumberger DM, et al. Brain stimulation in the treatment of late-life severe mental illness other than unipolar nonpsychotic depression. Am J Geriatr Psychiatry. 2014;22:216–40.

Loo CK, Mitchell PB, Croker VM, et al. Double-blind controlled investigation of bilateral prefrontal transcranial magnetic stimulation for the treatment of resistant major depression. Psychol Med. 2003;33(1):33–40.

Loo CK, Alonzo A, Martin D, et al. Transcranial direct current stimulation for depression: 3-week, randomised, sham-controlled trial. Br J Psychiatry. 2012;200:52–9.

Luber B, McClintock SM, Lisanby SH. Applications of transcranial magnetic stimulation and magnetic seizure therapy in the study and treatment of disorders related to cerebral aging. Dialogues Clin Neurosci. 2013;15(1):87–98.

Luccarelli J, McCoy TH Jr, Seiner SJ, Henry ME. Maintenance ECT is associated with sustained improvement in depression symptoms without adverse cognitive effects in a retrospective cohort of 100 patients each receiving 50 or more ECT treatments. J Affect Disord. 2020;271:109–14.

Luo J, Zheng H, Zhang L, et al. High-frequency repetitive transcranial magnetic stimulation (rTMS) improves functional recovery by enhancing neurogenesis and activating BDNF/TrkB signaling in ischemic rats. Int J Mol Sci. 2017;18(2):455.

Ma SM, Ni JX, Li XY, et al. High-frequency repetitive transcranial magnetic stimulation reduces pain in postherpetic neuralgia. Pain Med. 2015;16(11):2162–70.

Manenti R, Cotelli M, Miniussi C. Successful physiological aging and episodic memory: a brain stimulation study. Behav Brain Res. 2011;216(1):153–8.

Manenti R, Cotelli M, Robertson IH, Miniussi C. Transcranial brain stimulation studies of episodic memory in young adults, elderly adults and individuals with memory dysfunction: a review. Brain Stimul. 2012;5(2):103–9.

McIntyre RS. Ketamine and esketamine for treatment-resistant depression: response to Reus, Mattes, and Schatzberg. Am J Psychiatry. 2021;178(12):1130–2. https://doi.org/10.1176/appi.ajp.2021.21060653r.

McIntyre RS, Rosenblat JD, Nemeroff CB, et al. Synthesizing the evidence for ketamine and esketamine in treatment-resistant depression: an international expert opinion on the available evidence and implementation. Am J Psychiatry. 2021;178(5):383–99.

Meyer JP, Swetter SK, Kellner CH. Electroconvulsive therapy in geriatric psychiatry. Psychiatr Clin N Am. 2018;41:79–93.

Meyer JP, Swetter SK, Kellner CH. Electroconvulsive therapy in geriatric psychiatry: a selective review. Clin Geriatr Med. 2020;36(2):265–79.

Milev RV, Giacobbe P, Kennedy SH, et al. Canadian Network for Mood and Anxiety Treatments (CANMAT) 2016 clinical guidelines for the management of adults with major depressive disorder: section 4. Neurostimulation treatments. Can J Psychiatry. 2016;61(9):561–75.

Molero P, Ramos-Quiroga JA, Martin-Santos R, et al. Antidepressant efficacy and tolerability of ketamine and esketamine: a critical review. CNS Drugs. 2018;32(5):411–20.

Morrison RL, Fedgchin M, Singh J, et al. Effect of intranasal esketamine on cognitive functioning in healthy participants: a randomized, double-blind, placebo-controlled study. Psychopharmacology. 2018;235(4):1107–19.

Muller J, Pentyala S, Dilger J, Pentyala S. Ketamine enantiomers in the rapid and sustained antidepressant effects. Ther Adv Psychopharmacol. 2016;6(3):185–92.

Murrough JW, Wan LB, Iacoviello B, et al. Neurocognitive effects of ketamine in treatment-resistant major depression: association with antidepressant response. Psychopharmacology. 2013;231:481–8.

Nahas Z, Li X, Kozel FA, et al. Safety and benefits of distance-adjusted prefrontal transcranial magnetic stimulation in depressed patients 55–75 years of age: a pilot study. Depress Anxiety. 2004;19(4):249–56.

Nardone R, Tezzon F, Höller Y, et al. Transcranial magnetic stimulation (TMS)/repetitive TMS in mild cognitive impairment and Alzheimer's disease. Acta Neurol Scand. 2014;129(6):351–66.

Navarro V, Gasto C, Torres X, et al. Continuation/maintenance treatment with nortriptyline versus combines nortriptyline and ECT in late life psychotic depression: a 2-year randomized study. Am J Geriatr Psychiatry. 2008;16:498–505.

Ochs-Ross R, Daly EJ, Zhang Y, et al. Efficacy and safety of esketamine nasal spray plus an oral antidepressant in elderly patients with treatment-resistant depression-TRANSFORM-3. Am J Geriatr Psychiatry. 2020;28(2):121–41.

Pallanti S, Cantisani A, Grassi G, et al. rTMS age-dependent response in treatment-resistant depressed subjects: a mini-review. CNS Spectr. 2012;17(1):24–30.

Park MJ, Kim H, Kim EJ, et al. Recent updates on electro-convulsive therapy in patients with depression. Psychiatry Investig. 2021;18(1):1–10.

Peterchev AV, Wagner TA, Miranda PC, et al. Fundamentals of transcranial electric and magnetic stimulation dose: definition, selection, and reporting practices. Brain Stimul. 2012;5(4):435–53.

Phillips JL, Norris S, Talbot J, et al. Single and repeated ketamine infusions for reduction of suicidal ideation in treatment-resistant depression. Neuropsychopharmacology. 2020;45(4):606–12.

Popova V, Daly EJ, Trivedi M, et al. Efficacy and safety of flexibly dosed esketamine nasal spray combined with a newly initiated oral antidepressant in treatment-resistant depression: a randomized double-blind active-controlled study. Am J Psychiatry. 2019;176(6):428–38.

Rabey JM, Dobronevsky E, Aichenbaum S, et al. Repetitive transcranial magnetic stimulation combined with cognitive training is a safe and effective modality for the treatment of Alzheimer's disease: a randomized, double-blind study. J Neural Transm (Vienna). 2013;120:813–9.

Rachid F. Maintenance repetitive transcranial magnetic stimulation (rTMS) for relapse prevention in with depression: a review. Psychiatry Res. 2018;262:363–72.

Rami-González L, Salamero M, Boget T, et al. Pattern of cognitive dysfunction in depressive patients during maintenance electroconvulsive therapy. Psychol Med. 2003;33(2):345–50.

Rhebergen D, Huisman A, Bouckaert F, et al. Older age is associated with rapid remission of depression after electroconvulsive therapy: a latent class growth analysis. Am J Geriatr Psychiatry. 2015;23(3):274–82.
Rosen BH, Kung S, Lapid MI. Effect of age on psychiatric rehospitalization rates after electroconvulsive therapy for patients with depression. J ECT. 2016;32(2):93–8.
Rosenberg O, Shoenfeld N, Kotler M, Dannon PN. Mood disorders in elderly population: neurostimulative treatment possibilities. Recent Pat CNS Drug Discov. 2009;4:149–55.
Rossi S, Hallett M, Rossini PM, et al. Safety, ethical considerations, and application guidelines for the use of transcranial magnetic stimulation in clinical practice and research. Clin Neurophysiol. 2009;120:2008–39.
Rusjan PM, Barr MS, Farzan F, et al. Optimal transcranial magnetic stimulation coil placement for targeting the dorsolateral prefrontal cortex using novel magnetic resonance image-guided neuronavigation. Hum Brain Mapp. 2010;31(11):1643–52.
Rybak YE, Lai KSP, Ramasubbu R, et al. Treatment-resistant major depressive disorder: Canadian expert consensus on definition and assessment. Depress Anxiety. 2021;38(4):456–67.
Sabesan P, Lankappa S, Khalifa N, et al. Transcranial magnetic stimulation for geriatric depression: promises and pitfalls. World J Psychiatry. 2015;5:170–81.
Serra M, Gastó C, Navarro V, et al. Maintenance electroconvulsive therapy in elderly psychotic unipolar depression. Med Clin (Barc). 2006;126(13):491–2.
Shiozawa P, da Silva ME, Cordeiro Q. Transcranial direct current stimulation for treating depression in a patient with right hemispheric dominance: a case study. J ECT. 2015;31(3):201–2.
Singh JB, Fedgchin M, Daly E, et al. Intravenous esketamine in adult treatment-resistant depression: s double-blind, double-randomization, placebo-controlled study. Biol Psychiatry. 2016;80(6):424–31.
Smith GE, Rasmussen KG, Cullum M, et al. A randomized controlled trial comparing the memory effects of continuation electroconvulsive therapy versus continuation pharmacotherapy: results from the consortium for research in ECT (CORE) study. J Clin Psychiatry. 2010;71:185–93.
Solé Pedullés C, Bartres-Faz D, Junque C, et al. Repetitive transcranial magnetic stimulation effects on brain function and cognition among elders with memory dysfunction. A randomized sham-controlled study. Cereb Cortex. 2006;16(10):1487–93.
Spaans HP, Sienaert P, Bouckaert F, et al. Speed of remission in elderly patients with depression: electroconvulsive therapy v. medication. Br J Psychiatry. 2015;206(1):67–71.
Stek ML, van der Wurff FB, Hoogendijk WJ, Beekman AT. Electroconvulsive therapy for the depressed elderly. CSRS. 2003;2015:CD003593.
Stoppe A, Louzã M, Rosa M, et al. Fixed high-dose electroconvulsive therapy in the elderly with depression: a double-blind, randomized comparison of efficacy and tolerability between unilateral and bilateral electrode placement. J ECT. 2006;22(2):92–9.
Subramanian S, Lenze EJ. Ketamine for depression in older adults. Am J Geriatr Psychiatry. 2021;29(9):914–6.
Tang VM, Blumberger DM, Dimitrova J, et al. Magnetic seizure therapy is efficacious and well tolerated for treatment-resistant bipolar depression: an open-label clinical trial. J Psychiatry Neurosci. 2020;45(5):313–21.
Tatti E, Rossi S, Innocenti I, et al. Non-invasive brain stimulation of the aging brain: state of the art and future perspectives. Ageing Res Rev. 2016;29:66–89.
Tielkes CEM, Comijs HC, Verwijk E, Stek ML. The effects of ECT on cognitive functioning in the elderly: a review. Int J Geriatr Psychiatry. 2008;23:789–5.
Trevizol AP, Goldberger KW, Mulsant BH, et al. Unilateral and bilateral repetitive transcranial magnetic stimulation for treatment-resistant late-life depression. Int J Geriatr Psychiatry. 2019;34(6):822–7.
Tripathi S. In: Tripathi S, editor. Manual of geriatric anesthesia, vol. 1. New York: Springer; 2013.
Van der Wurff FB, Stek ML, Hoogendijk WJ, Beekman AT. The efficacy and safety of ECT in depressed older adults: a literature review. Int J Geriatr Psychiatry. 2003;18:894–904.
Van Dierman L, van den Ameele S, Kamperman AM, et al. Prediction of electroconvulsive therapy response and remission in major depression: meta-analysis. Br J Psychiatry. 2018;212:71–80.
Van Schaik AM, Comijs HC, Sonnenberg CM, et al. Efficacy and safety of continuation and maintenance electroconvulsive therapy in depressed elderly patients. Am J Geriatr Psychiatry. 2012;20:5–17.
Veraart J, Smith-Apeldoorn SY, Spaans HP, Kamphuis J, et al. Is ketamine an appropriate alternative to ECT for patients with treatment resistant depression: a systematic review. J Affect Disord. 2021;281:82–9.
Wagenmakers MJ, Oudega ML, Vansteelandt K, Spaans H-P, et al. Psychotic late-life depression less likely to relapse after electroconvulsive therapy. J Affect Disord. 2020;276(1):984–90.
Wu Y, Xu W, Liu X, et al. Adjunctive treatment with high frequency repetitive transcranial magnetic stimulation for the behavioral and psychological symptoms of patients with Alzheimer's disease: a randomized, double-blind, sham-controlled study. Shanghai Arch Psychiatry. 2015;27(5):280–8.
Xia G, Gajwani P, Muzina DJ, et al. Treatment-emergent mania in unipolar and bipolar depression: focus on repetitive transcranial magnetic stimulation. Int J Neuropsychopharmacol. 2008;11(1):119–30.
Xie J, Chen J, Wei Q. Repetitive transcranial magnetic stimulation versus electroconvulsive therapy for major depression: a meta-analysis of stimulus parameter effects. Neurol Res. 2013;35:1084–91.
Zarate CA, Singh JB, Carlson PJ, et al. A randomized trial of an *N*-methyl-D-aspartate antagonist in treatment-resistant major depression. Arch Gen Psychiatry. 2006;63(8):856–64.
Zibman S, Pell GS, Barnea-Ygael N, et al. Application of transcranial magnetic stimulation for major depression: coil design and neuroanatomical variability considerations. Eur Neuropsychopharmacol. 2019;45:73–88.

Psychotherapeutic Interventions 15

Erin Cassidy-Eagle and Rita Hitching

Abstract

Psychotherapeutic strategies need to adapt to the geriatric patient, rather than the other way around. In the United States, the population of adults aged 65 and older is projected to increase from 40.3 million to 72.1 million from 2010 to 2030. Older adults with mental health conditions and major neurocognitive disorder (MNCD) contribute disproportionately to rising healthcare costs. Yet, the number of geriatric mental health specialists is inadequate (Institute of Medicine, The mental health and substance use workforce for older adults. In: Whose hands? Washington, DC: The National Academies Press, 2012), making alternative treatment models a necessity. This chapter reviews common psychotherapeutic strategies which provide alternatives to excessive medication treatment or unnecessary interventions:

- Meeting the patient where he/she/they are, both geographically and psychologically
- Adapting to each individual's unique limitations, needs, and potential reluctance
- Incorporating a mix of modalities and activities which engage the patient
- Promoting as therapists those people who already interact with the patient
- Encouraging choice, independence, and an individual's unique perspectives

Psychotherapies for older adults need to accommodate to different social-environmental contexts, rather than only to the *older age* of the patients (Knight BG, Psychotherapy with older adults, 3rd ed., 2004). Older adults have shown a preference for self-management strategies that fit with their lived experiences, such as increasing their socialization or prayer, but also express willingness to consider professional services like psychotherapy in more severe cases (Nair et al., Gerontologist 60:e93–e104, 2020). Older adults living in the community rated combination (therapy + medication) as more acceptable and preferable over medication alone (Hanson and Scogin, J Gerontol B Psychol Sci Soc Sci 63:P245–P248, 2008). Psychological treatments that are effective in young adults are equally effective in older adults (Scogin and McElreath, J Consult Clin Psychol 62:69–74, 1994). There is a need to

E. Cassidy-Eagle (✉)
Department of Psychiatry and Behavioral Services, Stanford University School of Medicine, Palo Alto, CA, USA
e-mail: ecassidy@stanford.edu

R. Hitching
University of Newcastle, Newcastle, NSW, Australia

H. H. Fenn et al. (eds.), *Age-Adjusted Psychiatric Treatment for the Older Patient*,
https://doi.org/10.1007/978-3-031-53976-3_15

foster greater participation, access, and better outcomes for the growing proportion of aging individuals.

Case Example

A 79-year-old woman fell and fractured her hip, limiting her ambulation. At the family's insistence, she moved into an assisted living apartment. The daughter noticed a change in demeanor, energy, mood, and motivation within one month of the move. The patient did not often go to the dining room for meals and instead ate snacks in her room. She avoided other residents, even after the restrictions for COVID lifted and the rate of infection diminished drastically. She participated in physical therapy only *intermittently* and left early with the excuse that she was too tired, although she was noted to have good stamina before the move. The patient had little interest or joy in her prior activities, such as reading, and she began to talk about "the end," although there was no terminal illness or chronic, progressive disease.

At the request of her daughter for more check-ins, an onsite care manager began to visit regularly and have brief meals with her in the dining room. The topics focused first on death, salvation, and whether suicide was appropriate. Discussions evolved into her legacy, her grandchildren, and their accomplishments. The patient was able to identify some previously enjoyed activities and was encouraged to take small steps to reengage in new opportunities. Within 6 weeks, the patient began to share meals with others and joined a mahjong club. Grandchildren visited, and over the next year, many depressive symptoms diminished.

Adaptive Psychotherapeutics

Evidenced-based psychotherapies found effective with younger adults can show similar success with older patients, albeit with accommodations for scheduling, sensory limitations, and energy level. A *maturity-specific challenge model* acknowledges the greater wisdom of older adults and the challenges of chronic illness, loss of function, and grieving (Knight 2004). The Contextual Adult Lifespan Theory for Adapting Psychotherapy (CALTAP) is a transtheoretical and transdiagnostic approach (Knight and Pachana 2015), which incorporates the cohort (its cultural norms and experiences), social context (e.g., community-based versus residential care), and specific challenges associated with aging, as well as perceptions and reactions of the therapist.

Older adults bring a lifetime of experience to the task of optimal aging. The therapist, likely with fewer life experiences, must recognize these abilities and acknowledge these strengths as part of collaborative work. Although the theories of behavior change may differ between various orientations, in practice the collaborative work between therapist and patient is often best supported by integrating tools from more than one model. Psychotherapy can focus on aspects of the older patient's life, not all of which accrue to older age. Indeed, chronological age may be the *least* important issue in conceptualizing a case. This approach is embraced in *positive psychology*, which emphasizes the older individual's strengths (Seligman and Csikszentmihalyi 2000) and their resilience, reminiscence, life review, and wisdom.

Psychotherapeutic Modalities

Psychodynamic therapy, cognitive behavioral therapy (CBT), behavioral activation (BA), problem-solving therapy (PST), interpersonal psychotherapy (IP), and motivational interviewing (MI) have been around the longest and have evolved. Dialectical behavior therapy (DBT), acceptance and commitment therapy (ACT), and mindfulness-based therapies (e.g., mindfulness-based stress reduction/MBSR, being one variant) have developed more recently. The latter approaches shift the focus of therapy away from changing thoughts and emotions to *observation and acceptance*. Most approaches also include psychoeducation to facilitate a deeper understanding of the biopsychosocial context of the identified targets for change. Each therapeutic approach is discussed below.

Psychodynamic Approaches

Iterations and duration of psychodynamic psychotherapy have been found effective for a range of psychiatric conditions (Shedler 2010), including weekly sessions, time-limited (brief psychodynamic therapy), or open-ended duration. Exploring developmental experiences that shaped the patient can elucidate factors that carry over to present-day functioning and relationships. There is evidence that exploring the following topics, among others, can improve depressive symptoms in older adults (Shedler 2010; Thompson et al. 1987):

- Affect and expression of emotion
- Attempts to avoid distressing thoughts and feelings
- Identification of recurring themes and patterns
- Past experience and developmental issues
- Interpersonal relations
- The therapist-patient relationship
- Fantasy life

Brief psychodynamic therapy has been compared favorably to CBT for older adults with major depression; studies of outcome showed equivalent symptom improvement (Gallagher-Thompson and Steffen 1994). A longitudinal, effectiveness study reviewed psychodynamic psychotherapy for older adults aged 60–89 years old. Chart notes documented symptoms at 3-month intervals over more than 4 years and revealed large, positive effects of the intervention (effect size = 0.8) with little deterioration over time (Roseborough et al. 2013). Although manuals and protocol-based psychotherapy interventions have emerged, psychodynamically oriented skills may still benefit any therapeutic interaction given their focus on insight and consideration of developmental experiences that can be the basis of some emotional problems later in life. Models of psychodynamic approaches that integrate techniques and tools introduced in cognitive behavioral therapy (CBT; described in more detail below) have emerged. In a recent book by Busch (2019), a framework of problem behaviors and how to facilitate behavior change were reviewed. This approach incorporates an analysis of the problematic behavior, as well as the context and developmental origins. Next, the model includes working with the patient to identifying alternative behaviors that, through trial and error in a series of homework assignments, can bring about lasting change (Busch 2019).

Cognitive Behavioral Therapy (CBT)

This widely used therapeutic modality was developed by Aaron Beck, MD, a psychodynamically trained psychiatrist, to treat chronic depression. It recognizes a *negative cognitive triad* (negative view about oneself, one's experiences, and the future) (Beck 1979) and confronts unrealistic thoughts with real-world validity, encouraging a shift in perspective and a more balanced view of oneself or a situation. This *cognitive reframing* can result in a reduction in depressive symptomatology. A broader model of CBT incorporates thoughts, behaviors, feelings, and physical health (Steffen et al. 2022).

The efficacy of CBT for depression is supported by considerable research findings. A meta-analysis reviewed 16 methodologically rigorous studies of adults of all ages, focusing on effect sizes that contrast outcomes for CBT with outcomes for various control conditions across disorders. Moderate to large effect sizes were found with CBT for unipolar depression and other psychiatric conditions (e.g., generalized anxiety disorder, posttraumatic stress disorder, social phobia) (Butler et al. 2006). A Cochrane review reported that CBT was superior to active control interventions for depression in older adults (Wilson et al. 2008).

CBT for older adults was also reviewed in a meta-analysis of 17 studies that compared a psychological treatment with an active control condition (Cuijpers et al. 2006). Moderate to large effect sizes (Cohen's $d = 0.72$ on average) for psychotherapy with older adults (Cuijpers et al. 2006) were similar to effect sizes reported by Butler et al. (2006) for adults in general.

In sum, there is a strong evidence supporting CBT as an effective form of psychotherapy for older adults, particularly those who prefer non-pharmacological treatments, with results comparable to studies of younger adults. Duration of CBT is typically 12–16 sessions, intended to be discrete and goal-oriented, with or without pharmacotherapy; its long-term success includes identifying unhelpful thought patterns and learning techniques to modify them. Caveat: before a course of CBT, cognitive capacity may need assessment, especially the ability to learn new ways of thinking and engage in new behaviors and the ability to discuss thoughts in detail.

Behavioral Activation (BA)

This brief, effective, empirically validated treatment for depression of mild-to-moderate severity builds upon a foundation of CBT theory, including frail and medically ill older adults. It derives from the principle that behavioral change can impact thoughts and emotions and can be implemented by a range of care providers (i.e., social work, primary care physicians) after brief training. One study reported noticeable mood improvement after 2–4 weeks (Armento et al. 2012; Hopko et al. 2009). Several meta-analyses have documented the effectiveness of BA as a solo treatment for depression, including studies with older adults (Au et al. 2015; Cuijpers et al. 2007; Gum et al. 2016; Kanter et al. 2010; Samad et al. 2011).

BA has been found cost-effective, delivered by supervised non-specialty clinicians (Raue et al. 2019) and by mental health professionals (Dimidjian et al. 2011; Richards et al. 2016). Its flexibility and self-guided qualities are particularly suited for a minimalist approach.

Various adaptations of BA protocols for older adults (Pasterfield et al. 2014) focus on ameliorating loneliness and isolation (Polenick and Flora 2013). Common strategies include decreasing avoidance and depression-fueling behaviors (e.g., physical inactivity, social isolation, time spent ruminating) and increasing the number and types of pleasant activities and engagement strategies (e.g., exercising, spending time with family and friends, attending and engaging in community-based activities).

BA can facilitate a therapeutic experience for those who are socially isolated with few positive experiences in daily life (Polenick and Flora 2013). To facilitate success, it is helpful to talk through anticipated obstacles and problem-solve challenges or avoidance behaviors that might get in the way. Setting specific goals that are measurable, achievable, realistic, and timebound (think SMART goals) can be an extremely useful approach. Family members, friends, or caregivers can support the patient to enhance the chances of successful engagement in BA.

Problem-Solving Therapy (PST)

Reduction of negative physical and mental health outcomes can be pursued by increasing skill in problem-solving. PST focuses on identifying problems (i.e., who, what, when, what has been tried, do you have control?) which generate possible solutions and encourage implementation. After possible solutions or new coping strategies are used, the discussion focuses on results. Overarching goals include helping the patient to see problems as solvable, increasing self-efficacy, and bolstering ability to initiate effective solutions. The therapist does not generate the solutions but utilizes the Socratic method to elicit ideas from the patient (Kropf et al. 2017). Evidence has found PST effective for older adults with depression (Kirkham et al. 2016), as well as older depressed patients with executive dysfunction and other comorbid disabilities (Kiosses and Alexopoulos 2014).

Interpersonal Therapy (IPT)

Attachment theory underpins this modality and recognizes the impact of interpersonal stressors such as grief and loss, role transitions, interpersonal disputes, and interpersonal sensitivity, all common in the geriatric age group. The prevalence of loneliness in older adults has been exacerbated by a pandemic, which underscores how social skills can enhance social connections. IPT for the depression that can result from isolation, along with other root causes, often examines all of ones' relationships as they are the mechanism for symptom expression as well as possible healing. One study of IPT reported significant reductions in suicidal ideation, depressive symptoms, and improvement in meaning in life, social adjustment, and perceived social support, among other variables related to well-being (Heisel et al. 2015). A review of studies utilizing IPT with older adults (Miller 2006) found it to be efficacious alone and in combination with pharmacotherapy and reported its being explored for use in patients with cognitive impairment.

Motivational Interviewing (MI)

This modality consists of a structured discussion around specific changes, whether starting or stopping behaviors (e.g., use of substances or a new health-related behavior). The goal is to motivate engagement in the work needed for success. The therapist addresses the patient's feelings of ambivalence and helps develop a sustainable action plan. Fundamental principles typically covered include expressing empathy, developing discrepancy, rolling with resistance, and supporting self-efficacy (Kropf et al. 2017). Studies focused on older patients have explored the effect of office-based MI on prescription opioid adherence among older adults with chronic pain ($N = 30$). Over a 4-week study of MI, older adults showed a significant reduction in the risk of opioid misuse and alcohol consumption and reduced pain intensity (Chang et al. 2015). Although some studies were good examples of successful implementation, there are mixed results in use of MI with older adults. For example, one large study with community-dwelling older adults found MI lacking as it was difficult for participants to identify treatment goals that are amenable to the behavior change process. Care providers also felt it was hard to implement given the level of training they had received (Rietkerk et al. 2021).

Acceptance and Commitment Therapy (ACT)

This "third-wave behavioral intervention" focuses on the internal experience. ACT grew out of the practice of accepting thoughts and emotions without actively trying to change them, shifting the target of therapy away from trying to *change* ideations. The theoretical model stipulates that the cause of suffering is attachment to unhelpful thoughts, lack of psychological flexibility, lack of connection to our core values, and lack of contact with the present moment (Hayes et al. 1999). The six key ACT processes include defusion, acceptance, attention to the present moment, perspective taking, values, and committed action.

ACT has been found effective in older adults with mixed depression and anxiety (Petkus and Wetherell 2013), decreasing worry and depression in older adults suffering from generalized anxiety disorder (Wetherell et al. 2011a, b) as well as pain interference, depression, and pain-related anxiety (Wetherell et al. 2011a, b). ACT has also been implemented in groups of older veterans who showed improvement in symptoms of depression (Jacobs et al. 2018).

Dialectical Behavior Therapy (DBT)

Developed to treat suicidal behavior (Linehan 1987), this modality addresses acceptance and tolerance of distressing feelings and emotions. Few studies have focused on older adults, but one showed feasibility and effectiveness for personality disorders and depression (Lynch et al. 2007).

Mindfulness-Based Therapies

Similar to ACT, these therapies focus on how individuals relate to and accept their thoughts and emotions, instead of active efforts to change them. The targeted techniques are applied individually or in groups to teach mindfulness in various activities and meditation. Mindfulness-based stress reduction (MBSR) emphasizes a mind-body connection to enhance awareness of bodily sensations, surrounding environment, and mental states. Therapists encourage patients to observe thoughts and emotions in a nonjudgmental way with a focus on staying nonreactive. Psychoeducation, meditation exercises, and sometimes yoga practice are included. Therapy courses are 10 weeks as designed by Kabat-Zinn (1982) but can vary in duration depending on targeted outcomes. Research with older adults has found MSBR to lower depression scores and increase mindfulness skills, acceptance, and overall quality of life (Mathur et al. 2016). MSBR can also decrease worry and improve aspects of cognitive functioning, specifically memory and recall (Lenze et al. 2014).

Group Therapy

Individual psychotherapy is not always feasible nor always more effective than group therapy. Groups not only harness the power of social connection but offer a cost-effective and efficient means to reach a broad range of older patients who might otherwise be unable to access care.

Several studies have found psychotherapy treatment groups, for older adults suffering from a range of mental health conditions, effective in alleviating suffering. In a group of depressed elderly, an RCT of eight sessions of cognitive-behavioral *group* therapy (STEpS), conducted while participants were wait-listed for individual therapy, was effective and improved both depression and health-related quality of life ratings (Ruesch et al. 2017). A systematic review of studies examining the efficacy of group therapy for depression in older adults found significant improvements in mood across a range of settings, protocols, and participant characteristics (Tavares and Barbosa 2018). Groups are also effective vehicles for facilitating psychoeducational interventions for larger groups. For example, psychoeducational groups for older adults have successfully focused on treating mixed anxiety and depression in community-dwelling older adults (Bains et al. 2014) and healthy lifestyle behaviors to support optimal brain health in a population of veterans (Verstaen et al. 2020).

Therapeutic Interventions for Major Neurocognitive Disorder (MNCD)

The worldwide prevalence of MNCD is between 2 and 9% (Farina et al. 2020) and is predicted to double every 20 years. The US Preventive Service Task (US Preventive Services Task Force et al. 2020) report noted that dementia affects between 2.4 and 5.5 million Americans; prevalence increases with age. The 47 million people with MNCD worldwide is expected to increase to 131 million by 2050 (Arvanitakis et al. 2019) (Fig. 15.1).

Behavioral and psychiatric symptoms have been estimated in up to 98% of people with MNCD (Magierski and Sobow 2016; Phan et al. 2019). Such neuropsychiatric symptoms (NPS) increase morbidity and mortality, family and caregiver burden, nursing home placement, and healthcare system strain (Bessey and Walaszek 2019; Burley et al. 2020; Kales et al. 2014; Liu et al. 2017; Polenick et al. 2020; Terracciano et al. 2020).

Nonpharmacological treatment strategies are the first line of intervention for neuropsychiatric symptoms (NPS) associated with mild neurocognitive disorder and MNCD. Psychotherapeutic modalities for MNCD can be categorized into four primary domains (Fig. 15.2): *cognition*, *emotion*, *behavior*, and *stimulation* (Carrion et al. 2018). Psychotherapeutic approaches need to adapt to individuals with different economic and cultural backgrounds, familial situations, living situations (e.g., home, assisted living facility, psychiatric hospital), geographies, and mobilities. The D-I-C-E process for developing indi-

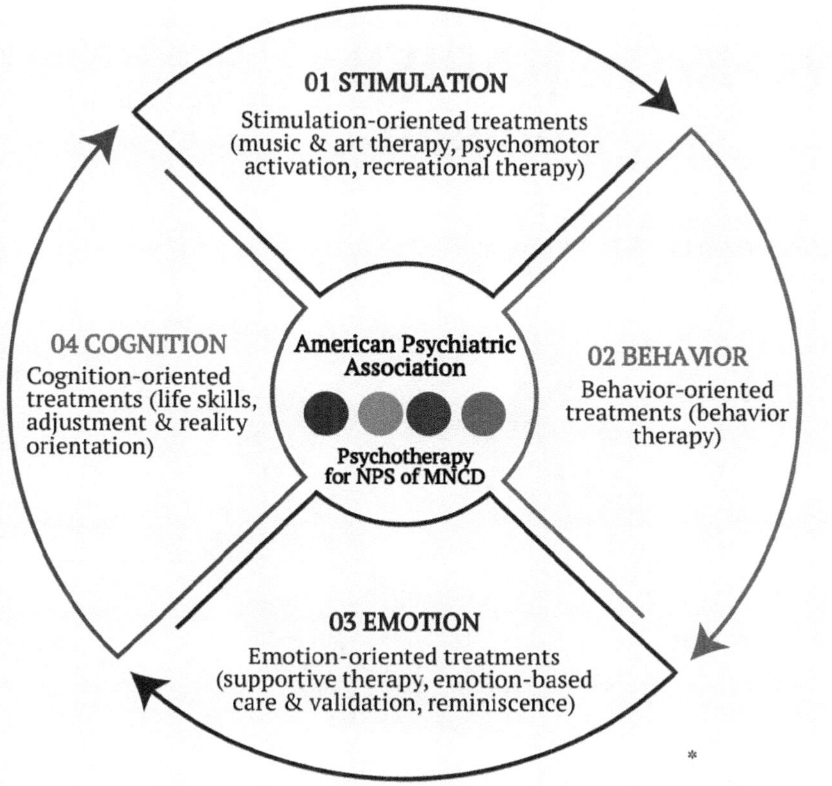

(Rita Hitching, MSc)

Fig. 15.1 Psychotherapeutic interventions for neuropsychiatric symptoms (NPS) of major neurocognitive disorder (American Psychiatric Association) (Rita Hitching, MSc)

vidualized strategy for behavioral and psychological symptoms of dementia (BPSD) is described in Chap. 5 (Kales et al. 2014).

Approaches that employ telehealth and digital technologies may be cost-effective and help fill gaps in access. Therapeutic strategies detailed in the reference to follow include a range of non-pharmacological interventions, including physical exercise, sleep treatments, nutritional treatments, meditation, and multisensory treatments. Treatments are adapted to meet the level of cognitive impairment and functioning of the patient and can be designed to incorporate caregivers and necessary environmental modifications (Sikkes et al. 2021).

The benefit from psychotherapeutic interventions for MNCD can be bolstered by assessment of the following:

- Cognitive impairment: which tailors the group to the individual's limitations and needs.
- Physical comorbidities, language limitations, or sensory deficits (e.g., hearing or speech impediments), medication adverse effects, depression or anxiety, and pain.
- Early-onset psychiatric conditions and pre-existing mental disorders (PMD) need to be identified and treated (Kuring et al. 2020).
- Depression and anxiety, which may not necessarily be sequelae of dementia, although they can be prodromes and symptoms of NPS. Depression is underdiagnosed (Starkstein et al. 2018).
- Overlap of symptoms in depression and MNCD, such as poor concentration, apathy, sleep, and appetite changes, need monitoring as treatment course may differ based on etiology (Leyhe et al. 2017).

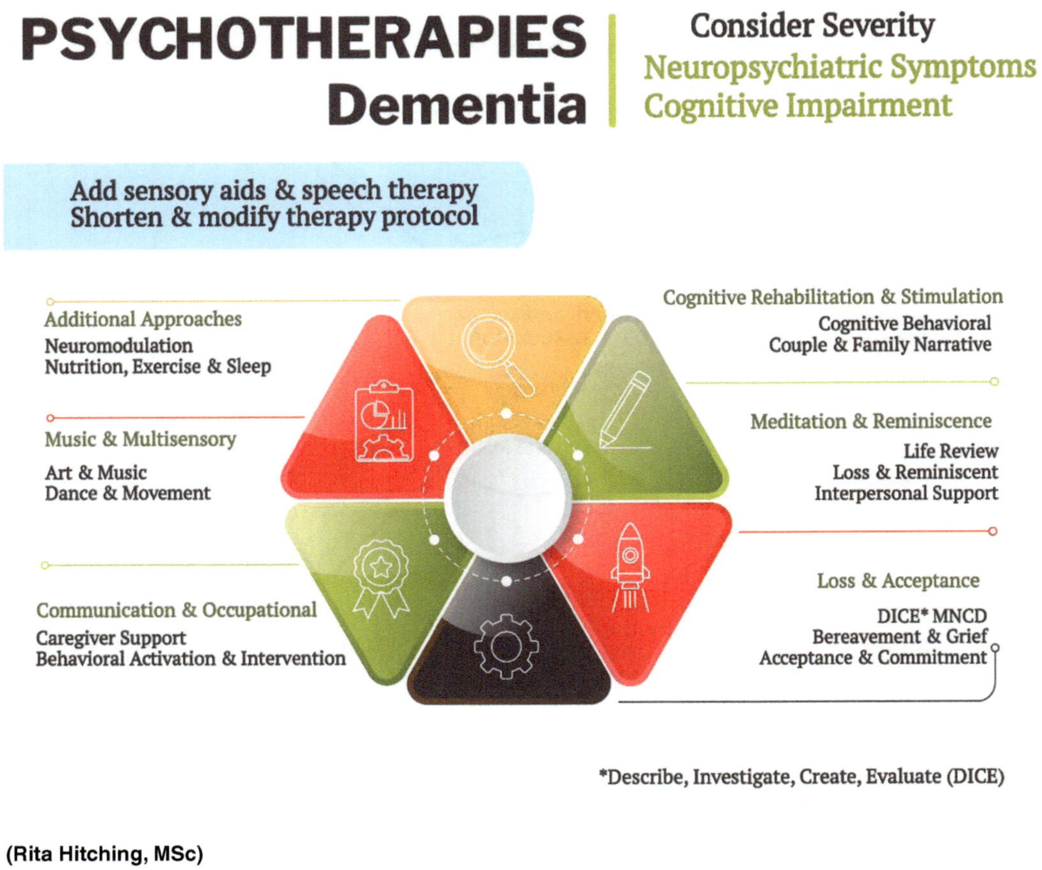

Fig. 15.2 Psychotherapeutic interventions for MNCD (Rita Hitching, MSc)

- The need for adaptations to accommodate fatigue (shortening sessions), language deficits (memory cards), sensory limits (hearing and visual aids), and learning (e.g., text reminders for homework activities) (see Chap. 16).

Cognitive Rehabilitation and Stimulation

Treatment focused on retaining social, emotional, and functional abilities impacted by cognitive dysfunction, especially those that interfere with activities of daily living (ADLs), can delay the transition to assisted living settings or acute hospitalization. Cognition-based therapies such as problem-solving therapy (PST), cognitive behavioral therapy (CBT), and life review therapy (LRT) have all been found to benefit NPS in mild cognitive impairment, while helping family and caregivers manage what for them is “a different person” (Cuijpers et al. 2014). An RCT of patients with mild cognitive impairment (mCI) and MNCD reported the effectiveness of CBT, cognitive rehabilitation, and reminiscence therapy, with significant improvement to depression symptoms, often persisting 6 months posttreatment (Tonga et al. 2021).

Conclusions

The young-old and oldest-old, with significant physical limitations or without, with cognitive impairments, or none, can all engage in therapeutic interactions and activities that can improve quality of life. To apply these techniques effectively, an understanding of the patient's strengths, limitations, coping mechanisms, cognition, and physical environment may be more important than chronological age. Telehealth, mobile digital applications, and web-based psychoeducation and interventions will likely enhance access to psychotherapeutic approaches in the future.

Age-Adjusted Recommendations

- Acknowledge the strength and resilience of the geriatric patient.
- Recognize efforts to change, regardless of how small.
- Collaborate with other clinicians, family, and caregivers.
- Encourage the maintenance and development of social networks to combat isolation.
- Adapt interventions to the patient: where to meet, how long, and goals.
- Accommodate to age-related changes in sensory, cognitive, and physical functioning (e.g., brighter rooms, accommodate assistive devices, print materials in 14-point font, simplify instructions).
- Minimize transitions of location and social group, and support aging in place where possible.
- Meet the patient on her/his/their terms and set expectations to address practical topics, for example, budgeting and logistics.
- Recognize that chronological age may not determine outcome.
- Avoid stereotypes and assumptions based on age.

References

Armento ME, McNulty JK, Hopko DR. Behavioral activation of religious behaviors (BARB): randomized trial with depressed college students. Psychol Relig Spiritual. 2012;4(3):206–22.

Arvanitakis Z, Shah RC, Bennett DA. Diagnosis and management of dementia: review. JAMA. 2019;322(16):1589–99.

Au A, Gallagher-Thompson D, Wong MK, et al. Behavioral activation for dementia caregivers: scheduling pleasant events and enhancing communications. Clin Interv Aging. 2015;10:611–9.

Bains MK, Scott S, Kellett S, Saxon D. Group psychoeducative cognitive-behavioral therapy for mixed anxiety and depression with older adults. Aging Ment Health. 2014;18(8):1057–65.

Beck AT. Cognitive therapy of depression. New York: Guilford Press; 1979.

Bessey LJ, Walaszek A. Management of behavioral and psychological symptoms of dementia. Curr Psychiatry Rep. 2019;21(8):66.

Burley CV, Livingston G, Knapp MR, et al. Time to invest in prevention and better care of behaviors and psychological symptoms associated with dementia. Int Psychogeriatr. 2020:1–6.

Busch FN. Psychodynamic approaches to behavioral change. Washington, DC: American Psychiatric Association; 2019. p. 53.

Butler AC, Chapman JE, Forman EM, Beck AT. The empirical status of cognitive-behavioral therapy: a review of meta-analyses. Clin Psychol Rev. 2006;26(1):17–31.

Carrion C, Folkvord F, Anastasiadou D, Aymerich M. Cognitive therapy for dementia patients: a systematic review. Dement Geriatr Cogn Disord. 2018;46(1–2):1–26.

Chang YP, Compton P, Almeter P, Fox CH. The effect of motivational interviewing on prescription opioid adherence among older adults with chronic pain. Perspect Psychiatr Care. 2015;51(3):211–9.

Cuijpers P, van Straten A, Smit F. Psychological treatment of late-life depression: a meta-analysis of randomized controlled trials. Int J Geriatr Psychiatry. 2006;21(12):1139–49.

Cuijpers P, van Straten A, Warmerdam L. Behavioral activation treatments of depression: a meta-analysis. Clin Psychol Rev. 2007;27(3):318–26.

Cuijpers P, Karyotaki E, Pot AM, et al. Managing depression in older age: psychological interventions. Maturitas. 2014;79(2):160–9.

Dimidjian S, Barrera M, Martell C, et al. The origins and current status of behavioral activation treatments for depression. Annu Rev Clin Psychol. 2011;7:1–38.

Farina N, Ibnidris A, Alladi S, et al. A systematic review and meta-analysis of dementia prevalence in seven developing countries: a STRiDE project. Glob Public Health. 2020;15:1878–93.

Gallagher-Thompson D, Steffen AM. Comparative effects of cognitive-behavioral and brief psychodynamic psychotherapies for depressed family caregivers. J Consult Clin Psychol. 1994;62(3):543–9.

Gum AM, Schonfeld L, Tyler S, Fishleder S, et al. One-visit behavioral intervention for older primary care patients with mild to moderate depressive symptoms. South Med J. 2016;109(8):442–7.

Hanson AE, Scogin F. Older adults' acceptance of psychological, pharmacological, and combination treat-

ments for geriatric depression. J Gerontol B Psychol Sci Soc Sci. 2008;63(4):P245–8.
Hayes SC, Strosahl KD, Wilson KG. Acceptance and commitment therapy: an experiential approach to behavior change. New York: Guilford Press; 1999.
Heisel MJ, Talbot NL, King DA, Tu XM, et al. Adapting interpersonal psychotherapy for older adults at risk for suicide. Am J Geriatr Psychiatry. 2015;23(1):87–98.
Hopko DR, Robertson SM, Carvalho JP. Sudden gains in depressed cancer patients treated with behavioral activation therapy. Behav Ther. 2009;40(4):346–56.
Institute of Medicine. The mental health and substance use workforce for older adults. In: Whose hands? Washington, DC: The National Academies Press; 2012.
Jacobs ML, Luci K, Hagemann L. Group-based acceptance and commitment therapy (ACT) for older veterans: findings from a quality improvement project. Clin Gerontol. 2018;41(5):458–67.
Kabat-Zinn J. An outpatient program in behavioral medicine for chronic pain patients based on the practice of mindfulness meditation: theoretical considerations and preliminary results. Gen Hosp Psychiatry. 1982;4(1):33–47.
Kales HC, Gitlin LN, Lyketsos CG, Detroit Expert Panel on Assessment and Management of Neuropsychiatric Symptoms of Dementia. Management of neuropsychiatric symptoms of dementia in clinical settings: recommendations from a multidisciplinary expert panel. J Am Geriatr Soc. 2014;62(4):762–9.
Kanter JW, Manos RC, Bowe WM, Baruch DE, et al. What is behavioral activation? A review of the empirical literature. Clin Psychol Rev. 2010;30(6):608–20.
Kiosses DN, Alexopoulos GS. Problem-solving therapy in the elderly. Curr Treat Options Psychiatry. 2014;1(1):15–26.
Kirkham JG, Choi N, Seitz DP. Meta-analysis of problem solving therapy for the treatment of major depressive disorder in older adults. Int J Geriatr Psychiatry. 2016;31(5):526–35.
Knight BG. Psychotherapy with older adults, 3rd ed. 2004.
Knight BG, Pachana NA. Psychological assessment and therapy with older adults. Oxford: Oxford University Press; 2015.
Kropf N, Cummings SM, Cummings S. Evidence-based treatment with older adults: theory, practice, and research. Oxford: Oxford University Press; 2017.
Kuring JK, Mathias JL, Ward L. Risk of dementia in persons who have previously experienced clinically-significant depression, anxiety, or PTSD: a systematic review and meta-analysis. J Affect Disord. 2020;274:247–61.
Lenze EJ, Hickman S, Hershey T, Wendleton L, et al. Mindfulness-based stress reduction for older adults with worry symptoms and co-occurring cognitive dysfunction. Int J Geriatr Psychiatry. 2014;29(10):991–1000.
Leyhe T, Reynolds CF, Melcher T, Linnemann C, et al. A common challenge in older adults: classification, overlap, and therapy of depression and dementia. Alzheimers Dement. 2017;13(1):59–71.
Linehan MM. Dialectical behavioral therapy: a cognitive behavioral approach to parasuicide. J Personal Disord. 1987;1(4):328–33.
Liu S, Jin Y, Shi Z, Huo YR, et al. The effects of behavioral and psychological symptoms on caregiver burden in frontotemporal dementia, Lewy body dementia, and Alzheimer's disease: clinical experience in China. Aging Ment Health. 2017;21(6):651–7.
Lynch TR, Cheavens JS, Cukrowicz KC, Thorp SR, et al. Treatment of older adults with co-morbid personality disorder and depression: a dialectical behavior therapy approach. Int J Geriatr Psychiatry. 2007;22(2):131–43.
Magierski R, Sobow T. Serotonergic drugs for the treatment of neuropsychiatric symptoms in dementia. Expert Rev Neurother. 2016;16(4):375–87.
Mathur S, Sharma MP, Bharath S. Mindfulness-based cognitive therapy in patients with late-life depression: a case series. Int J Yoga. 2016;9(2):168–72.
Miller MD. Using interpersonal therapy (IPT) with older adults today and tomorrow: a review of the literature and new developments. Curr Psychiatry Rep. 2006;10(1):16–22.
Nair P, Bhanu C, Frost R, Buszewicz M, et al. A systematic review of older adults' attitudes towards depression and its treatment. Gerontologist. 2020;60(1):e93–e104.
Pasterfield M, Bailey D, Hems D, McMillan D, et al. Adapting manualized behavioural activation treatment for older adults with depression. Cogn Behav Therap. 2014;7:e5.
Petkus AJ, Wetherell JL. Acceptance and commitment therapy with older adults: rationale and considerations. Cogn Behav Pract. 2013;20(1):47–56.
Phan SV, Osae S, Morgan JC, Inyang M, et al. Neuropsychiatric symptoms in dementia: considerations for pharmacotherapy in the USA. Drugs R D. 2019;19(2):93–115.
Polenick CA, Flora SR. Increasing social activity attendance in assisted living residents using personalized prompts and positive social attention. J Appl Gerontol. 2013;32(5):515–39.
Polenick CA, Struble LM, Stanislawski B, Turnwald M, et al. "I've learned to just go with the flow": family caregivers' strategies for managing behavioral and psychological symptoms of dementia. Dementia (London). 2020;19(3):590–605.
Raue PJ, Sirey JA, Dawson A, Berman J, et al. Lay-delivered behavioral activation for depressed senior center clients: pilot RCT. Int J Geriatr Psychiatry. 2019;34(11):1715–23.
Richards DA, Ekers D, McMillan D, Taylor RS, et al. Cost and outcome of behavioural activation versus cognitive behavioural therapy for depression (COBRA): a randomised, controlled, non-inferiority trial. Lancet. 2016;388(10047):871–80.
Rietkerk W, de Jonge-de Haan J, Slaets JP, Zuidema SU, et al. Increasing older adult involvement in geriatric assessment: a mixed-methods process evaluation. J Aging Health. 2021;33(7–8):482–92.

Roseborough DJ, Luptak M, McLeod J, Bradshaw W. Effectiveness of psychodynamic psychotherapy with older adults: a longitudinal study. Clin Gerontol. 2013;36(1):1–16.

Ruesch M, Helmes A, Bengel J. Cognitive behavioral group therapy for patients with physical diseases and comorbid depressive or adjustment disorders on a waiting list for individual therapy: results from a randomized controlled trial. BMC Psychiatry. 2017;17(1):340.

Samad Z, Brealey S, Gilbody S. The effectiveness of behavioural therapy for the treatment of depression in older adults: a meta-analysis. Int J Geriatr Psychiatry. 2011;26(12):1211–20.

Scogin F, McElreath L. Efficacy of psychosocial treatments for geriatric depression: a quantitative review. J Consult Clin Psychol. 1994;62(1):69–74.

Seligman ME, Csikszentmihalyi M. Positive psychology. An introduction. Am Psychol. 2000;55(1):5–14.

Shedler J. The efficacy of psychodynamic psychotherapy. Am Psychol. 2010;65(2):98–109.

Sikkes SA, Tang Y, Jutten RJ, Wesselman LM, et al. Toward a theory-based specification of non-pharmacological treatments in aging and dementia: focused reviews and methodological recommendations. Alzheimers Dement. 2021;17(2):255–70.

Starkstein SE, Mizrahi R, Power BD. Depression in Alzheimer's disease: phenomenology, clinical correlates and treatment. Int Rev Psychiatry. 2018;20(4):382–8.

Steffen AM, Gallagher-Thompson D, Thompson LW. Treating ater-life depression: a cognitive-behavioral therapy approach, therapist guide. 2nd ed. Oxford: Oxford University Press; 2022.

Tavares LR, Barbosa MR. Efficacy of group psychotherapy for geriatric depression: a systematic review. Arch Gerontol Geriatr. 2018;78:71–80.

Terracciano A, Artese A, Yeh J, Edgerton L, et al. Effectiveness of powerful tools for caregivers on caregiver burden and on care recipient behavioral and psychological symptoms of dementia: a randomized controlled trial. J Am Med Dir Assoc. 2020;21(8):1121–1127.e1.

Thompson LW, Gallagher D, Breckenridge JS. Comparative effectiveness of psychotherapies for depressed elders. J Consult Clin Psychol. 1987;55(3):385–90.

Tonga JB, Saltyte Benth J, Arnevik EA, Werheid K, et al. Managing depressive symptoms in people with mild cognitive impairment and mild dementia with a multicomponent psychotherapy intervention: a randomized controlled trial. Int Psychogeriatr. 2021;33:217–31.

US Preventive Services Task Force, Owens DK, Davidson KW, Krist AH, et al. Screening for cognitive impairment in older adults: US Preventive Services Task Force recommendation statement. JAMA. 2020;323(8):757–63.

Verstaen A, Rau HK, Trittschuh EH. Healthy aging project-brain: a psychoeducational and motivational Group for Older Veterans. Fed Pract. 2020;37(7):309–15. https://www.ncbi.nlm.nih.gov/pubmed/32908334.

Wetherell JL, Afari N, Ayers CR, Stoddard JA, et al. Acceptance and commitment therapy for generalized anxiety disorder in older adults: a preliminary report. Behav Ther. 2011a;42(1):127–34.

Wetherell JL, Afari N, Rutledge T, Sorrell JT, et al. A randomized, controlled trial of acceptance and commitment therapy and cognitive-behavioral therapy for chronic pain. Pain. 2011b;152(9):2098–107.

Wilson KC, Mottram PG, Vassilas CA. Psychotherapeutic treatments for older depressed people. Cochrane Database Syst Rev. 2008;(1):CD004853.

Telemedicine and Digital Mental Health Technologies

16

Christine E. Gould, Ana Jessica Alfaro, Ira Yenko, and Rita Hitching

Abstract

The enlarging need for clinicians with specialized geriatric expertise in the USA (Institute of Medicine (IOM) 2012; Wiechers et al. 2019) can hopefully be met through telemedicine and digital technologies, supplemented by remote video consultation to home-based and long-term care settings (Gentry MT et al., Am J Geriatr Psychiatry 27:109–27, 2019). This chapter reviews technologies which may facilitate prompt screening and assessment of older individuals by minimizing the time for a provider to receive clinical information (Fortuna 2019). Frequent subspecialty consultation and remote digital monitoring can foster *earlier* recognition of emerging psychiatric issues and reduce complications that result from delay of care. Timely review of medication regimens along with de-prescribing can avoid unnecessary or excessive treatment, the essence of an *age-adjusted* approach. Figure 16.1 summarizes the use of assistive technology in geriatric care, including the role of wearable devices, home monitoring systems, pandemic proof, and remote care and the considerations for telemedicine.

C. E. Gould (✉)
VA Palo Alto Health Care System, Geriatric Research, Education and Clinical Center (GRECC), Palo Alto, CA, USA

Department of Psychiatry and Behavioral Services, Stanford University School of Medicine, Palo Alto, CA, USA

VA Palo Alto Health Care System, Psychology Service, Palo Alto, CA, USA
e-mail: Christine.Gould@va.gov

A. J. Alfaro
VA Palo Alto Health Care System, Geriatric Research, Education and Clinical Center (GRECC), Palo Alto, CA, USA

Department of Psychiatry and Behavioral Services, Stanford University School of Medicine, Palo Alto, CA, USA

I. Yenko
VA Palo Alto Health Care System, Geriatric Research, Education and Clinical Center (GRECC), Palo Alto, CA, USA

R. Hitching
University of Newcastle, Newcastle, NSW, Australia

H. H. Fenn et al. (eds.), *Age-Adjusted Psychiatric Treatment for the Older Patient*,
https://doi.org/10.1007/978-3-031-53976-3_16

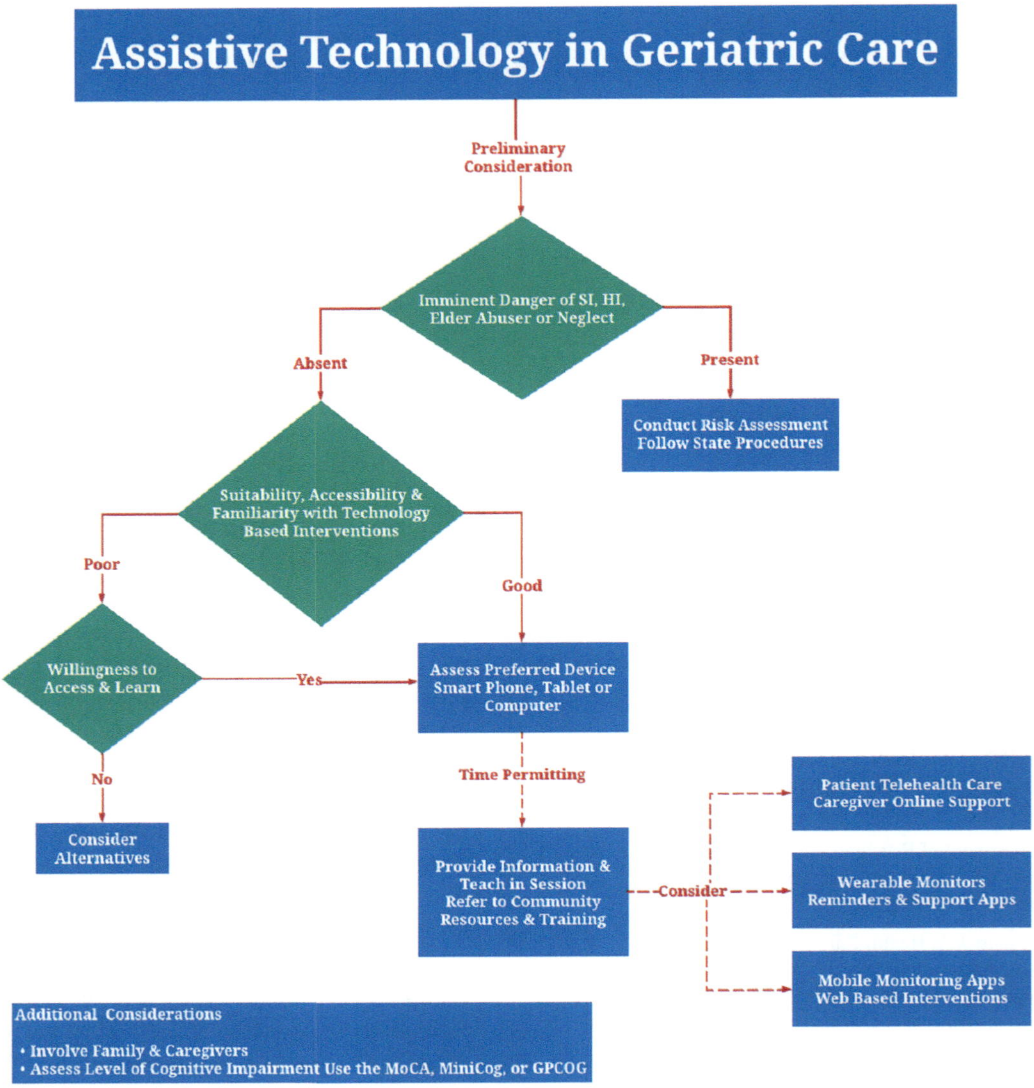

(Rita Hitching, MSc)

Fig. 16.1 Decision tree for assistive technology

Case Example: Telemedicine, Access to Information, and Timely Medication Adjustment

An 88-year-old nursing home resident with major neurocognitive disorder (MNCD) and behavioral disturbance was crying, disruptive, and agitated at night. The geriatric psychiatry consultant was limited to telemedicine visits, which provided unexpected benefits: nursing staff and caregivers gave up-to-moment information about behavior, two daughters and nursing staff were patched into video calls, and the consultation contacts happened weekly. Medication trials and adjustments were instituted promptly. As-needed doses of lorazepam and nightly dose of zolpidem were tapered and discontinued. Over 8 weeks, a regular nightly dose of either 12.5 mg or 25 mg quetiapine was started, and the nighttime emotional outbursts became less frequent. Daughters and staff gradually became less anxious and more reassured by predictable, timely consultations; the number and frequency of emergency calls declined.

Discussion: Telemedicine consultation improved access to immediate assessments and medication adjustments for treatment of BPSD.

Barriers to Implementation of Telemedicine and Digital Technologies

Despite numerous advantages to using communication technology, the following barriers persist:

1. The cost of devices (i.e., computers, smartphones, tablets) and Internet service (i.e., home Internet, broadband, data plan) may exclude many older adults. However, federal and state-funded programs provide access to cellphones for qualifying low-income consumers (Federal Communications Committee 2020). Shared devices can be used in long-term care setting but must be sanitized and monitored.
2. Geriatric individuals with access to communication technology may not have experience, training, or support resources (Gould et al. 2020a) to use the technology effectively or may be apprehensive of digital platforms (Andrews et al. 2019). Local technology training in public libraries, senior centers, and community colleges is one solution (Damodaran et al. 2014).
3. Sensory impairments and diseases are roadblocks. Hearing loss limits understanding synthetic voices, while tremors or motor dysfunction may prevent the use of touch screens (Kuerbis et al. 2017). Poor tactile sense and dexterity impede the use of a computer mouse or small touch screens (e.g., Fisk et al. (2009)). Visual impairment hinders navigation of a webpage or mobile application (app), which uses small fonts or displays which are not sharply contrasted (Fisk et al. 2009). Adaptations that increase accessibility are standard in many technological devices, for example, adjustable font and stylus pens.
4. Cognitive deficits can interfere with learning new technology. Repetition, handouts, and trials with the device during teaching sessions can make a difference. Hands-on instruction to the caregiver or family member may be the first step in order to introduce technology into the patient's healthcare system and set up synchronous telehealth visits. The patient can then be included and practice can proceed at the patient's pace. Programs or apps can help relax or distract the cognitively impaired from anxious, dysphoric, or agitated states.

Telemedicine

A natural experiment prompted by a pandemic has accelerated access to care. Until 2020, the Center for Medicare Services (CMS) restricted telemedicine reimbursements primarily to the provision of care in rural areas. After the onset of the COVID-19 pandemic, CMS provided waivers for services to be delivered to the home (Centers for Medicare and Medicaid Services 2020) as well as audio-only services (temporarily). The reimbursements promoted the adoption of *synchronous* telemedicine, which permit a simultaneous exchange of information and delivery of services through video telemedicine appointments.

Asynchronous services allow for the sharing of information (e.g., laboratory reports and diagnostic imaging) and delivery of interventions for low to moderate levels of psychiatric symptoms via technology, e-consults, secure messaging with patients, electronic health (eHealth) interventions, and mobile health (mHealth) apps (see Fig. 16.1). Home sensors and wearable body sensors can monitor health conditions and disease states or detect new problems, such as the onset of cognitive impairment. Asynchronous telemedicine, such as home monitoring, wearable devices, and mHealth, may, however, often go underutilized partially due to low provider awareness. Reimbursement for these services and the overall adoption of stepped care approaches is not well established, particularly in countries with *decentralized* healthcare systems, such as the USA (e.g., Gould et al. 2019a).

Telemedicine Assessments and Technology-Assisted Monitoring

Remote telemedicine assessments and home monitoring solutions, including timely cognitive assessment, detection of falls, and monitoring of mood, have been demonstrated through the following:

- Video-based telemedicine cognitive assessments
- Computerized cognitive assessments
- Experience-sampling methods
- Wearable sensors and home monitoring

Telehealth Cognitive Assessment (See Chap. 4)

Synchronous videoconferencing, or telemedicine, has proven acceptable to patients and caregivers (Gentry et al. 2019). Studies of telemedicine have reported diagnostic accuracy comparable to in-person examinations (Barth et al. 2018). Research on telehealth-based cognitive assessments has shown the reliability of videoconferencing techniques for the administration of specific cognitive measures (Galusha-Glasscock et al. 2016; Grosch et al. 2015) and neuropsychological assessments (Wadsworth et al. 2018).

Clinical judgment remains important in video-based cognitive assessments and can guide how to gather data needed for an accurate assessment. Telephone screening remains a supplementary tool in the assessment of cognitive status (Smith et al. 2009) as information obtained via telephone correlates well with in-person clinic visit data (Mundt et al. 2007).

Suitability of Brief Cognitive Screening Instruments in Telemedicine

The Montreal Cognitive Assessment (MoCA): This reliable and effective screening measure for mild cognitive impairment (MCI) and Alzheimer's related dementia (Nasreddine et al. 2005) has been used in telemedicine assessments. The MoCA has been adapted for administration via video (MoCA 8.1) with the same total and cutoff scores as the *paper MoCA*, albeit slight variations on question content and administration. An electronic version on tablets (eMoCA) was demonstrated to detect changes in cognitive function (Snowdon et al. 2015). Yet *deficient technological skills* can impact performance on the eMoCA, specifically visuospatial tasks (Wallace et al. 2019). Technological fluency must be considered first, and, if necessary, assessment of visuospatial tasks deferred.

The MoCA has been adapted for individuals with *visual* impairments (MoCA-B) to omit items needing visual input. Thus, the MOCA-B can be administered via telephone as well. The sensitivity and specificity for the MoCA-B have remained excellent in the detection of Alzheimer's disease, though its ability to detect mild cognitive impairment (MCI) appeared slightly reduced (Wittich et al. 2010).

Mini-Mental State Exam (MMSE): Video administration has been reported as valid (Ciemins et al. 2009). One study which compared *in-person* to *video-based* administration of the MMSE and the cognitive subscale of the Alzheimer's Disease Assessment Scale (ADAS-cog) in patients with Alzheimer's disease reported no significant differences in performance for most patients based on administration modality or cognitive assessment tool over 24 months (Carotenuto et al. 2018). For patients with pronounced cognitive deficits, videoconferencing slightly overestimated the level of cognitive impairment; videoconferencing is reliable to document cognitive stability or decline and to measure treatment effects in mild to moderate MNCD (for further discussion, see Chap. 4).

Suitability of Comprehensive Cognitive Testing in Telemedicine

Comprehensive neuropsychological assessment, also termed tele-neuropsychology, has been administered through videoconferencing

Table 16.1 Tele-neuropsychology: potential impediments and suggestions

Potential limiting factor	Examples of limitations	Suggestion
Access to technology	No computer, webcam, speakers, etc.; no Internet or poor Internet reliability	Assess access to technology and fluency during preinterview. Clinical judgment determines whether to attempt assessment via video
Fluency with technology	Limited ability to fluently engage with the technology	Involve someone to aid with setup or implementation. Provide instructions/handouts on relevant technology
Ecological and patient factors	Environment: Internet reliability, ambient lighting, timing (day), volume, privacy, safety, and comfort Patient: Fatigue, alertness, mood, effort, and motivation	Prior to testing, use videoconferencing to conduct an informal assessment of environmental conditions and patient factors, noting any issues with privacy, safety, and sensory difficulties. Address issues accordingly. Develop plan for disconnection (e.g., telephone call)
Test factors	Test factors include question formatting or test material presentation which may not be appropriate for telehealth	Use validated alternate forms (e.g., eMoCA, Boston Naming Test-15). Use screen-share to display high-quality figures, text, or images

(Martin-Khan et al. 2012). Videoconferencing was compared to standard face-to-face administration in a population of cognitively impaired (i.e., mild cognitive impairment, Alzheimer's disease) and healthy older adults. Videoconferencing was found comparable to face-to-face administration in distinguishing cognitively impaired from non-impaired individuals. This finding supports the construct validity of a tele-neuropsychology-based assessment (Cullum et al. 2014). Table 16.1 summarizes potential impediments, individual limitations, and suggestions to adapt test administration. These barriers may adversely impact cognitive performance.

Computerized Cognitive Assessments

Internet-based and computerized cognitive assessments rely on fewer provider resources (i.e., administration time, scoring), compared with face-to-face assessments, and improve timing, precision (Bilder 2011), efficiency, and implementation (Gibbons et al. 2008). Internet-based testing allows greater control over pacing, less scrutiny by a test administrator, and is acceptable to patients (Hansen et al. 2015). A major impediment is the low level of provider control over ecological factors (e.g., Internet reliability) that could affect performance (Parsons 2016). One web-based cognitive assessment (Cogniciti) developed by Troyer et al. (2014) demonstrated good feasibility, reliability, and validity in identifying preservation or impairment of cognition in middle-aged and older adults. Among older adults, Internet-based neuropsychological batteries such as WebNeuro (Silverstein et al. 2007) demonstrated good validity versus neuropsychological tests measuring similar cognitive constructs (Hansen et al. 2015).

Technology to Monitor Functioning, Supplement Treatment, and Avoid Adverse Events

Various technologies can provide moment-to-moment experience sampling and monitoring, which avoid pitfalls such as recall and memory bias (Scollon et al. 2009). Remote patient monitoring reduces costs (Malasinghe et al. 2019), supports aging-in-place, and facilitates detection of adverse events (e.g., cardiac arrythmias, falls). Aging adults may embrace technologies (e.g., apps, wearable devices) that facilitate independent living (Hein et al. 2010) although some may raise concerns about privacy and security, considerations when recommending technologies to patients (Torous and Roberts 2017).

Mobile App-Based Experience Sampling Method (ESM)

Mobile technologies facilitate *real-time* data entry and tracking by the user in response to a prompt (Van Berkel et al. 2017). This method of data collection captures an individual's experiences (thoughts, states, events) within the context of daily life (Csikszentmihalyi and Larson 2014) and can supplement monitoring and treatment. ESM-enabled mobile apps survey individuals throughout the day about specific behaviors, medication adherence, or mood states with the capability of gathering both subjective and objective data. ESM is reported to be more sensitive to change and more accurate in older adults versus traditional self-report assessments (Moore et al. 2016).

Wearable Sensors and Home Monitoring Technologies

Activity trackers and wearable sensors (e.g., FitBit, Apple watches) collect behavioral and physiological data such as step count (accelerometer), heart rate, falls (gyroscopes), sleep patterns (accelerometer and heart rate/rhythm), or location-based data (Global Positioning System [GPS]). These devices support remote patient monitoring (RPM) and may improve quality of life, encourage healthy behaviors, and reduce burden on the healthcare system (Tun et al. 2021). Clinicians can use these devices to monitor symptoms and set treatment and lifestyle goals; the export feature may instantly transfer encrypted data to a secure dashboard accessible only to the clinician, allowing real-time feedback.

Technology can enhance age-appropriate medical care by reducing time to crucial interventions, hopefully lowering the risk of prolonged disability and/or complications. Remote patient monitoring (RPM) via wearable devices can also help manage post-acute and chronic diseases (i.e., diabetes, chronic obtrusive pulmonary disease, congestive heart failure, chronic wounds, atrial fibrillation) and speed care delivery. One life-or-death example is the use of wearable devices to detect cardiac arrhythmias by estimating heart rate using photoplethysmogram (PPG) sensors that detect changes in tissue blood volume. RPM often focuses on physical health conditions rather than psychiatric conditions, but benefits to the latter can result from overlapping symptoms and bidirectional effects.

The increasing numbers of older adults living alone or without family members and the high cost of assisted-living situations can spur the use of RPM to support aging-in-place (Ní Scanaill et al. 2006). Remote monitoring in-home (i.e., ambient) and wearable devices (i.e., sensors) can provide some functions of an assisted living or care facility at reduced cost, with real-time detection of activities of daily living or falls and prompt response (De Vito et al. 2020). Ambient or noncontact sensors detect motion, pressure, sound, and object contact. These noncontact sensors can be combined with video and/or wearable sensors with GPS to provide monitoring. Integration of wearable sensors into home devices and mobile applications has revolutionized how data are collected. Ethical concerns about privacy, data security, and patient autonomy remain. Table 16.2 describes four examples of RPM.

Table 16.2 Applications of remote patient monitoring (RPM)

Problem	Solution	Barriers	Benefits
Falls	Wearable personal emergency response systems (PERS)[a]	Unreliable batteries	Tailored therapies and preventative action
• Associated with injury and death (Al-Shaqi et al. 2016) • Falls without immediate assistance led to 50% increased mortality (Rashidi and Mihailidis 2013)	• User presses button to alert others (Bulling et al. 2014) • Accelerometer elucidates type and impact of fall (Zhang et al. 2014)	• False-positives with sudden jolts or movements • Ineffective for falls resulting in loss of consciousness • Not wearing the device/not pressing alarm	• Accelerometer data may lead to tailored therapies • Preventative adaptations to the environment or lifestyle changes may diminish falls (Aghajan et al. 2007) • Strong sensitivity for simulated and real-life falls (Rantz et al. 2018)
Wandering	Remote patient monitoring (RPM)[a]	Cost	Rapid response and saves resources
• A behavioral symptom of major neurocognitive disorder (MNCD) that distresses families and places the patient at risk (Lai Kwan et al. 2019)	• Small device (e.g., shoe inserts, patches, watch) • Alert sent if wearer ventures beyond a set perimeter • If GPS enabled tracks location of the wearer	• Expensive to purchase and maintain support	• Allows for prompt location of disoriented/lost aged adults • Saves significant community resources
Medication monitoring	Motion sensors equipment	Motivation and use	Reminders and prompts
• Medication adherence difficulties potentially due to cognitive impairment	• Sensors alert when a medicine cabinet is opened	• Devices are dependent on the resident interacting with them as well as cameras monitoring the home (Franco et al. 2010)	• A reminder call or text to the patient (e.g., take missed medication)
ADL and IADLS Monitoring	Smart home	Motivation and interaction	Encourages independence
• Monitor activities of daily living (ADLs) and instrumental activities of daily living (IADLs) for older individuals living alone	• Robotic smart home technologies (e.g., Wi-Fi-connected cameras in refrigerator)	• In-home devices depend on interaction and cameras monitoring the home (Franco et al. 2010)	• Supports independent living • Information can lead to reminders to eat or remote turn-off of stove

[a] Alternatives to wearables to monitor wandering or falls: in-home devices, tracked remotely, that rely on sensors being triggered (e.g., bed pads, area rugs, door openings)

Telemedicine and Technology-Delivered Treatment

Synchronous Telemedicine Interventions

Tele-mental health (TMH) and synchronous telemedicine services encompass evaluation, consultation with patients and teams, and interventions (e.g., medication management, psychotherapy). Large, controlled trials (e.g., Ruskin et al. (2004)) have demonstrated equivalent outcomes for telemedicine compared to face-to-face visits.

A review of 76 articles examined the feasibility, acceptability, and efficacy of synchronous TMH services in older adults; most studies focused on cognitive assessment and a few studies examined psychotherapy for older adults, caregivers, or nursing home consultation (Gentry et al. 2019). Research generally demonstrates the equivalence between telehealth-delivered and in-person psychotherapies such as problem-solving therapy (Choi et al. 2014) or behavioral activation (Egede et al. 2015). In summary, high-quality randomized psychotherapy and caregiver intervention trials are limited, but psychotherapy via TMH has been reported as effective as in-person therapy.

A "hub-and-spoke" model of synchronous telehealth can deliver services from larger clinic hubs to smaller clinic spokes (Lum et al. 2020) or may deliver telehealth directly into the patient's home (e.g., Moo et al. 2020). A survey found that geriatric psychiatry services were highly satisfactory to patients (Hantke et al. 2020). TMH increases access to synchronous geriatric psychiatry services, but its reach is limited by the number of providers able to deliver it.

Some phone and video interactions blend synchronous and asynchronous approaches. For example, a combination of video-delivered content and telephone support for MNCD caregivers was found effective when delivered with behavioral coaching compared with education conditions (Steffen and Gant 2016). A video-delivered intervention with telephone support for late-life anxiety *reduced* anxiety, depressive, and somatic symptoms, compared with a wait-list control condition (Gould et al. 2019b).

Internet Interventions

Internet interventions provide a mix of video-delivered content, practices, and other interactive techniques which target psychiatric issues. These programs generally are delivered as automated interventions that advance (i.e., unlock new content) as the user completes each module. Some Internet interventions include human support from a therapist, peer, or another provider.

Internet-delivered CBT (iCBT) studies with older adults have focused on depression, anxiety, or PTSD (e.g., Dear et al. 2015; Knaevelsrud et al. 2017). A meta-analysis of Internet intervention studies (Xiang et al. 2020) of older adults with depression found a large within-group effect ($d = 1.27$) that diminished slightly ($d = 1.18$) when including only studies with comparison conditions.

Access to Internet interventions varies by country and healthcare system. In the United Kingdom, evidence-based programs with support among older adults (McMurchie et al. 2013) such as *Beating the Blues* (Proudfoot et al. 2004) are available as part of the National Health System. In contrast, within the USA, *Beating the Blues* is only available to patients with select insurers. While many tools are targeted toward younger and middle-aged users, the aged may also benefit, especially as the available options increase. Information about available programs can be found on several websites:

- Dartmouth College Center for Technology and Behavioral Health provides information about available programs: https://www.c4tbh.org/program-reviews.
- Evidence-informed, free courses are available through the Veterans Health Administration: https://www.veterantraining.va.gov/.
- Muñoz et al. (2018) have advocated for free online mental health interventions available as massive open online courses (MOOCs): https://i4health.paloaltou.edu/digitalapothecary.html.

Mobile Mental Health Apps

Mental health symptoms can be addressed through apps. Designed for smartphones and tablets, these apps range from behavioral coaching and psychotherapy to medication reminders. Most mental health apps contain psychoeducation, interactive coping skills, and tools to practice (e.g., mindfulness exercises, relaxation techniques, guided imagery). Engaging users to use coping strategies in real time can increase opportunities for learning (Bakker et al. 2018). Further, aging adults seem motivated to use digital technology for mental health, promote self-reliance, avert loneliness, and improve mood (Andrews et al. 2019; Gould et al. 2020a).

Factors to consider in recommending a mental health app are the following:

1. The patient's ability to manage a situation which the app cannot: if symptoms worsen or whom to reach in a crisis (e.g., suicide hotline). A high-risk patient may need backup resources, such as a safety plan and weekly individual psychotherapy.
2. The patient's motivation and likelihood of adherence.
3. Finances: Many aging adults cannot accommodate unexpected data charges and may need help to understand account statements, contracts, or information about their data plan.
4. The rationale and goals for a particular app: aging adults are less likely to avoid technology when the benefits are explained, and a support system is identified.
5. Knowledge of mobile devices (e.g., differences between Wi-Fi and data plans) should be assessed and bolstered. Gould et al. (2020b) developed and evaluated materials on how to download apps, the basics of mobile device use, and overviews for some common VA mobile apps. Materials should be written clearly, with step-by-step instruction (Kuerbis et al. 2017).
6. Capacity to make an informed decision about the use of a MHapp.
7. The potential benefits and risks of mobile technologies; often a balance between patient autonomy and the benefit of clinical care (Torous and Roberts 2017).
8. Security features and privacy issues: Cautions should be conveyed about public Wi-Fi connection, benefits of passcode protection, password confidentiality, and the importance of reading End User License Agreements.

Few studies examining the benefits of MHapps include aging adults. A small study reported that an app-based intervention to promote self-management of chronic conditions among older adults (n = 10; M age = 68.8 years) with serious mental illness was feasible, acceptable, and potentially helpful in improving outcomes (Fortuna et al. 2018). Gould et al. (2021) investigated the use of an eight-week app intervention called Meru Health program in community-dwelling middle-aged and older adults (n = 20; M age = 61.7 years) with elevated depressive symptoms. The Meru Health program includes app-based video instructional content, guided practices (e.g., mindfulness), and access to therapist support via in-app messaging or phone calls. The app also included moderated discussion for about 5–10 group members about their thoughts and experiences as they work through the program as a cohort. The program was found feasible and acceptable, with the potential to reduce psychiatric symptoms among middle-aged and older adults (Gould et al. 2021).

Factors such as cognition may guide the use of these technologies in the future. Comprehensive recommendations to enhance the utilization of mobile technology in late life, such as the timing of the intervention (morning or afternoon rather than evening) and transparency (ease of use), have been proposed (Kuerbis et al. 2017). Recommendations highlighted the importance of a supportive learning environment with enough time to explore, examine, and experiment with their device at their own pace (Kuerbis et al. 2017). The evaluation framework developed by the American Psychiatric Association aims to guide providers through considerations when deciding on an app. PsyberGuide also provides reviews of commercially available apps (https://www.psyberguide.org). As research expands the understanding of the efficacy of MHapps in older adults, mobile health assessment and interventions will offer more options for delivering mental health services.

Social Robots

Social robots, such as robotic animals, provide nonpharmacological interventions for behavioral symptoms of MNCD and loneliness. Robotic animals in long-term care settings attempt to reduce agitation and anxiety and improve quality of life. A cluster RCT of PARO (for personal assistive robot), a robotic seal, reported greater engagement and lower agitation for those using PARO compared with the plush toy (Moyle et al. 2017). A follow-up analysis of the PARO group found that it was effective for residents with lower levels of agitation and cognitive impairment compared with those with higher levels (Jones et al. 2018).

Cost and Access

Understanding insurance reimbursement for new technologies and need for Medicare support will be crucial for healthcare providers in the future.

Figure 16.3 summarizes the components of assistive technology in geriatric care, including the role of wearable devices, home monitoring systems, pandemic proof, and remote care, and the necessary considerations for telemedicine.

Conclusions

Telemedicine and digital mental health technologies can provide timely and efficient assessment, monitoring, and management of psychiatric and neurocognitive disorders in late life. Technology, however, requires learning time and effort by patient and clinician, as well as attention to security/privacy issues. The clinician must assess (1) access to technology, (2) technology literacy, (3) cognition, and (4) availability of others to assist. Figure 16.2 summarizes the assistive technology in geriatric care and the consideration of individual patient suitability.

Future integration of technology into care may include the use of peer specialists and healthcare professionals (Fortuna et al. 2018). Guideline development will help realize the full potential of technology; the application of telemedicine and digital technologies may address the demand for geriatric mental healthcare.

Retrospective studies of the 2003 SARS epidemic found that rates of suicide among aging adults spiked during the period of the epidemic (Yip et al. 2010). During COVID, a proliferation of existing digital services and resources, in addition to new services, supported mental health among older adults. Mobile apps like *COVID Coach* were quickly developed to help support self-care within the comfort of one's home. The natural experiment of COVID bodes well for future similar situations, in which frequent telephone contact with significant others and resources like the *Senior Friendship Line*, can promote social support, a sense of belongingness, and healthy coping (Friendship Line California n.d.). Figure 16.3 summarizes how telehealth facilitates care delivery and its benefits.

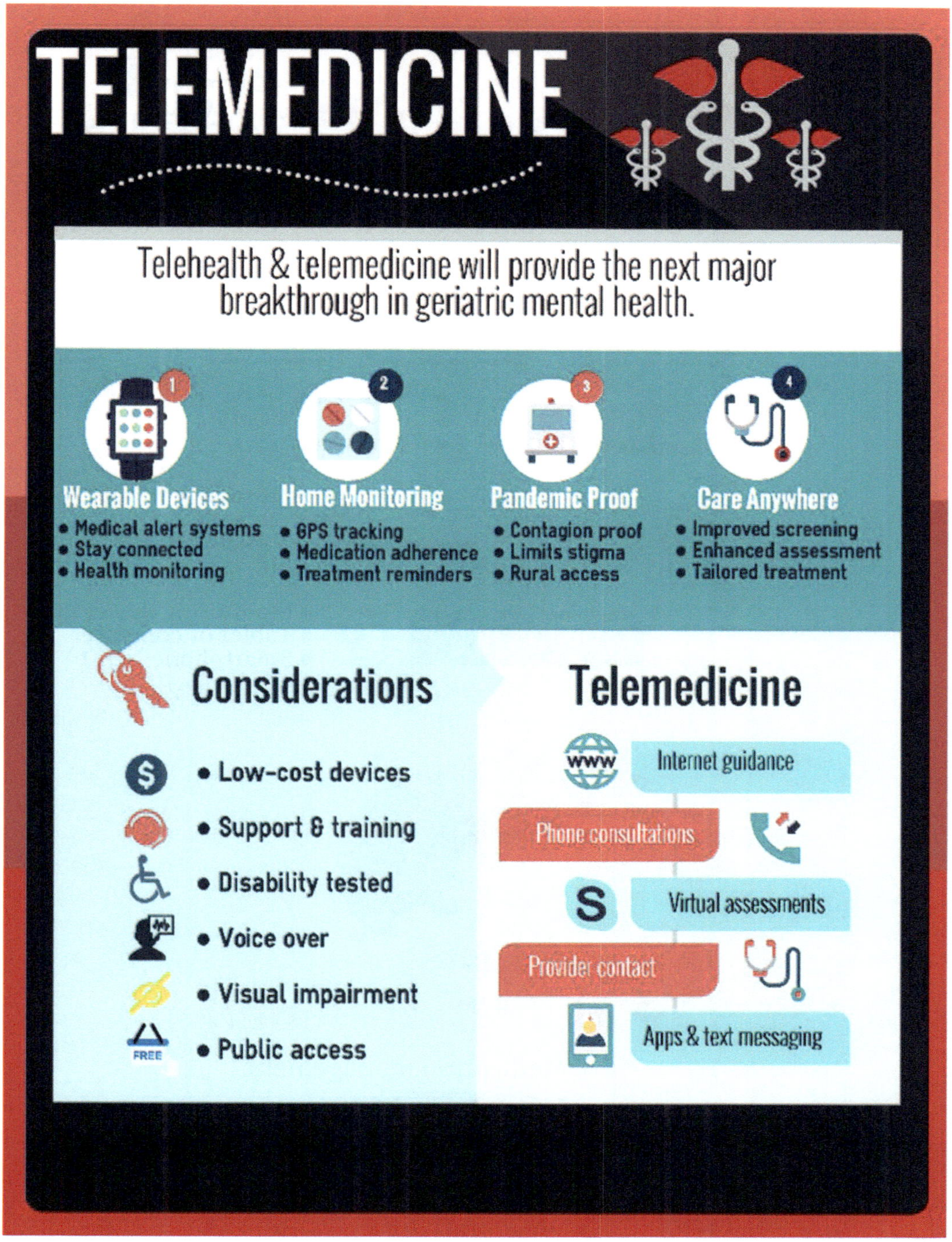

(Rita Hitching, MSc)

Fig. 16.2 Advantages of telemedicine technology in geriatric mental healthcare (Rita Hitching, MSc)

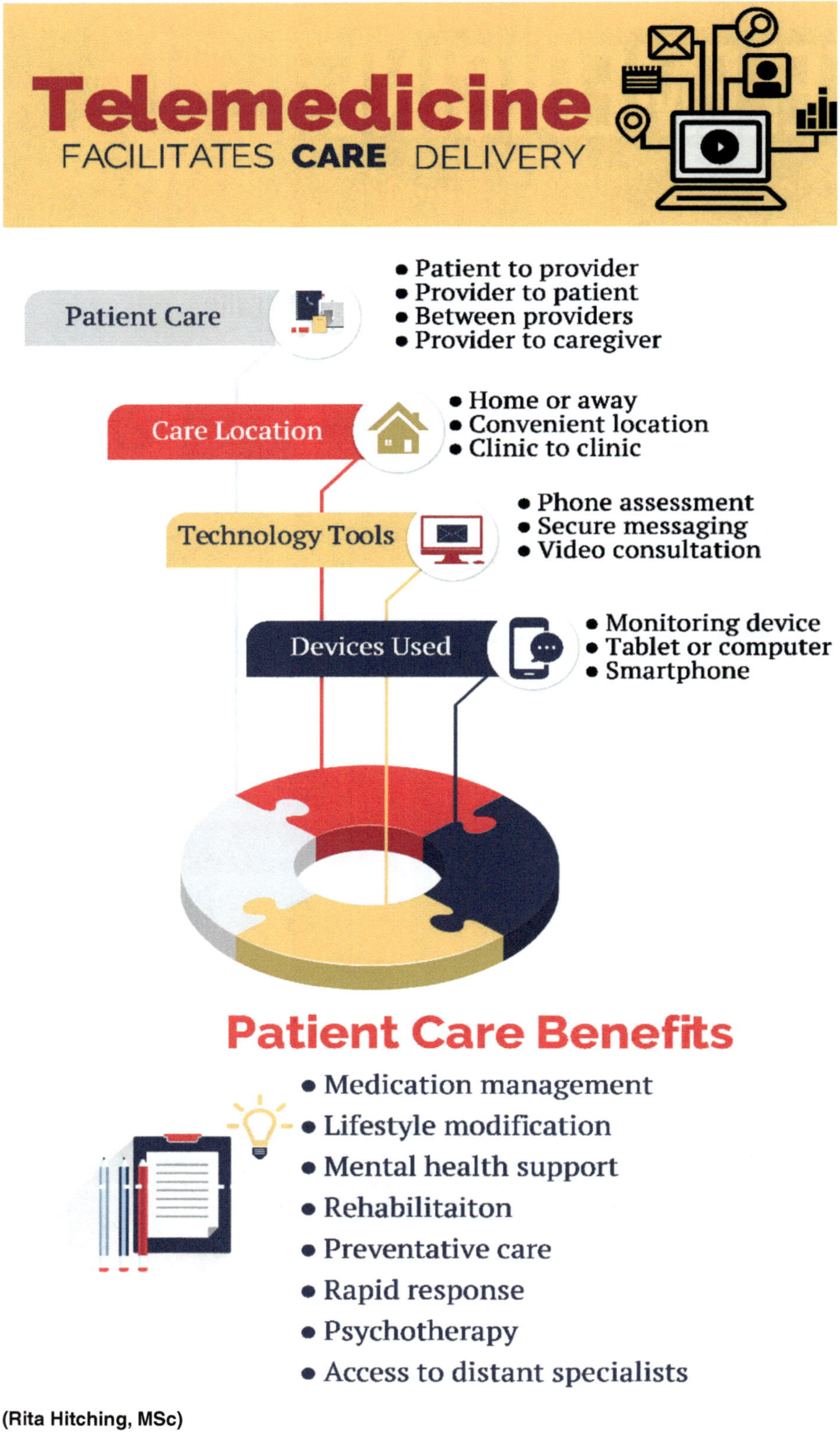

Fig. 16.3 Components of telemedicine care delivery (Rita Hitching, MSc)

Age-Adjusted Recommendations

- Explain to patient/families how technology and close monitoring of health information may facilitate timely access to specialist care, support services, and tailored treatment.
- Engage caregivers of patients with mild to severe cognitive impairment; introduce new technologies to the family or caregiver *first*.
- Determine access to requisite equipment and ability to use technology: use detailed questioning of available technology devices.
- Assess technology literacy and recognize that it is modifiable.
- Minimize barriers with user handouts, drop in technology sessions, or practice video sessions before telehealth appointments.
- Assess cognition and other limitations before deploying technology.

Acknowledgments Dr. Gould was supported by a Career Development Award (IK2 RX001478; PI: Gould) from the US Department of Veterans Affairs Rehabilitation Research and Development Service. Views expressed in this article are those of the authors and not necessarily those of the Department of Veterans Affairs or the Federal Government.

References

Aghajan H, Augusto JC, Wu C, et al. Distributed vision-based accident management for assisted living. Proceedings of the 5th International Conference on Smart Homes and Health Telematics, Nara, Japan. 21–23, 2007.

Al-Shaqi R, Mourshed M, Rezgui Y. Progress in ambient assisted systems for independent living by the elderly. Springerplus. 2016;5:624.

Andrews JA, Brown LJ, Hawley MS, Astell AJ. Older adults' perspectives on using digital technology to maintain good mental health: interactive group study. J Med Internet Res. 2019;21(2):e11694.

Bakker D, Kazantzis N, Rickwood D, Rickard N. A randomized controlled trial of three smartphone apps for enhancing public mental health. Behav Res Ther. 2018;109:75–83.

Barth J, Nickel F, Kolominsky-Rabas PL. Diagnosis of cognitive decline and dementia in rural areas—a scoping review. Int J Geriatr Psychiatry. 2018;33(3):459–74.

Bilder RM. Neuropsychology 3.0: evidence-based science and practice. J Int Neuropsychol Soc. 2011;17(1):7–13.

Bulling A, Blanke U, Schiele B. A tutorial on human activity recognition using body-worn inertial sensors. ACM Comput Surv. 2014;46:1–33.

Carotenuto A, Rea R, Traini E, et al. Cognitive assessment of patients with Alzheimer's disease by telemedicine: a pilot study. JMIR Ment Health. 2018;5(2):e31.

Centers for Medicare and Medicaid Services. Medicare telemedicine health care provider fact sheet. 2020. https://www.cms.gov/newsroom/fact-sheets/medicare-telemedicine-health-care-provider-fact-sheet. Accessed 23 June 2020.

Choi NG, Marti CN, Bruce ML, et al. Six-month postintervention depression and disability outcomes of in-home telehealth problem-solving therapy for depressed, low-income homebound older adults. Depress Anxiety. 2014;31(8):653–61.

Ciemins EL, Holloway B, Coon PJ, et al. Telemedicine and the mini-mental state examination: assessment from a distance. Telemed J E Health. 2009;15(5):476.

Csikszentmihalyi M, Larson R. Validity and reliability of the experience-sampling method, in flow and the foundations of positive psychology. Dordrecht: Springer; 2014. p. 35–54.

Cullum CM, Hynan LS, Grosch M, et al. Teleneuropsychology: evidence for video teleconference-based neuropsychological assessment. J Int Neuropsychol Soc. 2014;20(10):1028–33.

Damodaran L, Olphert CW, Sandhu J. Falling off the bandwagon? Exploring the challenges to sustained digital engagement by older people. Gerontology. 2014;60(2):163–73.

De Vito AN, Sawyer RJ, LaRoche A, et al. Acceptability and feasibility of a multicomponent telehealth care management program in older adults with advanced dementia in a residential memory care unit. Gerontol Geriatr Med. 2020;6:233372142092498.

Dear BF, Zou JB, Ali S, et al. Examining self-guided internet-delivered cognitive behavior therapy for older adults with symptoms of anxiety and depression: two feasibility open trials. Internet Interv. 2015;2(1):17–23.

Egede LE, Acierno R, Knapp RG, et al. Psychotherapy for depression in older veterans via telemedicine: a randomised, open-label, non-inferiority trial. Lancet Psychiatry. 2015;2(8):693–701.

Federal Communications Committee. Lifeline support for affordable communications. 2020. www.fcc.gov/consumers/guides/lifeline-support-affordable-communications. Accessed 28 June 2020.

Fisk AD, Rogers WA, Charness N, et al. Designing for older adults: principles and creative human factors approaches. 2nd ed. Boca Raton: CRC Press; 2009.

Fortuna KL, DiMilia PR, Lohman MC, et al. Feasibility, acceptability, and preliminary effectiveness of a peer-delivered and technology-supported self-management intervention for older adults with serious mental illness. Psychiatry Q. 2018;89(2):293–305.

Franco C, Demongeot J, Villemazet C, Vuillerme N. Behavioral telemonitoring of the elderly at home: detection of nycthemeral rhythms drifts from location data. Proceedings of the IEEE 24th International Conference on Advanced Information Networking and Applications Workshops. Perth, WA, Australia. pp. 759–766, 2010.

Friendship Line California. n.d.. https://www.ioaging.org/friendship-line-california. Accessed 23 July 2020.

Galusha-Glasscock JM, Horton DK, Weiner MF, Cullum CM. Video teleconference administration of the repeatable battery for the assessment of neuropsychological status. Arch Clin Neuropsychol. 2016;31(1):8–11.

Gentry MT, Lapid MI, Rummans TA. Geriatric telepsychiatry: systematic review and policy considerations. Am J Geriatr Psychiatry. 2019;27(2):109–27.

Gibbons RD, Weiss DJ, Kupfer DJ, et al. Using computerized adaptive testing to reduce the burden of mental health assessment. Psychiatr Serv. 2008;59(4):361–8.

Gould CE, Kok BC, Ma VK, et al. Veterans Affairs and the Department of Defense Mental Health apps: a systematic literature review. Psychol Serv. 2019a;16(2):196–207.

Gould CE, Kok BC, Ma VK, et al. Video-delivered relaxation intervention reduces late-life anxiety: a pilot randomized controlled trial. Am J Geriatr Psychiatry. 2019b;27(5):514–25.

Gould CE, Loup J, Kuhn E, et al. Technology use and preferences for mental health self-management interventions among older veterans. Int J Geriatr Psychiatry. 2020a;35(3):321–30.

Gould CE, Loup J, Scales AN, et al. Development and refinement of educational materials to help older veterans use VA mental health mobile apps. Prof Psychol Res Pr. 2020b;51(4):414–23.

Gould CE, Carlson C, Ma F, et al. Effects of a mobile app-based intervention for depression in middle-aged and older adults: mixed methods feasibility study. JMIR Form Res. 2021;5(6):e25808.

Grosch MC, Weiner MF, Hynan LS, et al. Video teleconference-based neurocognitive screening in geropsychiatry. Psychiatry Res. 2015;225(3):734–5.

Hansen TI, Haferstrom ECD, Brunner JF, et al. Initial validation of a web-based self-administered neuropsychological test battery for older adults and seniors. J Clin Exp Neuropsychol. 2015;37(6):581–94.

Hantke N, Lajoy M, Gould CE, et al. Patient satisfaction with geriatric psychiatry services via video teleconference. Am J Geriatr Psychiatry. 2020;28(4):491–4.

Hein A, Winkelbach S, Martens B, et al. Monitoring systems for the support of home care. Inform Health Soc Care. 2010;35:157–76.

Jones C, Moyle W, Murfield J, et al. Does cognitive impairment and agitation in dementia influence intervention effectiveness? Findings from a cluster-randomized controlled trial with the therapeutic robot, PARO. J Am Med Direct Assoc. 2018;19(7):623–6.

Knaevelsrud C, Böttche M, Pietrzak RH, et al. Efficacy and feasibility of a therapist-guided internet-based intervention for older persons with childhood traumatization: a randomized controlled trial. Am J Geriatr Psychiatry. 2017;25(8):878–88.

Kuerbis A, Mulliken A, Muench F, et al. Older adults and mobile technology: factors that enhance and inhibit utilization in the context of behavioral health. Ment Health Addict Res. 2017;2(2):1–11.

Lai Kwan C, Mahdid Y, Motta Ochoa R, et al. Wearable technology for detecting significant moments in individuals with dementia. Biomed Res Int. 2019;2019:6515813.

Lum HD, Nearing K, Pimentel CB, et al. Anywhere to anywhere: use of telehealth to increase health care access for older, rural veterans. Public Policy Aging Rep. 2020;30(1):12–8.

Malasinghe LP, Ramzan N, Dahal K. Remote patient monitoring: a comprehensive study. J Ambient Intell Humaniz Comput. 2019;10:57–76.

Martin-Khan M, Flicker L, Wootton R, et al. The diagnostic accuracy of telegeriatrics for the diagnosis of dementia via video conferencing. J Am Med Dir Assoc. 2012;13(5):487.e19.

McMurchie W, Macleod F, Power K, et al. Computerised cognitive behavioural therapy for depression and anxiety with older people: a pilot study to examine patient acceptability and treatment outcome. Int J Geriatr Psychiatry. 2013;28(11):1147–56.

Moo LR, Gately ME, Jafri Z, Shirk SD. Home-based video telemedicine for dementia management. Clin Gerontol. 2020;43(2):193–203.

Moore RC, Depp CA, Wetherell JL, Lenze EJ. Ecological momentary assessment versus standard assessment instruments for measuring mindfulness, depressed mood, and anxiety among older adults. J Psychiatr Res. 2016;75:116–23.

Moyle W, Jones CJ, Murfield JE, et al. Use of a robotic seal as a therapeutic tool to improve dementia symptoms: a cluster-randomized controlled trial. J Am Med Direct Assoc. 2017;18(9):766–73.

Mundt JC, Kinoshita LM, Hsu S, et al. Telephonic remote evaluation of neuropsychological deficits (TREND): longitudinal monitoring of elderly community-dwelling volunteers using touch-tone telephones. Alzheimer Dis Assoc Disord. 2007;21(3):218–24.

Muñoz RF, Chavira DA, Himle JA, et al. Digital apothecaries: a vision for making health care interventions accessible worldwide. Mhealth. 2018;4:18.

Nasreddine ZS, Phillips NA, Bédirian V, et al. The Montreal Cognitive Assessment, MoCA: a brief screening tool for mild cognitive impairment. J Am Geriatr Soc. 2005;53(4):695–9.

Ní Scanaill C, Carew S, Barralon P, et al. A review of approaches to mobility telemonitoring of the elderly in their living environment. Ann Biomed Eng. 2006;34(4):547–63.

Parsons TD. Telemedicine, mobile, and internet-based neurocognitive assessment. In: Clinical neuropsychology and technology. Cham: Springer; 2016. p. 99–111.

Proudfoot J, Ryden C, Everitt B, et al. Clinical efficacy of computerised cognitive-behavioural therapy for anxiety and depression in primary care: randomised controlled trial. Br J Psychiatry. 2004;185(1):46–54.

Rantz M, Skubic M, Miller S, Krampe J. Using technology to enhance aging in place; Proceedings of the international conference on smart homes and health telematics, Singapore, 169–176, 2018.

Rashidi P, Mihailidis A. A survey on ambient-assisted living tools for older adults. IEEE J Biomed Health Inform. 2013;17:579–90.

Ruskin PE, Silver-Aylaian M, Kling MA, et al. Treatment outcomes in depression: comparison of remote treatment through telepsychiatry to in-person treatment. Am J Psychiatry. 2004;161(8):1471–6.

Scollon CN, Prieto CK, Diener E. Experience sampling: promises and pitfalls, strength and weaknesses in assessing well-being. Dordrecht: Springer; 2009. p. 157–80.

Silverstein SM, Berten S, Olson P, et al. Development and validation of a world-wide-web-based neurocognitive assessment battery: WebNeuro. Behav Res Methods. 2007;39(4):940–9.

Smith MM, Tremont G, Ott BR. A review of telephone-administered screening tests for dementia diagnosis. Am J Alzheimers Dis Other Dement. 2009;24(1):58–69.

Snowdon A, Hussein A, Kent R, et al. Comparison of an electronic and paper-based Montreal Cognitive Assessment tool. Alzheimer Dis Assoc Disord. 2015;29(4):325–9.

Steffen AM, Gant JR. A telehealth behavioral coaching intervention for neurocognitive disorder family carers. Int J Geriatr Psychiatry. 2016;31(2):195–203.

Torous J, Roberts LW. The ethical use of mobile health technology in clinical psychiatry. J Nerv Ment Dis. 2017;205(1):4–8.

Troyer AK, Rowe G, Murphy KJ, et al. Development and evaluation of a self-administered online test of memory and attention for middle-aged and older adults. Front Aging Neurosci. 2014;6:335.

Tun SYY, Madanian S, Mirza F. Internet of things (IoT) applications for elderly care: a reflective review. Aging Clin Exp Res. 2021;33(4):855–67.

Van Berkel N, Ferreira D, Kostakos V. The experience sampling method on mobile devices. ACM Comput Surv. 2017;50(6):1–40.

Wadsworth HE, Dhima K, Womack KB, et al. Validity of teleneuropsychological assessment in older patients with cognitive disorders. Arch Clin Neuropsychol. 2018;33(8):1040–5.

Wallace SE, Brown EV, Simpson RC, et al. A comparison of electronic and paper versions of the Montreal Cognitive Assessment. Alzheimer Dis Assoc Disord. 2019;33(3):272–8.

Wittich W, Phillips N, Nasreddine ZS, Chertkow H. Sensitivity and specificity of the Montreal Cognitive Assessment modified for individuals who are visually impaired. J Vis Impair Blind. 2010;104(6):360–8.

Xiang X, Wu S, Zuverink A, et al. Internet-delivered cognitive-behavioral therapies for late-life depressive symptoms: a systematic review and meta-analysis. Aging Ment Health. 2020;27:1–11.

Yip PS, Cheung YT, Chau PH, Law YW. The impact of the epidemic outbreak: the case of the severe acute respiratory syndrome (SARS) and suicide among older adults in Hong Kong. Crisis. 2010;31(2):86.

Zhang Q, Su Y, Yu P. Assisting an elderly with early dementia using wireless sensors data in smarter safer home. Proceedings of the 15th IFIP WG 8.1 International Conference on Informatics and Semiotics in Organisations, Shanghai, China, 398–404, 2014.

Part V

Special Topics

Medical-Legal Topics 17

Mike Kelly, Leah McGowan, and Howard H. Fenn

Abstract

Medical-psychiatric-legal issues are often inescapable in the treatment of geriatric patients. An elderly patient's capacity to make decisions about a work-up ranges in risk, for example, from whether to pursue a X-ray with radio-opaque, contrast medium with adverse impact on kidney function, to a brain biopsy. Treatment decisions can range, for example, from capacity to give informed consent to an antidepressant that can interfere with libido, to open heart surgery to repair an expanding aortic aneurysm.

Although some of these tasks fall within the purview of social workers or other specialists, early recognition by the clinicians who diagnose and direct medical treatment can help avoid more complicated medical-legal problems later and can facilitate smooth delivery of necessary medical and psychiatric care.

The specific statutes that control medical practice, standard of care, definitions of capacity, guardianship, informed consent, involuntary psychiatric treatment, mandatory reporting, and other issues differ between jurisdictions; this chapter offers an overview of the basic concepts behind these topics and principles common to the majority of jurisdictions across the USA and other countries that strive to adhere to an individual's right to make decisions over one's own body. Topics discussed here also include *decision-making capacity over financial matters and estates (testamentary capacity), surrogate decision-making such as conservatorships and guardianships, identification of elder abuse, recognition of vulnerability to undue influence, and mandatory reporting requirements.*

Case Example: Role Confusion of Clinician

An 88-year-old man with heart failure (ejection fraction 33%), chronic renal insufficiency (GFR of 30), and stenosis of both carotid arteries suffered his third stroke in 2 years. He was now dysarthric and intermittently confused and could no longer ambulate. A Montreal Cognitive Assessment (MoCA) scored at 19/30 on hospital admission, and an unspecified dementia was diagnosed by the admitting physician. After a

M. Kelly
Coalinga State Hospital, Coalinga, CA, USA

L. McGowan (✉)
McGowan Family Law, P.C.,
Woodside, CA, USA

H. H. Fenn
VA Health Care System, Palo Alto, CA, USA

Department of Psychiatry and Behavioral Sciences,
Stanford University, Stanford, CA, USA
e-mail: hhfenn@aol.com, howard.fenn@va.gov

H. H. Fenn et al. (eds.), *Age-Adjusted Psychiatric Treatment for the Older Patient*,
https://doi.org/10.1007/978-3-031-53976-3_17

2-week hospitalization, the patient was discharged to live with one of his four daughters, who then initiated a change in the beneficiaries on his five million dollar trust, to make her the sole beneficiary.

This daughter made three video recordings of the patient in the 2 weeks prior to the beneficiary change. In each video, from off-camera, she asked him if he knew who she was and if he agreed with the *change in beneficiaries*. The patient appeared frail, barely alert, gave brief *yes* answers, and nodded his head, apparently in assent to all questions. Daughter asked him if *she* provided what he needed. She said, "I take good care you right?" He nodded. She asked if it was fine to *not* have other siblings visit him, as she said "… it is better for your mental health."

The patient died within one month of the video recordings. At the daughter's request, the treating family physician for over 20 years submitted a letter stating that the patient had demonstrated full decision-making capacity and consented to change the trust. The change in beneficiaries was challenged by the other three daughters and an expert forensic geriatrician was retained, who rebutted the contention that the deceased had mental capacity to revise the trust. A suit alleging elder abuse was also filed against the daughter who was the new beneficiary.

The primary *treating* physician was deposed twice (once by each side) and was subpoenaed to testify at trial for 2 days, during which the expert witness challenged the thoroughness and expertise of the primary care physician's determination of full capacity. The treating physician was also questioned on the stand about any potential benefit she obtained from the change in beneficiaries, as she was a friend of the deceased's new beneficiary and had received gifts in the past from that daughter.

Discussion: This treating primary care physician was enlisted to support one side of a contentious family inheritance dispute. The neutral role of treater was therefore compromised, and this contributed to unnecessary involvement in litigation, stressful testimony in court, and alienation from the patient's family. A retrospective evaluation of the deceased's capacity to execute a change in the trust should have been conducted by an *independent* expert evaluator who would have provided expert testimony.

Assessment

The formal tools used for assessment of capacity range from scales designed to measure a person's ability to engage in activities of daily life, to formal neuropsychological testing. A variety of assessment instruments also provide objective measures of decision-making abilities. The American Bar Association (ABA) and American Psychological Association (APA) co-authored a series of handbooks for use by attorneys, judges, and clinicians on the appropriate use of capacity assessment for older adults in clinical settings (available for free download at http://www.apa.org/pi/aging/programs/assessment.index.aspx) (American Bar Association and American Psychological Association n.d.).

Aging adults with cognitive decline, even those without any psychiatric comorbidities, tend to display more impairment of capacity compared to healthy controls (Huthwaite et al. 2006; Kim et al. 2001; Okonkwo et al. 2008). These impairments tend to be greatest in the domain of *understanding* choices, followed by the domains of *reasoning* and *appreciation* of the decision (Moye and Marson 2007).

Often used interchangeably, the terms *capacity* and *competency* refer to an individual's ability to make informed decisions. *Capacity* often refers to the assessment *by a clinician* of a patient's abilities to make decisions about their healthcare, living situation, and finances. *Competency* often refers to the judicial determination, in court or other administrative hearing, by a magistrate, judge, or jury, of the individual's *legally established* or *adjudicated* ability to exercise a decision. *Competency* often can be based in part on clinical evidence and information about a patient's *cognitive and emotional functioning*.

Various decision-making tasks differ in complexity, outcome, and gravitygravity, and therefore depend on different cognitive abilities to carry them out. The thresholds of evidence needed to demonstrate capacity may differ between tasks and by controlling law in varying legal jurisdictions.

The spectrum of decisions ranges from those that require the straightforward capacity to understand and consent to medications, as assessed by the clinician, to more complex evaluations, such as to undergo a radical mastectomy or decide the beneficiaries of a large estate. Potentially serious outcomes of any decisions may invite or require specific evaluation by specialists, especially by experts who are not part of any ongoing treatment.

Capacity is a situation-specific determination made by clinicians (Mishkin 1989), which rests upon four abilities:

- To communicate a choice
- To apprehend relevant information
- To understand medical consequences
- To reason logically about treatment choices (Appelbaum 2007)

Documentation of the patient's cognitive status and *capacity* for decision-making may be used as evidence (de facto) upon which a Trier of Fact or jury issues a de jure determination.

Competence is a judicial determination about a patient's cognition regarding a specific issue, or generally. In criminal law, a legal Trier of Fact (judge, jury, magistrate, tribunal) may determine that an individual is able to tell the difference between right and wrong, with greater criminal culpability generally if the accused is determined to have exercised decision to commit a criminal act *not influenced* by a mental disorder. In civil law, a legal body may determine that an individual is incapable of making basic life decisions and therefore in need of a conservatorship, guardianship, durable power of attorney for healthcare (DPAHC), or other surrogate decision-makers.

Common domains of decision-making include the capacity to consent to the following:

- Medication use
- Medical and surgical procedures
- ECT and other invasive modalities
- Operation of a motor vehicle
- Legal contracts
- Choice of living situation
- Composition or revision of wills and trusts (testamentary)
- Commission or participation in a criminal act
- Hospitalization
- End-of-life management, withdrawal of treatment, or related interventions
- Administration of involuntary medications or involuntary hospitalization (commitment), which may also rest on the individual's capacity to care for himself/herself or provide food, clothing, and shelter

Advance Directives

These legal instruments allow patients to make healthcare decisions while they have the requisite decisional capacity. The directive may be implemented if and when the patient later *loses* decisional capacity. As long as the individual retains capacity, the advance directive can be revised or revoked. The possible medical decisions that are controlled by the advance directive differ by jurisdiction and may or may not include psychiatric treatment. Advance directives can express personal treatment preferences (e.g., decision directives or living wills) or create proxy directives (e.g., durable power of attorney). As early as possible, a clinician should encourage development of an advance directive in situations of terminal illness, advanced age, chronic disease, possible cognitive decline, or hereditary conditions with potential dire consequences. The limitations of an advance directive include the challenge of anticipating specifics of medical decisions that may arise in the future, which also involve the uncertainty of how one may feel in the face of particular, and unforeseen, sets of choices. Another limitation involves the difficulty of implementing an advance directive if family members or others strenuously oppose the directed care.

The clinician with knowledge of any future treatment within her or his expertise should begin discussion of the need for an advance directive by the following:

- Describing realistic clinical scenarios and healthcare decisions which the patient or family may confront.
- Explaining the options in detail and ensure understanding.
- Answering questions about specific medical interventions and decisions which may arise.
- Inviting family and caregivers into the process, with patient's permission.
- The Patient Self-Determination Act (1990) in the USA requires hospitals, skilled nursing facilities, home health agencies, hospice programs, and health maintenance organizations to:
  - Inform patients about their right to make decisions concerning their medical care.
  - Periodically inquire as to whether a patient executed an advanced directive and document the patient's wishes regarding their medical care.
  - Refrain from discriminating against individuals who have executed an advance directive.
  - Ensure that legally valid advance directives and documented medical care wishes are implemented.
  - Provide educational programs for staff, patients, and the community on ethical issues concerning patient self-determination and advance directives (Levin 2015).

Proxy Directives

Patients may designate others to make care decisions through proxy directives (known also as Durable Power of Attorney). Proxy directives designate a particular individual to make financial and/or medical decisions for a person if he or she ever lacks capacity. States have statutes that authorize a proxy directive or "durable power of attorney for health care." These codes specify when the power of attorney will take effect, which is usually when the patient's physician determines that he or she lacks decision-making capacity. At that point, the physician must obtain informed consent from the designated proxy. The document that the patient signs will allow another individual, who is designated, to make healthcare decisions on his or her behalf in the event of incapacity—a durable power of attorney for healthcare (DPOAHC).

Decision Directives/Living Wills

Decision directives, known also as living wills, allow patients to outline preferences for healthcare treatment. Like the proxy directives described above, they typically become effective when a patient lacks decisional capacity. Patients can use living wills to declare their wishes regarding the use of life-sustaining treatment in the event they become terminally ill or permanently unconscious. The living will, therefore, authorizes physicians to follow instructions regarding medical treatment that was previously designated by the patient.

Only a patient can revoke her or his own living will. A patient can change or revoke the living will at any time when she or he is capable of making the decision to change the living will. Living wills may not be changed once a person loses decision-making capacity. Unfortunately, a patient's living will may not envision all potential scenarios or take into account advances in medical science that might change prognoses. A patient can designate a healthcare proxy and still outline preferences for treatment. In instances where a patient has both a durable power of attorney and a decision directive, the decision directive has priority.

Testamentary Documents

Educating patients about the availability of testamentary documents such as advance directives (for the patient's own healthcare) and wills (for dispossession of assets) can avoid situations of undue influence and exploitation and provide an opportunity for the individual to make more choices.

Conservatorship, Guardianship, and Surrogates

A court or legal authority may appoint a guardian, conservator, or surrogate decision-maker to act on behalf of a person if the Trier of Fact or judicial authority determines the person lacks decision-making capacity in personal or financial affairs, such as inability to find housing, pay bills, or avoid wandering. This process is intended to ensure that vulnerable individuals who lack capacity are protected from exploitation and neglect, in situations where mechanisms such as advanced directives, proxy directives, or decision directives are not available or not working. The Uniform Guardianship and Protective Proceedings Act (Uniform Adult Guardianship and Protective Proceedings Jurisdiction Act (2007) n.d.) details the procedures for the appointment of guardians and conservators for incapacitated persons.

A *guardian* is qualified pursuant to court appointment and has custody of the individual lacking capacity. Typically, guardianships of the person involve the appointment of someone to make decisions that are not financial in nature, such as healthcare and housing (Schouten 2017). Guardianships of the estate may be appointed to manage financial affairs. Certain jurisdictions use the term "guardianship" to signify both financial and nonfinancial decision-making power, while other states refer to this as a "conservatorship." Guardianship essentially denies a person who lacks capacity, the legal right to engage in decision-making. When a guardian is appointed, the individual lacking capacity may not enter contracts, manage funds, file lawsuits, vote, or consent to surgery.

Limited guardianships may be effective for persons who lack decision-making capacity in one domain (e.g., healthcare decision-making) but retain decision-making capacity in another (e.g., finances). This type of guardianship protects the incapacitated individual within the domain of incapacity while retaining the individual's authority and autonomy to make decisions within other functional domains where decision-making remains intact.

A *conservator* is appointed by a court to manage business affairs and the estate of the individual lacking capacity over these issues. The law assumes that, unless proven otherwise, individuals with appointed guardians or conservators *also* lack *testamentary* capacity, the capacity to make a will. However, because finances and estates often arouse disagreements, testamentary capacity can be challenged. The question may be brought by family or patient to the treating clinician who may be placed in an awkward position of supporting or opposing the patient or family. A formal evaluation and evidentiary report are often best conducted by an independent, non-treating expert evaluator.

Guardians and conservators make decisions on behalf of the individual lacking capacity based upon either of two standards:

- The *best interest standard* by which the appointed person acts in accord with the best interest of the incapacitated person.
- The *substituted judgment standard* whereby the appointed persons must make choices based on what they think the incapacitated person *would have chosen* prior to becoming incapacitated. Advance directives can provide evidence of the incapacitated person's wishes.

The individual subject to limitations on self-determination may experience lowered self-esteem, passivity, and feelings of inadequacy and incompetency. Because of this potential for adverse psychological effects, courts are instructed to impose the least restrictive but safe mechanism for alternative decision-making (Judicial Determination of Capacity of Older Adults in Guardianship Proceedings (n.d.)).

Elder Abuse

First referenced during the 1970s (Burston 1975), elder abuse remains underreported in a variety of settings (Cooper et al. 2008; Moore 2016). It can encompass physical abuse, verbal or psychological abuse, sexual abuse, neglect, and financial exploitation (Lachs and Pillemer 2015).

Prevalence data suggests that roughly 10% of older adults are victims of abuse over a 12-month period. Considered together, these types of abuse occur in approximately 10% of older adults over a 12-month period with neglect being the type most commonly reported to adult protective services (Cooper et al. 2008). Victims of abuse are often afraid to disclose what they have experienced. Suspected victims should be interviewed in a comfortable, nonthreatening environment.

Identifying elder abuse can be a particular challenge among aging persons with multiple medical comorbidities (e.g., bruising on a patient's arms can be attributed to a fall). Medical malpractice has also been identified as a potential source of elder abuse. For instance, in Bergman v. Chin (1999), a San Francisco physician was determined to be negligent for failing to adequately treat the pain of an 85-year-old cancer patient. Clinicians need to remain cognizant of the fact that an older adult's lack of communication should not automatically indicate a lack of pain or discomfort.

In most jurisdictions, clinicians are *mandated reporters*, which means they are obligated to report suspected elder abuse. Mandated reporters are not typically held liable for reports of abuse made in good faith; failure to report or interfering with a report of elder abuse is a misdemeanor in many states, however. Adult protective services agencies help geriatric individuals who are victims of abuse by providing investigatory, protective, and supportive services through state or county funding. Family members and elder victims may be willing to report abuse when queried. But mental health clinicians must also avoid the role of a detective, gathering evidence against a suspect, at the expense of clinical care.

Types of elder abuse include the following:

- *Abandonment* is defined often by withdrawal or desertion by someone who has assumed responsibility for the care of an adult presumed incapable of care.
- *Psychological:* The act of promoting emotional pain or distress by verbal or nonverbal behavior.
- *Financial exploitation* or material exploitation: Illegal or unauthorized or improper use of an older adult's property or financial assets.
- *Physical abuse*: Actions that can affect injury to body, pain, or impairment.
- *Neglect*: Lack of fulfillment of obligations to care for older adult.
- *Sexual abuse*: Nonconsensual sexual interaction with an older adult (adapted from the National Center on Elder Abuse. http://www.ncea.aoa.gov).

High levels of stress among those who care for geriatric individuals have been associated with elder abuse and neglect. One study involving 481 nurses and healthcare assistants found that high levels of stress coupled with poor working relationships among team members were associated with provider burnout, elder abuse, and neglect (Andela et al. 2018). The demands on caregivers for persons with MNCD increased during the COVID-19 pandemic (Cohen et al. 2020). Vigilance for potential elder neglect and abuse is appropriate.

Undue Influence

Vulnerability to undue influence deserves attention in part due to the prevalence of MNCD in society, longer life spans, and communication technologies through which a vulnerable individual can be abused. Scams, email and text phishing, and false documents can lead to theft of funds, disbursement of assets in wills, or false contracts. Some jurisdictions have codified and defined the elements under which undue influence is likely to occur:

- A confidential relationship with opportunity for influence; the will, or other testament would not have otherwise been changed but for undue influence.
- Influence on someone, with a disposition or inclination.
- Suspicious circumstances around the creation of a will.

Characteristics which suggest *vulnerability* to undue influence include the following:

- Impaired cognition or impaired emotional capacity
- Sensory or cognitive impairment
- Grief and loss
- Substance use or dependence
- Special relationship with a caregiver, suitor, de facto partner, or spouse, who is younger and more cognitively intact than the alleged victim
- Dependence (physical or emotional) of the alleged victim or testator upon the alleged influencer

Undue influence can be difficult to detect and challenging to prove. The abusive behavior of an influencer does not typically occur in view of others or yield direct evidence of abuse or neglect (e.g., video recordings, eyewitness accounts, etc.). Circumstantial evidence indicative of undue influence is often the only type of evidence available. Examples include the following:

- Unanticipated changes to a loved one's will (e.g., will changed when testator is near death)
- A setting in which the testator is allowed only limited access to loved ones (e.g., influencer keeps loved one separate from rest of family)
- Restricted communications (e.g.., influencer manages correspondence, text messages, etc.) and/or cognitive or health limitations which make the testator dependent on the influencer for information and sustenance

Courts often rely on indirect evidence to determine whether undue influence was exercised or capacity was not intact. Clinical notes might be used as evidence if a patient's will is contested. A thorough and well-documented assessment of a geriatric patient's mental status can be helpful in the event that undue influence is later suspected.

The case example above suggested that the deceased testator was vulnerable to assent to leading questions and was not allowed the opportunity to object or voice genuine wishes. The alleged influencer (daughter) acknowledged the imposition of limited access to other family members who might have offered alternative information to the vulnerable individual.

Mandatory Reporting

The clinician must adhere to reporting requirements in the jurisdiction of practice. These codes generally mandate reporting common clinical situations, including the following:

- Elder abuse and neglect (e.g., the California Welfare and Institutions Code Section 15630-15632 (elder abuse reporting)
- Capacity to operate a motor vehicle
- The diagnosis of major neurocognitive disorder (MNCD), other cognitive impairment, seizure disorder, or other etiologies for intermittent loss of consciousness
- Risk of harm to others

Conclusions

Medical-legal issues, understandably, may rank low on the list of priorities for the busy clinical team. Yet these concerns are often unavoidable in the treatment of the geriatric patient, especially one who has cognitive limitations, and whose medical and psychiatric conditions are complex and serious. The clinician who recognizes the emergence of cognitive decline can educate patient and families about competency, capacity to exercise good judgement, decision-making, and the need for advance directives or surrogates to manage future medical decisions.

Attending to these issues early in evaluation and treatment can head off later more complex problems that may interfere with the delivery of crucial medical care. Charting should include documentation of standard of care, assessment of the patient's decision-making capacity, and efforts to disclose information needed for informed consent. Where indicated, an assessment for, and reporting of, vulnerability to elder abuse or undue influence is needed.

In sum, knowledge of, and adherence to, the statutes which control medical treatment in the jurisdiction of care for the aged patient, and other medical-legal issues, can clarify the physician's role as treater, can facilitate smooth delivery of healthcare, and can strengthen the treatment alliance with patient and family.

Age-Adjusted Recommendations

- Document the assessment of *capacity to consent* to medical/surgical procedures and medications, as well as discussions of the risk-benefit ratio of treatments proposed.
- Assess and document capacity for *refusal* of essential medical care, where consequences of not treating are consequential or life-threatening.
- Identify decision-making surrogates, conservators, proxies, and guardians early in treatment.
- With the patient's assent or expressed consent, enlist family and trusted others in crucial medical decision-making.
- Refer families and patients who request medical-legal opinion involving litigation and involving financial, contracts, and estate issues to *independent* expert evaluators who are not involved in providing treatment or clinical consultation. This avoids confusing the role of treater with the role of legal advocate.
- Document evidence of elder abuse or vulnerability to undue influence.
- Report clinical information (such as dementia and capacity to drive) as required by law.
- Recognize that informal notes, clinical records, reports, and verbal comments may be discoverable in case of litigation, and authors of clinical information can be compelled to testify in legal proceedings.
- Unless otherwise contracted, recognize that the clinician's role in litigation is only to provide *clinical evidence and* not to provide an opinion as an expert witness.
- Review pertinent statutes which regulate and control medical practice in your jurisdiction.

References

American Bar Association and American Psychological Association. Assessment of older adults with diminished capacity: a handbook for psychologists. n.d.. http://www.apa.org/pi/aging/programs/assessment/capacity-psychologist-handbook.pdf.

Andela M, Truchot D, Huguenotte V. Work environment and elderly abuse in nursing homes: the mediating role of burnout. J Interpers Violence. 2018;36(11–12):5709–29.

Appelbaum PS. Assessment of patients' competence to consent to treatment. NEJM. 2007;357(18):1834–40.

Bergman v. Chin. 1999.

Burston GR. Letter: Granny-battering. BMJ. 1975;3(5983):592.

Cohen G, Russo MJ, Campos JA, Allegri RF. Living with dementia: increased level of caregiver stress in times of COVID-19. Int Psychogeriatr. 2020;32(11):1377–81.

Cooper C, Selwood A, Livingston G. The prevalence of elder abuse and neglect: a systematic review. Age Ageing. 2008;37(2):151–60.

Huthwaite JS, Martin RC, Griffith HR, et al. Declining medical decision-making capacity in mild AD: a two-year longitudinal study. Behav Sci Law. 2006;24:453–63.

Judicial Determination of Capacity of Older Adults in Guardianship Proceedings. A handbook for judges. n.d.. https://www.apa.org/pi/aging/resources/guides/judges-diminished.pdf. Accessed XX.

Kim SYH, Caine ED, Currier GW, et al. Assessing the competence of persons with Alzheimer's disease in providing informed consent for participation in research. Am J Psychiatry. 2001;158(5):712–7.

Lachs MS, Pillemer KA. Elder abuse. NEJM. 2015;373(20):1947–56.

Levin S. H.R.4449—101st congress (1989–1990): Patient Self Determination Act of 1990. 2015. https://www.congress.gov/bill/101st-congress/house-bill/4449.

Mishkin B. Determining the capacity for making health care decisions. In: Issues in geriatric psychiatry, vol. 19. Basel: Karger Publishers; 1989. p. 151–66.

Moore S. See no evil, hear no evil, speak no evil? Underreporting of abuse in care homes. J Adult Prot. 2016;18:303.

Moye J, Marson DC. Assessment of decision-making capacity in older adults: an emerging area of practice and research. J Gerontol B Psychol Sci Soc Sci. 2007;62(1):3–11.

Okonkwo OC, Griffith HR, Belue K, et al. Cognitive models of medical decision-making capacity in patients with mild cognitive impairment. J Int Neuropsychol Soc. 2008;14(2):297–308.

Schouten R. Mental health practice and the law. 1st ed. Oxford: Oxford University Press; 2017.

Uniform Adult Guardianship and Protective Proceedings Jurisdiction Act (2007). n.d.. http://www.uniformlaws.org/shared/docs/adult_guardianship/UAGPPJA_2011_Final Act_2015feb4.pdf.

18 Nutraceuticals, Dietary, and Herbal Supplements

Talia Puzantian

Abstract

The use of over-the-counter supplements and nutraceuticals by aging adults over age 60 in the United States is common, with a 67% increase over 10 years (Mishra S, Dietary supplement use among adults: United States, 2017–2018. NCHS Data Brief, no 399. Hyattsville: National Center for Health Statistics, 2021). Over half of USA adults use at least one dietary supplement and use grows in advancing age, with an estimated 74.3% of those 60 and older taking dietary supplements (Mishra S, Dietary supplement use among adults: United States, 2017–2018. NCHS Data Brief, no 399. Hyattsville: National Center for Health Statistics, 2021). The *number* of supplements used also is greater with age, with a quarter of older adults taking four or more supplements. The most frequently used are multivitamin-mineral supplements, vitamin D, omega-3 fatty acids, calcium, and vitamin B12. Due to the paucity of evidence, clinicians may be unprepared to answer questions or make recommendations about these products. This chapter offers an overview of what is known regarding the efficacy and safety of various common supplements which have purported benefits for psychiatric symptoms and syndromes in aging adults. Improving and maintaining overall health are the most commonly reported reasons for taking supplements (Bailey RL, JAMA Intern Med 173:355–361, 2013). As people age, they tend to burn fewer calories, be less physically active, gradually lose lean muscle mass, need fewer calories, and experience decreased appetite. Therefore, aging adults may need more nutrients via supplementation to maintain proper health. Aging adults also report specific motivations for using supplements such as heart, bone/joint, or eye health (Bailey RL, JAMA Intern Med 173:355–361, 2013). This broadens the range of products typically used by the geriatric population to include not only dietary supplements but also medicinal herbs (sometimes referred to as phytoceuticals or phytochemicals) and other "natural products." See Table 18.1.

T. Puzantian (✉)
Keck Graduate Institute School of Pharmacy and Health Sciences, Claremont, CA, USA
e-mail: tpuzantian@kgi.edu

H. H. Fenn et al. (eds.), *Age-Adjusted Psychiatric Treatment for the Older Patient*,
https://doi.org/10.1007/978-3-031-53976-3_18

Table 18.1 Supplements commonly used by older adults

Phytoceutical/nutraceutical	Target disease/condition
Antioxidants (vitamin E, vitamin C, polyphenols)	Cancer, heart disease, and neurodegenerative disease
B vitamins (folate, B6, B12)	Heart disease and neurocognitive disorders
Calcium and vitamin D	Osteoporosis, cancer, and diabetes mellitus
Coenzyme Q10	Inflammation and endothelial dysfunction
Epigallocatechin-3-gallate (EGCG)	Cancer
Fiber (soluble and insoluble)	Diabetes mellitus and constipation
Glucosamine, chondroitin, and collagen	Osteoarthritis
Lutein, zeaxanthin, and lycopene	Macular degeneration
Multivitamins and minerals	Overall health maintenance
Omega-3 fatty acids (fish oil, DHA, EPA)	Inflammation, heart disease, and stroke
Plant stanols/sterols	Elevated blood cholesterol and heart disease
Prebiotics and probiotics	Diarrhea and gut health
Whey protein	Sarcopenia (muscle mass and strength)
Zinc	Immunity and macular degeneration

Adapted from Gupta and Prakash (2015)

Case Example

A 77-year-old male, semiretired licensed practical nurse, was referred to his primary care physician by a dental hygienist who noticed that the patient showed excessive bleeding in his gums. The patient became apprehensive about repeated bleeding and as a result avoided brushing his teeth regularly. The patient was being treated for atrial fibrillation with warfarin, 3 mg daily, and had a stable INR ranging between 2.0 and 2.5.

The primary care physician explored the patient's use of nutraceuticals and found that he had been taking Ginkgo (Ginkgo biloba) for cognitive complaints for about one year at an excessive dose. When the Ginkgo was discontinued, the bleeding of gums resolved.

Psychiatric consultation for a neurocognitive disorder was sought. Upon psychiatric evaluation, the patient complained of difficulties in short-term memory, word-finding, and cognitive processing speed. He had mild chronic insomnia, anxiously depressed mood, no suicidal ideation, nor psychotic symptoms. MSE revealed dysphoric, non-melancholic, non-tearful affect, PHQ-9 of 12, and MoCA of 22/30 with 1/5 recall memory and 1/3 serial subtractions. A trial of mirtazapine 7.5 mg bedtime led to improved sleep, mood, and cognitive performance. After 5 weeks of treatment, the MoCA was 25/30 and subsequent PHQ-9 was 5.

Discussion: Careful history taking and clinical suspicion elicited information about the use of a nutraceutical which was responsible for adverse effects not previously recognized.

Overview of Commonly Used Nutraceuticals and Supplements

These types of over-the-counter products are *not* regulated by the USA Food and Drug Administration (FDA) to the same extent as prescription or traditional over-the-counter *medications*. Since they are not intended to "prevent, treat, or cure disease", they fall under the Dietary Supplement Health and Education Act (DSHEA) of 1994. There is no requirement for rigorous clinical trials assessing efficacy or safety to market these products (Pew Charitable Trusts 2017). The DSHEA only requires that manufacturers and distributors ensure that their products are not adulterated or misbranded and gives the USA FDA authority to take action against any adulterated or misbranded marketed products. The FDA has exercised this authority and taken such action. For example, in 2019, FDA brought action against companies that were making false claims for more than 58 products that purported to prevent, treat, or cure Alzheimer's disease (Food and Drug Administration (FDA) 2018).

Due to the paucity of evidence, clinicians may find they are unprepared to answer questions or make recommendations when facing patients' inquiries about these products. What follows is a summary of what is known regarding the efficacy and safety of various common supplements which have purported benefits for psychiatric symptoms and syndromes seen in aging adults (Table 18.1).

Evidence for Use

Compared to traditional FDA-approved medications, supplements are less rigorously studied, and their clinical trials vary widely in quality. Small sample size, poorly designed methodology, homogeneity of population studied (typically, healthy younger adults), and short trial duration are major limitations to determining efficacy for older adults. Nevertheless, a well-informed healthcare professional can help older adults make more deliberate decisions when considering the use of supplements.

Supplements for Depressive and Anxiety Disorders

Surveys of USA adults have indicated that 40–50% with moderate mental distress or self-reported "depression" used complementary medicines in the previous year (Rhee et al. 2017; Kessler et al. 2001). However, studies usually included healthy or younger adults rather than aging adults.

- **Inositol** is a naturally occurring isomer of glucose, is derived from diet, and is involved in serotonin, dopamine, and glutamate neurotransmission. Its purported benefits include improvement of bipolar disorder, depressive disorders, premenstrual dysphoric disorder (PMDD), obsessive-compulsive disorder (OCD), panic disorder, and posttraumatic stress disorder (PTSD). Studies are small with mixed findings. A meta-analysis found no statistically significant benefit, including either as monotherapy or adjunct for major depressive disorder; a nonsignificant trend toward benefit was seen only for depressive symptoms in PMDD (Mukai et al. 2014). Its use is generally not recommended because studies have not demonstrated evidence of efficacy (Sarris et al. 2022). Although well tolerated, it is not recommended due to insufficient evidence of efficacy.
- **Kava** originates from the roots of *Piper methysticum*, a plant native to the South Pacific where it is consumed as a beverage for religious, medicinal, and recreational purposes. In Western countries like the USA, it is available as capsule, tablet, and concentrated liquid elixir formulations. Its proposed mechanism of action is GABA modulation and reuptake inhibition of norepinephrine and dopamine (Sarris et al. 2011). Initial reports of anxiolytic effects were favorable, but more recent studies and a meta-analysis did not find a significant difference compared to placebo (Ooi et al. 2018); its use in anxiety disorders is therefore not recommended (Sarris et al. 2022). Common adverse effects include headache and sedation. The numerous reports of severe hepatotoxicity and liver failure, most often with long-term use, represent a significant safety concern. Some have suggested that contaminants were responsible for cases of liver failure; however, it is also known that certain kavalactones are toxic (White 2018). Dermopathies, reversible eruptions typically on the arms and upper back, have also been reported with regular kava use.
- **Lavender** (*Lavandula angustifolia*) may be a reasonable option for generalized anxiety disorder (Sarris et al. 2022). A large randomized, double-blind, controlled study showed that a proprietary blend of linalool, linalyl acetate, and other compounds from the lavender plant had better efficacy than both placebo and paroxetine 20 mg/day on the Hamilton Anxiety Rating Scale (Kasper et al. 2014). Secondary measures of depression, sleep, and quality of life also fared better with the lavender preparation. A smaller study found lavender to have comparable efficacy to lorazepam 0.5 mg/day in patients with generalized anxiety disorder (Woelk and Schläfke 2010). Both studies used a proprietary blend marketed as *Silexan*, a prescription product in other countries. In the USA, it is available over the counter as *CalmAid*. One systematic review and meta-analysis of the effects of lavender on anxiety deemed the majority of studies to be of poor quality (Donelli et al. 2019). Oral *Silexan* seemed effective, but the benefits of topical oil and inhalation preparations were less robust and difficult to assess due to methodological

limitations. Adverse effects are mild and include nausea, mild headaches, and lavender-flavored burping. Lavender has some weak estrogenic effects, possibly significant only in prepubertal individuals.

- **L-Methylfolate** is a metabolite of dietary folic acid necessary for the synthesis of neurotransmitters including serotonin, dopamine, and norepinephrine. Dietary folate is transformed to L-methylfolate by methylenetetrahydrofolate reductase (MTHFR), an enzyme for which some people may have a genetic polymorphism that impedes conversion. Several studies support the use of either folate or L-methylfolate (for those who cannot convert) as adjuncts to antidepressants for depressive disorder (Alvarez-Mon et al. 2021). As with other supplements, the data on outcomes are not robust. However, the use of L-methylfolate is well tolerated and safe, so it may be a reasonable adjunct in depressive disorders (Sarris et al. 2022).
- **Omega-3 fatty acids** are essential polyunsaturated fatty acids (PUFAs) found in many fish and certain nuts and seeds (Alvarez-Mon et al. 2021). Supplementation with omega-3 fatty acids as augmentation in depressive disorders appears beneficial in some studies; however, most meta-analyses have not shown robust effects (Asher et al. 2017; Hallahan et al. 2016; Sarris et al. 2016; Schefft et al. 2017). Network meta-analyses found higher response rates with SSRI or St. John's wort compared to omega-3 fatty acids as monotherapy (Asher et al. 2017). Trials of omega-3s in combination with SSRIs resulted in greater response rates than either intervention alone (Asher et al. 2017). In studies showing most robust benefit, the formulation was predominantly more eicosapentaenoic acid (EPA) than docosahexaenoic acid (DHA) in content (Hallahan et al. 2016; Sarris et al. 2022). The Canadian Network for Mood and Anxiety Treatments (CANMAT) recommend omega-3s as second-line monotherapy for mild to moderate depressive disorder and second-line adjunctive for moderate to severe depressive disorder (Ravindran et al. 2016). The American Psychiatric Association Task Force on Complementary and Alternative Medicine in Major Depressive Disorder also support the use of omega-3s as an adjunct (Freeman et al. 2010). Typically, omega-3s are well tolerated, with mostly mild gastrointestinal side effects including nausea, diarrhea, and fishy taste, but there have been rare reports of manic episode induction and bleeding risk.
- **S-Adenosyl-L-methionine, or SAMe**, is an endogenous amino acid metabolite made from methionine derived from diet. It regulates key functions in living cells by, among other mechanisms, serving as a methyl donor involved in the signaling and production of monoamines including dopamine, serotonin, and norepinephrine. A large number of studies of SAMe in depressive disorder have shown evidence of efficacy, more so as augmentation rather than monotherapy, although studies had significant methodological limitations (Asher et al. 2017; Sharma et al. 2017; Sarris et al. 2022). SAMe is generally well tolerated but can cause gastrointestinal upset, insomnia, irritability, restlessness, and activation in some patients. Manic and hypomanic episode induction may be more of an issue with the injectable formulation used in Europe.
- **St. John's wort** (*Hypericum perforatum)* is a perennial plant, with active components in the flowering buds that may inhibit the reuptake of monoamines and have weak monoamine oxidase inhibition activity. In randomized controlled trials for treatment of depressive disorders, it has demonstrated benefit over placebo and effects equal to low-dose TCAs and low-dose SSRIs (Asher et al. 2017; Ravindran et al. 2016; Freeman et al. 2010). The positive results have been found for milder depressive disorders. A study in moderate to severe depressive disorder did not show benefit over placebo or sertraline (Hypericum Depression Trial Study Group 2002). When used, it should be as monotherapy, standardized to a dose of 0.2–0.3% hypericin or 5–6% hyperforin (Sarris et al. 2022). St. John's wort is well tolerated in most, although some patients may experience

gastrointestinal upset, headache, photosensitivity, and skin irritation. Serotonin syndrome and manic episodes have been reported rarely, and St. John' wort should not be combined with serotonergic agents.

- Caution should be exercised in patients taking other medications due to the high risk for drug-drug interactions. St. John's wort is a strong cytochrome P450 inducer (especially CYP3A4 which is responsible for the metabolism of half of medications but also CYP2C9, CYP2C19, CYP1A2, and P-glycoprotein) (Mannel 2004). It can reduce serum levels of many other medications, leading to significant clinical effects including, among others, antiviral resistance in HIV patients, insufficient anticoagulation, transplant rejection, and contraception failure.
- **Tryptophan (or L-tryptophan)** is an essential amino acid that is converted to 5-HTP in the body and plays a role in the synthesis of serotonin. It is not synthesized endogenously but must be supplied through diet. It was theorized that intake of this neurotransmitter precursor may potentiate antidepressant effects. The majority of studies are inadequately powered and inconclusive. Neither a randomized controlled trial nor a systematic review has yet provided clear evidence of efficacy as an adjunct in depressive disorder; hence its use is not recommended (Ravindran et al. 2016; Sarris et al. 2022). Tryptophan is generally well tolerated with mild side effects including drowsiness, gastrointestinal distress, dry mouth, and blurry vision. Thousands of cases of eosinophilia myalgia syndrome in the late 1980s led to a recall; however, the reaction was likely due to contaminants specific to batches from a Japanese manufacturer, rather than tryptophan itself.
- **Vitamin D** is derived from sunshine, dietary intake, and supplementation. Dietary sources provide D2 (ergocalciferol) from plant sources such as mushrooms and soy milk and D3 (cholecalciferol) from animal sources such as tuna, swordfish, and salmon. D3 is more potent and generally the preferred form for supplementation. Vitamin D insufficiency and deficiency (serum levels of 25-hydroxyvitamin D below 30 ng/mL) are commonly seen with older adults, particularly if they are housebound or living in nursing homes. Inadequate levels of vitamin D have been associated with symptoms of depressive disorder, but whether supplementation may be *beneficial* in patients with depressive disorder is unclear (Parker et al. 2017). Vitamin D deficiency increases the risk of delirium in older patients (Chouët et al. 2020). Some studies, with significant methodological limitations, have suggested benefit from vitamin D supplementation in depressive disorder (Sarris et al. 2022). However, several meta-analyses do not support its use beyond those patients with insufficiency or deficiency. Vitamin D supplementation is well tolerated. As a fat-soluble vitamin, toxicity is possible but would generally require much higher dosing than that typically used for supplementation. See Table 18.2.

Supplements Used for Insomnia

Insomnia and disrupted sleep are common complaints of aging adults. However, the use of prescribed medications often comes with the risk of tolerance, dependence, and withdrawal, as well as increased risk for falls, fractures, and/or cognitive impairment. Over-the-counter medications approved for treating insomnia may also be problematic. Antihistaminergic agents (e.g., diphenhydramine, doxylamine) have secondary anticholinergic effects that cause troubling adverse effects including dry mouth, constipation, blurred vision, and cognitive impairment (delirium and/or major neurocognitive disorder). The following supplements for insomnia have some appeal:

- **Melatonin** is an endogenous hormone, produced typically in darkness and released by the pineal gland to control the sleep-wake cycle. Supplementation with exogenous melatonin has been extensively studied and has shown benefit in sleep quality and in sleep-

Table 18.2 Supplements used for depressive and anxiety disorders

Supplement	Reported use(s)	Usual dosage range	Evidence of efficacy	Safety concerns
Inositol	Depressive disorders Anxiety disorders OCD PTSD	Up to 12 g per day	Mixed findings; meta-analysis showed no statistically significant benefit, not recommended	Well tolerated, flatulence, nausea, and abdominal pain
Kava	Anxiety disorders	120 mg/day for up to 3 months	Mixed, inconclusive findings, not recommended	Hepatotoxicity and dermatitis
Lavender *(Silexan, CalmAid)*	Generalized anxiety disorder	80–160 mg po QHS	As effective as lorazepam 0.5 mg/day and more effective than paroxetine 20 mg/day; less support for topical oils and inhalations	Well tolerated, lavender-flavored burping, and weak estrogenic properties (avoid under age 18)
L-methylfolate (*Deplin*, others)	Depressive disorders	15 mg po QD	May reduce depressive symptoms as adjunctive	Well tolerated
Omega-3 fatty acids	Depressive disorders	500–2000 mg po QD or divided BID-TID	Studies show benefit of preparations with >60% EPA as adjunctive to antidepressants in milder depressive disorders	Well tolerated, nausea, loose stools, fishy taste, bleeding, and manic episode
S-Adenosyl-L-methionine (SAMe)	Depressive disorders	400–800 mg po BID	More than 50 studies show promising benefit mostly as augmentation, but studies mostly of poor quality	Nausea, diarrhea, agitation, manic episode, hypomanic episode, and serotonin syndrome
St. John's wort	Depressive disorders	300 mg po TID (standardized to 0.2–0.3% hypericin or 5–6% hyperforin)	May be effective in mild depression; used as monotherapy only	Drug-drug interactions, serotonin syndrome, manic episode, and photosensitivity
Tryptophan/5-hydroxytryptophan (5-HTP)	Depressive disorders	Tryptophan: 500–2000 mg po divided BID-TID 5-HTP: 200–300 mg divided BID-QID	Minimal evidence to support use, not recommended	Well tolerated, serotonin syndrome, and eosinophilia-myalgia syndrome (current products are likely safe)
Vitamin D	Depressive disorders	1000–5000 IU po QD	Potential benefit most likely in those with insufficiency or deficiency	Well tolerated and toxicity rare

onset insomnia but likely is not helpful for sleep maintenance (Fatemeh et al. 2022). A recent systematic review of a dozen meta-analyses found significant but small improvements in objective measures of sleep (Low et al. 2020). At usual doses, it is well tolerated. At higher doses, some patients may experience vivid dreams or morning grogginess.

- **Valerian**, from the root of *Valeriana officinalis*, was first described by Hippocrates. Its mechanism of action is not clear, but it likely binds to GABA receptors. Studies of its use for anxiety disorders did not demonstrate benefits over placebo. Multiple reviews and meta-analyses of insomnia studies, the majority of which had significant methodologic limitations, found conflicting findings. Evaluating these studies is difficult as some studies used valerian in combination with other herbal products including passionflower (*Passiflora*

Table 18.3 Supplements used for insomnia

Supplement	Reported use(s)	Usual dosage range	evidence of efficacy	Safety concerns
Melatonin	Insomnia	1–5 mg po HS	May reduce the time to fall asleep and improve subjective feeling of sleep quality	Well tolerated but grogginess and vivid dreams possible at higher doses
Valerian	Insomnia	300–600 mg po HS	Inconsistent findings and may help subjective feeling of sleep quality only	Well tolerated and avoid combining with other CNS depressants

incarnate), lemon balm (*Melissa officinalis*), and hops (*Humulus lupulus*). *Objective* measures of sleep were not improved; however, some studies suggested that valerian may improve *subjective* sleep quality (Lelli et al. 2021). Common side effects include sedation and dizziness. Its combination with other CNS depressants, including alcohol and benzodiazepines, should be avoided due to the potential for additive effects. See Table 18.3.

Supplements for Neurocognitive Disorders

Gradual decline of cognitive capabilities is an inherent part of aging. Mild cognitive impairment (MCI) in some aging adults will progress to major neurocognitive disorder (MNCD)/dementia, often accompanied by behavioral and psychological symptoms of dementia (BPSD). There are no medications proven to permanently prevent the progression of neurocognitive decline. However, supplements purported to prevent cognitive decline or improve cognitive function is burgeoning.

- **Ginkgo** (*Ginkgo biloba*), a tree native to China and the oldest living tree species, has been used medicinally for over 1000 years with purported neuroprotective effects. Over 400 clinical trials have evaluated its medicinal uses, with a great majority examining its effects on cognition. Evidence of its efficacy for treating MNCD/dementia (both Alzheimer's disease and vascular dementia) is inconsistent. In a systematic Cochrane Database review, three of four studies did not show benefits compared to placebo (Birks and Grimley Evans 2009). For prevention of MNCD/dementia, studies enrolled patients with normal cognition or MCI; studies also evaluated whether ginkgo could enhance memory in adults with normal cognitive functioning. Studies with more robust methodology showed no improvement in memory function in those with impairment, no reduction in dementia risk in cognitively healthy adults or those with MCI, nor memory enhancement in cognitively intact adults (DeKosky et al. 2008; Solomon et al. 2002; Tewari et al. 2018). Ginkgo is generally safe and well tolerated with only gastrointestinal upset or headaches in some patients. It has significant antiplatelet and antithrombotic effects and therefore poses a risk for increased bleeding in patients taking aspirin, nonsteroidal anti-inflammatory drugs, warfarin, antiplatelet agents, factor Xa inhibitors, and serotonergic antidepressants.
- **Ginseng** (*Panax ginseng*) is a traditional medicine used for over 2000 years as a remedy for fatigue, weakness, and aging (Tewari et al. 2018). Ginseng's mechanism of action likely involves immunomodulatory effects which may be neuroprotective (Tewari et al. 2018). Trials with ginseng are limited by small sample size and poor methodology. A meta-analysis determined that therapeutic effects in MNCD/Alzheimer's disease were inconsistent among the studies (Tewari et al. 2018). Ginseng is well tolerated; insomnia and rash are reported as the most common side effects. Similar to ginkgo, ginseng can also pose a bleeding risk and should not be combined with other agents that increase this risk. See Table 18.4.

Table 18.4 Supplements used for neurocognitive disorders

Supplement	Reported use(s)	Usual dosage range	Evidence of efficacy	Safety concerns
Ginkgo	MNCD/ dementia	120–240 mg po divided BID-TID	Multiple negative trials in healthy adults and inconsistent findings in adults with cognitive impairment	Serotonin syndrome, bleeding, stroke/TIA, and arrhythmias
Ginseng	MNCD/ dementia	1–2 g (root) or 200–400 mg (extract) po daily divided BID-TID	Inconsistent findings and not recommended	Well tolerated, insomnia, rash, and bleeding risk

Safety

Since dietary and nutritional supplements are not regulated, there is no requirement for evaluating or testing the products either before or after they are marketed. As a result, their risks are often not recognized or discussed, unlike the informed consent sought for prescribed FDA-regulated products. Therapeutic efficacy, safety evidence, and information regarding toxic chemicals, adulterants, and ingredients are often not listed on the label.

While the FDA has requirements for good manufacturing practices (GMP) for dietary supplements, adherence is a concern. Federal inspectors cited 71% of facilities manufacturing supplements for not following GMP; each company received an average of seven deficiencies (Long 2013). The FDA does act when products are adulterated or misbranded and maintains a Dietary Supplement Ingredient Advisory List, intended to alert the public and healthcare providers when ingredients are discovered that require investigation (Food and Drug Administration (FDA) 2022). However, even after the FDA recalled supplements due to adulteration with pharmaceutical ingredients, 66.7% remained available for purchase with banned ingredients for at least 6 months after the recalls (Cohen et al. 2014).

In addition to this FDA oversight, the US Pharmacopeia (USP) contributes to the safe use of these unregulated products by setting quality standards for supplements (United States Pharmacopeia 2016). The USP provides guidance on the "4 Ps of Quality":

- Positive identity: Is the product in the bottle what it states on the label?
- Potency: Are the ingredients in the amount listed on the label?
- Purity: Does the product include unwanted, potentially unsafe ingredients (e.g., heavy metals, pesticides, mold, active pharmaceutical ingredients)?
- Performance: Is the product manufactured in a way that will be absorbed and distributed appropriately and effectively?

The USP Verification Program entails manufacturing facility audits, manufacturing quality control reviews, and laboratory testing of samples to evaluate conformance to the 4 Ps quality standards. Participation is voluntary but manufacturers that participate receive the "USP Verified" mark on their products, offering some reassurance to buyers.

Another safety concern is that aging adults may be at greater risk for adverse effects. With decreased renal and hepatic clearance, half-lives of medications, substances of abuse, metabolites, and supplements are typically longer. Aging adults may also have greater tissue and receptor sensitivity, thereby heightening effects such as sedation, dizziness, or orthostasis. There is a greater risk for drug-drug interactions, since the number of medications usually increases with age and the likelihood of clinically significant interactions rises with the number of agents. Often, information on drug-drug interactions with supplements is lacking, and guidance is based on theoretical concerns or case reports.

Clinically significant effects due to interactions between drugs and supplements include the following:

- Increased bleeding risk, especially when combined with anticoagulants, factor Xa inhibitors, antiplatelets, NSAIDs, SSRIs, SNRIs, TCAs, trazodone, and buspirone
  - The "5Gs": ginkgo, ginseng, ginger, garlic, and green tea
  - Omega-3 fatty acids
- Cytochrome P450 interactions
  - St. John's wort is a potent inducer and may decrease levels and efficacy of many medications.
- Serotonin syndrome from serotonergic antidepressants or other serotonergic medications combined with the following:
  - St. John's wort, SAMe, and tryptophan
- Additive CNS depressant effects from alcohol, benzodiazepines, opioids, or other depressants combined with the following:
  - Kava and valerian

Communication with Patients and Their Support Systems

Many patients do not disclose their supplement use to healthcare providers, and clinicians may not ask. Some patients are reluctant to disclose for fear of disapproval or may consider use of nutraceuticals not related or relevant to their medical care. Healthcare practitioners may not consider the topic important to the treatment, or they may be hesitant due to lack of knowledge and experience and inability to address patient's questions. One study reported that less than a quarter of supplements used were recommended by a healthcare provider (Bailey et al. 2013).

To bridge this communication gap:

- Utilize resources to become more knowledgeable and share with interested patients:
  - National Institutes of Health National Center for Complementary and Integrative Health https://www.nccih.nih.gov/
  - National Library of Medicine Medline Plus https://medlineplus.gov/druginfo/herb_All.html
  - Natural Medicines Comprehensive Database (requires subscription): https://naturalmedicines.therapeuticresearch.com/
  - Consumer Lab (requires subscription): https://www.consumerlab.com/
  - Pew Trusts Dietary Supplements: https://www.pewtrusts.org/en/research-and-analysis/fact-sheets/2017/10/dietary-supplements-what-are-they-and-how-are-they-regulated
  - FDA Supplement Your Knowledge: https://www.fda.gov/food/information-consumers-using-dietary-supplements/supplement-your-knowledge
- Incorporate supplement use into intake questionnaires, history taking, and routine follow-ups with patients.
- Develop individualized recommendations about supplement use:
  - Is there quality evidence to support use?
  - Is the patient's condition likely to benefit relative to the evidence (e.g., mild vs. severe depressive disorder)?
  - Are there vitamin or mineral deficiencies present either due to poor appetite or intake or systemic medical conditions that would support supplement use?
  - Is the supplement safe for the patient (based on what is known for adverse effects and drug interactions)?
  - Are there alternative interventions which may be more appropriate for the patient?
- Help patient choose appropriate brand, formulation, and dose of supplement:
  - USP verification (look for the USP Verified Mark on products)
  - NSF supplement certification https://www.nsf.org/consumer-resources/articles/supplement-vitamin-certification
  - Consumer lab testing https://www.consumerlab.com/
  - Adhere to reputable brands

Conclusion

Over 80,000 supplement and nutraceutical products result in over $40 billion in annual sales in the USA (Pew Charitable Trusts 2017). Patients perhaps consider them safer than medication or may turn to them if conventional treatments are not helpful or not tolerated. Such substances are also easier to access than a conventional medication and may be less expensive. But supplements may not provide benefit and may not be free from harm. Healthcare practitioners who gather details of supplement and nutraceutical use can incorporate this information into the larger medication regimen while monitoring for evidence of benefits as well as adverse effects. If benefits are unclear, or the patient is experiencing adverse effects, clinicians should encourage discontinuation. These practices strengthen the patient-practitioner alliance, improve the risk-benefit ratio, and support an *age-adjusted* approach to care.

Age-Adjusted Recommendations

- Demonstrate knowledge of the benefits, risks, and use of supplements and nutraceuticals; this builds a trustful therapeutic alliance.
- Determine the patient's use of, duration of, and dosing of any substances taken regularly.
- Search for and study adverse effects of specific supplements and the potential for significant drug interactions.
- Recognize that understanding a patient's regimen of nutraceuticals fosters *further exploration and further disclosure* and increases patient's *receptivity* to recommendations.
- Avoid a judgmental or dismissive attitude toward non-prescribed substances.
- Ask to see containers of substances in use and examine their ingredients.

References

Alvarez-Mon MA, Ortega MA, García-Montero C, et al. Exploring the role of nutraceuticals in major depressive disorder (MDD): rationale, state of the art and future prospects. Pharmaceuticals. 2021;14(8):821.

Asher GN, Gartlehner G, Gaynes BN, et al. Comparative benefits and harms of complementary and alternative medicine therapies for initial treatment of major depressive disorder: systematic review and meta-analysis. J Altern Complement Med. 2017;23(12):907–19.

Bailey RL, Gahche JJ, Miller PE, et al. Why US adults use dietary supplements. JAMA Intern Med. 2013;173(5):355–61.

Birks J, Grimley Evans J. Ginkgo biloba for cognitive impairment and dementia. Cochrane Database Syst Rev. 2009;1:CD003120.

Chouët J, Sacco G, Karras SN, et al. Vitamin D and delirium in older adults: a case-control study in geriatric acute care unit. Front Neurol. 2020;11:1034.

Cohen PA, Maller G, DeSouza R, Neal-Kababick J. Presence of banned drugs in dietary supplements following FDA recalls. JAMA. 2014;312(16):1691–3.

DeKosky ST, Williamson JD, Fitzpatrick AL, et al. Ginkgo biloba for prevention of dementia: a randomized controlled trial. JAMA. 2008;300(19):2253–62.

Donelli D, Antonelli M, Bellinazzi C, et al. Effects of lavender on anxiety: a systematic review and meta-analysis. Phytomedicine. 2019;65:153099.

Fatemeh G, Sajjad M, Niloufar R, et al. Effect of melatonin supplementation on sleep quality: a systematic review and meta-analysis of randomized controlled trials. J Neurol. 2022;269(1):205–16.

Food and Drug Administration (FDA). Unproven Alzheimer's disease products. 2018. https://www.fda.gov/consumers/health-fraud-scams/unproven-alzheimers-disease-products. Accessed 2 June 2022.

Food and Drug Administration (FDA). Dietary supplement products & ingredients. 2022. https://www.fda.gov/food/dietary-supplements/dietary-supplement-products-ingredients. Accessed 10 June 2022.

Freeman MP, Fava M, Lake J, et al. Complementary and alternative medicine in major depressive disorder: the American Psychiatric Association task force report. J Clin Psychiatry. 2010;71(6):669–81.

Gupta C, Prakash D. Nutraceuticals for geriatrics. J Tradit Complement Med. 2015;5(1):5–14.

Hallahan B, Ryan T, Hibbeln JR, et al. Efficacy of omega-3 highly unsaturated fatty acids in the treatment of depression. Br J Psychiatry. 2016;209(3):192–201.

Hypericum Depression Trial Study Group. Effect of Hypericum perforatum (St John's wort) in major

depressive disorder: a randomized controlled trial. JAMA. 2002;287(14):1807–14.
Kasper S, Gastpar M, Müller WE, et al. Lavender oil preparation silexan is effective in generalized anxiety disorder: a randomized, double-blind comparison to placebo and paroxetine. Int J Neuropsychopharmacol. 2014;17(6):859–69.
Kessler RC, Soukup J, Davis RB, et al. The use of complementary and alternative therapies to treat anxiety and depression in the United States. Am J Psychiatry. 2001;158(2):289–94.
Lelli D, Cortese L, Pedone C. Use of plant-derived natural products in sleep disturbances. Adv Exp Med Biol. 2021;1308:217–24.
Long J. FDA GMP inspectors cite 70% of dietary supplement firm.s 2013. https://www.naturalproductsinsider.com/regulatory/fda-gmp-inspectors-cite-70-dietary-supplement-firms. Accessed 6 June 2022.
Low TL, Choo FN, Tan SM. The efficacy of melatonin and melatonin agonists in insomnia—an umbrella review. J Psychiatr Res. 2020;121:10–23.
Mannel M. Drug interactions with St John's wort: mechanisms and clinical implications. Drug Saf. 2004;27(11):773–97.
Mishra S, Stierman B, Gahche JJ, Potischman N. Dietary supplement use among adults: United States, 2017–2018. NCHS Data Brief, no 399. Hyattsville: National Center for Health Statistics; 2021.
Mukai T, Kishi T, Matsuda Y, Iwata N. A meta-analysis of inositol for depression and anxiety disorders. Hum Psychopharmacol. 2014;29(1):55–63.
Ooi SL, Henderson P, Pak SC. Kava for generalized anxiety disorder: a review of current evidence. J Altern Complement Med. 2018;24(8):770–80.
Parker GB, Brotchie H, Graham RK. Vitamin D and depression. J Affect Disord. 2017;208:56–61.
Pew Charitable Trusts. Dietary supplements: what are they and how are they regulated? 2017. https://www.pewtrusts.org/en/research-and-analysis/fact-sheets/2017/10/dietary-supplements-what-are-they-and-how-are-they-regulated. Accessed 2 June 2022.
Ravindran AV, Balneaves LG, Faulkner G, et al. Canadian Network for Mood and Anxiety Treatments (CANMAT) 2016 clinical guidelines for the management of adults with major depressive disorder: section 5. Complementary and alternative medicine treatments. Can J Psychiatry. 2016;61(9):576–87.
Rhee TG, Evans RL, McAlpine DD, Johnson PJ. Racial/ethnic differences in the use of complementary and alternative medicine in US adults with moderate mental distress. J Prim Care Community Health. 2017;8(2):43–54.
Sarris J, LaPorte E, Schweitzer I. Kava: a comprehensive review of efficacy, safety, and psychopharmacology. Aust N Z J Psychiatry. 2011;45(1):27–35.
Sarris J, Murphy J, Mischoulon D, et al. Adjunctive nutraceuticals for depression: a systematic review and meta-analyses. Am J Psychiatry. 2016;173(6):575–87.
Sarris J, Ravindran A, Yatham LN, et al. Clinician guidelines for the treatment of psychiatric disorders with nutraceuticals and phytoceuticals: the World Federation of Societies of Biological Psychiatry (WFSBP) and Canadian Network for Mood and Anxiety Treatments (CANMAT) taskforce. World J Biol Psychiatry. 2022;23:424–55.
Schefft C, Kilarski LL, Bschor T, Köhler S. Efficacy of adding nutritional supplements in unipolar depression: a systematic review and meta-analysis. Eur Neuropsychopharmacol. 2017;27(11):1090–109.
Sharma A, Gerbarg P, Bottiglieri T, et al. S-Adenosylmethionine (SAMe) for neuropsychiatric disorders: a clinician-oriented review of research. J Clin Psychiatry. 2017;78(6):e656–67.
Solomon PR, Adams F, Silver A, et al. Ginkgo for memory enhancement: a randomized controlled trial. JAMA. 2002;288(7):835–40.
Tewari D, Stankiewicz AM, Mocan A, et al. Ethnopharmacological approaches for dementia therapy and significance of natural products and herbal drugs. Front Aging Neurosci. 2018;10:3.
United States Pharmacopeia. Choosing a quality supplement. 2016. https://qualitymatters.usp.org/choosing-quality-supplements. Accessed 2 June 2022.
White CM. The pharmacology, pharmacokinetics, efficacy, and adverse events associated with kava. J Clin Pharmacol. 2018;58(11):1396–405.
Woelk H, Schläfke S. A multi-center, double-blind, randomised study of the lavender oil preparation silexan in comparison to lorazepam for generalized anxiety disorder. Phytomedicine. 2010;17(2):94–9.

Correction to: Neuromodulation Therapies

Amer M. Burhan, Daphne Goveas, Sama Thiab, and Mervin Blair

Correction to:
Chapter 14 in: H. H. Fenn et al. (eds.), *Age-Adjusted Psychiatric Treatment for the Older Patient*, https://doi.org/10.1007/978-3-031-53976-3_14

The affiliation for the author Mervin Blair was published incorrectly and has been corrected as below in the revised publication in the front matter (list of contributors section) and chapter opening page of Chapter 14.

Current Affiliation Content:
Mervin Blair
Psychiatry at University of Toronto,
Ontario Shores Centre for Mental Health Sciences, Whitby, ON, Canada
Lawson Health Research Institute/Parkwood Institute, London, ON, Canada

Updated Affiliation Content:
Mervin Blair
Ontario Shores Centre for Mental Health Sciences, Whitby, ON, Canada
Lawson Health Research Institute/Parkwood Institute, London, ON, Canada

The updated version of this chapter can be found at https://doi.org/10.1007/978-3-031-53976-3_14

H. H. Fenn et al. (eds.), *Age-Adjusted Psychiatric Treatment for the Older Patient*,
https://doi.org/10.1007/978-3-031-53976-3_19

Index

H. H. Fenn et al. (eds.), *Age-Adjusted Psychiatric Treatment for the Older Patient*,
https://doi.org/10.1007/978-3-031-53976-3

C

D

U

V

W

Z

GPSR Compliance

The European Union's (EU) General Product Safety Regulation (GPSR) is a set of rules that requires consumer products to be safe and our obligations to ensure this.

If you have any concerns about our products, you can contact us on ProductSafety@springernature.com

In case Publisher is established outside the EU, the EU authorized representative is:

Springer Nature Customer Service Center GmbH
Europaplatz 3
69115 Heidelberg, Germany

Batch number: 10732809

Printed by Printforce, the Netherlands